Textbook of Community Health for Nurses

Third Edition

Dr. G.N. Prabhakara MD
Principal and Professor of PSM
SDM College of Medical Sciences and Hospital
Manjushree Nagar, Sattur
Dharwad 580 009

PEEPEE
PUBLISHERS AND DISTRIBUTORS (P) LTD.®

Textbook of Community Health for Nurses

Published by
Pawaninder P. Vij and Anupam Vij

Peepee Publishers and Distributors (P) Ltd.
Head Office: 160, Shakti Vihar, Pitam Pura, Delhi-110 034 (India)

Correspondence Address:
7/31, First Floor, Ansari Road, Daryaganj
New Delhi-110 002 (India)
Ph: 41512412, 9811156083
e-mail: peepee160@yahoo.co.in
e-mail: peepee160@gmail.com
www.peepeepub.com
join us on facebook.com/pp.publishers

First Edition: 2004
Second Edition: 2009
Third Edition: 2014
Reprint: 2020

ISBN: 978-81-8445-109-2

Preface for the Second Edition

I am happy and thankful to readers for the opportunity for the succeeding edition following earlier edition and reprint.

Nursing profession has been identified as an indispensable entity in the care of the sick, injured and healthy; it has further been extended to the health of the community. So much so NURSING PRACTICE has altered a great deal since Nightingale era, not only because of the remarkable changes in medical knowledge but also because of the social changes of our modern society.

An effort has been made to incorporate all theoretical, practical and field aspects of nursing packed into this **"Textbook of Community Health for Nurses"** which is very much needed in the field both for Trainers and Trainees.

Besides, whole aspect required by the Nursing Council of India and All Affiliated Universities of Health Sciences in India has also been incorporated to make the text more comprehensive and to meet the requirement of the Nursing Professional as well as the students of Nursing Course.

In maintaining a textbook of this nature, author felt necessary to preserve a balance between the old and the new techniques; and some nursing skills / procedures have, on occasion to be retained alongside newer ones; because nevertheless they are still practised in village, taluk and district level nursing care procedures.

The text covers in-depth some of the units like Nursing Research, Therapeutic adoption of normal diet, Human sexuality, Non communicable diseases, Nursing component, Nursing education, Nursing administration which hitherto not readily available in texts, but being taught by the tutors at institutional level.

Full help, appreciation, corrections, guidance of life partner Mrs. Malathi Prabhakara, Ex-Scientist, Technology Transfer, Industrial Development and Consultancy, CFTRI (Council of Scientific and Industrial Research) is gracefully acknowledged.

Source of inspiration and helping hand in additions and corrections by son Dr. Bharat M.P. is acknowledged.

I thank all Tutors, Nursing Professionals and Nursing students who are indirectly the source of inspiration in shaping this updated textbook for the Noble Profession.

I place my sense of gratitude to Poojya Dr. D Veerendra Heggade Dharmadhikari of Srikshetra Dharmasthala, Dr YS Rai, Dean and Dr. Niranjan Kumar, Medical Director, SDM College of Medical Sciences and Hospital, Dharwad.

Efforts of Mr. Pawaninder P Vij, Director, Peepee Publishers and Distributors (P) Ltd., Delhi in giving a good and appreciable shape to my modest work as ***TEXTBOOK OF COMMUNITY HEALTH FOR NURSES*** is acknowledged with heartfelt thanks.

Dr. G.N. PRABHAKARA

Preface for the First Edition

Nursing profession has been identified as an indispensable entity in the care of the sick, injured and healthy; it has further been extended to the care of sick, injured and health of the community. So much so NURSING PRACTICE has altered a great deal since Nightingale era, not only because of the remarkable changes in medical knowledge but also because of the social changes of our modern society.

An effort has been made to incorporate information on all theoretical, practical and field aspects of nursing packed into this **"Textbook of Community Health for Nurses"** which is very much wanted in the field both by Trainers and Trainees.

Besides, whole aspect required by the Nursing Council of India and All Affiliated Universities of Health Sciences in India has also been incorporated to make the text more comprehensive and to meet the requirement of the Nursing Professional as well as the students of Nursing Course.

In maintaining a textbook of this nature, author felt necessary to preserve a balance between the old and the new techniques; and some nursing skills / procedures have, on occasion to be retained alongside newer ones; because nevertheless they are still practised in village, taluk and district level nursing care procedures.

The text covers in-depth some of the units like Nursing Research, Therapeutic adoption of normal diet, Human sexuality, Non communicable diseases, Nursing component, Nursing education, Nursing administration which hitherto not readily available in texts, but a tutor used to teach at institutional level.

Full help, appreciation, corrections, guidance of life partner Mrs. Malathi Prabhakara, Ex-Scientist, Technology Transfer, Industrial Development and Consultancy, CFTRI (Council of Scientific and Industrial Research) is gracefully acknowledged.

Source of inspiration and helping hand in additions and corrections of son Dr. M.P. Bharat, Future Health Professional in Human Resource Development and Patient Care; and Dr. Soumya Kumar, Future Educational Professional in Human Resource Development and Student Care, are acknowledged.

I thank all Tutors, Nursing Professionals and Nursing students who are indirectly the source of inspiration in shaping this textbook for the Noble Nursing Profession.

Efforts of Mr. Pawaninder P. Vij, Director, Peepee Publishers and Distributors (P) Ltd., New Delhi in giving a good and appreciable shape to my modest work as **TEXTBOOK OF COMMUNITY HEALTH FOR NURSES** are acknowledged with heartfelt thanks.

Dr. G.N. PRABHAKARA

Contents

Abbreviations

ABER Annual Blood Examination Rate
AC Air Conditioning
ACL Anthroponotic Cutaneous Leishmaniasis
ADI Acceptable Daily Intake
ADS Anti Diphtheria Serum
AFB Acid Fast Bacilli
AFI Annual Falciparum Incidence
AFP Acute Flaccid Paralysis
AIDS Auto Immune Disorder Syndrome
AIIH & PH All India Institute of Hygiene and Public Health
AIIMS All India Institute of Medical Sciences
AIR All India Radio
AM Arithmetic Mean
ANM Auxiliary Nurse Midwife
ANP Applied Nutrition Programme
APH Ante Partum Haemorrhage
APHA American Public Health Association
API Annual Parasite Incidence
APT Alum Precipitated Toxoid
ARC AIDS Related Complex
ARDS Adult Respiratory Distress Syndrome
ARI Acute Respiratory Infection
ARS Anti Rabies Serum
ASO Anti Strepolycin O titre
ATS Anti Tetanus Serum
AV Audio Visual
AZT Zidovudine
BASIC Beginners All Purpose Symbolic Instruction Code
BB Border Line
BBT Basal Body Temperature
BC Before Christ
BCG Bacilli Chalmette Guirae
BD Two times a day (Bis in Die)
BDCS Border District Cluster Strategy
BDO Block Development Officer
BEE Block Extension Educator
BHC Benzyl Hexa Chloride
BL Borderline Lepromatous
BMR Basal Metabolic Rate
BNP Balawadi Nutrition Programme
BOAA Beta Oxlyl Amino Alanine
BOD Biological Oxidation Demand
BP Blood Pressure
BPL Beta Proprio Lactone
BR Birth Rate
BIS Bureau of Indian Standards
BT Borderline Tuberculoid
CARE Co-operative for Assistance and Relief Everywhere (American relief)
CCF Congestive Cardiac Failure
CCH Central Council of Health
CCP Code of Criminal Procedure
CDD Control of Diarrhoeal Diseases
CDP Community Development Programme
CDPO Child Development Project Officer
CET Corrected Effective Temperature
CF Correction Factor
CFI Community Fluorosis Index
CFR Case Fatality Rate
CFTRI Central Food Technological Research Institute
CHC Community Health Centre
CHD Coronary Heart Disease
CHEB Central Health Education Bureau
CHO Carbohydrate
CHS Central Health Service
CI Confidence Interval
CL Cutaneous Leishmaniasis
CME Cyto Megalo Virus Entity
CMR Child Mortality Rate
CNS Central Nervous System
COBOL Common Business Oriented Language
COD Chemical Oxygen Demand
COPRA Consumer Protection Act
CPD Cephalo Pelvic Disproportion
CPM Critical Path Method
CPR Cardio Pulmonary Resuscitation
CPR Couple Protection Rate
CSF Cerebro Spinal Fluid
CSI Child Survival Index
CSSM Child Survival and Safe Motherhood
CSW Commercial Sex Worker
CT Computerised Tomography Scan
CTC Central Technical Committee
CV Coefficient of Variation

CVS	Cardio Vascular System
dT	Diphtheria Tetanus adult
DALE	Disability Adjusted Life Expectancy
DALY	Disability Adjusted Life Year
DANIDA	Danish International Development Agency
DAS	Disability Assessment Schedule
DAVP	Directorate of Audio and Visual Publicity
dB	Deci bell (noise level)
dBA	Acceptable noise level
DDT	Di chloro Di Pheyl Trichloro Ethane
DEC	Di Ethyl Carbamazine
DF	Day light Factor
DF	Deep Freezer
DF	Degree of Freedom
DG	Director General
DGHS	Director General of Health Services
DH & FWO	District Health and Family Welfare Officer
DHF	Dengue Haemorrhage Fever
DI	Development Index
DIO	District Immunisation Officer
DMPA	Depot Medroxy Progesterone Acetate
DNA	Deoxy ribo Nucleic Acid
DOTS	Directly Observe Treatment Short Course
DPT	Diphtheria Pertussis and Tetanus
DR	Death Rate
DT	Diphtheria Tetanus
DTC	District Tuberculosis Centre
DWACRA	Development of Women and Children in Rural Areas
EAEC	Entero Aggregative E Coli
EAS	Employment Assurance Scheme
EC	Exposure Code
ECG	Electro Cardio Graphy
ECT	Electro Convulsive Therapy
ED	Epidemic Disease Hospital
EDTA	Ethylene Di amine Tetra Acetic Acid
EEG	Electro Encephalogram
EHCP	Environmental Health Criteria Programme
EHEC	Entero Haemorrhagic E Coli
EIA	Enzyme Immuno Assay
EIEC	Entero Invasive E Coli
ELISA	Enzyme Linked Immuno Sorbent Assay
EPEC	Enteropathogenic E Coli
EPI	Expanded Programme of Immunisation
EPID	Epidemiology
ESIS	Employees State Insurance Scheme
ETEC	Entero Toxigenic E Coli
FABM	Fertility Awareness Based Methods
FAO	Food and Agriculture Organisation
FFHC	Freedom From Hunger Campaign
FORTRAN	Formula Translation
FP	Family Planning
FPO	Fruit Products Order
FSH	Follicle Stimulating Hormone
FT	Formal Toxoid
FTA-ABS	Fluorescent Treponemal Antibody Absorbed Test
FW	Family Welfare
G	Gram
GAD	Generalised Anxiety Disorder
GBD	Global Burden of Disease
GDM	Gestational Diabetes Mellitus
GDP	Gross Domestic Product
GE	Gastro Enteritis
GFR	General Fertility Rate
GI	Gastro Intestinal
GI	Granuloma Inguinale
GNP	Gross National Product
GOBI	Growth monitoring Oral rehydration Breast feeding and Immunisation
GOI	Government of India
HAB	Hepatitis B virus
HALE	Health Adjusted Life Expectancy
HAV	Hepatitis A virus
Hb	Haemoglobin
HBS Ag	Hepatitis B Surface Antigen
HBIG	Hepatitis B Immunoglobulin
HBS	Handicaps, Behaviour and Skills Schedule
HCG	Human Chorionic Gonadotrophin
HDI	Human Development Index
HFA	Health for All
HIS	Heat Stress Index
HIV	Human Immunodeficiency Virus
HKNS	Hind Kushth Nivaran Sangh
HRD	Human Resource Development
HRIG	Human Rabies Immunoglobulin
HS	Health Supervisor
HSV	Herpes Simplex Virus
HTST	High Temperature and Short Time Method
HUDCO	Housing and Urban Development Corporation
HUS	Haemolytic Uraemic Syndrome
Hz	Hertz
IAP	Indian Academy of Paediatrics
IAY	Indira Awaz Yojana
ICCDE	International Commission for Certification of Dracunculiasis Eradication
ICCU	Intensive Coronary Care Unit
ICCW	Indian Council for Child Welfare
ICD	International Classification of Diseases
ICDS	Integrated Child Development Services

ICF	International Classification of Functioning, Disability and Health
ICIDH	International Classification of Impairment Disabilities and Handicaps
ICMR	Indian Council of Medical Research
ICRP	Indian Council of Radiological Protection
ICU	Intensive Care Unit
IDD	Iodine Deficiency Disorders
IDU	Intra venous Drug User
IEC	Information Education and Communication
IFA	Iron Folic Acid
IGT	Impaired Glucose Test
IHD	Ischemic Heart Disease
ILO	International Labour Organisation
ILR	Ice Lined Refrigerator
IM	Intra Muscular
IMA	Indian Medical Association
IMCI	Integrated Management of Childhood Illness
IMR	Infant Mortality Rate
INC	Intra Natal Care
INH	Iso Niazid Hydrazine
IOL	Intra Ocular Lens
IP	Incubation Period
IPC	Indian Penal Code
IPCU	Intensive Paediatric Care Unit
IPD	In Patient Department
IPP	India Population Project
IPPI	Intensive Pulse Polio Immunisation
IPV	Injectable Polio Vaccine
IQ	Intelligent Quotient
IRC	International Red Cross
IRDP	Integrated Rural Development Programme
ISI	Indian Standard Institute
IU	International Unit
IUD	Intra Uterine Device
IV	Intra Venous
JE	Japanese Encephalitis
JIT	Just In Time Planning
JRY	Jawahar Rojgar Yojana
KAP	Knowledge Attitude and Practice
KFD	Kyasanur Forest Disease
KMF	The Kasturba Memorial Fund
LAM	Lactational Amenorrhoea Method
Lb	Pound
LB	Live Births
LBW	Low Birth Weight
LCU	Leprosy Control Unit
LDC	Lower Division Clerk
LDCOC	Low Dose Combined Oral Contraceptives
LDU	Low Density Lipoprotein
LE	Life Expectancy
LFT	Liver Function Test
LGV	Lympho Granuloma Venerium
LH	Luteinizing Hormone
LL	Lepromatous Leprosy
LMO	Lady Medical Officer
LOA	Left Occipito Anterior
LP	Lumbar Puncture
LRI	Lower Respiratory tract Infection
LSD	Lysergic Acid Diethylamide
MAB	Man and Biosphere Programme
MB	Multi Bacillary
MBO	Management By Objectives
MCH	Maternal and Child Health
MCL	Muco Cutaneous Leishmaniasis
MCQ	Multiple Choice Question
MDT	Multi Drug Regimen
MI	Myocardial Infarction
MIG	Measle Immuno Globulin
MI	Milli Litre
MLEC	Modified Leprosy Elimination Campaign
MMR	Mass Miniature Radiography
MMR	Maternal Mortality Rate
MMR	Measles Mumps and Rubella
MP	Mandal Panchayat
MP	Malaria Parasite
MPF	Multi Purpose Food
MPO	Modified Plan of Operation
MPW	Multi Purpose Worker
MR	Magnetic Resonance Scan
MRL	Maximum Residual Limit
MRP	Material Requirement Planning
MTP	Medical Termination of Pregnancy
MUAC	Mid Upper Arm Circumference
MWS	Million Wells Scheme
MYP	Mid Year Population
NACO	National AIDS Control Organisation
NBO	National Building Organisation
NCD	Non Communicable Disease
NCHS	National Center of Health Statistics
NCI	Nursing Council of India
NET EN	Norethysterone Enanthate
NFPP	National Family Planning Programme
NGO	Non Governmental Organisation
NHD	Natural History of Disease
NICD	National Institute of Communicable Diseases
NICU	Neonatal Intensive Care Unit
NID	National Immunisation Days
NIDDCP	National Iodine Deficiency Disorder Control

Programme
NIHAE National Institute of Health Administration and Education
NIMH National Institute for Mentally Handicapped
NIMHANS National Institute of Mental Health and Neuro Science
NIN National Institute of Nutrition
NIOH National Institute for the Orthopaedically Handicapped
NLEP National Leprosy Eradication Programme
NMCP National Malaria Control Programme
NMEP National Malaria Eradication Programme
NNAPP National Nutritional Anaemia Prophylaxis Programme
NNT Neo Natal Tetanus
NPC National Productivity Council
NPCB National Programme for the Control of Blindness
NPU Net Protein Utilisation
NRR Net Reproduction Rate
NTI National Tuberculosis Institute
NTP National Tuberculosis Control Programme
OBG Obstetrics and Gynaecology
OC Oral Contraceptive
OCD Obsessive Compulsive Disorder
OHP Over Head Projector
OK All right (Ol Kright)
OPD Out Patient Department
OPV Oral Polio Vaccine
ORS Oral Rehydration Solution
ORT Oral Rehydration Therapy
OSCE Objective Structured Clinical Examination
OSPE Objective Structured Practical Examination
OT Operation Theatre
OTC Orientation Training Camp
PI Plasmodium
PAS Para Amino Salicylic Acid
PASCAL Software Language
PB Pauci Bacillary
PCM Protein Calorie Malnutrition
PCT Presumptive Coliform Test
PEM Protein Energy Malnutrition
PEP Post Exposure Prophylaxis
PERT Programme Evaluation and Review Technique
PET Pre Eclamsic Toxaemia
PF Provident Fund
PFA Prevention of Food Adulteration Act
PG Post Graduate
PGL Person with Gland Lesion
PHC Primary Health Centre
PID Pelvic Inflammatory Diseases
PIB Press Information Bureau
PKDL Post Kalaazar Leishmaniasis
PKU Phenyl Ketone Urea
PL Permissible Limit
PMF Progressive Massive Fibrosis
PMR Perinatal Mortality Rate
PNC Post Natal Care
POP Progesterone Only Pill
PPBS Planning Programming Budgeting System
PPBS Post Prandial Blood Sugar
PPC Post Partum Programme
PPD Purified Protein Derivative
PPE Personal Protection Equipment
PPF Public Provident Fund
PPH Post Partum Haemorrhage
PPI Pulse Polio Immunisation
PPM Parts Per Million
PQLI Physical Quality of Life Index
P_4SR Predicted four hours Sweat Rate
PT Presumptive Treatment
PTAH Purified Toxoid in Aluminium Hydroxide
PTAP Purified Toxoid in Aluminium Phosphate
PUFA Poly Unsaturated Fatty Acids
r Correlation
RBC Red Blood Corpuscle
RBS Random Blood Sugar
RCA Research Cum Action
RCE Regional College of Engineering
RCH Reproductive Child Health
RCT Randomized Controlled Trial
RDA Recommended Dietary Allowance
RhIG Rh Isoimmunoglobulin
RIG Rabies Immunoglobulin
RMP Registered Medical Practitioner
RNA Ribo Nucleic Acid
RNTCP Revised National Tuberculosis Control Programme
RR Respiratory Rate
RT Radical Treatment
RTI Reproductive Tract Infection
SAPEL Special Action Projects for the Elimination of Leprosy
SAR Secondary Attack Rate
SARS Severe Acute Respiratory Syndrome
SC Status Code or Schedule Caste
SD Standard Deviation
SE Standard Error

SEARO	South East Asian Regional Office
SET	Survey Education and Treatment
SFR	Slide Falciparum Rate
SIDA	Swedish International Development Agency
SITA	Suppression of Immoral Traffic Act
SMR	Standard Mortality Rate
SNP	Special Nutrition Programme
SPR	Slide Positive Rate
SPSS	Statistical Packages for Social Sciences
SSPE	Sub acute Sclerosing Pan Encephalitis
STD	Sexually Transmitted Diseases
STLS	Senior Tuberculosis Laboratory Supervisor
STO	State Level Tuberculosis Officer
STS	Senior Treatment Supervisor
TL	Teaching and Learning
TAB	Typhoid A and B
TAF	Toxoid Antitoxin Floccule
TAI	Tuberculosis Association of India
TB	Tuberculosis
TBA	Traditional Birth Attendant
TCC	TB Chemotherapy Centre
TIA	Transient Ischemic Attack
TIG	Tetanus Immuno Globulin
TL	Tubal Ligation
TL	Tuberculoid Leprosy
TORCHES	Toxoplasmosis Rubella. Herpes infection and Syphilis
TPHA	Treponema Palladium Haemagglutination Assay
TRS	Technical Report Series
TRYSEM	Training of Rural Youth for Self-Employment
TSH	Thyroid Stimulating Hormone
TT	Tetanus Toxoid
TU	Tuberculoid Unit
TV	Tele Vision
TV	Trichomonas Vaginalis
UBS	Urban Basic Service
UDC	Upper Division Clerk
UFMR	Under Five Mortality Rate
UFWC	Urban Family Welfare Centre
UHT	Ultra High Temperature
UIP	Universal Immunisation Programme
UK	United Kingdom
UN	United Nation
UNDP	United Nations Development Programme
UNEP	United Nations Environmental Programme
UNFPA	United Nations Fund for Population Activities
UNICEF	United Nations International Children Fund
UNO	United Nation Organisation
URI	Upper Respiratory Infection
USA	United States of America
USAID	Unites States Agency for International Development
USG	Ultra Sono Graphy
UT	Union Territory
UV	Ultra Violet Rays
VDRL	Venereal Disease Research Laboratory
VHG	Village Health Guide
VL	Visceral Leishmaniasis
VP	Village Panchayat
VPD	Vaccine Preventable Diseases
VSC	Voluntary Surgical Contraception
VVM	Vaccine Vial Monitor
VZIG	Vericella Zoster Immunoglobulin
WBC	White Blood Corpuscle
WHO	World Health Organisation
WTO	World Trade Organisation
YHL	Years of Healthy Life
YLD	Years Lived with Disability
YLL	Years of Life Lost
ZCL	Zoonotic Cutaneous Leishmaniasis
ZP	Zilla Parishad

1

Historical Background of Nursing

Nursing profession contributes to the revolutionized health care delivery system recognizing national health goals, participating in its implementation. It aims at:

- Recognizing health needs
- Planning quality health care
- Provision of quality health care
- Collaboration with other professions

To all those who begin their Nursing Training, history of Nursing provide the necessary background to understand the spirit of the course. The word Nursing means nourishing. Therefore it has come to mean tending and helping all who need it, especially the sick. The object of training nurses is to provide an adequate service more effectively, to tend the sick and to help in the preservation and promotion of the health of the community in general and of the nation in specific.

Nursing activity concept has come up in recent times. The representative language (e.g., KRSS—Knowledge Representation Syntax), Integration language (e.g., GRAIL—Galen Representation and Integration language), Tools (e.g., Ontylog) are the main ones

Recent times focus on nursing diagnosis, signs, symptoms, problems, prevention, promotion and maintenance are emphasized as Activity Focus.

BACKGROUND

Health is influenced by an array of demographic, socioeconomic, political and environmental factors that are constantly changing. Major obstacles to health are poverty and deteriorating economic conditions. The demand for trained nurses has been increasing due to: social and political crises, ageing process of the population and deteriorating environmental factors. Despite improvement in health care, there is a wide gap between health service givers and consumers; more so between trained nurses and the needy population. Hence, effective use of human resource, inter-sectoral cooperation and community participation which builds up partnership between individual and community is called for, to bridge the gap.

Nursing is the key component of health care in all socio-economic setting. It ranges from carrying out high Technology investigations like aortogram to low technology first contact care like O.R.S. preparation.

CORE ELEMENT

Virginia Henderson's definition offers a sound foundation for describing nursing service as it relates to all Health care situations:

"The unique function of the nurse is to assist the individual, sick or well, in the performance of those activities contributing to health or its recovery (or to a peaceful death) that She/He would perform unaided if She/He had the necessary strength, will or knowledge and to do this in such a way as to help man/woman regain independence as soon as possible."

Functional description of Nursing is as follows:

- Nursing helps individual, family and group to determine and achieve their physical, mental and social potential in the context of their environment in which they live. It includes promotion of health and prevention of illness. Nursing plan to give care of ill, rehabilitation of disabled and compassion at dying.
- Encourage self reliance and self determination for active involvement of individual in all aspects of health care.
- Nursing is an Art and Science, requiring understanding and application of specific knowledge and skills. They are derived from humanities, physical science, social science, medical science and biological science.

Nursing Care Covers

- Managing physical and mental health in Health and Disease.
- Monitoring and ensuring the quality of health care practice.
- Organizing and managing Health care system.
- Caring and helping the well, the ill and the dying.
- Teaching the art and Science of nursing for self care, family guidance.
- Managing situations that are changing rapidly.
- Advanced educational preparation, coupled with practical experience, enabling nurse to practice at an advanced level.
- Innovators and participants in complementary and traditional approaches to health care.
- No enforcement of boundaries between professions and even within nursing profession allows no conflict and no restriction for a better nursing care.

CONTEXT OF NURSING

Nursing practice is influenced by the context in which it takes place. The force field for nursing practice is illustrated in figure 1.1.

Thus, economic resource, demography, environment, politics, social factors and cultural factors have an impact on nursing practice.

NURSING REGULATORY BODY

Time has come for governance of nursing practice, Nursing education and Functioning of Health care system under law. Effective contribution of nursing care is possible by a Regulatory body like Nursing Council at National Level.

HISTORICAL ASPECT

Nursing in Early Centuries

Many illness of today are found recorded in early centuries and history has shown the existence of these illnesses. Ancient India is first to give a place of honors to 'VAIDYA' who treats and to 'SUSHRUSHA' who nurse. Nurse at that time was an attendant. There is no mentioning of any specially trained attendant or skilled nursing. Other countries notable in history are Egypt, Assyria and Greece, where honoring in civil life that cared for sick was common practice. However attending to sick was inextricably

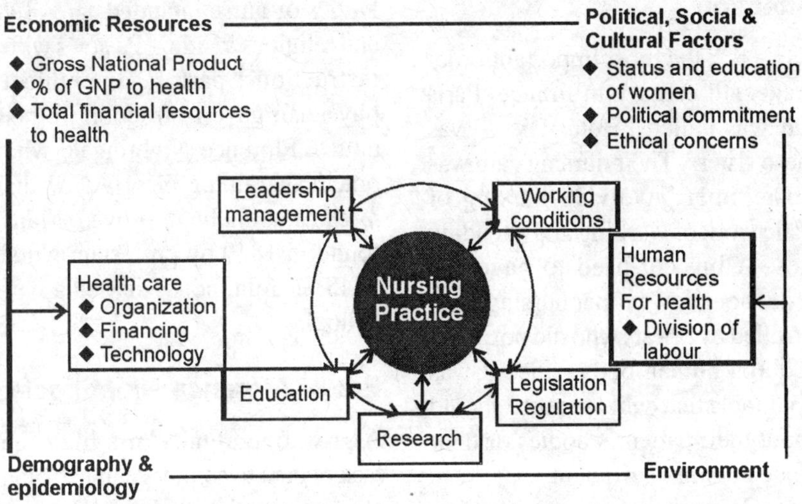

Fig. 1.1: Force field for nursing practice

mingled with religious practices. Sickness was thought of as the work of evil spirits and due to wrath of Gods.

There was a transition in the attitude from attributing illness to work of evil with the birth of Greek physician "Hippocrates" in fourth century B.C. who pointed out that illness is due to disorder function of the body and is due to disobeying the laws of health. This still serves as a model in nursing profession. His pupil, assistants, woman of the household and woman of slaves used to assist in nursing care of the sick.

In late early centuries the word "Midwife" is heard. It was a hereditary family profession. During seventeenth century the word "Man Mid-Wife" came to existence.

Nursing in Christian Era

Biblical notation gave the very humblest living creature's nursing equal to service to God. It connotes the duty and privilege of strong, to bear the burdens of the weak. Here we see the spiritual need of the sick was met with. We see the first organized visiting service to the sick by the order of Deaconesses, working with the Deacons under the Bishops. During fourth century St. Jerome's followers included nursing among Christian duties and were not an order. Many monasteries had houses for nuns and monks. It was under the control of Abbess (Elderly Christian woman). Their wide knowledge and able administration is found recorded in the history.

In 12th century we come across famous order of "the Knights Hospitallers" of St.John of Jerusalem. This lead to hospital maintenance in Jerusalem, Rhodes and Malta. "Serving Brothers" were named for nursing. Below this hierarchy, "Subsidiary women" found nursing in "Hospitallers langue".

In 16th century nursing profession was totally suppressed. Traditional Healers predominated and no nursing care takers are observed in the history.

In 19th century, there was rejuvenation of nursing activities with group activity particularly with "St. John Ambulance Association" and "Voluntary Nursing Corps".

French Connection

"Augustinian Sisters", the most important order is seen in seventeenth century in France. Paris Hospital which was called "Hotel-Dieu" was managed by these sisters. Their nursing care was an over crowd regimen involving nursing of patients, domestic work of washing and attending religious duties. A big cot used to have 5-6 patients which did not allow proper nursing care. They were controlled by priests who did not allow them to know about human body, since it was not considered suitable that celibate nurse should know much about their patient's bodies or their illness. This made nursing inefficient.

The Nursing Community grew with First Superior of the Sisters of Charity "Mile. Le Gras". She helped Vincent DePaul (French priest) to take a house in Paris, gathered country girls to train nursing. Thus a voluntary visiting service by influential ladies formed "Dames de charite". These ladies nursed the sick at home, at hospital, at home for aged, home for insane and even in battle field. There is a record of teaching instructions, by reading, by writing and use of arithmetic.

Dark Age of Nursing

After "Dames de charite" in 17th century nearly for 150 years there was little progress which is called Dark Age of Nursing. In early 19th century, progressive leaders in science and profession awakened public conscience to "Nurse care of the sick". With great advance in medicine, surgery and science during later half of 19th century, real nursing service was started.

Pre Nightingale Reformation

Upbringing to be Deaconesses by training young women of good character is recorded in history of nursing which was by a German pastor and his wife (Theodore and Frederica Fliedner). Duties of nurse included care of young children and religious visiting. Pastor's wife gave practical instructions; pastor gave ethical lectures and physician gave instruction in their professional duties. Florence Nightingale who received this practical training clearly saw that nursing and hygiene could be improved. Many activities are found in 1840 by protestant Nursing Sisters. In 1845 St. John house started a Nursing Training School.

Era of Florence Nightingale

A great opportunity of a life of preparation for task of care to soldiers came to Nightingale when she was asked the help by War Secretary, Sidney Herbert. She then took a band of nurses out to the Crimea to give nursing care to soldiers. She had good education and from high social strata. She had great opposition from home for the above task. She set standards of practical nursing, hospital administration, which still serves as a model. She took charge of a small hospital at

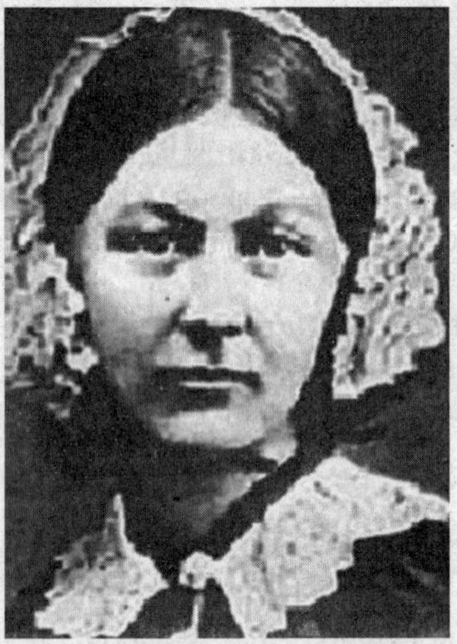

Fig. 1.2: Miss Florence Nightingale
Pioneer of Modern Nursing
Born on : 12th May, 1820
Died on : 13th August, 1910

war time. In the army to be a "Nurse of a reliable character" was a great challenge and Red tape obstructed her on all sides. Army doctors resented presence of a woman. Much worse, was the inability to face dreadful condition of war by women.

Her bravery in facing all constraints and nursing the sick soldiers made her an angel, another leading light and national heroine. Voluntary contributions by private soldiers to the tune of £ 9000 lead her to start "Nightingale Training School" at St.Thomas Hospital, where nurses were trained.

In addition to laying the firm foundations of modern system of nurse training, Florence Nightingale was responsible for the total reorganization of civil hospitals and military hospitals. She brought out many reformations including improving sanitation and hygiene of Indian Army. Her pledge is vivid even today (Appendix II).

NURSING ORGANIZATIONS

"British Nurse Association" was the first organized body of trained nurses in 1887. The Founder was Miss Gordon Manson (Matron of St. Bartholomew's Hospital). She is widely known under the name Mrs. Bedford Fenwick (after marrying Dr. Bedford Fenwick).

In 1894 Matron's Council of Great Britain and Matron's Council of Ireland were formed. In 1901, First International Congress of Nurses was held at Buffalo.

Leaders of nursing profession started college of nursing in 1916. A new bill was sponsored by Health Ministry and became "the Nurses Registration Act", in 1919.

In India, with the establishment of "Lady Reading Health School" (in 1918) preparation of nursing workers started. Bhore committee appointed by British Government (1946) and Mudaliar Committee appointed by Indian Government (1961) recommended replacement of untrained and partially trained nurses by trained Nurses. As first model in Nursing Education, a college of Nursing was established in Delhi in 1946. It is well known as R.A.K. College of Nursing in post Independent India.

Importance of nursing care in the community was thus visualized in India and following chronological progress is seen :

1947 - The Indian Nursing Council Act, 1947 was promulgated in Dec. 1947.
- The Indian Nursing Council was constituted.

1951 - A special subcommittee of Council, 1949, was appointed to study syllabus for General Nursing and Midwifery.

1953 - A guide for teachers and examiners in relation to Health subject was approved by the council.

1954 - Special provision for Male Nurse was made with (2/6) prescribed course of duration of 3 months in place of Nursing for women.
- Integration of Public Health in Nursing done.
- Minimum standards were laid down for recognition of nursing colleges.

1956 - Curriculum was developed for Nursing Colleges.
- Resolutions by Florence Nightingale Committee of Trained Nurses Association of India was accepted.

1963 - Revision of syllabus done.
- Guidance for School of Nursing by WHO made available.

1982 - Second Revision of syllabus done.
- Workshop reports of syllabus were accepted for National uniformity for:
  a. Staff
  b. Extension service

c. Physical facility.
d. Clinical Facility
e. Hostel
f. Number of Hours of Teaching (Appendix I).

2002 - Directed to the development of standard for professional nursing as envisaged in National Health Programme 2002.

NURSING UNDER W.H.O.

Attainment of Health by all - a set out preamble of constitution of WHO gave a starter to Nursing services all over the world. Positive health demarcated the line of action by Nurse to serve both well and ill in the community. Right to Medical care and Right to Nursing care are implied in the Fundamental Human Rights.

A changing trend in community care (from individual care) gave birth to community Health Nursing. It ranged from speciality hospital, Teaching hospital, District Hospital, Taluk Hospital, Community Health Centres, Primary Health centres and sub centres in the Nation and nursing service started as Team approach to health care.

W.H.O. approved the goal of Primary Health care and Health For All. International council of Nurses made these as priority issues. These concepts restructured the Health services. (Both urban and rural) M.P.W. (female) for a sub centre to a cover a population of 5000 was made mandatory. The Nursing council of India revised the curriculum for training of A.N.M. A scheme of village Health Guide to provide First Contact Care to a population of 1000 was started. Training of Indigenous Dais for safe deliveries was emphasized. Thus Nursing care had gone beyond the horizon to serve the community for promotion of health and care of the people wherever they live and wherever they work.

First, Second and Third level of care (Primary, Secondary and Tertiary Care) brought the nurses to home, school, health centres and varied (other) centres across the country.

In the words of W.H.O., "Millions of nurses throughout the world hold the key to an acceptance and expansion of Primary Health care, because they work closely with people." Here, we see a powerful potential for improvement of quality of human life.

NURSING BEYOND THE YEAR 2000

W.H.O. study group on Nursing beyond the year 2000, tried to include the need for continuing assessment of change of Community Health. The recommendations have 3 strategic aims.

- A new multisectoral systems approach to health care delivery and full collaboration of health care personnel at all levels.
- A shift in the focus of workforce development in nursing and midwifery to reflect country's health needs, with particular emphasis on vulnerable groups.
- Revitalization and reorientation of nursing and midwifery education and practice to meet the challenges of the future.

NURSING AND MENTAL HEALTH

Nursing, presently, is more than a custodian care of mentally sick persons. They are governed by Acts of parliament, the Lunacy Act, Mental treatment Act and Mental Deficiency Act. Even attending person need training and much more so a nurse who gives Psychiatric nursing, Mental hospitals do no longer have padded cells, strait jackets, locked doors, but have therapeutic cells, jackets and doors. With this change, nursing council and nursing colleges shall procure mental health training before final award of certificate and registration under Nursing Council to practice.

Nursing profession holds highest responsibility in discharging 75% of medical, surgical, obstetrical treatment and 100 percent of Community Nursing care. It occupies a strategic position in health care of well and ill and is committed to achieve the goal, Health for all beyond 2000.

FURTHER REFERENCES

1. Henderson V—Basic Principles of Nursing care, London International council for Nurses (Latest).
2. Nursing Practices—WHO TRS No. 860.
3. Indian Nursing Council—Regulations for General Nursing and Midwifery 1986.
4. Ordinances of University of Health Sciences in Nursing.
5. Evaluation of Type Definition for representing nursing activities—Suzanne Bakken *et al.* California (1999).

2

Sociology

INTRODUCTION

Two basic animal instincts, hunger and sex among lower animals are for individual survival as well as for species survival. Human being has the same instinct but has transformed himself physically, mentally, physiologically and culturally to rule as Master of Animal Kingdom. This art of adding experience has helped him to shape a better tomorrow. In man, biological forces are tuned to required desires through social standards which guide him. These two forces namely social standards and biological forces result in human behaviour, which is performed by him in everyday life.

The word sociology is derived from *socios* meaning society and *logos* meaning study.

Sociology along with human anthropology, psychology and psychiatry form Behavioural Sciences since they determine and influence human behaviour or how he conducts himself in the society.

Let us take an illustration in Nursing care:

Sham aged 22 years admitted for surgery hernia. He is admitted in surgical ward bed number 4. Surgeon, Matron and head nurse all give instructions like:

- Get blood test for bed number 4 hernia case.
- Do not give night meal to hernia case for surgery tomorrow.
- From which place bed number 4 case has come?

Thus all along, attending surgical and nursing profession has never called him by name. Patient even gets discharged as hernia case. Just calling him by name Sham would have brought out very good nurse-patient relationship. Even when Sham was eager to know the length of incision, what do they do on operation table etc., which remain unanswered, would have been attended to by conducting herself/himself as professional nurse.

This is how sociology as behavioural science helps in understanding sick, disabled and even dying. Present concept of understanding "well being" is also of utmost importance for an effective nursing care in the community.

DEFINITION

One has to think away from usual routines for proper understanding of sociology. To illustrate, a sister greets you in the ward "Good morning".

It has symbolic value for your social activity. It provides occasions for your social interaction. In human society it is an accepted norm and not a misbehaviour. Moreover, if you are greeted you have commanded respect and regards in your position and you have lifestyle choice to greet her by any means like:

a. Bowing your head.
b. Raising your right hand to give a partial salute.
c. Raising your left hand to say "Hoi", and rarely.
d. Say "*namaste*" with both palms putting together.

A study of sociology, thus, provides an insight into the understanding of activities that seem to concern our society, our family, our hospital (organization) etc.

The word sociology was coined by French author Auguste Comte (1798-1857) from his original word "Social Physics". His law was that human efforts to understand world in ordinary words, always passes through theological, metaphysical and positive stage as they are supernatural stage, natural stage and scientific stage.

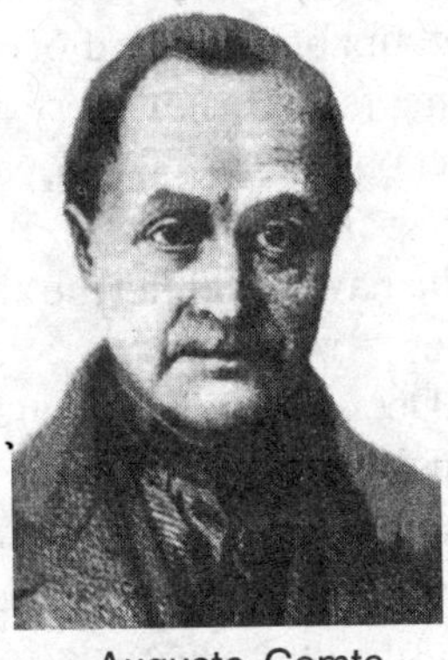

Auguste Comte

He defined Sociology as "the investigation of the laws of action and reaction of different parts of social system or social institutions and analysis of society as a unit for progress, change and development."

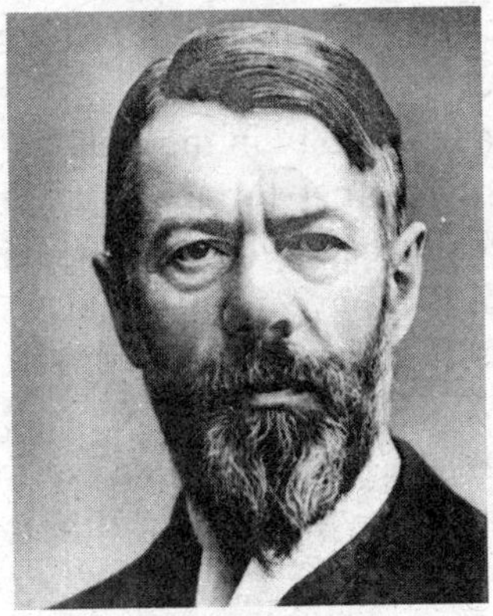

Max Weber

Emile Durkheim defined sociology "as the study of social facts".

Karl Marx points out that sociology is science that deals with social changes primarily by economic influences. Max Weber (1864-1920) points out "the study of organization of social and economic life according to the principles of efficiency and on the basis of technical knowledge". Thus broader definition of sociology includes four elements viz., (i) Social institutions, (ii) interaction between these institutions, (iii) Family forms a unit of study in sociology, and (iv) it focuses attention on social acts and social relationships.

NATURE AND SCOPE

Complexity of subject matter makes it hard to understand the nature of sociology. There are many social institutions which are related to each other in different ways giving room for social system. How we live and interact in a society is depicted in sociology. Functioning of family, school, industry, hospital, nursing home, health centre are the areas forming parts of the study of sociology.

Wide scope exists in understanding sociology. In a hospital Nurse-Doctor relationship, Nurse-Patient relationships which have common and distinctive features are found to be built up as "Social Act".

Medical sociology in the field of sociology has area of interest for the study of health, disease, health behaviour and social-medical interactions. We have many social diseases like tuberculosis, leprosy, sexually transmitted diseases, AIDS. Though they are caused by biological agent, we are turning our interests to study social, behavioural and cultural factors in disease occurrence. A nurse needs to be appraised of both biological and behavioural causation of well-being or ill-being in human beings.

IMPORTANCE OF SOCIOLOGY

From the point of nursing profession one has to understand the social aspect of disease, how it is influenced by certain predisposing and perpetuating factors, how to make nursing profession understandable, acceptable and even affordable by the community. Sociology can help to improve health service facility by:

a. Awareness of cultural differences.
b. Assessment of effects by national politics, and
c. Can lead to self enlightenment or increased self understanding.

USES OF SOCIOLOGY IN NURSING

There are many seen and unseen utility of knowledge of sociology. They can be enumerated as under:

a Rights of individual is understood
b. Responsibility for health increases
c. Family pattern influencing health is understood
d. Cultural pattern influencing health and disease is perceived
e. Role of social structure is made visible
f. Social problems are analysed
g. Social agencies that are available become visible.

MAN AND SOCIETY

Health or disease in man is determined by his social environment. Social and structural factors have direct bearing on the nature of illness. Social problems like poverty, poor sanitation, illiteracy influence man on his positive health. A patient whether in a hospital or at home has his own habits, customs and beliefs. This new outlook has brought a closer link to man and society.

Influencing factors are shown in figure which determine man's health in his society (Fig. 2.1).

Health is determined by four major variables in a society. They are:

a. Social circumstances like employed, earning etc.
b. Social predispositions like accident, family history of diabetes etc.
c. Ecological factors like values, culture etc.
d. Social opportunities like accessibility availability etc.

These are in-turn influenced by demographic, political and religious factors.

INDIVIDUAL

W.H.O. has expressed that "The enjoyment of the highest attainable standard of health is one of the fundamental rights of every human being without distinction of race, religion, political belief, economic or social condition". All countries including India have accepted the above and the right to health.

Universal Declaration of Human Rights under Article 30 consists:

"all human beings are born free and equal in dignity and rights... Everyone has the right to a standard of living adequate for the health and well being of himself and his family, including food, clothing, housing, medical care, necessary social services, right to security in the event of unemployment, sickness, disability, widowhood, old age or other lack of livelihood in circumstances beyond his

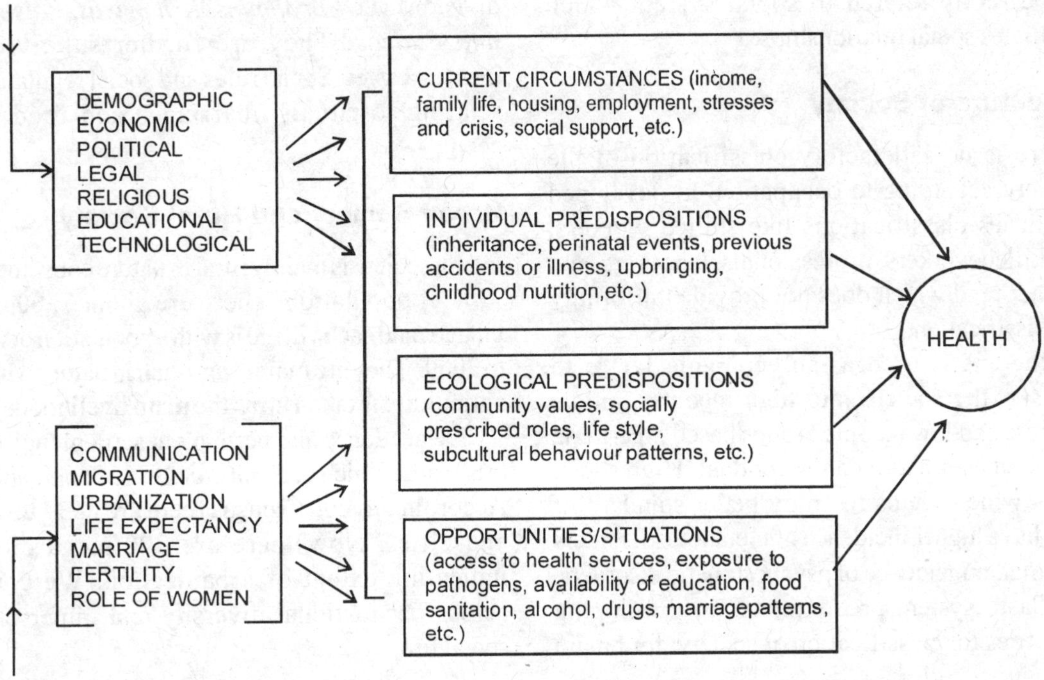

Fig. 2.1: Social factors in health

control......Motherhood and childhood are entitled to special care and assistance. All children born in or out of wedlock shall enjoy the same social protection.

Constitution of India has given guarantee of fundamental rights of individual:

a. The right to equality.
b. The right to freedom and expression
c. The right against exploitation
d. The right to freedom of practice and propagation of religion.
e. The right of minorities to conserve their culture.
f. The right to property.
g. The right to constitutional remedies for the enforcement of fundamental rights.

RESPONSIBILITY FOR HEALTH

This involves mutual adjustment and understanding by individual, his society, his community and his state.

Though society assures availability of services, it is the individual who should hold responsible for personal health. They include healthy habits in terms of diet, rest, care of skin, care of teeth, immunization, reporting of sick and service utilization.

SOCIETY

Man has always lived in group which is partially or fully organized, which we call as society. Man cannot live without society. It maintains a standard or laid down principles. Every individual maintains a social relationship which regulates the human behaviour. Here we notice social regulation, Law and Customs. Effort of an individual is either motivated or is hindered by social norms which stipulate either right or wrong.

More advanced science; professional activities are taken up or not acknowledged by a society. Thus morbidity, mortality and achievements are directly related to social system which regulates social relationships.

Structure of Society

There is no satisfactory classification of the society according to occupation. In developed countries classifications like skilled workers, unskilled workers, professionals, labourers etc., are adopted which does not provide uniformity in classification.

Income is used as an economic factor to classify the society into high income, middle income and low income groups based on criteria of income earned by an individual. High social class which seems to enjoy better standard of life, have higher incidence of metabolic disorders and higher incidence of psychosomatic disorders.

Caste system predominates in developing countries for classification of society; four main divisions viz. - *Brahmins, Kshatriyas, Vaishyas and Sudras*. They are further subdivided into sub castes. Social rules and social regulations relating to rituals, marriages and food are seen.

Urban Society and Rural Society

Indian society is mainly rural in nature constituting 72% of population. There are about 7, 00,000 villages and each village is with a population of 500 to 2000. They are mainly agrarian in nature where agriculture is taken up as the main livelihood.

Large, dense and permanent settlement form urban area which accounts for 28% of population. According to 2001 census there are 8637 towns and cities. Now there are 300 mega cities indicating extent of urbanization. We come across occupational diversity and impersonal social life.

Table 2.1: Difference between urban and rural society

	Rural Society	Urban Society
Disease Pattern	Infections	Metabolic diseases Cancer diseases
Socio-economic characteristics		
Domicile	Rural	Urban
Family	Joint family	Single family
Occupation	Mainly agriculture	Mainly Industry
Per Capita Income	Low	High
Literacy	Low	High
Standard of living	Low	High
Medical Care	Low	High
Demography		
Population	Young more	Older more
Problem	Of paediatric age	Of old age
Birth Rate	High	Low
Death Rate	High	Low
Growth Rate	High	Low
I.M.R.	High	Low
M.M.R.	High	Low
Life Expectancy	Low	High
Health Problems	Infection Malnutrition	Obesity Non communicable disease
Health Manpower	Shortage of manpower	More than adequate

There is wide difference between urban and rural society in terms of health aspect, like disease pattern, socio-economic characteristics, demography, availability of health man power, health status and nature of health problem (Table 2.1).

Social Mobility

Indian society is a "closed-class" system. There is restricted movement of social ladder. People changing their religion, caste and race are not commonly found. Recently, urbanization and civilization is making people accept social mobility on the basis of gaining wealth or on the basis of achievement.

COMMUNITY

W.H.O. has defined community as "group of individuals and families living together in a defined geographic area, usually comprising of a village, a town, or a city". The community usually has shown common interests.

Community implies some common characteristic features. They are:

- People live in a defined geographic area.
- People live together with certain social regulations
- They show cooperative effort in day to day life.
- They establish requisite sub-organisations like hospital, bank, store, school, college, market, industry etc.

Human network is found established in a given community. At a given point of time we see all categories of people with different spectrum from health point of view. At a given point of time we find healthy group, apparently healthy group, sick but ambulatory group, sick hospitalized, chronic, dying and dead.

Communities have varied economic functions. Directly or indirectly industries or occupation groups them for the purpose of categorisation. They are:

- Primary occupation like agriculture, forestry, fishing, mining etc.
- Secondary occupation like fabricating auto industry production etc.
- Tertiary occupation like education, health services, recreation club etc.

Community is also grouped under following categories:

a. *Rural community:* Villages form a specified boundary, specified independent occupation, specified administrative setup.
b. *Standard urban area:* A town with a population of 50,000 having encroachment of rural community with mutual socio-economic link.
c. *Urban agglomeration:* A few cities with good growth with delineated boundary.
d. *Urban community:* Population density is seen more than 400 people per square kilometre and is declared urban area by Government.
e. *Cosmopolitan community:* Mega cities with above 3 *lakh* population, specified geographic boundary, defined under city corporations.

NATURE OF SOCIETY AS BIOSOCIAL SYSTEM

Biosocial system of society is made up of value, customs, tradition and conventions. That system keeps a standardized ways of action to survive longer and face time tested odd situations. Natural calamities, man made conflicts have made this biosocial system to survive the test of time. Each biosocial system will have varied social system like primitive, civilized and moderately rigid in terms of sociological manifestations. A society can be with well advanced science and technology and show open class societies mainly thriving on achievement and progress.

Biosocial system of society is influenced by:

– Civil unrest

- Social problems including crime
- Unemployment
- Overgrowth of population.

Evolution of Society

Evolution of society is determined by literacy, standard of living and population movement.

Urbanization and civilization are bringing revolutionary changes in a society where we see over density of population and a shift from primary occupation to a secondary and tertiary occupation.

Special type of urbanization has developed called metropolitanisation where central city shows economic dominance over surrounding cities.

These evolutionary changes bring following changes in a society. They are:

- Demographic changes
- Economic changes
- Behavioural changes
- Health changes.

SOCIAL PROBLEMS

All of us follow social norms which is the outcome of socialization, which we are used to doing so. All social norms are accompanied by sanctions that promote conformity and protect against non conformity. A sanction is any reaction from others to the behaviour of an individual or a group that is meant to ensure compliance with a given norm. There are some individuals who refuse to live by the rules that majority of us follow. We come across alcoholism, drug users, S.T.D. Juvenile delinquency, prostitution, violent criminals. These people do not conform to a given set of norms that are accepted by significant number of people in a community. Some have health implications in the community.

Alcoholism

It is a global problem; over the past 50 years production, consumption and abuse has grown to such an extent to cause civil unrest. With the changes in social order alcohol is being considered a symbol of civilization resulting in alcoholism. Mild to serious health problems resulting from alcoholism are:

- Looses balance by poor reasoning due to alcohol content in the blood
- Peptic ulcer and gastritis
- Cirrhosis of liver
- Hypertension
- Heart failure
- Urinary disturbance
- Impotence and sterility
- Foetal damage.

Social implications of alcoholism are as under:

- Crime
- Murder
- Prostitution
- Family negligence
- Unemployment
- Indebtedness
- Malnutrition
- Delinquent child
- Traffic accidents
- Other psychosocial problems.

Health education and awareness programme can check the menace due to alcoholism. There are de-addiction centres to rehabilitate alcoholics. Simultaneously they need good and continuous counselling.

Drug Users

Repeated intake of habit forming drugs cause drug addiction (now it is called substance abuse). Patient show violent behaviour, nausea, vomiting and other severe allergic manifestations if a given drug is not made available. This is called physical dependence. Gradually drug users increase their dose intake indicating the development of tolerance. Finally even they commit crime (compulsion) to procure drug.

Social factors which seem to influence drug abuse are:

- Accessibility to young generation
- Broken homes
- Disturbed home environment
- Escapism from tense life and frustrated life.

Common drugs seem to produce drug abuse are:

Narcotics	–	Morphine
		Heroin
		Codeine
		Opium
Marijuana	–	Hashish
		Ganja
		Bhang
Hallucinogens	–	L S D
		Mescaline
Hypnotics	–	Barbiturates
Tranquillisers	–	Chlorpromazine
		Equanil
Stimulants	–	Amphetamine
		Cocaine

Case management include:

- Drug identification
- Detoxication in hospital environment
- Counselling
- Rehabilitation
- Change of environment in some cases
- Psychotherapy in some cases.

Social therapy includes:

- Individual health education
- Target group awareness

Legislative procedure available:

- Narcotic drug and psychotropic substance Act, 1985 to combat source.

S.T.D.

This is associated with development of slum and shanty town. Industrialization influence sexually transmitted diseases.

S.T.D. and prostitution are inter-related. In early days 5 classical venereal diseases viz. syphilis, gonorrhoea, chancroid, lympho-granuloma venereum and granuloma Inguinale used to top the list. Now more than 20 different entities are included in the list of S.T.D. Among new entrants Genital Chlamydial infection, Genital herpes, Genital human papilloma infection, and A.I.D.S. found to be predominating.

Social causes of STD are many and following are commonly seen in pre-disposing to infection:-

- Prostitution
- Possible high financial return
- Conducive lifestyle of urbanisation
- Idea of independence leading to behavioural change
- Alcoholism
- Broken homes.

Case detection by screening, full course of treatment of diagnosed cases, health education of the community seems to be practicable intervention strategies.

Juvenile Delinquency

Delinquent means any person who deviates from his or her normal behaviour, thus committing theft, sexual offence, murder, burglary, etc.

Juvenile delinquency means problem with children. Broken homes, poverty, feeble minded children precipitate the child to commit an offence. Here juvenile crime is confined to a boy below 16 years and a girl below 18 years of age.

Social measures like improving family life, free schooling for education, child guidance and other social welfare services are aimed at preventing juvenile delinquency. The Children Act 1960, provide legislative measures through orphanage, foster home, adoption, borstals and remand homes. Of late Juvenile Justice Act 1986 has made provision for rehabilitation of juvenile delinquent.

Prostitution

It is one of the old known social evils very commonly by broken homes, illegitimate love making and easy money as sex worker. Poverty seems to lead a woman to prostitution.

This is closely related with sexually transmitted diseases and AIDS.

Social regulation and a good culture in the family can reduce its incidence. The suppression of Immoral Traffic Act in women and girls (SITA) 1956, now called as the Immoral Traffic (prevention) Act 1986, covers men and women who are exploited for commercial purpose.

Violent Criminals

Various causes including lack of social regulations in the family and mental illness due to organic lesions found to produce violent criminals. Little different to crime, we have Deviant. The concept of deviance is much broader than that of crime which refers to non-conformist conduct that breaks the law.

Unmarried Mothers

It is insignificant in developing countries like India. But teenage mothers out of wedlock issues are becoming social problems.

They require guidance, counselling and nursing care.

Physically Challenged

This category comprising of blind, deaf, physically handicapped, crippled with leprosy, mental retardation is included under social problem.

Rehabilitation services with health care, education of blind, deaf, physical rehabilitation, vocational training are being undertaken to meet the above social challenges.

DIFFERENCE BETWEEN SOCIETY AND COMMUNITY

Society is group of people who settle down permanently and organize themselves. This shows a social system with demonstratable social relationships between individuals. Here behaviour of individual is regulated by social regulations. Society changes from time to time as a dynamic process. It incorporates one or more community.

Community is a social group determined by a markable boundary. It shows common values and common interests. It demarcates a geographical area to map out a village, a town, a city or a nation. Community is a network of human relationships; it is a major functioning unit of society; our house is located in a community. Our children are educated in a community. Human basic needs are met in the community.

SOCIAL SYSTEM

Social system enrolls individual, family, community and society at large. It provokes many social institutions. Social system is seen, as Weber put it, "in all human behaviour in so far as the acting individual attaches subjective meaning to it".

Societies differ from each other and they simulate each other in a social system.

The system has identifiable institutions like family, school, college, hospital, nursing homes, industry and the like. Thus it deals with societies and institutions.

Various identified social relationships are manifolds of social system.

Structure, Function and Mechanism of Social System:

Society, in a social system has its structure and stratification as under:

Social Anatomy

- Socioeconomic groups:
  Upper, Upper middle, Middle,
  Lower middle, Lower.
- Professional groups:
  Doctors, nurses, engineers etc.
- Religious groups:
  Hindu, Muslim, Christian etc.
- Caste groups:
  Four major with subgroups.
- Demographic groups:
  Young, Old, Male, Female, etc.
- Rural, Sub rural, Urban, Suburban etc.

Social Physiology

This explains ventilation (respiration), nutrition (gastrointestinal), waste disposal (excretion) and removal of offenders in the society (vital organ) just to depict manifold functions of society.

Social Pathology

It describes pathology of society like infant deaths, PEM etc., in the social system.

Social Diagnosis

Survey, screening, surveillance help us to identify social pathology and risk factors in health and disease.

Social Therapy

Personal or group health education, counselling, social welfare activities, social security measures for Social Therapy in social system.

ROLE, STATUS, RACE

Role

In social system we have many roles to play like son, daughter, brother, sister, teacher, lecturer, priest, mother, father, grandfather, grandmother and the like. This role play demarcates our relationships within a social system. Role confirms the behaviour of an individual to differentiate with others in the group. When it is given by virtue of age, sex, etc., it is called "Ascribed Role". By virtue of education, experience when done it is "Achieved Role". We play our role as nurses and doctors in health care services. When training is given to a nurse it is called "Role Induction".

Status

Status is an Achieved Role or Ascribed in the community or society. It can be head of the family, head of the state and head of the country. This is possible by social selection and is demarked with political activity. Status gives power to produce or to modify norms, values and customs. It is also called a social honour or prestige accorded to a person by society. Such status groups follow their normal life style and behavioural pattern. According to sociologists status may be positive or negative. Group leader is a positive status; Outcast is negative status.

Race

On the basis of biologically grounded features, many competencies are assigned to a group or to individuals who demonstrate a set of social relationships. Many attributes of biological origin help to differentiate a group which is called Race.

SOCIAL INTERACTION AND SOCIAL PROCESS

Social interaction includes both formal and informal situations in which people meet one another. In nursing college interaction between tutor and a nurse is formal social interaction. The same tutor and nurse when meet in a class social it becomes social interaction of informal type.

Social process is long term effective behaviour molding step which involve many formal and informal interactions. Child developing social norm and values at home with mother is a social process which is termed as socialization.

A positive outlook in social interaction and social process is seen with Cooperation, Completion, Accommodation and Assimilation. In Assimilation, values and norms of a dominant culture is taken up by a weak group in a society. During social process an acceptance of minority group by a majority group is through acceptance of norms of majority.

A negative outlook in social interaction is seen with conflict and isolation. A non interactive individual or a group is said to be isolated in the social process. Conflict is a sociological perspective of competition. When a group struggles to gain access to and to control resources, conflict is seen as a social process which allows tension and divisions.

SOCIALIZATION

It is a social process where man inducts his role as an individual in a family, society or community. He gains the knowledge of norms, values, sanctions and customs in the process of socialization.

TYPES OF SOCIALISATION

Primary Socialization

A child on developing awareness of social norms and values achieves a sense of self. This infant and childhood process is first time socialization. The child gets easily influenced and hence its development of sense of self determines the culture it gets.

Secondary Socialization

This is achieved by man when he gets exposed to outside family environment like school, neighbour etc., where he gets the second exposure to achieve sense of self. This further ties him up to the future social norms and values.

Re-Socialization

When a person has to mix up with other culture, other race that have customs other than his primary or secondary level, he starts acquiring that culture to become the member of that group. This is a needed sociological call. Typical example is when a boy or a girl from India goes to U.S.A. for higher studies, first few weeks of his or her adaptation to acquire new culture.

PROCESS OF SOCIALIZATION

It is a life-long process in man. It allows individuals to develop themselves and their potential to learn and to make adjustments.

Freud has postulated that dependency, fear; need for sympathy and love takes the child to social process of socialization where he/she may replicate the values and culture of parents and other relatives.

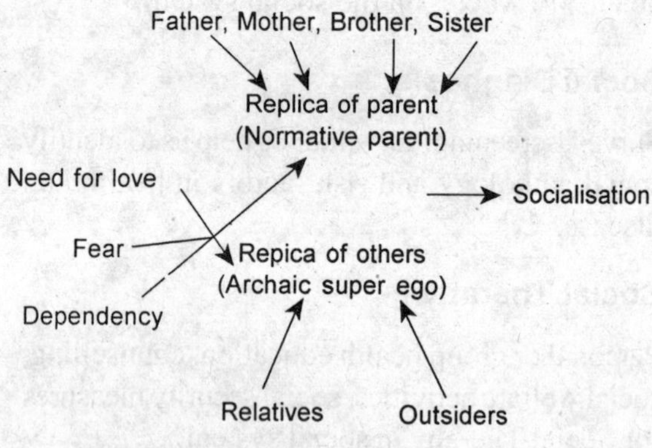

Fig. 2.2: Socialisation model after freud

Principle of socialization is used in nursing training where we do "role induction". During nursing training, set of norms are achieved by the student nurse here.

SELF IMPORTANCE OF SOCIALIZATION, INDIVIDUALIZATION

A person undergoes transformation through imitation, identification. This can be within the family (normative parent) or outside the family (archaic super ego). This has great relevance in making a required and good member of a society. Blending and fusion of personalities are looked upon with great care for personality development and for individualization.

Social Control

Human social behaviour is regulated by many factors. At family level we come across social regulations and in a society we see law and enactment. These are to regulate social behaviour towards normal. This has the control over deviation from normal.

Rewards and punishments control behaviour. Standardized social interactions become customs. Among them a few are stringent and are called mores. They become social regulations when we make them as formal one. Cultural standards in a society are termed as value orientation. Fashion is a typical example of value orientation in social control. Right way of doing things in society is called folkway. Most of the occasions folkways are done by reflex and do not carry vital importance.

In nursing profession we have many social controls for an effective training. Code of conduct and dress code is a formal social control enforced in nursing college. Similarly, nurses take an oath in an oath taking ceremony which can be regarded as formal social control of the institution.

SOCIAL GROUP

Any number of individuals when interact, when perceive creating a sense of "we", "they", social group is formed. There are many uses of social group.

They are to solve a problem, to reduce anxiety and tension, to attain a goal and to have cooperation.

Types of human groups are:

- Primary group
- Secondary group
- In-group
- Out-group
- Economic group
- Political group
- Religious group.

In a group consciousness of the members create certain commitment to conduct them for a required expectation.

Various theories are postulated in social group formation. They are:

1. Human wants nearness (proximity).
2. Cooperation to achieve goals (George Homans theory).
3. Sharing commonness (Newcomb theory).
4. Mutual comparison and reward (Theory of Tibut and Kelly).

A social group can be small or big. It can be temporary or permanent by nature.

Crowd, Public, Audience

These are temporary without common-ness. They are just emotional and do not have goal oriented activities. Colloquially it is called "mob" and mob mentality is described when there is no need, perseveration or interaction in a group.

FAMILY

Definition

"It is a group of individuals who are biologically related and live together, and eat from a common kitchen." House and social environment are shared by them and hence a family is called a "Social unit" or a "Cultural unit". By removing the word "biologically related", the unit becomes a "household".

Types of Family

Nuclear family: This is elementary family of married couple and their unmarried children.

Joint family: This has more than one married couple and their children, who live together in the same household.

Three generation family: When married son or daughter live with their parents along with their children.

Extended family: When old generation live, unmarried children live, polyandrous and polygamous couple live, married daughters live in father's house (matrilocal), married sons live in in-laws house (patrilocal) extended family is formed.

Family Cycle

There are four stages:

Stage 1 : Stage of formation when couple marry.

Stage 2 : Stage of growth when children are born.

Stage 3 : Stage of retraction when children marry and go away.

Stage 4 : Stage of disintegration when death of one or both parents occurs.

Functions of the Family

- Child birth and child rearing
- Sexual gratification
- Primary socialisation of individual occurs
- Social and mental stress are overcome
- Social and economic support is obtained
- Social interaction brings about new knowledge
- Each member has a role play and a job responsibility.

Family Problems

- Infertility, sterility
- Adoption
- Egoism
- Marital disharmony
- Broken family
- Poor social interaction
- Divorce
- Economic problem
- Malnutrition
- Alcoholism
- Conflict due to non adaptation of culture
- Susceptibility to diseases
- Chronic illness in the family. .

Marriage

It is a socially approved relation which allows sexual relationship between two individuals of opposite sex. Marriage forms basis of a family of procreation with an expectation that married couple will produce and bring up children.

Deviant marriage: Modern families are seen with homosexual marriages which do not serve the purpose of marriage. Similarly polygamy or polyandry is deviant marriage which forms extended families as seen in certain religions.

Modern Families

Pattern of family is getting changed due to accessibility and availability of social and economic sanctions. When both couple are earning members, child rearing is by a contract worker. Marriage is not a permanent bond and leaving to separate and live to separate are legally permitted by the Act of Divorce. Following outcome are seen in modern families:

- Lone parent household
- Remarriage
- Female partner to head the family
- Violence and abuse in the family
- Low accordance to family values.

Change in Indian Family

Slowly, size of the family, type of the family and composition of the family are changing due to varied social interactions and progressive urbanization and civilisation. Slowly, there has been reduction in joint family or three generation family. Average size of the family has come down from 6.3 to 3.1

This change has led to loosening of social regulation, no role of family in health and disease. Indian women, like western culture, face difficulty in reproductive and child health period, which used to be taken care by elderly women at home. Kinship in the family is slowly deteriorating. Nuclear family is predominant mainly because of industrialization of societies. Divorce rate is increasing giving room for reduced number of first marriages. Thus there is considerable diversity in family norms.

Legislation on Indian Marriage and Family

Family law, Hindu law cover the legal implications of divorce, remarriage, property dispute and care taker of offspring, which regulate the social problems from time to time.

As a policy measure age at marriage for a boy and girl have been fixed at 18 and 21 years respectively. This dictum is given as a family planning measure.

Civil marriage and registered marriage are allowed as per Marriage Act in India. As per Registration of Births, Deaths and Marriage Act, Registration of Marriage (even after civil marriage) is made mandatory.

Since social regulation is not found useful in social control over family issues, legislation on Indian marriage is put into action for allowing smooth and effective family pattern.

THE URBAN FAMILIES

Since population is getting concentrated in urban areas due to industrialization with varied occupation, urban family has molded to a pattern which needs consideration in a social system. This has lead to "urban crisis" which is a direct impact of increased exponential urban growth (now it is 3.09%).

Following table gives urban rural contrast:

Table 2.2: Urban-rural contrast for families

Item	*Rural*	*Urban*
Population	Thin	Dense
Occupation	Agriculture	Varied
Social dependence	Self reliant	Dependent
Social interaction	Primary	Secondary
Caste system	Dominant	Not dominant
Geographic boundary	Small	Big
Residence area	Not planned	Planned

Urban families are facing following economic, social and health problems:

- *Health problems:* Diarrhoea, STD, Hepatitis, Skin infection, malignancy.
- *Social problems:* Alcoholism, drug use, prostitution.
- *Environmental problems:* Road accidents, atmosphere pollution (Air, water, soil pollutions).
- *Economic problems:* Poverty.
- *Psychological problems:* Stress, anxiety, neurosis, suicides.

Above family problems are mainly:

a. Poverty induced and
b. Prosperity induced.

Healthy family movement is determined by social interactions and civic amenities.

They are: Small family norm.
Quality and Quantity of food.
Healthy environment.
Slum improvement measures.

SOCIAL STRATIFICATION

Social inequality is present in all types of communities. In some it may be by race, while in others it may be by caste.

Ranking of social activities according to values are age old phenomenon. This is a requirement for functioning of society. Another cause of social classification seems to be to hold position and power in a society.

Health Implications

a. Social class is related to certain types of diseases; malnutrition among low socio-economic and hypertension among high socio-economic group illustrate the relation.
b. Susceptible or risk group identification is possible.
c. Health service planning is possible.

Social Classification

By Occupation

We come across this classification in Britain (Registrar General of England).

Table 2.3: Socioeconomic classification by occupation

Social Class	*Occupation*
I	Professional
II	Managerial
III	Skilled
IV	Semiskilled
V	Unskilled

By Education

Illiterate, literate, primary, secondary, metric, graduation, post graduation are noted grouping for social classification.

Awareness, knowledge, practice with respect to health programme, disease are related to educational status.

By Pareek Method

For rural areas, Pareek has evolved a method by considering caste, occupation, education, social participation, land holding, housing, farm power, material possession and type of family. It is a form of scoring system for social stratification.

Income

Income alone is not considered for social classification. It gives value of socioeconomic grouping. However with other variables many methods are adopted in research methodology.

Prasad Classification

Per Capita Income (Rupee)

Social Class	*Prasad (1961)*	*Updated (1) for 1991*	*Updated (2) for 2001*	*Updated (3) for 2004*	*Updated (4) for 2008*
I	100 & above	1021 & above	20503 & above	29900 & above	37500 & above
II	50–99	510–1020	10230–20499	14600–29899	20600–37499
III	30–49	306–509	6,130–10,229	8600–14599	13600–20599
IV	15–29	154–305	3,076– 6,129	4490–8599	8500–13599
V	Below 15	Below 153	Below 3,075	Below 4490	Below 8500

1. Inflation index 206

Consumer index 4.96

$$C.F. = \frac{206 \times 4.96}{100} = 10.2176$$

Contd.

2. Inflation index	406	$C.F. = \frac{406 \times 5.05}{100} = 20.503$
Consumer index	5.05	
3. Inflation index	506	$C.F. = \frac{504 \times 5.94}{100} = 29.937$
Consumer index	5.94	
4. Inflation index	551	$C.F. = \frac{551 \times 6.8}{100} = 37.468$
Consumer index	6.8	

$$C.F. = \frac{(\text{Cost Inflation Index}) \times (\text{Current Price Index})}{100}$$

Note : C.F. (Correction Factor) based on Cost Inflation Index (GOI) of 551 (Feb 2008), Current Price Index of 6.8 (Feb 2008) are considered.

As per calculation:

100=00 of 1961 is equal to 1021=76 at 1991.
is equal to 20503=00 at 2001.
is equal to 29900=00 at 2004.
Is equal to 37,468=00 at 2008

Table 2.4: Prasad classification (Updated)

Kuppuswamy Classification (Modified)

	Item	*Score*	
A.	Education :	Professional, PG	7
		Graduate	6
		Inter	5
		High school	4
		Middle school	3
		Primary	2
		Illiterate	1
B.	Occupation :		
		Profession	10
		Semiprofession	6
		Clerk, shop, farm	5

Contd.

Contd.

		Skilled	4
		Semiskilled	3
		Unskilled	2
		Unemployed	1
C.	Income (Per Capita):		
		800 and above (14300 and above*)	12
		400–799 (9000 – 14229*)	10
		300–399 (8000 – 8999*)	6
		200–299 (6500 – 7999*)	4
		120–199 (4000 – 6499*)	3
		40–199 (2550 – 3999*)	2
		Below 40 (Below 2550*)	1

* The Gazette of India July 18, 2002 for current salary. Total Score : A + B + C

Social Class	Score (Total)
I	26-29
I I	16-25
I I I	11-15
IV	5-10
V	Below 5

Belonging and Achievement (Prabhakara, G.N. 1982, Urban-Slum)

	Score			
	0	1	2	3
House	Rented	Lease	Own	-
Room	Nil	1-2	3+	-
Toilet	Shared	Separate	-	-
Kitchen	Not separate	Separate	-	-
Vehicle	Nil	2 Wheeler (Mechanised)	2 Wheeler (Auto driven)	-
Radio/Tape records	Nil	Own one	Own two	-
Father's education (Head)	Illiterate	Primary	Secondary/ Technical	University
No. of living children	Seven	3-6	1-2	-

Social Class :

I	-	0-3
II	-	4-6
III	-	7-9
IV	-	10-12
V	-	13-15

By Caste

Classification by caste is no longer valid because of its sensitive and intricate nature. In India people do not easily change their caste or religion (Closed class). Movement of the social ladder by caste or religion is restricted and has influenced progressive movement. The movement in social ladder is called social mobility which brings about transformation. Social transformation is met with social resistance.

Presently, in India, social classification like upper caste, other caste, scheduled caste, scheduled tribe, other backward caste are in use for social welfare activities.

RURAL COMMUNITY IN INDIA

About 72.2% of population lives in rural community in over 700,000 villages. Govt. of India has 3-tier system of health care for primary health care through village health guide, *Aganwadi* worker and traditional birth attendant.

Health Profile of Villages

- *Health problems:* Infection, malnutrition, poor sanitation, shortage of health personnel.
- *Demography picture:* More young people with paediatric problem, high rates of birth, death, growth, infant mortality, maternal mortality and low life expectation.
- *Socioeconomic picture:* Joint family system with agriculture as occupation, low rates of per capita income, literacy rate, standard of living and medical care.

Changes in Indian Rural Life

Panchayat raj system has come into effect to uplift villages and for democratic decentralization. Three tier system of local self government is as under:

Gram Panchayat	-	at village level
Mandal Panchayat	-	at block level
Zila Panchayat	-	at District level

Gram panchayat is responsible for village improvement.

Cooperative movement has brought cooperatives in agriculture, bank, marketing to facilitate village upliftment.

Following G.O.I. programmes are approved from time to time for rural development and for social and economic growth. They are:

1. *Indira Awas Yojana* (IAY)—Shelter to shelterless.
2. *Jawahar Rozgar Yojana* (JRY)—Sustained employment.
3. Employment Assurance Scheme (EAS)—Assured employment.
4. Million Wells Scheme (MWS)—open irrigation wells.
5. Integrated Rural Development Programme (IRDP).
6. Development of Women and Children in Rural Areas (DWACRA).
7. Training of Rural Youth for Self Employment (TRYSEM).
8. Supply of Toolkits to Rural Artisans.
9. Land Reforms (Surplus land distribution).
10. Waste Land Development.
11. Old age pension scheme.
12. Rural women delivery allowance.

SOCIAL CHANGE

It is an alteration in basic structure of a social group. Social change is continuously occurring social phenomenon in life. They are now intense in modern era. There has been a tremendous shift from traditional system to modern social system.

Determinants

Following are the determinants of social change:

i. Demographic – Age, sex, occupation, education.

ii. Behaviour	– Suicide, homicide, delinquency, sexual offenses.
iii. Culture	– Values, custom, etc.
iv. Social structure	– Family pattern, Social control.

Influencing factors of social change:

- Physical environment
- Political environment
- Cultural environment.

Change in social system in modern period is mainly due to economic influence, political influence and cultural influence.

Cycle of social change is represented as under:

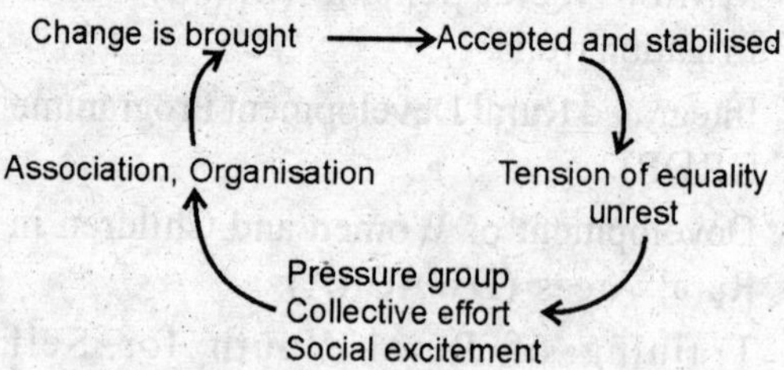

Fig. 2.3: Social change cycle

Social Change Indicators

- Development of Science and Technology
- Agriculture Development
- Modernisation of Industry
- Ecological changes.

STANDARDS OF LIVING

It refers to ways of living as shown by spending capacity and acquiring capacity. This depends on:

a. National income
b. Total production
c. Population growth
d. Educational level.

Standard of living is related to health and disease. High standard of living brings down diarrhoea, cholera, tuberculosis and improves standard health status in population. Standard of living determines birth rate, death rate, nutritional level and life expectancy.

CULTURE

Culture is defined as values, ceremonies and ways of life characteristic of a given social group. Culture is one of the most distinctive properties of human social association. Culture stands for mode of living, language, custom and belief. Hence it is socially acquired and learned behaviour.

Cultural diversity is seen with diversity of human behaviour and his practice. Small and big societies have monoculture and multicultural practice respectively. Subculture refers to a segment of population showing a change in cultural pattern.

Cultural pattern in India :	(example)
Health and disease	– It is by supernatural factor. It is by sin of past life.
Personal hygiene	– Bathing everyday done Apply oil before bath Pan, *supari*, lime eaten as custom *Hukka* smoking is a custom Walking barefoot common.
Environmental hygiene	– Open field defecation, using river water for ablution purposes, washing animals in the same source of water.
R.C.H.	– Certain foods are avoided in pregnancy, lactation, infancy. Delivery is conducted by untrained indigenous Dai. New born is not given colostrum:

Cow dung application to cut end of umbilical cord.
Skin branding for head-ache.

Nutrition – Higher caste do not eat non-vegetarian food.
– Some foods are hot.
– Some are cold.
– Eating garlic is a taboo.

Above illustration gives us the cultural pattern of people which have direct bearing on health activities.

Understanding of culture is important to bring about changes in habit, custom and belief of the community, with respect to health of the individual and community.

SOCIAL SECURITY

It is defined as "Security that society furnishes through appropriate organization, against risk to which people are exposed." Common risks are:

- Sickness
- Invalidity
- Maternity
- Old age
- Death

They are classified under 3 categories:

a. For industry workers
Indian Factory Act, 1948
E.S.I.S., 1948
Workmen Compensation Act, 1923
Central Maternal Benefit Act, 1961
Family Pension Scheme, 1971

b. For Civil Servants
Pension
Gratuity
P.F.
Family pension

c. For public
Insurance schemes
P.P.F.

Social Security Benefits are distributed through three channels. They are:

Social Assistance

It covers old age pension, widow pension, assistance to leprosy patients, F.P. Assistance, Old age homes, stipend for unemployed graduates, maternity assistance to the poor and senior citizen facility.

Social Defence

Like Punishment of criminals, Anti Dowry Act, Eradication of beggary, Welfare of prisoners, Alcohol prohibition, Gambling control, Prostitution control, Suicide counselling.

Social Insurance

Like ESI, Crop insurance, Accident insurance, Insurance for health.

SOCIAL AGENCIES

As part of social cultural tradition, there are many social welfare services as an integral part of community development. In the field of social welfare, it is estimated that there are about 60,000 voluntary organizations in India are doing yeomanly services. Coordination of social welfare is by Ministry of social welfare and central social welfare Board. They are categorized as:

a. All welfare activities
b. Women welfare
c. Child welfare
d. Specific disease control
e. Specific welfare activities.

FURTHER REFERENCES

1. An introduction to Sociology – Sachdeva, Bhushon (Kitab).
2. G.O.I. – Guide to community development.
3. Sociology – Giddens (Polity).
4. Sociology for Nurses by Dr. G.N. Prabhakara (Peepee).
5. The Gazette of India July 18, 2002.

3

Nurse and the Community

INTRODUCTION

Progress of nursing has reflected the social outlook of present century, so also Health centres, District Hospitals and Teaching hospitals.

In the beginning nurse has to adjust, at her entry, to new surroundings and should not get bewildered by many aspects of hospital life. Preconceived idea by nursing student about hospital and about nursing may bear little resemblance to reality. Hence the need of understanding the structure and function of hospital is essential.

Health care especially nursing care is a continuous exercise to be carried out day and night without interruption; for the sick there is no time interval. All departments are geared to serve the sick; many units and discipline like all specialties, dispensary, laboratory, X-ray, physiotherapy and ancillary staff like orderly, porter, domestic workers and so on. Hospital is a complex institution/organization and demands your attention that is not equaled in many other spheres.

Hospital serves as an in-house training to doctors, radiographers, Physiotherapists, Midwifes, Social workers, Medical postgraduates as well as undergraduate students including nursing students. Nursing profession has greater role to play not only in curative treatment/ arresting of disease, but also to restore the patient as far as possible to full activity. The co-operation of patient is required so that he can play his part in recovery and subsequent welfare, nursing profession has great role to play in getting the patient's co-operation.

Nursing has its role in hospital research. Experience and observation has helped health staff to give a confidence based specific treatment. Joseph Lister's "Antiseptic Surgery" has opened the door to great surgical advances. Such great examples are available to mitigate sufferings of mankind and truly are part of hospital services.

NURSE AND PATIENT

A somewhat sobering statement which is worth careful consideration is:

"Do the sick no harm":

This is from none other than Florence Nightingale. Constant vigilance is needed in nursing procedures in order that these may be carried out with the highest degree of competence.

Checking administration of dangerous drugs, measures to prevent cross infection, care of elderly, care of child, care of women in labor pain need substantial attention which are available only from nursing profession.

Anxiety and stress of patient need attention to overcome distressing effect on family life. To watch an experienced and sympathetic ward sister set about the task of allaying the fears of anxious relatives and establishing their confidence in the hospital and the staff is a most valuable lesson in good human relationships.

NURSING ETHICS

It is a code of moral behavior and rules of conduct related to Nursing. Compassion, sympathy, pleasant manners are required for successful management of a case.

Loyalty and obedience to authorities, recognition of experience of senior staff, maintaining confidentiality on affairs of patient are other aspects of ethical issues.

Trustworthiness and reliability are essential if the nurse is to develop a sense of responsibility as a member of nursing team.

It is the moral and ethical obligation of a nursing profession to offer one's service to a patient irrespective of social distinction, race, creed or caste.

Professional Etiquette

Certain rules of behavior for maintaining discipline and orderliness which are necessary for safety and welfare of patient is of prime importance.

While nursing staff are addressed with a title of Matron, sister, Nurse etc., Patients should be identified by their name and not by number or disease. Courtesy to visitors who visit their patients improve patient-nurse relationship and this extends to the good hospital environment. Courtesy shown to seniors matters much in nursing professional etiquette.

Major Principles of Nursing Ethics

1. Principle of doing good (Beneficence).
2. Serve the ill with fairness, equity and impartiality (Justice).
3. Patient can choose his choice of treatment (Respect for autonomy).
4. Principles of not harming patient (Non maleficence).

Formal Procedures in Nursing Ethics

Values and norms drawn are followed and ethical issued are considered while attending formal procedures in the following:

- Organ donations.
- Dealing with human life area, e.g. MTP.
- Living will.
- Advanced life directives in terminally ill and cancer patients.
- Dying declaration.

Professional Nursing Ethics

There are certain moral principles which guide nursing profession in day to day interaction with colleagues, patients, relatives of patient etc. They are:

a. CONTRACT: Fully attending till normalcy, is an utmost requirement. When a case is being handled, one has entered into a contract with patient to do all required professional act to bring him back to normal and not disallowing in the middle. It will become breach of contract.
b. CONFIDENTIALITY: In nursing profession it is obligatory to maintain strictly confidential about the physical and mental status of a patient.

Rational Use of Drugs

In nursing profession, need for use of discretion is very critical in administering the right dosage in right time and of required combination in order to relieve the patient's suffering or to avoid any distress and/or help the patient's speedy recovery.

RESEARCH

No Over Investigation

Unnecessary investigation which might bring discomfort to the patient and /or result in unnecessary expenditure should be avoided.

Animal Experiment

Humaneness animal ethical procedures are followed in Research, drug trial etc.

GUIDING PRINCIPLES IN NURSING CARE

Following are guiding principles for nursing profession:

- Compassion
- Confidentially
- Element of informed consent
- Obligation to treat
- Respect for persons
- Solidarity
- Well being or beneficence.

FURTHER REFERENCES

1. Prabhakara G.N. – Short Text Book of Professional Medical Ethics (Paras).
2. ICMR – Guidelines on Research involving Human subject.

4

Psychology

Psychology is concerned with human behaviours. Both physical factors and mental factors (Bodily action/function and mental action/function) interact with each other which are more complicated than a circuit and computer.

Man in his society is influenced by values, attitude, economic condition, interaction with other members of his family, co-workers in his working placement, his religious placement and other social systems. Social stratification and gender difference have limited the normal behaviour of people.

Man has set certain do's and don'ts in his setting. His behaviour is determined by these factors. Acceptance or a sanction for treatment also is determined by his behaviour.

In nursing care we come across following type behaviour which directs the individual towards acceptance or rejection of care.

a. Health Behaviour

Oral hygiene, care of teeth, care of genital organs, periodic health check up to identify risks at early phase, eating habit, sleeping habit, bowel habit etc., are examples of health behaviour. They help in prevention of many diseases. Monogamy and marital harmony is another example of health behaviour which prevents S.T.D. and AIDS.

b. Illness Behaviour

In early part of sickness home remedy from enquiry with friends, advices from elders are common. This is a natural reaction to subjective manifestations of a disease. On the contrary, health awareness helps in early diagnosis and prompt treatment.

c. Treatment Behaviour

Acceptance or no acceptance of activities suggested for disease form treatment behaviour. Some like oral, others parenteral (injections) at advice. Many are scared of surgery and go for medical treatment only. In nursing care, taking drugs or medicamentation as directed and return for follow-up and advice is regarded as good treatment behaviour.

DEFINITION

Psychology is "the study of human behaviour, the study of how people behave, the study of why they behave and which are within accepted norm".

SCOPE

Psychology is glued with every aspect of human life. It is seen in all types of human interaction. Understanding of human mind helps us to analyze intricacies involved in mental disorders. There are various branches of psychology which deal with day to day occurrence in human behaviour. These branches are:

- Social Psychology
- Educational Psychology
- Child Psychology
- Applied Psychology
- Psychoanalysis
- Medical Psychology (Psychiatry)
- Adult Psychology
- Women Psychology
- Elders Psychology.

APPLICATION TO NURSING

Psychology helps a nurse in understanding the need of a patient. Nurse can motivate patient for required helpful activity useful for recovery. She can make patient think and reason out in medical emergencies. Understanding emotions and feelings of the sick will be secret of success in effective nursing care. Psychotherapy may be required in cases of psychosomatic disorders like Asthma, Peptic ulcer, ulcerative colitis, hypertension etc.

METHODS

Methods adopted in Psychology, as a science of behaviour in abnormal behaviours and mental illnesses are:

- Psychoanalysis
- Psycho diagnosis
- Psychosocial Counselling
- Psychotherapy.

HUMAN BEHAVIOUR (BEHAVING ORGANISM)

Human behaviour is nothing but response to our surroundings. When we see a snake we run away; when we see a coin lying on the ground, we go near and pick that up, we hit a person who spit on us. Here snake, coin, spitting on the face are stimulus and running away, picking up and hitting are responses. It is an age old dictum that stimulus determines our behaviour.

Lower animals' responses are at lower level of functioning. Man responds at higher order of functioning and he uses integrated and coordinated responses.

Integrated Response

Man as a higher animal uses integrated and consolidated response as a response to stimulus. Habits and skills are used by reflex and emotions, feeling, tension are created as automated response. But man uses thinking, reasoning and perceptions which are intellectual response.

LEVELS OF FUNCTIONING OF STIMULI

Conscious Behaviour

As per the standards of and norms in social system man reacts to external stimuli like touch, smell which is determined by cerebral cortex. Student nurse standing and greeting the Matron is a reflex process but standardized code of behaviour which is stimulated by the sight of Matron.

Subconscious Behaviour

These arise within our body and level of functioning is thalamus of the brain. This response is in terms of emotions and feelings. Anger, Joy, Sympathy and Affection are responses from subconscious behaviours to natural occurrences. Death, Birth, Loss of leg by accident are typical examples to produce this behaviour.

Unconscious Behaviour

Opposite to conscious behaviour, man responds to certain stimuli, say without his knowledge. When a person witnesses "great suffering to die" he is bound to pronounce many things which did not happen at all. Very bad event in life despite associated with stimuli, when avoided, constitute unconscious behaviour.

Intellectual Behaviour

Thinking, reasoning and analysis of situation before response is a high order functioning. This type is diagnomonic to man as a behaving organism.

ATTENTION AND PERCEPTION

Attention and perception are two major mental activities. Attention is an alternate to observation. They have lead to many great discoveries. Theory of gravitation was formulated by Newton by his keen attention, fungal growth observed helped in the discovery of antibiotic "penicillin" by *Alexander Fleming*. Similarly signs and symptoms observed by Hippocrates laid the foundation of modern medicine.

Attention leads to thinking, reasoning and further to learning. Poor attention leads to poor learning.

Present concept of attention is that it is more careful observation. Primary red colour in "Inverted Red Triangle" of Family Planning symbol is only for drawing attention that Health care including Family Welfare Facilities are available.

Perception

It denotes "observe, recognize and discriminate". Vision, sound, taste, smell and touch help us to sense the stimulus. Thus perception is a behaviour where man interprets and appreciates. A heart attack patient who craves for fresh air to breath comes out with the perception that he gets good oxygen outside. Here motivation and need makes him to do so though there is no difference in the air existing inside and outside; but the fact is that he lacks oxygen which is due to heart attack (Myocardial Infarction).

Perception by Selection

By value orientation (Importance given), man perceives either accurately or otherwise. When a Nursing Superintendent instructs a nurse, she does the job with immediate effect giving due importance. Suppose the same instruction is given by a neighbour (a senior citizen), accepting and perceiving are different. There is no value orientation that it must be done with immediate effect.

Following diagram depicts a perception set up:

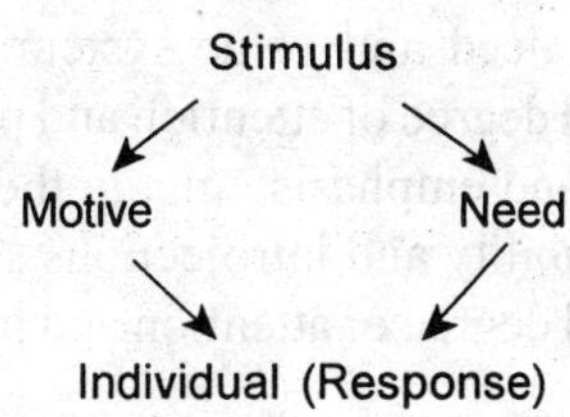

Fig. 4.1: Perceptual organization

Perception Emphasis

There are many parts of perception say early, middle and final parts. When man gives emphasis to Final part it is an emphasis or perceptual accentuation.

Perception Stabilized

A person, who has experienced chest pain (angina pectoris) after a mild heart attack, always perceives and gets fear of another attack. Unless perception of patient is reorganized, his old perception does not break up so easily.

Perception Introjected

Many experiments have shown that memory of childhood has the ability of perception introjected. Neurosurgeon Penfield has shown that a scene "Fire was engulfing parents" by a child is made available as perception but is taken off, as this being unperceivable.

Determinants of attention and perception are:

a. Neurological causes.
b. Psychological causes
c. Sensory organ damage (loss of smell, hearing etc.).
d. Mental disorders cause false perception called illusion.
e. Mental disorders causing hallucinations which are gross error of perception.

Duration and Degree of Attention and Perception

Motivation, need and value system affect the duration and degree of attention and perception. Selectivity and emphasis enlarge the duration, where as stability and introjections shorten the duration and degree of attention and perception.

Sensory Perceptions

Perception takes place with the help of sensory organs. Accordingly they are:

- Visual
- Auditory
- Olfactory
- Muscular
- Cutaneous perception
- Taste perception.

MOTIVATION

It is the driving force in human psychology. Man is driven to any social action by an inner force. Motivation thus is a best determinant of behaviour. There are two sides of motivation. They are:

- Positive motivation (Right-doing- behaviour).
- Negative motivation (Wrong-doing-behaviour).

Occasionally manipulation is confused with motivation. MANIPULATION is acquiring phenomenon for a developed desire and urge.

Definition

Motivation is the desire, acquired to gratify the needs. It includes all activities and need which are directed to acquire gratification.

Needs and Drives

Human needs are Basic, Additional and Health needs. Some psychologists include luxury as a type of need.

To acquire and gratify above needs man has 2 major types of drives—One is innate and the other acquired.

Range and Classification of Needs and Drives

Needs are classified as under:

a. **Social need:** They are mainly desired needs like love, affection, recognition, education etc., which pertains to social nature of man.
b. **Economic need:** To fulfil the want of economic security is topmost need of the day.
c. **Ego need:** Self respect, power, position and status are present updated item under needs.
d. **Biological need:** They are mainly survival needs like water, food, shelter etc.
e. **Psychological need:** Sympathy, concern, attachments, influence are under psychological needs.

DRIVES which are called motive are classified under:

a. **Innate drive**: They are desires to gratify the biological needs.
   i. **Primitive innate drive:** Has come from ancestors and are reflex oriented. To charge a man who beats you is similar to animal instinct.
   ii. **Reflex innate drive:** Hunger contraction motivates to acquire food. Typical example is seen with Dog experiment by Pavlov.
   iii. **Universal innate drive:** Some innate drives are common in human beings like acquiring a house, to become a good singer, like to have a baby boy, like to have an auto drive vehicle and so on.
b. **Acquired Drive:** During the process of socialization, child or adult acquires certain drives which are learned during social acts. A boy who wants a show off acquired by observing others, dresses up most fashionably to meet a girl. This is an acquired drive to meet a psychological need.

Certain common social motives are always seen in a community. A girl without lower limb and upper limb is seen with a related behaviour to depend on another normal girl. This does not allow any other alternative but to have an acquired drive of "common social motive".

Biological Motives

In Health Science we expect people to be self reliant on health related matters. This is expected of them to achieve improvement of health by their own effort (Community participation). There are many issues related to biological motives. They are:

- Mother to attend antenatal clinic.
- Child to be brought for immunization.
- Eligible couple to practice contraception.
- Use potable water to prevent water borne diseases.

Theories of Motivation

i. Habit formed out of trial and satisfaction produce motivation.

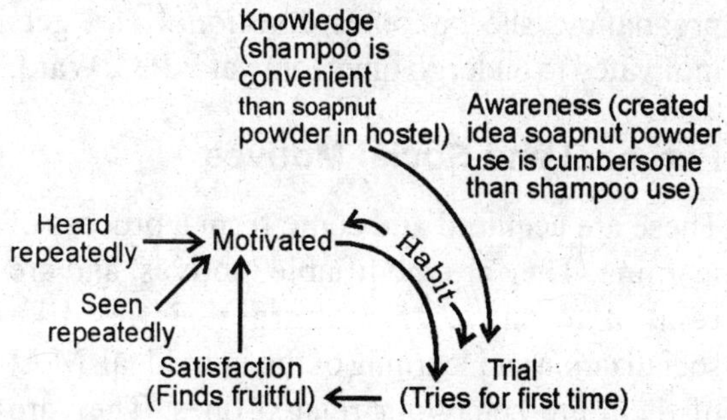

Fig. 4.2: Trial –satisfaction—trial cycle

ii. Curiosity produces intense behaviour of motivation.
iii. Self life experience produces a stable motivation.

Stages of Motivation

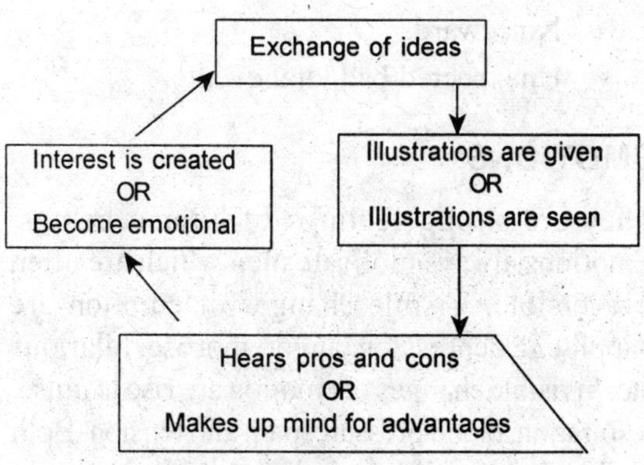

Fig. 4.3: Stages of motivation

Typical example of stages of motivation is seen with a mother who has delivered recently in a hospital. Her peers exchange the idea of post partum tubectomy which is easiest and comfortable. She sees other mothers getting satisfied with Post Part Centre programme, she finds more advantages if she avoids future pregnancy; she becomes emotional and gets motivated to undergo tubectomy at P.P.C. Ward.

Personal and Social Motives

These are acquired and come from a process of learning. They are modifiable motives, and are related to subjective characteristics like socialization and learning of the individual. Most of them are behaviour related ones. They are explained under "common social motives" above.

Conflict in Motives and Resolution

Motivation is deterred by many factors in psychosocial atmosphere of an individual or a group. These factors may take off the motive which is called resolution.

Common conflicts noted in the process are:

- No good personal relations.
- No good approach or free discussion.
- Shortfall in guidance, support and encouragement.
- No reward.
- Unexpected bad vital event.

EMOTIONS

They are strong feelings of human beings. Emotions always motivate men which are often irreversible. Visible changes of emotion are happiness, depression, anger, morose, hilarious etc. Invisible changes of emotion are rise in pulse, respiration, blood pressure, pain and tension. Both visible and invisible emotions usually return to normal with rest and relaxation.

Types of Emotions

Specific Emotions:
Anger, Fear, Hate, Love.

Non-specific Emotions:
Grief, Joy, Jealous, Lust, Moodiness, Pity, Sorrow, Sympathy.

Emotions are major barriers of communication. Only after "Pass-off" period of emotion, patient can talk freely and there is chance of effective nurse-patient interaction for nursing procedures.

Definition

Emotion is defined as "Sudden force surfacing in the mind in response to a situation."

States of Emotion

There are 2 states of emotion:

i. Positive state–Pleased, Joyous, Loved, Satiated etc.
ii. Negative state–Sad, Sorrow, Anger, Hatred, fearful etc.

Emotion as a Motive

Emotion expressed becomes a motive to gratify the needs. A nurse falling unconscious at work attracts attention. Her friends get emotional to see her state of affair. It is a motive for quick interaction. Duty nurse is motivated to attend to her at her best out of emotional attachment to her professional colleague.

Both positive and negative emotions are found useful as motives in Health Care services.

- Example of positive emotion as a motive: Very low birth interval with low birth weight, repeated infection of new born emotionally makes a mother to get motivated. She accepts "Spacing" as contraceptive method for the sake of health of new born.

- Example of negative emotion as motive: Showing a clinical case of Tetanus to a mother who used to resist TT for school children, explaining her that TT as the only weapon to prevent Tetanus. Emotions of fear and concern in the mother allow her child to get TT by negative motivation.

General Theory of Emotion

Emotion and culture are associated. Differences of emotions in various societies are seen. Culture determines the way of expression of emotions.

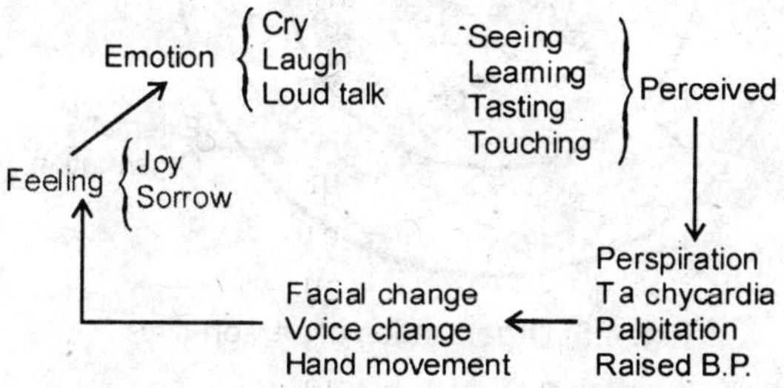

Fig. 4.4: General theory of emotion

Emotion and Health

Various disorders are seen associated with emotions. These vary with Age, Sex and other demographic variables.

Adults – Loss of concentration
– Loss of appetite
– Increased accidents
– Loss of sleep
– Palpitation

Women – Anorexia nervosa
– Amenorrhoea
– Pseudo pregnancy

Children – Tantrums
– Abdominal pain
– Spasms
– Tics
– Aggressiveness

Control of Emotions

Children – Love
– Affection
– Appreciation.

Adults – Happy family life
– Reassurance
– Cultivating hobbies
– Habit of Reading
– Recreation
– Adaptation of Philosophy of life
– Understanding ones own limitations
– Development of sense of humour.

PERSONALITY

Since personality determines human behaviour and human behaviour is molded by personality, they are inter-related. Personality of health professional influence prognosis of sick and hospitalized.

Definition

Personality is defined as body pattern which are influenced by status role etc., externally and by thinking, desire, goals and motivation etc., internally and all these lead to an aspect of selfhood.

Types

According to Swiss psychiatrist Carl Jung (1875-1961), there are 2 types of human personalities.

i. *Extrovert:* A person always exhibits his feelings, easily mixes, active, deemed practical and dare devil in action.
ii. *Introvert:* A person always shy, keeps himself aloof, reserved.
iii. *Mixed:* A combination of extrovert and introvert.

Development of Personality

Following factors help in development of personality. They are:

i. Heredity (Parent's reflection)
ii. Physical environment
iii. Social environment
iv. Gratified basic needs
v. Attained educational level.

In human cycle, stages of a given cycle influence the development of personality.

i. Infant and childhood – Primary socialization
ii. School age child – Secondary socialization
iii. Adolescent – Adventure, Romance, Love
iv. Adults – Mature and balanced
v. Old age – Changes due to senescence.

Components of Personality

i. Physical components:
Height, Weight, Skin colour, Face.
ii. Emotional components:
Anger, Fear, Guilt, Jealousy, Love, Worries.
iii. Intelligence components:
High IQ.
iv. Behaviour component:
Kind, Affectionate, Aggressive, Submissive, Balanced.

Personality Trait

It is defined as a stable personality manner and the tendency to behave in such a manner for a given social interaction. By 5 year 10 months, the child develops basic personality trait. In adulthood some traits are cultivated and some are concealed. Some of the examples of personality traits are:

- Kindliness
- Reliability
- Sense of humour
- Loyalty
- Tactfulness
- Willingness to help
- Good manners
- Cheerfulness.

Organization of Personality

It is summarized by the following diagram:

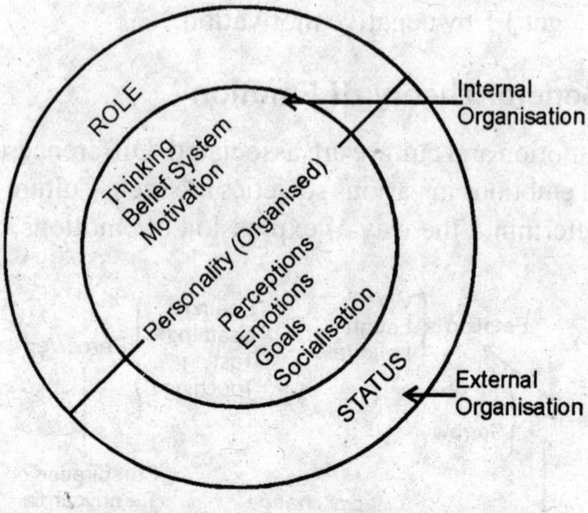

Fig. 4.5: Organization of personality

Theories in Personality

i. Theory of Self:
It is basic feature of personality. Learning in the family setting and use of language contribute to development of personality. Socialization within the family and foundation of attitude outside the family determine "self". Self is symbolized with surname, family title etc. Membership and class position extends the development of self.

ii. Kardiner's basic personality structure Theory:

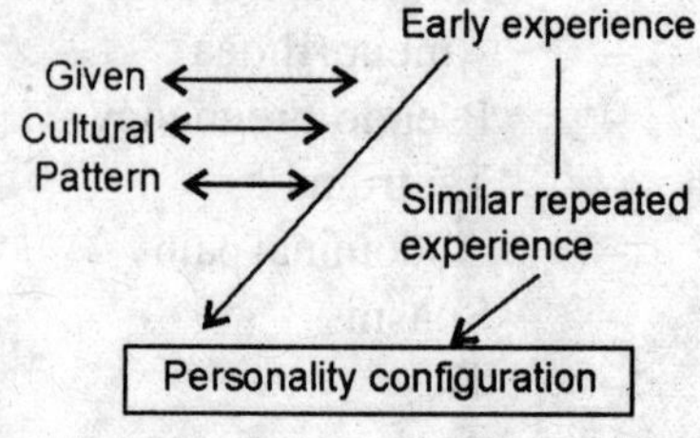

Fig. 4.6: Kardiner's theory of basic personality

iii. Man in early life has a common and fundamental experience—which is reflected as "Personality structures" and is a common phenomenon in any given society.
iv. Individuals will have many common elements in their personality that are common.
v. Early experience in life (of individual) varies from society to society. Hence personality norms also vary from society to society.

Role of Character in Personality

Character implies moral worth of an individual. It is different from personality. Character of an individual is variable from time to time whereas personality does not. Often conduct and character are synchronized. How a person conducts himself in a society is described in terms of character, though they mean differently.

Role of Will in Personality

Determination of an individual forms a will. Willingness leads to a way in characterization. Thus, will and character are interdependent on each other; will is transient and flexible which do not mould personality.

LEARNING

Learning is a psychosocial process that is required for survival and human progress. It is not equivalent to education but imply acquiring knowledge, skills, habit formation and perception development. Human intelligence has lead to lot of change in learning. Age old observation and service at *Gurukula* for a learning which used to take years of exposure, has been reduced to a shorter spell of time where learning is processed even independently. Conscious learning is an adopted behaviour, where as unconscious learning is a conditional behaviour.

Definition

Learning is an active and continuous process which results in relatively permanent behavioural change in man. This is reflected through thinking, feeling, doing and attitude of a learner. It is also an outcome of one's interactive experience with his surrounding.

Law of Learning

Learning has come up through all stages of human development - Birth, Marriage, Family - formation, Service, Health, Sickness, Disability and even death. Learning is appropriated for survival and progress. It is for habit formation and perception development. Law of learning attains an individual to face any psycho-social interaction by reflex and do not allow him to succumb to injury or death.

Nature of Learning

A good deal of animal experiment and human experiment conducted by psychologists has brought out following aspects of learning:

a. Reflex learning
b. Learning by trail and error
c. Learning by observation
d. Learning by imitation
e. Learning by doing
f. Learning by remembering
g. Learning by mental exploration
h. Learning by any combination.

Principles of Learning

Various theories of learning have evolved certain principles which are applied in learning activities to enhance learning.

The *Principles* of Learning are:

a. Human learning is guided by many set goals to achieve either at a shortest time or on a long term.

b. Human needs in terms of Physiological, safety, social, esteem, self actualization and aesthetic needs are strong reasons for learning.
c. Life oriented education through observation and participation form the basis of learning.
d. It is a voluntary process involving thinking, feeling and doing. Hence it involves the learner actively.
e. Basic styles of learning in man have been surface learning, deep learning and strategic learning.
f. There should be learning with an understanding which is called meaning orientation in learning.
g. Learning leads to knowledge and in turn should lead to application of mind.
h. Learning should be for a real life situation and real life problem solving.
i. Learning should begin from known and should proceed to unknown.
j. Reinforcement of learning is possible by feedback process.

Types of Learning

Present concept of classification in learning is called "Taxonomy in Education".

There are 3 main types of learning. They are:

Bloom's Cognitive Domain

This is the area of intellectual skills. Learning is by acquiring, recalling and recognizing a thing or an item. This is represented Figure 4.7.

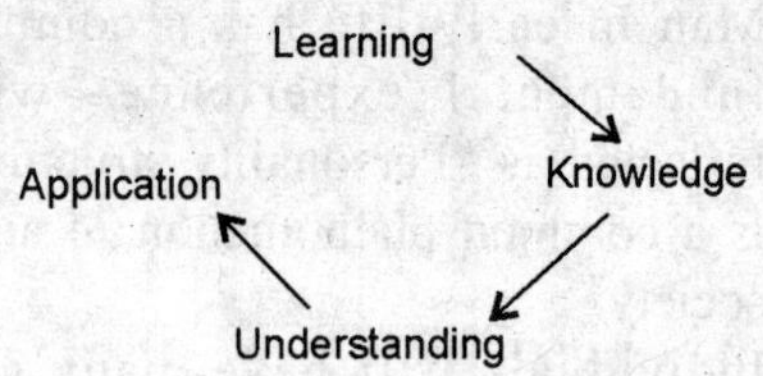

Fig 4.7: Bloom's Cognitive domain of learning

Bloom and Krathwohl's Affective Domain

This is the areas of learning communication skills. It deals with interpersonal relationships. Learning is considered by interest, attitude, values, appreciations and adjustment. This is represented as: (Fig. 4.8)

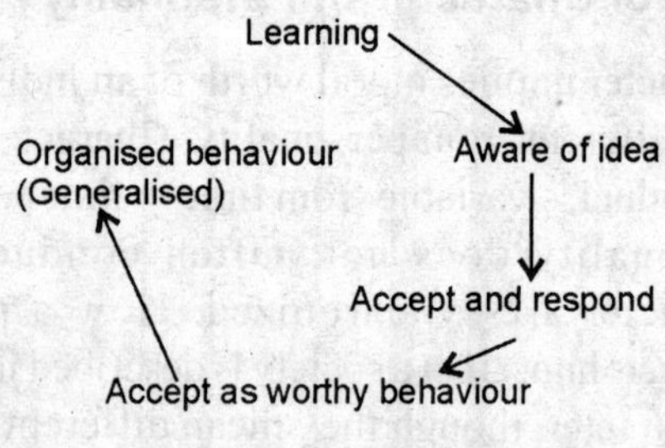

Fig. 4.8: Affective domain of Bloom and Krathwohl

Krathwohl's Psychomotor Domain

This is the area of practical skill learning. It involves mind and perception. Further human neuromuscular coordination determines this behaviour of learning. It is represented as under:

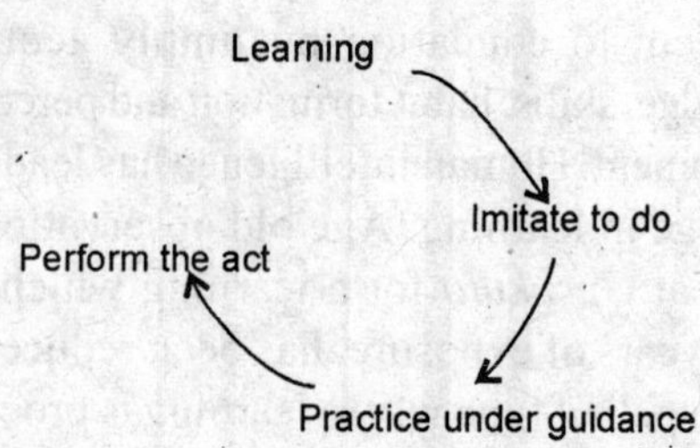

Fig. 4.9: Krathwohl's psychomotor domain

Examples of above types of learning:

a. **Knowledge Gain (Cognitive Domain):**
- Nurse defines hypertension.
- She enumerates APGAR scoring.
- She understands normal menses to decide ideal contraceptives.

b. **Communication skill (Affective domain):**
- Nurse understands anxiety of person going to O.T. room for operation.
- She gives reassurance to patient on the issue of scheduled operation.
- She helps to overcome emotion of the patient to cooperate in O.T.

c. **Practical Skill (Psychomotor domain) :**
- Nurse learns and does cardio pulmonary resuscitation.
- Nurse learns and gives enema to a patient as pre operative procedure.

Conditions for Effective Learning

Following conditions influence effective learning:-

i. Physical health
   e.g. Sick, Deaf, Blind, Dumb

ii. Mental health
   e.g. Worry, anxiety

iii. Learning situation
   e.g. Facility, distance, material

iv. Motivation
   e.g. Success, reward, gain

v. Intelligence
   e.g. Low I.Q.

vi. Age
   e.g. Very young, very old.

Theories of Learning

Learning is a character which differentiates human with other creatures. Man has great ability of learning. Various theories are postulated which are as under:

Conditioning Theory

According to Pavlov Theory of Conditioning Response, learning involves a series of conditional responses. This is not relevant to the main learning process of nursing education.

Connectionism Theory

According to Thorndike Theory of Connectionism, learning is based on strengthening of bonds between stimuli and response. This is well represented by a diagram.

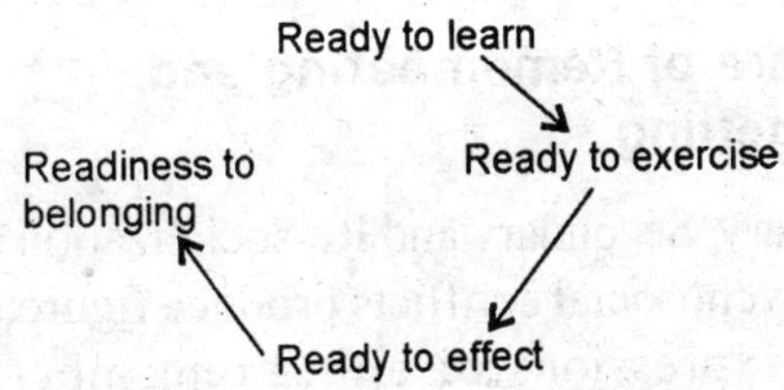

Fig. 4.10: Connectionism theory of learning

Field Theory

According to Gestalt, Theory of field considers the realization of truth for the given situation. Learning in context is superior to learning in isolated parts.

Learning Model Theory

According to Ausubel, theory of learning model uses steps of problem solving for learning. It is better suited to nursing course where clinical problem solving is used in case presentation and discussion.

REMEMBERING AND FORGETTING

Thomas Addison has aptly said that "What we want to remember we easily forget and what we want to forget we easily remember" in his novel essay "Art of Forgetting". Personality determines the way of remembrance and forgetting. Priority, closeness and benefit make the person to remember effectively. Remote items, general and nonbeneficiary make the person to forget easily.

Types of Remembering and Forgetting:

- Innate or reflex based
- Routine based
- Inter related social based
- Vital event based
- Response based.

Nature of Remembering and Forgetting

Primary, Secondary and Re-socialization as well as Psychosocial conflicts produce figure, words and expressions of either remembering or forgetting. These Psychosocial words are always purposive in nature. They try to serve a purpose of a life situation. When man wants solace he remembers and forgets an event of considerable importance. Each minute man gets flash of ideas which cannot be equated to remembrance.

Religious discourse from *Ramayana, Geeta, Quran, Bible* are time immemorial slabs of remembrances learnt by heart with a purpose. This remembrances and recitation itself can help an individual to forget unwanted memories of painful events.

Thus remembering and forgetting are complimentary to each other.

Causes of Forgetting

i. **Intentional forgetting:** When an individual do not want to involve or participate he embraces the art of forgetting.
ii. **Natural forgetting:** When an individual has not made proper record of event and has taken casually he is likely to forget the event.
iii. **Medical amnesia:** When individual gets neurological manifestations and nerve disorders he succumbs to forgetting as in head injury and Alzheimer's disease.
iv. **Senile cause:** Senescence causes forgetfulness.

Methods of Memory:

i. Recitation or Learning by heart.
ii. Practical doing and undoing (Trial and Error).
iii. Observation and recording.
iv. Using Mnemonic, Phrases, anecdotes, and proverb or life situations.
v. Personal exposure to experience.
vi. Group interactions.

THINKING AND REASONING

In man's perception, memory and imaginations have given way to thinking. As a higher order of mental process there is a psychosocial analysis in brain called Reasoning.

Routine, skill use, performance of an activity create an opportunity for thinking.

Thinking may produce pleasant or violent aspect of thoughts. Outwardly expression of thinking is called *extrovert and* expressionless thinking is called *introvert*. Bizarre thinking produces psychopaths in the society.

Types of Thinking

i. **Objective thinking:** Here there is logical association between events and symbols. It is a disciplined imagination. Objective thinking leads to many scientific innovations and discoveries.
ii. **Wishful thinking:** Evading tendency of man leads to wishful thinking. It is also called Fantasies. This represents future anticipation of an individual. Very common wishful thinking area Health and Wealth. Among adolescents it is romance that makes wishful thinking.

iii. **Imaginative thinking:** Day dreaming and thinking of impossibilities like magic world or wonder world is imaginative thinking. This does not serve any purpose in life except spending time in an unfruitful way.

iv. **Creative thinking:** It refers to thoughts brought out by an effective learning where there is scope for new ideas, new discoveries and new inventions. Creative thinking is a common word used in dress making, art, painting etc.

Development of Thinking

Education and commitment leads to development of objective thinking and creative thinking. Psychosocial norms should facilitate the process of required thinking and avoiding unrequired thinking. Unrequired thinking lead to worrying which is not a health process. Hence required thinking should be allowed in an atmosphere of good psychosocial environment.

Camp life, attending religious discourses, well developed hobbies regulates a covert activity of objective thinking. "Best thinking is to forget everything" make you and allow you to effectively regulate ways of your thinking.

Reasoning

It is a highest stage of human thinking where he tries to solve problems in life which may be simple or complicated. Thinking and allowing the use of intelligence brings about reasoning. Careful reasoning disallows fallacies.

Types of Reasoning

i. Primitive reasoning comes from conventional outline. Problem solving in daily routine are from primitive reasoning where individual's experience, family experience and society experience play a vital role.

ii. Psychosocial reasoning comes from understanding of behaviour, personality and inter-personal relationships.

iii. Scientific reasoning is based on demonstrable scientific reasons in a reasoning.

Problem Solving Methods:

Thinking and reasoning are used in solving both simple and complicated issues in life situations. Collection and arrangement of information on a subject, drawing conclusions and testing conclusions are methods used in Practical problem solving methods.

Examples of Problem Solving by Reasoning and Thinking:

a. You are on a call to conduct normal home delivery in a house situated nearer the sub centre. When you visit the house, woman is in first stage of labour and there is rupture of amniotic fluid. Discuss your nursing line of management.

b. An elderly woman at home has fallen and has sustained fracture of neck of femur (Right side). Reason out your first line of management of this elderly woman at home.

c. In Labour room, you have conducted a normal delivery and the woman with newborn is to be shifted to postnatal ward. You are expected to assess the mother before shifting. Describe your nursing procedure.

Here the nurse is expected to explain post partum techniques to be performed; viz., Assessing the mother by (a) Palpating the Fundus and bladder (b) Evaluate the Lochia (c) Inspect the perineum (d) Inspect and palpate the breasts to confirm normalcy before shifting.

INTELLIGENCE

Intelligence is an aspect of personality. The act of intelligence include the process of:

Perceiving — Knowing — Reasoning — Remembering

It is defined as "an ability to see meaningful relationships between interrelated matters".

Patient's subjective manifestations, patient's objective manifestations are to be observed, interpreted and a meaningful decision is drawn by nursing profession.

General Intelligence in Nursing

Taking over charge, handing over charge, morning assessment before clinical round, attending to duty doctor's instructions, drug administration, sample dispatch for investigation, getting report collected, recording 4th hourly pulse, respiration recording 6th hourly, body temperature recording 12th hourly, blood pressure recording etc., are commonly done routine nursing which is managed with general intelligence.

Special Intelligence in Nursing

Assisting in heart transplant operation, performing kidney dialysis, case management in ICU, ICCU, IPCU and emergency nursing care require special intelligence.

Concept of Mental Age in Intelligence

According to Benet and Simen (1896) who developed the concept, Mental age is determined by year wise acquired and adopted tests which measures aptitude. Accordingly the outcome of test describes the mental age or intelligence by skill. It did not include details of the lowered or altered mental acumen to group the child under normal for age or not normal for the age. A 7 year child passing intelligent skill test of child aged 6 years does not mean that the child is dull. Thus Mental age determination serves as a relative expression in psychoanalysis.

Concept of Problem Solving in Intelligent Test:

According to Terman who used abstract ideas for solving problems indicated that mental age is possibly determined. But it did not elicit adoptive behaviour and motor ability properly.

Concept of Intellectual Development Consideration for Mental Age:

According to Gessel who included four criteria to assess Mental age described (a) Motor ability (b) Language development (c) Adoptive behaviour and (d) Personal social behaviour. Gessel agrees that his concept has to be standardized.

Intelligence Tests

Individual Performance Test

Understanding of language, general understanding, reasoning are used to measure psychological process of individual performance. Here time fixation is not a factor. There are specifications in test set to formulate evaluation of (a) Young children (b) Illiterates (c) Feeble mindedness (d) Monolinguist.

I.Q. Tests are applied which a concept of mental age is improved upon to obtain a Quotient by chronological age.

$$\text{I.Q.} \ \frac{\text{Mental Age}}{\text{Chronological age}} \times 100$$

Normal I.Q. ranges from 90 to 100 in our set up. When mental age and chronological age is same it comes to 100 which is an average, e.g.

$$\text{I.Q.} \ \frac{\text{Mental Age}}{\text{Chronological age}} \times 100 \ \frac{12 \text{ years}}{12 \text{ years}} \times 100 = 100$$

According to level of I.Q. grouping of individual is done which is as follows:

Level of Intelligence	I.Q.
Genius	140 and above
Very superior	120 – 139
Superior	110 – 119
Normal	90 – 109
Low normal	80 – 89
Border line	70 – 79
Moron	50 – 69
Imbecile	25 – 49
Idiot	0 – 24

I.Q. measures the quality and potential intelligence. Higher performance is closely related to higher I.Q.

Adult intelligence is analyzed based on item analysis. According to Thurstone, adult intelligence includes 8 components and item analysis of these 8 components proves efficient method of intelligence analysis.

They are:

i. Memory of words and ideas.
ii. Ability of finding out principles.
iii. Ability of using principles in solving problems.
iv. Ability of expression with appropriate words.
v. Ability of verbal comprehension.
vi. Familiarity of elementary arithmetic.
vii. Ability to perceive objects.
viii. Flexibility and quickness of thought.

Group Performance Tests

Just as on examination, group test is administered to a group giving a specified time to complete. Here questions administered, tests the ability of group for perceiving, knowing, reasoning and remembering. Scoring system is adopted for giving ranking for best performance.

Uses of I.Q. Test in Psychology:

- Arrangement of special education to low I.Q. individuals.
- Selection of able individuals for a given task performance.
- To test the eligibility of individual for an entry to a formal or informal education.
- Help in work allotment according to ability of individual.
- Common entrance tests for the selection to professional colleges.
- Help in educational guidance.
- Help in Therapeutic prognosis.

Wing's Comprehensive Skill Test

It is a standardized measure of behaviour, psychological function and social performance. This is known as HBS Test. (Wing's comprehensive handicaps, Behaviour and skills schedule). It details the scale for special abilities and disabilities. It is used as a Research tool in Psychoanalysis. A further extension of HBS is DAS where (Disability Assessment Schedule) mobility communication and Social interaction are measured in service contests.

EDUCATIONAL PSYCHOLOGY

From the early historic times, imparting knowledge from one generation to the next has been in vogue where man is making conscious attempt to train children and adults. In recent times the implication and relevance of education has undergone a revolutionary change due to the scientific and technological progress.

Proper education of child starts from birth and the child is ready for formal education by 5 completed years. At this stage he is ready for learning only elementary things.

Meaning

Imparting sound education at different age levels is an arduous task because intelligence development and level of ability is found to vary from age to age. Children of same age are not alike in their mental capacity. The scientific study on individual differences has revealed that there are significant differences in the rate of mental growth and that different functions in the same child will grow at different rates. Vijay aged 9 years is found able to solve arithmetic problems where as his elder sister Asha aged 12 years cannot solve arithmetic problem though she is more intelligent than Vijay. These variations in capacity render the problem of teaching even more difficult than it would otherwise be.

Personality and character is produced by education and education give place for more complex social adjustments and social responsibilities. Psychologists feel that education is for socioeconomic survival.

Scope and Aims

In order to fit into our society man has to learn certain ways of life, as needed by a particular society. Thus, objectives of education are determined by conditions outside the field of psychology.

In the field of education, psychologist does not determine what is to be done. He points out the methods to be used in order to attain the desired result with the greatest degree of efficiency. In educational psychology main emphasis have been laid on child psychology, learning, special methods and personality. Of late, need for study of mental hygiene in educational psychology has been recognized and introduced in the study.

According to Kelly, purposes of educational psychology are as under:

- To give knowledge on the nature of the child.
- To give an understanding of the nature, aims and purpose of education.
- To give an understanding of the scientific methods and procedures which have been used in arriving at the facts and principles of educational psychology.
- To present the principles and techniques of learning and teaching.
- To give training in methods of measuring abilities and achievements in school subjects.
- To give knowledge on the growth and development of children.
- To assist in the better adjustment of children and help to prevent their maladjustment.
- To study the educational significance and control of emotions.
- To give an understanding of the principles and techniques of character training.

Relation with Other Spheres

Children are admitted to the formal schooling at or after the age of 5 years. There may not be any psychological reasons behind this. It is to secure a more homogenous group who can show similar grades by intelligent tests.

However, many drop-outs are noticed from the school. Apart from psychological problems, there are non psychological causes of drop outs. Philosophy, religion, politics, economics determine the scope and aims of education. School curricular which is older than psychology decides and determines the aims and objectives of education.

Extra curricular activities are necessary for an all rounded education. This will help in getting social adjustment for the child.

Procedures and methods are found to influence education. They are based on principles of psychology.

Individuals choose different careers which will vary according to the interests, abilities and vocational plans of the students.

Teaching Methods

According to Monroe and Marks there are nine general teaching methods and are applicable to a wide variety of subjects. They are:

- The Lecture Method: Didactic and Active Lecturing.
- The Recitation Method: Question by teacher answer by pupil based on textbook.

- Object Teaching: Observation of objects followed by comment by teacher.
- Development method: Skillful question to help students to think through and clear up ideas.
- The Laboratory Method: Work with guidance in Laboratory.
- The Project Method: Minimum Teacher guidance, only group activity, student selection.
- The Problem Method: Problem assigned by teacher.
- Socialized Recitation: Democratic atmosphere by discussion in groups.
- Teach and Test until mastery (Unit –Mastery plan).

Individual Differences

It is obvious that people are physically different. Motor and Sensory functions also differ greatly in individuals. Based on individual difference in intelligence men are classified into genius, normal, idiot etc.

But scientific observation has made it clear that all are qualitatively alike mentally, but differ in the degree of efficiency with which different functions work. Mind of a genius is similar to that of an idiot. But genius learns more easily, remembers easily and solves difficult problems.

Individual differences may be divided within a group, into group differences including age, sex, income, social status and race etc.

In one of the studies I.Q. of 100 nurses were analyzed & following are the observations:

Mean I.Q. = 102

S.D of I.Q. = 4.3

They are found distributed in the following manner: (Fig. 4.11)

Since 99% of nurses in a normal distribution fall within ± 3 SD, 99% nurses will have I.Q between 89.1 and 114.9

$$\bar{x} \pm 3 \text{ S.D.} = \bar{x} + 3\,[4.3] = \bar{x} \pm 12.9$$
$$= 102 \pm 12.9$$

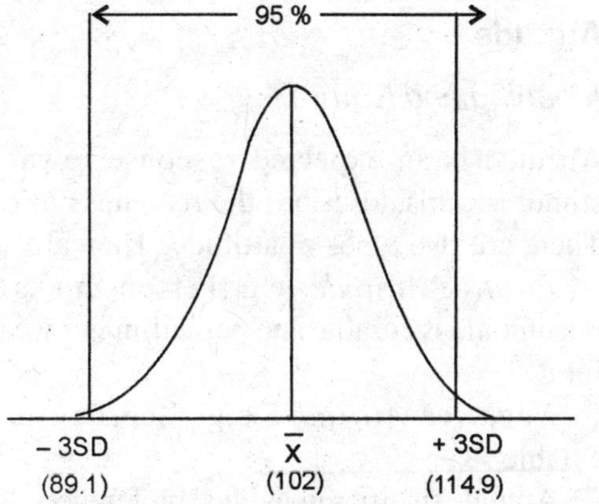

Fig. 4.11: Normal distribution of I.Q. of 100 nurses

Therefore,

$$102 - 12.9 = 89.1$$
$$102 + 12.9 = 114.9$$

To get practical range of mental capacity of nurses, their age can be multiplied by 0.89 to get lower limit of distribution and by 1.15 to get upper limit of distribution.

Above finding points out that 99 out of 100 nurses will be having a range of I.Q between 89.0 and 115. Those who are below 90 can be improved by modified and intensive teaching and training.

Heredity and Environment:

They can influence individual differences like colour, vision, Rate of memory, learning, deducing and reasoning. Group differences like age, sex etc. are usually influenced by environmental factors.

How individual difference is caused?

All individual posses same grade of ability in learning, comprehension, performance etc. This leads us to deduce that all minds are qualitatively alike. But they are different in the degree of efficiency with which different functions work.

Learning process, remembering process and solving the problem by low I.Q. individual can be upgraded to the level of high I.Q. person by principles and stages enunciated by educational psychologists.

Attitude

Meaning and Nature

Attitude is an expected response towards a stimulus. This describes the readiness to react. There are two types of attitude. They are:

Positive Attitude: e.g. Person thinks that pneumonia is curable and penicillin is a weapon for it.

Negative Attitude: e.g. Leprosy is not curable.

Attitude signifies individual preferences. They are acquired by social interactions and observed experiences. Attitude survey and attitude measurements are included in recent epidemiological approaches.

Development

Attitude is developed by experience and it is the effect of environmental stimuli. Attitudes are conditioned by the growth of intelligence.

Following are examples of attitude development:

- Young child has limited capacity for understanding world and so incapable of forming attitude.
- 7 years child can observe a picture and make out what is taking place in the picture. But it cannot interpret the reason for happening in the picture.
- 12 years child can interpret the reason for what happening in a picture.
- Adolescence is marked especially by the maturation of sex emotions.

Factors Influencing the Development of Attitude Age

- Home influences
- The social environment
- School environment
- Movie, TV serial
- Teacher
- The curriculum
- Teaching methods
- Group memberships
- Associations.

Measurement of Attitude

Suitable scales are available to measure attitude.

A check list prepared can be used to measure the attitude of nurses, as shown below (as a model).

Table 4.1: Attitude measurement scale

S.l.	*Items*	*Liked*	*Not liked*	*Not answering*
1.	Present Nursing College Fee			
2.	Theory Classes by Tutors			
3.	Demonstration by Matron			
4.	Dress Code of Nurse			
5.	Shift Duty by Nurse			
6.	SUPW by Nurse Student etc.			

Instruction: Place a check mark for your reaction.

The Teacher

Personality of teacher: One of the most important factors in the mental hygiene of education is teacher's personality and Behaviour. He should show a sense of fairness and justice, tact, sense of humour, good teaching skill, disciplinary practice etc.

Professional Growth of Teacher

A good teacher should show professional skill and be ready to clarify any doubts in a pleasant manner with pupils. Teacher should define precisely just what is expected of a class and that this is done well in advance for better performance.

Teacher should exercise democracy in teaching and be flexible in dealing with students.

One of the professional tasks is evaluation without bias which is most troublesome point in teacher-pupil relationships.

Incentive, Rewards for Teacher

Length of service is positively correlated with salary scale of school system. Special care is allowed for the family life of a teacher with a good House Rent and city compensation allowances. Care is taken to see they are not overworked. In-service training helps the teacher to achieve greatest degree of skill and allows him for a promotion.

Characteristics of an Effective Teacher

According to Robbins, following are characteristics of an effective teacher:

i. Make the course interesting.
ii. Knows subject matter of the course.
iii. Shows enthusiasm.
iv. Has the material well organized.
v. Encourage student participation.
vi. Uses practical illustration.
vii. Has real sense of humour.
viii. Has friendly personality.
ix. Shows interest in the students.
x. Has pleasant voice.
xi. Neatly dressed.
xii. Has a poised and business like attitude.

Teacher-Learner Relationship

In educational psychology Teacher-student relation is built up by above mentioned characteristics of an effective teacher. This is also a prime element for a positive attitude in education.

Evaluation

Meaning

Evaluation implies a system of values to be attained by education. It is the judgement of the degree of success. It determines whether predetermined educational objectives have been achieved. It implies that there exist objectives and an appropriate measurement is used.

Steps

Several factors like purpose of evaluation, domain sought to be tested, number of students, feasibility are considered in following the steps of evaluation.

Steps of evaluation are represented as follows:

Objective defined
Teaching provided
Measuring instrument is selected
Test is administered
Marking is decided
Test is scored
Result is analyzed
Decided on the result

Fig. 4.12: Steps of evaluation

In educational psychology personality tests, group tests are done with a purpose of evaluation of effect and outcome of education.

Tools of Evaluation

In health science institutions, Board of affiliated University suggests the following tools for education. They are:

- Essay type questions.
- M.C.Q.
- Oral examination.
- Objective Structured Clinical Examination.
- Practical examination.
- Short answer type questions.

HABIT

Habits are defined as accustomed way of doing things. They are acquired through repetitive act and are automatically exerted. Habits are exerted only under similar circumstances. They can become customs in due course to influence human behaviour. They may be grouped under:

i. Good habits
ii. Bad habits
iii. Healthy habits.

Principles involved in habit formation are:

- It starts from early childhood.
- Frequently repeated.
- Occurs in due course of time.
- Emotions create habits.
- They are under human control.

CONFLICTS

It is a powerful repulsive action between two courses of actions. They are configerated with emotions. Correct decision always keeps us away from conflicts. Conflicts cause emotional disturbances and leads to neurological disorders.

FRUSTRATIONS

When man is unable to meet his needs and desire, he ends up with frustrations. External causes are failure, defeat, unemployment and internal causes are poor health, low I.Q. etc.

Frustration can lead to nervous breakdown. Initially anger, dejection, hostility, suicidal tendencies are met with.

Frustration leads to drug abuse and alcoholism.

DEFENCE MECHANISMS

Problems, failures, difficulties make a man to employ certain Defence mechanism which help him to get a way to achieve happiness and success. Mentally healthy person use them to achieve success or happiness. These Defence mechanisms are:

a. Justifications of behaviour: (Rationalization)
   e.g. declaring grapes as sour.
b. Blaming others for fault: (Projection)
   e.g. Teachers are blamed for exam failure.
c. Enhancing self esteem by compensation: e.g. Poor in study show up as good sportsman.
d. Escapism:
   e.g. Pretend ill at examination.
e. Displacing the situation:
   e.g. Office problem reflected at home.
f. Follow childhood practice:
   e.g. Crying.

SOCIAL PSYCHOLOGY

It is a branch of psychology and deals with behaviour of individual in society. It studies attitude of individual towards culture and social values.

Group Behaviour:

Interaction and social behaviour of individual in a group is called group behaviour. Man's activities are regulated by custom, law and social obligations. Group is lead by a leader. It is responsible for solidarity of the group behaviour which is called "Group morale".

Group activity, group discussion, group opinion and group reaction are common psychosocial events in a society.

Group behaviour can lead to progressive reformation of society or can lead to civil unrest.

Social group is responsible for primary, secondary and re-socialization of an individual. Social attitudes are shared by others in the community.

FURTHER REFERENCES

1. Pasqual – Mental Health Nursing (Mosby).
2. NIMHANS Manual 1998.
3. Kapoor – Text book of Psychiatry Nursing.
4. Henry, Ernes – General Psychiatry (Eurosia).
5. Crow, Crow – Educational Psychology (EPH).
6. Robert S. Ellis – Educational Psychology (CAEWP).
7. Sociology for Nurses by Dr G.N. Prabhakara (Peepee).

5

Elementary Statistics and Nursing Research

Introduction

Primary objective of statistics is to provide reliable, relevant and up-to-date data to nursing profession to carry out day to day technical and scientific routine. Statistics are of following types:

i. Health statistics which mainly deals with normal health aspect.
ii. Medical statistics which deals with data of case management.
iii. Vital statistics which deals with data pertaining to vital events like births, deaths etc.
iv. Biostatistics which deals with data of Biological and Biosciences.

These data are presently called "Health information" and the system or

Organization which works for it is called "Health Information System".

Definition

WHO has defined statistics as:

"A mechanism for the collection, processing, analysis and transmission of information required for organizing and operating health science and also for research and training".

Mainly, Statistics has a major role and is of great importance in National Health System. It has become a basic tool of management in public health.

Following terminologies are commonly used in elementary statistics:

Data: They are discrete observations and do not carry any meaning.

Information: They are tabulated data which give meaning.

Intelligence: They are transformed information based on social and political value.

Characteristics:

Each individual is characterized by certain physical characters like age, sex, weight, Hb%, B.P., WBC count etc., Similarly there are some socioeconomic characters like occupation, literacy, Income. These qualities are called characteristics. These characteristics are grouped under 2 categories:

i. *Attributes:* Characters that are not measurable are called attributes. eg., sex, death, survival etc., The person having attribute is countable and attribute as such is not countable.

ii. *Variable:* Characteristics that are measurable are called variables, e.g. Height, Hb%, etc.

Importance

Importance of statistics are enumerated as under:

a. It is a guide for Nursing care services.
b. It is a tool for research.
c. It is a measure of health status of a community.
d. It identifies health problems.
e. It identifies health needs.
f. It helps in providing a Scientific basis for recording, collection, compilation, presentation and analysis.
g. For comparing health status between Individual to Individual
   Society to Society
   Hospital to Hospital
   Community to Community
   District to District
   State to State
   Country to Country
h. For planning and Health Administration.
i. It helps in finding out:
   - Impact of a health programme and health management.
   - Success or failure of an operation.
j. It helps in health programme evaluation.
k. It is a key to all Health administration.

Statistics and Health Science

Application of statistical principles and methods are necessary, not only for understanding of biological and medical sciences but also for effective practice in health professions. Biological, Clinical and laboratory data are variable and hence need statistics for understanding and interpretation.

In health science a course on statistics is necessary because:

- Decisions on diagnosis, prognosis and therapy are based on concepts of probability.
- Interpretation of tests, observations and measurements require knowledge of variations of physiological, observer and information.
- Epidemiological facts are necessary for controlling or preventing disease.
- Health workers who are primary data generators should know about statistics.
- Describing health level, health trend and health resources are possible through interpretations and inferences.
- Statistics in health sciences foster critical and analytical mind which are required during the course and later in professional practice.

Parameters

Parameter is a characteristic which describe population. When we say average size of family in India is 5.3, IMR in India is 71 per thousand LB, they indicate parameters.

When a sample is described by a unit it is called statistic. In a sample study of a village in Agra showed average family size as 6.0 and IMR of the same village as 74 per thousand LB, then characteristic describing this sample is statistic. Parameter is always single for a universe when compared to statistic which are many (for many samples).

Estimates

Estimates are observed values of a sample or a population. We select, for example, 50 nurses for their Hb%. We have average Hb% of Nurse Population. Mean Hb% of 50 Nurses is 10.8 G% and population mean of nurse population is 11.6 G%.

10.8 and 11.6 are single numbers. They are called Point Estimates.

Point Estimates:

Suppose we want range of Hb% in 50 nurse sample and in nurse population. This is called *Range estimates* commonly called, confidence interval (C.I.).

Point estimate in 50 nurse sample:

It is 10.8 G% because sample mean is best estimate of population mean.

Range estimate in 50 nurse samples:

Let us say S.E is 0.7 and interval with 2 times S.E. (it is 1.96) below and above the mean will be,

10.8 ± 2SE (correctly 10.8 ± 1.96 SE)

10.8 ± 2(0.7)

= 10.8 ± 1.4

Lowest is 10.8 – 1.4 = 9.4

Highest is 10.8 + 1.4 = 12.2

So range estimate is (C.I.) = 9.4 to 12.2 Hb%

In Statistical estimate we always use mean (point estimate) and Range (confidence interval). It can be represented as:

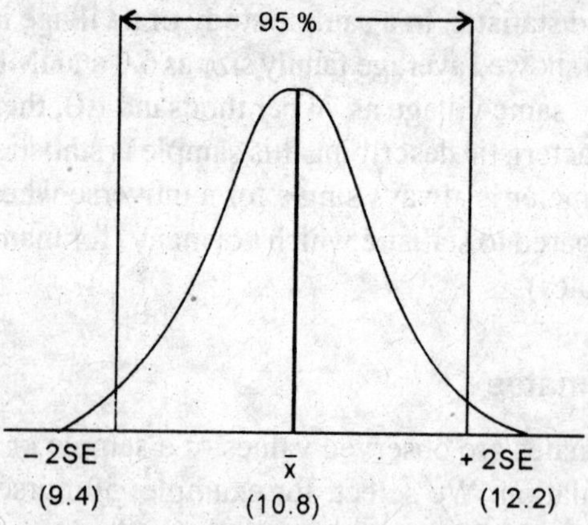

Fig 5.1: Statistical Estimates

Descriptive Statistics

Descriptive statistics are used to describe or characterise data by summarising them into more understandable terms without loosing or disturbing much of the information.

Examples:

Pie diagram
Bar chart
Frequency polygon
Mean, Median, Mode.

Inferential Statistics

Inferential statistics consists of a set of statistical techniques that provide predictions about population characteristics based on information in a sample taken from the population.

Example:

By Hb% data of 50 nurses given above under estimates we can infer as under:

- 50 nurses selected is a sample of study.
- Mean Hb% is 10.8.
- Confidence interval (Range estimate) is 9.4 to 12.2.

We infer from the sample study that mean Hb% of nurse Population is 10.8 and C.I. is 9.4 to 12.2 (± 1.96 SE). So we have predicted values for nurse population by sample nurse population. It is called inferential statistics.

Scale of Measurement

Measurement is the assignment of numerical to objects or events according to a set of rules. For example chest measurements of nurses are done with measuring tape which is calibrated by cms or inches.

According to Stevens (1946) there are 4 types of measurement scales for variables.

They are as under:

Nominal Scale

When people, object or event are categorized say A, B, C, D etc., or 0, 1, 2, 3, 4, etc., we are assigning a number or a letter as labels. It is categorical scale.

Examples:

Sex:	0	=	Female
	1	=	Male
Hygiene:	0	=	Worst
	1	=	Bad
	2	=	Good

Ordinal Scale

When characteristics are put into categories which give meaning, but distance between the categories are not properly known, it is ordinal scale. For example in final B.Sc. Nursing *Asha, Rita and Zinat* secured I, II and III Ranks respectively. This does not tell us by how many marks they differ?

Examples:

Socioeconomic class:			
	1	=	Low
	2	=	Middle
	3	=	High
I.Q.	0	=	Idiot
	1	=	Moron
	2	=	Normal
	3	=	Genius

Interval Scale

When characteristics have, fixed and equal distance between them, we refer it as interval scale.

		(Divisible unit)	(No Gap)
Fahrenheit Temperature		98° F	98.2 F
		99° F	98.3 F
		100° F	98.4 F
Inch scale	1"	2.5 cm	
	2"	5.0 cm	

Examples of discrete "interval scale"

	(Gap is there) (Indivisible unit)
Para	1
	2
	3
Family members	4
	5
	6

Ratio Scale

It is a precise level of measurement. Here characteristics have equal intervals.

Zero in the scale is determined by nature (not arbitrary). Ratio scale has characteristics of interval scale. But has a true zero point as its origin.

Example:

I.Q.	Mental age/Chronological age
D.F.	Indoor illumination/outdoor illumination
NPU	N2 retained/N2 intake
Quetlet index	Weight/ Height
Calorie Coefficient etc.	

DATA PRESENTATION

Raw Data, the Array, Frequency Distribution

Mass of raw data is available when they are collected. They do not mean anything for a profession to infer. No useful information is immediately evident from a mass of raw data. They are the array of number, words and response. These collected data need to be organised in such a way that the information they contain clearly reveals the pattern of variation.

It is required to understand the structure of data and characteristics of data before application of precise analysis. In all fields including nursing profession. There is need for understanding the purpose and ways of reducing and presenting data. When the data is grouped in tabular form based on a particular characteristic which occurs in a particular data set, it is called frequency table. It is illustrated in the table below:

Table 5.1: Frequency table showing PEM cases according to age in a sample survey

Age group (year)	*Tally mark*	*Frequency*
< 1	III	4
1-4	𝍸 𝍸 𝍸 𝍸 𝍸 𝍸 IIII	34
5-9	𝍸 𝍸	10
10-14	II	2
	Total	50

Frequency table is prepared by determining the range, tallying the frequencies.

Steps of Tabulation of Data:

Tabulation is the first step before data is analysed or interpreted. Following principles are followed in Tabulation.

i. Each table should have a number.
ii. Each should have self explanatory and brief title.
iii. Care is taken to give clear and specific legend.
iv. Clear rows and columns are made.
v. It must be according to size or according to importance.
vi. Number and percentage should be closer.
vii. It should not be too large.
viii. It should not be too small.
ix. Uniform class interval is maintained, except in case of age distribution where standard grouping of variable class interval is allowed.

Coding and Editing

Coding and editing are required for proper interpretation. When collected data is entered with a decision of entering through code like 1, 2, 3 or A, B, C or X, Y, Z care should be taken for proper entry and proper interpretation.

Example:

All male		=	01
All Female		=	02
Single		=	01
Married		=	02
Widowed		=	03
Awareness	Yes	=	X
No =	Y		

At edition, care is taken to group or regroup a variable for proper interpretation. This does not allow original meaning.

Example:

Para 0, 1, 2, 3, 4, 5 is grouped to
Para – Nil
Para – 1 to 2
Para – 2 to 4
Para – 4 +

Demographic Data

Before we can assess the magnitude of the health problem posed by a disease or impact of intervention we must have an idea of the size of the community we are dealing with, its composition with respect to various demographic characteristics and the magnitude of changes in relation to vital events.

Demographic data relates to health and illness of population for a community diagnosis.

They include:

- Population characteristics – size, age, sex etc.
- Health profile – risk factors.
- Environmental factors–Socio-economic aspect.
- Morbidity, Mortality, Fertility.

- Birth, Death, migration
- Reticulation – Boundary of census, unit etc.

Tabulation of Mortality

Crude and specific deaths, disease and cause specific deaths, Age and Sex specific deaths are considered for mortality data tabulation.

Tabulation of Morbidity

Disability, handicap, impairment, incidence, prevalence, population at risk, rate, ratio and population are considered for morbidity data tabulation.

Tabulation of Other Data

Fertility, current users, transition, relevance, Health measures are considered for other data tabulation.

Principles of Graphical Representations

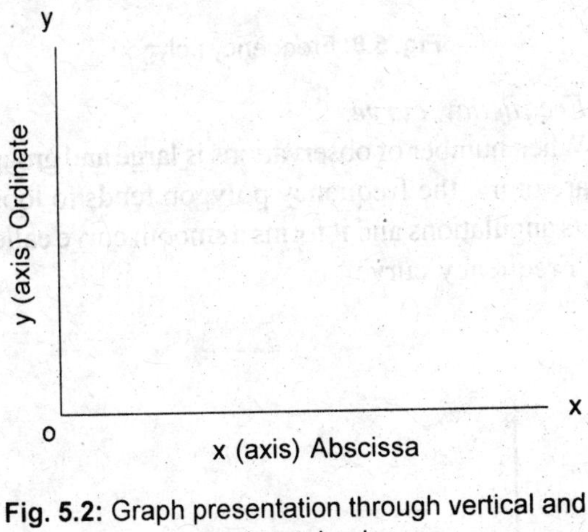

Fig. 5.2: Graph presentation through vertical and horizontal axis

We always use 2 axis and label them X and Y starting from zero to form vertical and horizontal presentation. 'X' axis is marked with group, score, class interval whereas 'Y' axis is marked with frequencies. Ratio between 'X' and 'Y' axis can be 3:2, 4:3 or 5:3 for proper presentation.

Diagrams

In addition to table and graph, diagrams are used which furnish a good impression of numbers and about idea. Real grasp of overall picture is possible by diagram. They are of course drawn based on set principles.

Bar diagram

They are common and easiest diagrams for data presentation. They indicate the frequency of a character. Spacing between bars should be equal or more than half of the width of the bar. These are 3 types:

- Simple Bar
- Multiple Bar
- Component Bar.

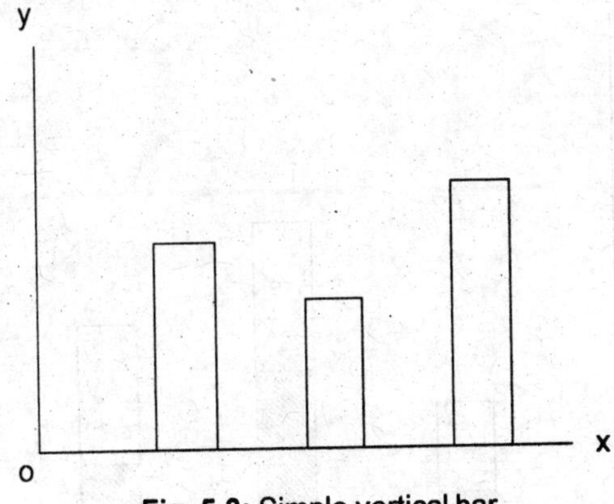

Fig. 5.3: Simple vertical bar

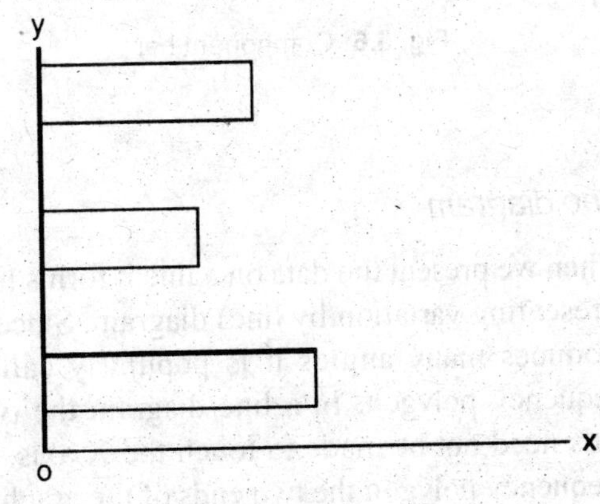

Fig. 5.4 : Simple horizontal bar

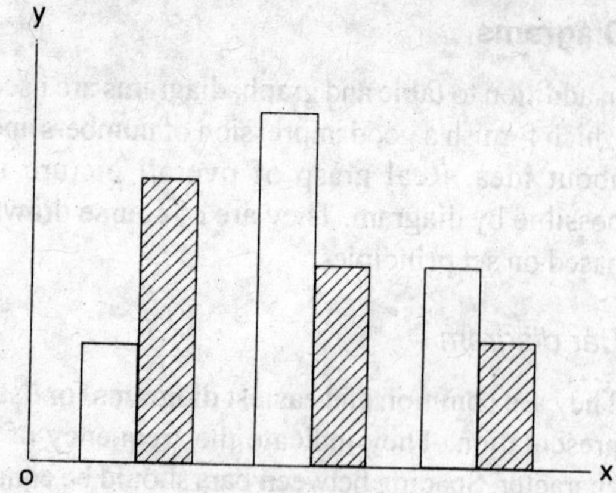

Fig 5.5: Multiple bar

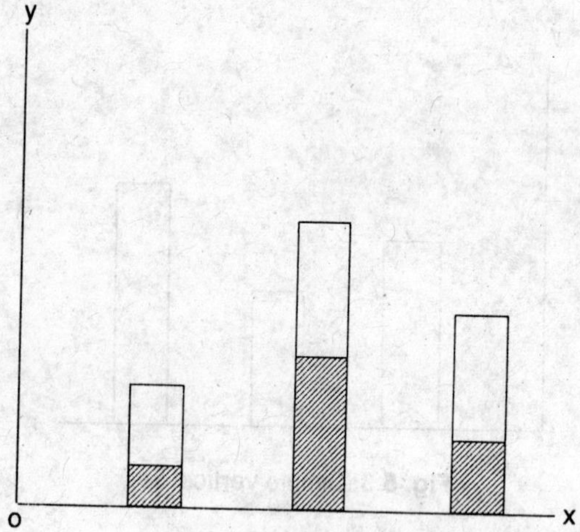

Fig. 5.6: Component bar

Line diagram

When we present the data on a line it forms line (presenting variation by line) diagram. Since it produces many angles it is popularly called frequency polygon. In a line diagram the two ends need not be made to touch the X axis. In Frequency polygon the two ends of the graph is allowed to touch X axis.

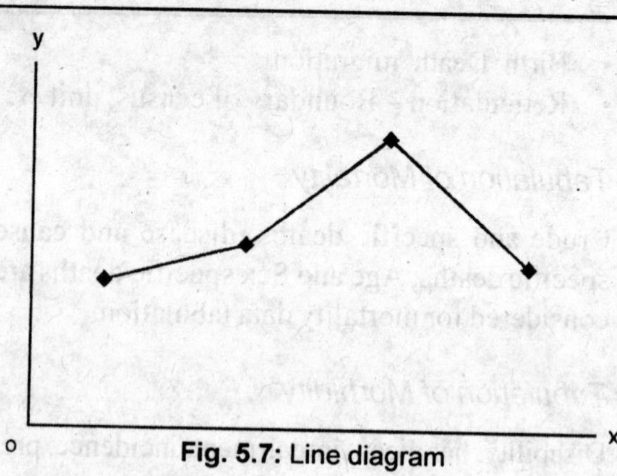

Fig. 5.7: Line diagram

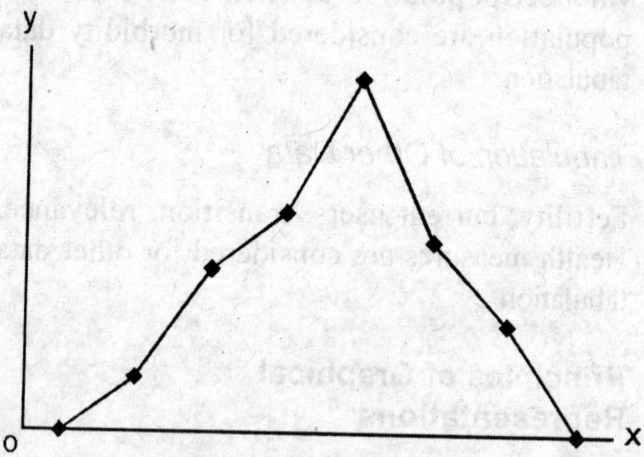

Fig. 5.8: Frequency polygon

Frequency curve:

When number of observations is large and groups are more, the frequency polygon tends to loose its angulations and it forms a smooth curve called "Frequency curve".

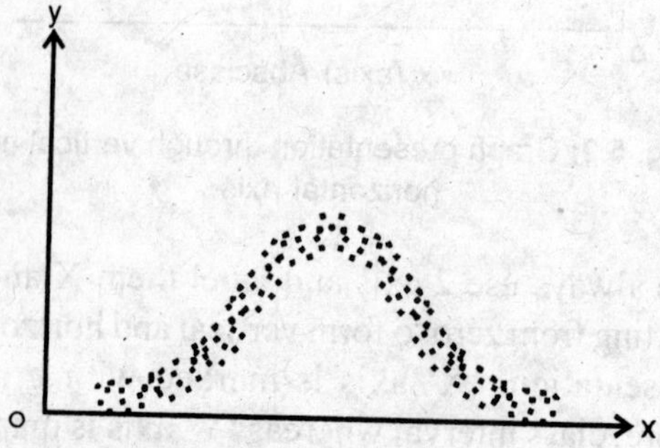

Fig. 5.9: Observations on axis

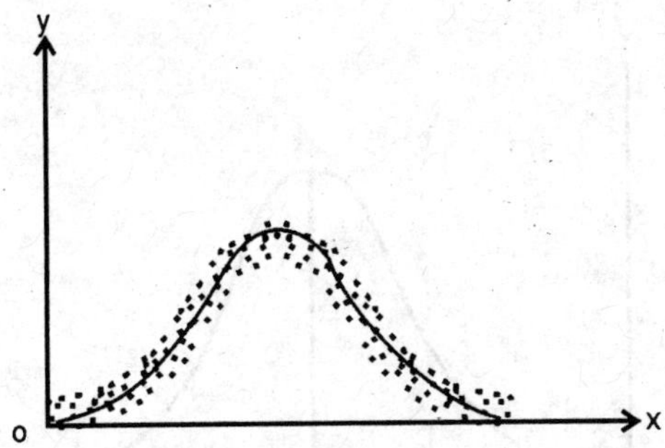

Fig. 5.10: Frequency curve

When a frequency curve form bell shape and symmetrical around the mean of the distribution, it is called normal curve. We can define symmetry as frequencies at equal distances from the mean on either side are the same.

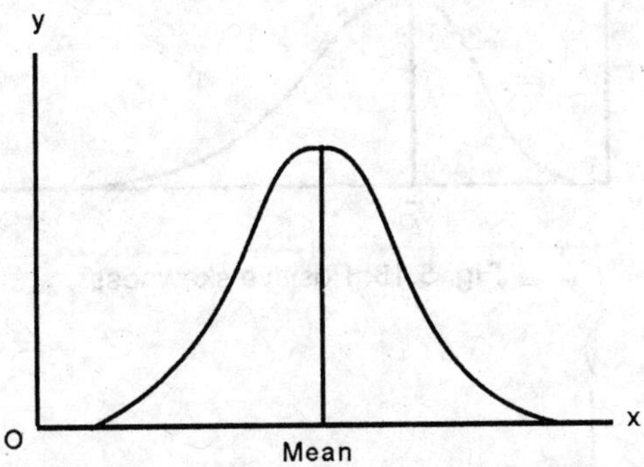

Fig. 5.11: Normal curve by line diagram

Pie diagram

It is a called *sector diagram* where frequencies of the groups are shown in circle. Degrees of angle are denoted by frequencies and area of sector.

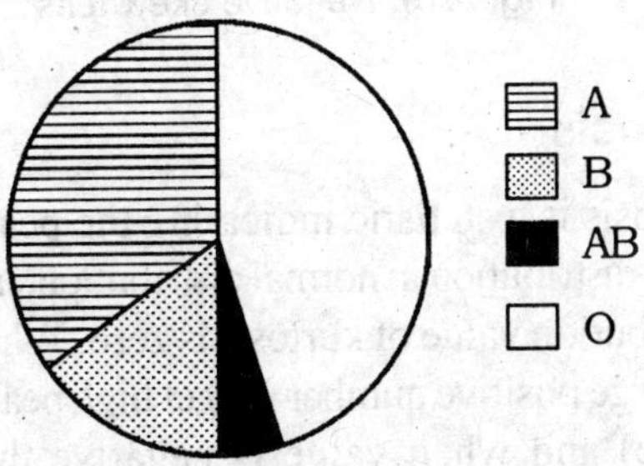

Fig. 5.12: Distribution of blood groups

Total area of Pie diagram should be 100 percent and each angle is calculated as under:

$$\text{Angle} = \frac{\text{Class frequency}}{\text{Total observtion}} \times 360$$

Dot diagram

It is called *scattered diagram* where data show the nature of correlation between 2 characters (e.g., Age and weight).

This can also be called correlation diagram.

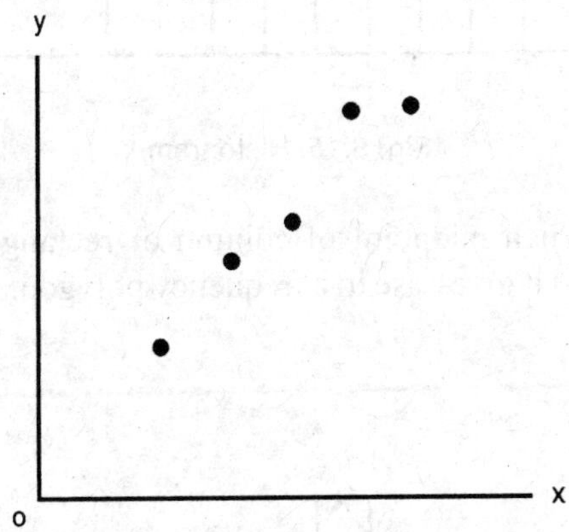

Fig. 5.13: Scatter (dot) diagram

Picture diagram

It is a method of illustration through picture (Figurative presentation).

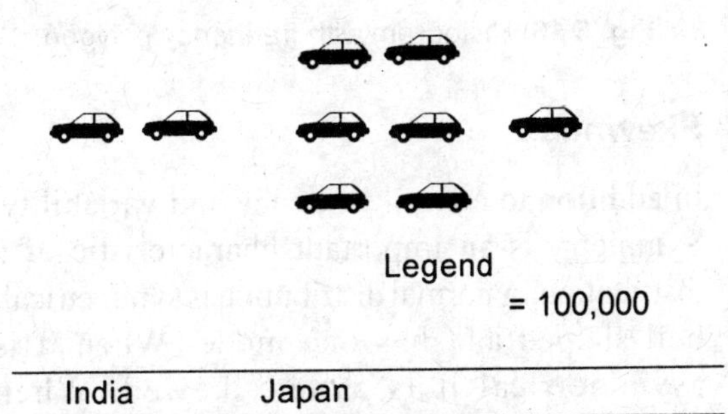

Fig. 5.14: Car production in India and Japan

Histogram

When data is represented in the form of column or rectangle it is called Histogram.

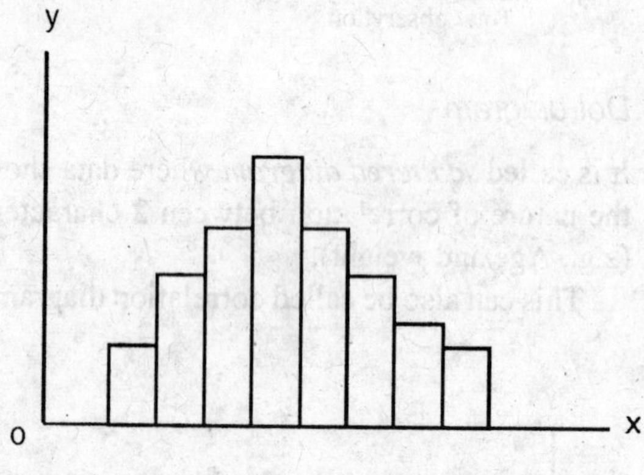

Fig. 5.15: Histogram

When midpoint of column or rectangle is joined it gives rise to a frequency polygon.

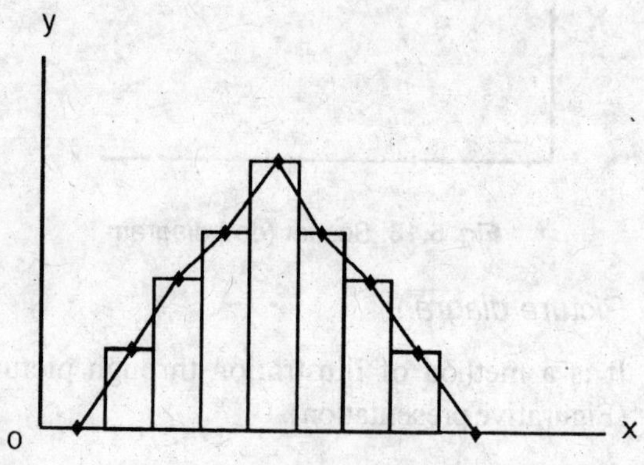

Fig. 5.16: Histogram with frequency polygon

Skewness

In addition to central tendency and variability, <u>Symmetry</u> is an important characteristic of a distribution. A normal distribution is symmetrical; bell shaped and has one mode. When it is asymmetrical it is called skewed. When frequencies are more on left of the distribution it is positive skewness; and it is negative when more frequencies are on right side of distribution.

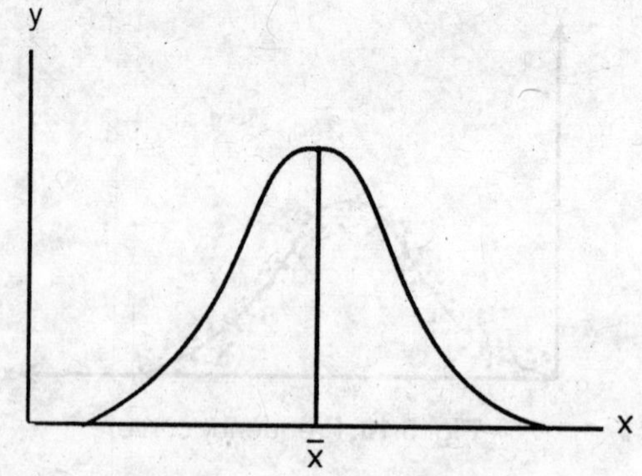

Fig. 5.17: Normal skewness

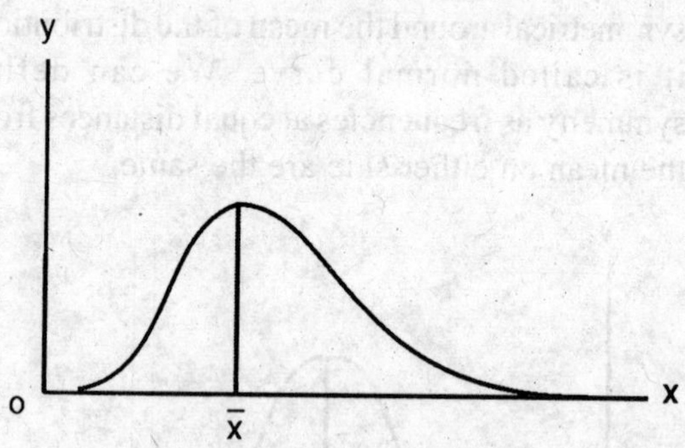

Fig. 5.18: Positive skewness

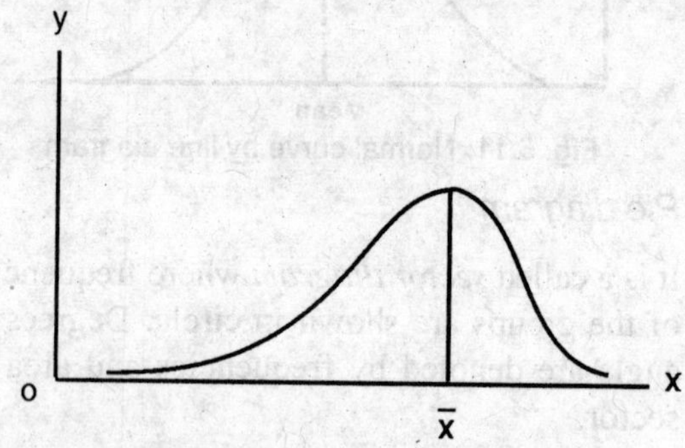

Fig. 5.19: Negative skewness

Kurtosis

Kurtosis is a statistic indicating the peakedness of the distribution in normal distribution. In normal distribution value of kurtosis is zero. When value is a large positive number we get high peak (Lepto kurtic) and when value is negative the curve becomes flat (Platy kurtic).

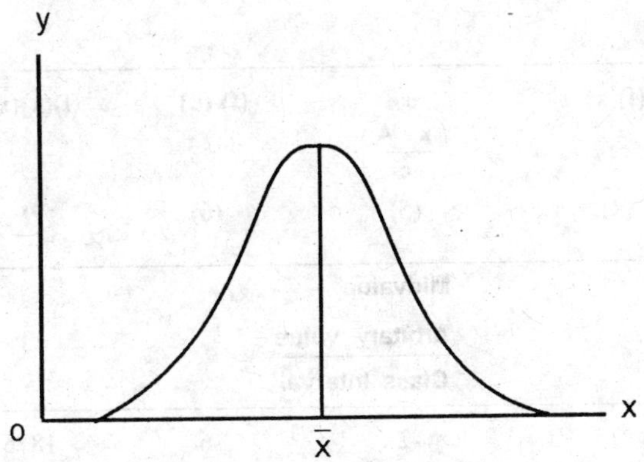

Fig. 5.20: Zero kurtosis in normal curve

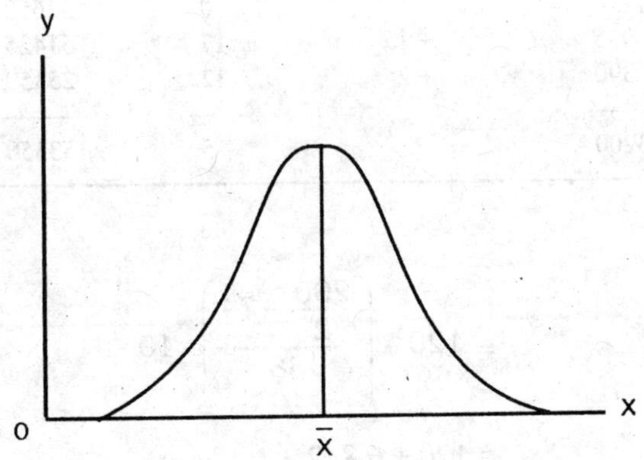

Fig. 5.21: Too peaked curve in leptokurtic curve

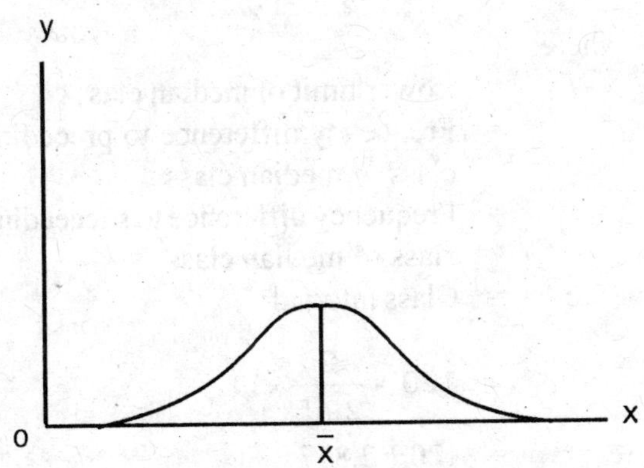

Fig. 5.22: Too flat curve in platy kurtic curve

MEASURES OF CENTRAL TENDENCY

Meaning and Importance

When the observations are clustered around a central value, it is called Central Tendency. Normally it is called an average. This average is different for different observations. For examples:

In Delhi average age of student who enters nursing course is 19 years.

In Mysore average age of student who enters nursing course is 22 years.

In the above 2 cases we observe many students cluster around 19 and 22 years at Delhi and Mysore. This clustering is measured by Measures of Central Tendency.

Computation of Mean, Median and Mode

For ungrouped data

10 nurses have I.Q. as follows:
158, 139, 120, 146, 111, 99, 114, 156, 111, 94.

Arithmetic Mean = 158 + 139 + 120 + 146+ 111 + 99 + 114 + 156 + 111 + 94

$$\text{Mean} = \frac{1248}{10} = 124.8$$

Median = We get mid value when they are arranged in an ascending order:
94, 99, 111, 111, 114, 120, 139, 146, 156, 158
↓

$$\text{Median} = \frac{232}{2} = 117$$

Mode = Most fashionable number or the number which repeats most is taken which is 111, is mode.

For grouped data

In a private hospital 70 nurses are working. Their age distribution is as follows:

Let us compute Mean, Median and Mode:

X	x	F	(f)(x)	u $\left(\frac{x - A}{c}\right)$	(f) (u)	(f)(x)(x)
(1)	(2)	(3)	(4)	(5)	(6)	(7)
Mid value	Age group	Frequency		Midvalue – Arbitary value / Class Interval		
25	20-30	3	75	-2	-6	1875
35	30-40	18	630	-1	-18	22050
A (45)	40-50	26	1170	0	0	52650
55	50-60	17	935	+ 1	17	51425
65	60-70	6	390	+ 2	12	25350
		70	3200		5	153350

Note: A = arbitrary value taken

Age group (Yr)	*Number of nurses*
20-30	3
30-40	18
40-50	26
50-60	17
60 and above	6
Total =	70

$$A.M. = \frac{\Sigma fx}{\Sigma f} = \frac{3200}{70} = 45.71$$

Median =

$$l + \left(\frac{\frac{n}{2} - F}{f}\right) \times C$$

where l = Lower limit of median class
n = Number of observation
F = Cumulative frequency
f = Frequency of median class
c = Class interval

$$= 120 + \left(\frac{\frac{200}{2} - 74}{38}\right) \times 10$$

$$= 120 + 6.842$$
$$= 126.84$$

$$\text{Mode} = l + \quad l + \left(\frac{f_2}{f_2 + f_1}\right) \times c$$

where:

l = Lower limit of median class
f_2 = Frequency difference to preceding class of median class
f_1 = Frequency difference to succeeding class of median class
c = Class interval

$$= 120 + \frac{2}{2+5} \times 10$$
$$= 120 + 2.857$$
$$= 122.857$$

Comparison and Uses of Mean, Median and Mode

Table 5.2: Comparative table of central values

Mean	*Median*	*Mode*
• Easy to calculate	• Easy to calculate	• Easy to calculate
• Easy to understand	• Not easy to understand	• Not easy to understand because not clearly defined
• Gets influenced by an abnormal value	• Not influenced by an abnormal value	• Not effected by an abnormal value
		• We get more than one mode

Mean is best known and most widely used average. The Median is not sensitive to extreme scores and is useful when the data are skewed. The mode is most frequently occurring value that has the largest frequency of scores.

MEASURES OF VARIABILITY (DISPERSION)

Meaning and Importance

When we collected I.Q. of 10 nurses and found out mean of I.Q. we wanted to know how each nurse varies in their I.Q. But Mean alone cannot give real picture of variation of I.Q.

Apart from knowing that I.Q. for each nurse is nearer to mean I.Q., we can know how the I.Q. for each nurse varies with each other through Measurers of Variability. They include Range, Mean Deviation, Standard Deviation, Coefficient of Variation, Quartile Deviation and Variance.

Measures

Range

It is the value between minimum and maximum.

Let us compare range for the following:

Nine nurses from each class were observed to have cash (in Rupees) as under:

Class	*Cash in Rs. with 9 nurses*								
	1	2	3	4	5	6	7	8	9
I year	40	40	40	40	40	40	40	40	40
II year	36	37	38	39	40	41	42	43	44
III year	1	9	20	30	40	50	60	70	80
IV year	0	0	0	0	0	0	0	0	360

	I year	**II year**	**IIIrd year**	**IV year**
Total cash	360.00	360.00	360.00	360.00
Mean	40.00	40.00	40.00	40.00
Range	40-40=0 Zero variation	-4 to + 4 44-36 = 8 variation is "8"	80-1=79 Variation is 79	No one represent mean 360-0 = 360 Variation is 360

Mean Deviation

Let us take I.Q. of 10 nurses to compute Mean Deviation.

158, 139, 120, 146, 111, 99, 114, 156, 111, 94

x	$(x-\bar{x})$
158	33.2
139	14.2
120	– 4.8
146	21.2
111	– 13.8
99	– 25.8
114	– 10.8
156	31.2
111	– 13.8
94	– 30.8

$\bar{x} = \frac{1248}{10} = 124.8$ $\quad \Sigma \left| x - \bar{x} \right| = 199.6$

$$\text{Mean deviation} = \Sigma \frac{\left| x - \bar{x} \right|}{10}$$

$$= \frac{199.6}{10} = 19.96$$

This is an average deviation from the mean.

Standard Deviation (S.D.)

For ungrouped data:

Let us compute S.D. for I.Q. of 10 nurses which are as under:

158, 139, 120, 146, 111, 99, 114, 156, 111, 94

x	$(x-\bar{x})$	$(x-\bar{x})^2$
158	33.2	1102.34
139	14.2	201.64
120	– 4.8	23.04
146	21.2	449.44
111	– 13.8	190.44
99	– 25.8	665.64
114	– 10.8	116.64
156	31.2	973.44
111	– 13.8	190.44
94	– 30.8	948.64

$\bar{x} = \frac{1248}{10} = 124.8 \quad \Sigma (x-\bar{x})^2 = 4861.6$

$$\text{S.D.} = \sqrt{\frac{\Sigma (x-\bar{x})^2}{n-1}} = \sqrt{\frac{4861.6}{9}} = 23.24$$

For grouped data

Let us take 70 nurses working in a private hospital according to their age.

Age year	*Number of nurses*
20-30	3
30-40	18
40-50	26
50-60	17
60 and above	6
Total =	70

Similar to computation of grouped data for mean, median and mode, we have to compute grouped data in the following way through finding out S.D. as given in next page:

X	x	f	(f)(x)	$\left(\frac{x - A}{c}\right)$ u	(f)(u)	(f)(x)(x)
(1)	(2)	(3)	(4)	(5)	(6)	(7)
Mid value	Age group	Frequency		Midvalue – Arbitary value / Class Interval		
25	20-30	3	75	-2	-6	1875
35	30-40	18	630	-1	-18	22050
A(45)	40-50	26	1170	0	0	52650
55	50-60	17	935	+ 1	17	51425
65	60-70	6	390	+ 2	12	25350
		70	3200		5	153350

Note: A = Arbitrary value taken.

$$\text{S.D.} = \sqrt{\frac{\Sigma fx^2}{n} - \left(\frac{\Sigma fx}{n}\right)^2}$$

$$= \sqrt{\frac{153350}{70} - \left(\frac{3200}{70}\right)^2}$$

S.D. = 10.05

Steps to calculate S.D. of ungrouped data:

- Find A.M. of I.Q.
- Find Mean Deviation of each $\left(x - \bar{x}\right)$
- Find square of each $\left(x - \bar{x}\right)^2$
- Find $\Sigma(x - \bar{x})^2$ i.e. sum of squares
- Find the square root of above with

D.F. n or n-1 as denominator.

i.e.= $\sqrt{\frac{\Sigma\left(x - \bar{x}\right)^2}{n}}$ or $\sqrt{\frac{\Sigma\left(x - \bar{x}\right)^2}{n-1}}$

Property and value of S.D.

Standard Deviation helps to find out the deviation of value from Arithmetic mean as a unit of variation. In other words, it explains symmetry or Asymmetry of normal curve (distribution).

± 1 S.D. means it cover 68 % values.
± 2 S.D. means it cover 95 % values.
± 3 S.D. means it cover 99 % values.

Apart from this, S.D. is useful in the following:

a. It is possible to know whether observed difference of I.Q. of a nurse is a real one or is by chance.
b. From S.D. we can calculate standard error which helps to compare sample value with universal value. (e.g. I.Q. of Delhi nurses to I.Q. of nurses in the world).
c. S.D. helps to calculate the size of sample for a study.

Coefficient of Variation (C.V.)

It is a measure of variability by using a coefficient obtained from the mean and standard deviation.

Let us compute C.V. for the following data: 42 nurses of I year showed the following mean and S.D. for their Height and Weight recorded at their medical examination.

Mean Height	=	160 cms
Mean Weight	=	55 kg
S.D. of Height	=	10 cms
S.D. of Weight	=	5 kg

$$C.V. = \frac{S.D.}{Mean} \times 100$$

$$C.V. \text{ of height} = \frac{10}{160} \times 100 = 6.25\,\%$$

$$C.V. \text{ of weight} = \frac{5}{55} \times 100 = 9.09$$

We can infer by the above finding as under:

i. Height of 42 nurses is more consistent than weight.

ii. Weight of 42 nurses is more variable than height.

Variance

The square of S.D is called variance. Variance is called as a measure of variability (Dispersion). Calculation of variation is similar to that of S.D except that it is without square root.

It is represented by 'V' or 'S^2'.

$$V = S^2 = \frac{\Sigma\left(x-\bar{x}\right)^2}{n} \text{ or } \frac{\Sigma\left(x-\bar{x}\right)^2}{n-1}$$

Quartile Deviation

Out of 100, if we take 25th, 50th, 75th values, they stand for quartile, which is denoted by Q_1, Q_2, and Q_3 respectively; 50th Quartile gives Median Value.

Let us compute Quartile Deviation from the following exercise.

Weight (kg)	*No. of nurses*
0-10	2
10-20	7
20-30	13
30-40	28
40-50	12
50-60	6
60-70	2

Above table is prepared with grouped data of weight of 70 circus troop people.

First we have to obtain cumulative value and represent graphically to obtain Median Quartile.

Frequency	*Cumulative Frequency*	
	Less than ogive	*More than ogive*
2	2	70
7	9	68
13	22	61
28	50	48
12	62	20
6	68	8
2	70	2

Now, let us prepare a cumulative frequency curve which is called "Ogive".

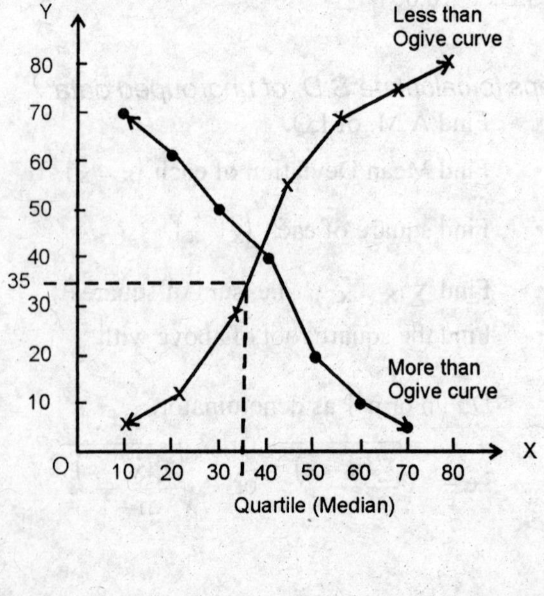

Q_2 = Median = 70/2 = 35

Similarly Q_1 = 25th percentile = 70/4 = 17.5
Q_3 = 75th percentile = 70/0 × ¾ = 52.5

CORRELATION

Meaning

Correlation is a technique to study relationships. The relationship is measured mathematically. However, a correlation that shows that two variable are related does not mean that one variable caused the other. It is not correct to infer causation from correlation alone. When we use "Zero-order correlation" this simply means the correlation between 2 variables.

According to Cohen (1987) correlation "r" = 0.10 is small effect, "r" = 0.30 moderate effect and "r" = 0.50 is large effect.

The Pearson correlation coefficient "r" allow us to state mathematically the relationship that exists between 2 variables. It ranges from + 1.00 through 0.0 to – 1.00 (perfect +ve, no relation and perfect negative relationship respectively).

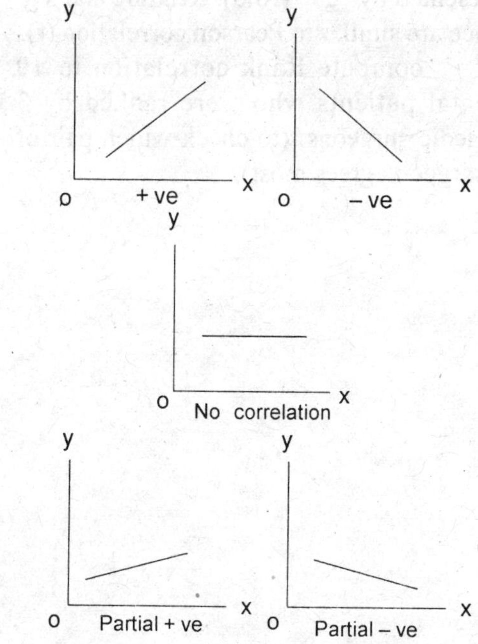

Fig. 5.23: Graphical representation of correlation

Types of Correlation

Following are types of correlation:

a. Positive – where r = 1.00.
b. Partial positive – when r = between 0.1 to 0.9.
c. Negative where r = -1.00.
d. Partial negative when r = between – 0.9 to – 0.1.
e. Linear – one variable is continuous and the other dichotomy type.
f. Non linear – not a linear relationship.
g. Rank – when data are from ranking.
h. Phi–When each of the variables is dichotomy.
i. Tetra choric – when data is set into four-fold table.
j. Spurious – it is a nonsense correlation.
k. Multiple – when many variables are tested.

Computation of Correlation Coefficient

Pearson Correlation

Let us calculate "r" to determine association if any, between fluoride content of drinking water and community fluorosis index.

Drinking water fluoride level mg/L	*Community Fluorosis index %*
0.8	0.1
1.3	0.4
1.5	0.8
1.9	0.6
2.3	0.7
2.3	1.1
2.4	0.8
2.6	1.1
3.5	1.6
3.6	1.3

x	y	(x − x)	$(x - x)^2$	(y − y)	$(y - \bar{y})^2$	$(x - \bar{x})\ (y - \bar{y})$
(1)	(2)	(3)	(4)	(5)	(6)	(7)
0.8	0.1	− 1.42	2.02	− 0.75	0.56	1.06
1.3	0.4	− 0.92	0.85	− 0.45	0.20	0.41
1.5	0.8	− 0.72	0.52	− 0.05	0.003	0.03
1.9	0.6	− 0.32	0.10	− 0.25	0.063	0.08
2.3	0.7	0.08	0.006	− 0.15	0.023	− 0.12
2.3	1.1	0.08	0.006	0.25	0.063	0.02
2.4 0.8	0.18	0.032	− 0.05	0.003	− 0.009	
2.6	1.1	0.38	0.144	0.25	0.063	0.095
3.5	1.6	1.28	1.638	0.75	0.563	0.96
3.6	1.3	1.38	1.904	0.45	0.203	0.62
22.2	8.5		7.22		1.74	3.296
$\bar{x} = 2.22$	$\bar{y} = 0.85$					

$$r = \frac{1}{n} \frac{\Sigma (x - \bar{x})(y - \bar{y})}{(SD_x)(SD_y)}$$

$$= \frac{1}{10} \frac{(3.296)}{(0.896)(0.439)}$$

$$r = \frac{0.3296}{0.3933} = 0.8380$$

There is +ve correlation between x and y.

i.e. there is an association between F_2 level and C. F. I.

Spearman Rank Correlation Test

When we get a ranked data, we can find out association by Spearman Rank correlation. This is represented by "ζ" (Rho). Reading and significance are similar to Pearson correlation (r).

Let us compute Rank correlation to 10 accidental patients who were ranked by 3 orthopaedic surgeons: (to check which pair of ortho surgeon agrees most).

Ortho surgeon	Accidents Patients									
	1	2	3	4	5	6	7	8	9	10
A	1	6	5	10	3	2	4	9	7	8
B	3	5	8	4	7	10	2	1	6	9
C	6	4	9	8	1	2	3	10	5	7

Ortho surgeon A (Score)	1	6	5	10	3	2	4	9	7	8	
Ortho surgeon B (Score)	3	5	8	4	7	10	2	1	6	9	
Difference (d_1)	– 2	1	– 3	6	– 4	– 8	2	8	1	– 1	Total
(d_1^2)	4	1	9	36	16	64	4	64	1	1	200

Spearman Rank Correlation (δ) = $\frac{1 - 6\,\Sigma\,(d_1)^2}{n(n^2 - 1)} = \frac{1 - 6\,(200)}{10\,(10^2 - 1)} = 1 - \frac{1200}{990}$

$= \boxed{-\,0.2120}$

Similarly Rank correlation coefficient between B & C, and between C and A are:

i. Between ortho surgeon B and C is - $\boxed{0.2970}$

ii. Between ortho surgeon C and A is - $\boxed{0.6364}$

Inferences:

Between ortho surgeon C and A there is good association. They agree most.

Use of Pearson's Correlation "r"

The association or relationship between two quantitavely measured variable help us to understand Biological variables which influence physiology and pathology of human body. Relation of 2 variables can be represented as under:

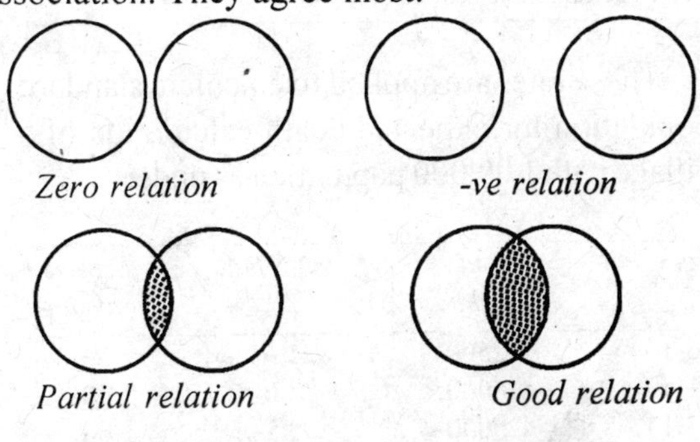

Fig. 5.24: Meaningfulness of "r"

Mathematically, square of correlation coefficient can measure meaningfulness of "r". overlapping (shaded area) indicates shared variance which can be found out mathematically as under:

If r = 0.30, $r^2 = 0.09$ which is 9% (that means 9% accounts for association and 81% do not).

If r = 0.80, $r^2 = 0.64$ which is 64% (Accountability is more than half).

MEASURES OF RELATIVE STANDARDS

Age Norms

Age adjustment or age standardisation removes the compounding effect of different age structure and gives a single standard rate. This helps in comparing of mortality experience in 2 population.

Direct Standardisation

Age	*Mid year population*	*Deaths in the year*	*Age specific death rate*
0-1	3000	65	21.6
1-4	5000	20	4.0
5-14	3000	10	3.3
15-44	21000	90	4.3
45 +	15000	200	13.3
	47000	385	

Crude death rate is 8.0

These rates are applied to calculate standard population for expected death calculation of a village with 1,00,000 population as under:

Age	*Std. population*	*A.S.D.R.*	*Expected death*
0-1	2500	21.6	54
1-4	10000	4.0	40
5-14	20000	3.3	66
15-44	43000	4.3	185
45 +	24500	13.3	326
	1,00,000		671

Standardised death rate for the village is:

$$\frac{671}{1,00,000} \times 1000 = 6.71$$

Crude death rate of 8.0 and Standardised death rate of 6.71 shows that effect of age structure is removed by standardisation.

Indirect Standardisation

Standard Mortality ratio is more common and useful form and is calculated by:

$$SMR = \frac{\text{Observed Deaths}}{\text{Expected Deaths}} \times 100$$

From above example it is

$$= \frac{385}{671} \times 100 = 57.4\,\%$$

Value below 100% is relatively favourable mortality and above 100% is unfavourable mortality.

Other Method

a. Calculation of index death rate.
b. Life table.
c. Regression techniques.
d. Multivariate analysis for standardisation.

Grade Norms

When a variable as such do not define a condition, we are forced to standardise that to a grade for proper inference. For example body weight is in Kg can be standardised by a few coefficients like:

a. Body mass index (Quetlet index) Weight/Height ^{2}
b. Ponderal index Height/Weight ^{2}
c. Broca index Height – 100
d. Lorentz's formula

$$\text{Height} - 100 - \frac{\text{Height} - 150}{(2\ (\text{women})\ \text{or}\ 4\ (\text{men})}$$

e. Corpulence index

Actual weight/Desired weight

Grade norms are required in many spheres like malnutrition grading etc.

Percentiles

Percentile allows us to describe a given score in relation to other scores in a distribution. It helps us to understand the relative position of a given score.

It is calculated by:

$$\frac{\text{No. of scores less than a given score}}{\text{Total number of scores}} \times 100$$

Example: A nurse (Rita) gets 90 marks out of 100 in a test where 50 nurse students took test. Out of 50 nurses a total of 40 had obtained less than 100 in the test. Then percentile of Rita is

$$\frac{40}{50} \times 100 \quad = \text{80th percentiles}$$

That means Rita scored higher than 80% of nurses (higher than her 40 classmates) and that 10 nurses in her class got higher than Rita.

25th percentile, 50th percentile, 75th percentile represent first quartile, second quartile (median) and third quartile respectively.

Standard Scores

They are ways of expressing a score in terms of its relative distance from the mean. A "Z" score is commonly used standard score. It is found out by:

$$Z = \frac{x - \bar{x}}{SD}$$

Example:

Average hospital days of stay (mean), in city A = 36 days. Mr. A stays in hospital for 50 days. SD of hospital stay available is 4.

$$\text{Then } Z = \frac{50\text{-}36}{4} \times 3.5$$

Using Z table we get 49.98 as value. So, percentile rank for Mr 'A' is 99 (50+49). That means Mr. A has stayed 50 days which is more (higher) than 99 other patients. Only one patient has stayed more days than Mr. A.

Standard score helps in the measurement of relative standards.

HEALTH INDICATORS

Concept, Importance

In order to evaluate the effectiveness and efficiency of a health treatment, health programme or health service, the extent of achievement of targets and objectives etc., we need the yardsticks called Health Indicators.

Health indicators measure health change, compare different stages of health and demarcate effective treatment. Inter-state and international comparison is possible through Health indicators.

In the nursing career, the need for monitoring health activities and level of health is possible by:

- Determining the extent to which nursing targets are being reached.
- Assessing the impact and effectiveness of nursing care given.
- Providing information for effective nursing care and reprogramming of nursing activities.

Expected requirement of Health indicators are:

i. *Feasibility:* The ability to obtain the data needed to compute the indicator.

ii. *Reliability:* The indicator should be reproducible if measured by different people under similar circumstances.

iii. *Relevance:* The extent to which an indicator contributes to the understanding of the phenomenon of interest.

iv. *Sensitivity:* The degree to which an indicator reflect changes in the phenomenon of interest.

v. *Specificity:* The ability of an indicator to reflect changes in only the specific phenomenon of interest.

vi. *Validity:* the degree to which an indicator is a true expression of the phenomenon of interest.

Examples for expected requirement of health indicators:

- Indicator for foetal loss is not feasible because foetal loss data are not collected.
- I.M.R is a reliable indicator.
- Median height for age among under five children is relevant for stunted growth.
- "All drugs are non expired in a store" is not a specific indicator of drug supply.
- Drug issued to a patient is not a specific indicator.
- Amount spent on drugs is not a valid health indicator.

Examples of health indicators that are found appropriate in nursing health care services.

I. *Health status indicators:*
- Percentage of L.B.W.
- I.M.R., child mortality Rate, under five mortality rate.
- Life expectation in years for a given age.
- MMR.
- Disease specific mortality rates.
- Disease specific morbidity rates.
- Disability rates.

II. *Indicator on the provision of nursing care:*
- Availability.
- Physical accessibility.
- Economic and cultural accessibility.
- Quality of care.
- Level of health awareness.
- Availability of safe water within walkable distance.
- Conducting delivery by trained Dais.
- Availability of essential drugs.

III. *Socioeconomic indicators:*
- Rate of population growth.
- Gross National and gross domestic product (GNP and GDP).
- Income distribution.
- Work availability.
- Adult literacy rate.
- Overcrowding (floor space per person)

IV. *Health policy indicators:*
- Level of political commitment.
- Allocation of adequate resources.
- Level of community involvement.

Rate, Ratio, Proportion

Magnitude of a disease, problem, event is expressed by rate, ratio and proportions. They are the basic tools in measurements of health and form common Health indicators.

a. Rate $= \dfrac{\text{Numerator}}{\text{Denominator}}$

per 100, 1000, or 10,000 etc.

An event is measured in a population over a period of time and expressed per 1000 constitute rate.

Example:

$$\text{Birth rate} = \frac{\text{No. of births in 1 year}}{\text{Mid year population}} \times 1000$$

Types of Rates are:

i. Crude Rates: e.g.: Death rate, birth rate.

ii. Specific Rates: e.g.: Age specific Death by TB.

iii. Standardised Rates: e.g.: Standardised Death Rate.

b. Ratio: Ratio is an expression of relation in size between 2 random quantities. It is the result of dividing one quality by another quantity.

Example:

Sex Ratio (933 females for 1000 males) in last census

Nurse population Ratio (0.8 : 10000) 2004 estimate

c. Proportion : It is a ratio which indicates the relation in magnitude of a part of the whole, and is in percentage.

Example:

Scabies in children is

$$\frac{\text{263 scabies children}}{\text{10,000 children population}} \times 100 = 2.6\%$$

i.e., 2.6 % children are scabies children.

Common Health Indicators

i. *Birth rate:* It is the number of live births during a year per 1000 mid year population.

$$\text{Birth rate} = \frac{\text{No. of live births in 1 year}}{\text{Mid year population}} \times 1000$$

It is 24.1 at present estimate.

ii. Death rate : It is the number of deaths per 1000 mid year population in 1 year.

$$\text{Death rate} = \frac{\text{No. of deaths in 1 year}}{\text{Mid year population}} \times 1000$$

It is 7.5 at present estimate.

iii. Growth rate : It is the difference between B.R and D.R and is expressed in percentage. It is now 1.7% at present estimate.

iv. Sex Ratio: It is the number of females per 1000 males. It is now 933.

v. Dependency Ratio: This is proportion of persons above 65 years and below 15 years who are dependent on adult earning members.

It is 64 in India at present.

vi. Family size: It is total number of members in a family. It is 3.0 as per estimate.

vii. Literacy rate: It is the number of literates (who can read and sign) (in his/her mother tongue) per 1000. It is now 65.38 as per 2001 census.

viii. Life expectancy: It is expectation of life at birth i.e average number of years which a person of that age may be expected to live. It is now 63.90 for men and 66.90 for women .

ix. Age at marriage: It is average age at which female marries and enters reproductive period of life. It is 20.1 years. Every 1 year increase in age at marriage brings down births by 4 to 5%.

x. General Fertility Rate: It is the number of live births per 1000 women in the age group of 15 to 49 years.

$$\text{G.F.R.} = \frac{\text{No. of LB in 1 year}}{\text{Mid year Female population 15-19 years}} \times 1000$$

It is 95.3 as per 2003 estimate.

xi. Total Fertility rate: It is the average number of children women would have if she were to pass through her reproductive age group. It is 3.0 at present.

xii. Gross reproduction rate: It is the average number of girls that would be born to women if she experiences the current fertility in her 15-49 age, assuring no deaths.

It is 1.4 in India as per 2003 estimate.

xiii. Net reproduction rate: It is the number of daughters who deliver girl child during her 15-49 age assuming no deaths.
It is 1.46 as per estimate.
N R R is a demographic indicator. Government of India has adopted an N R R of 1 by the year 2006 which was possible if couple protection rate was 60%.

xiv. Pregnancy rate: It is the number of pregnancies which include live birth, still birth, and not delivered by married women of 15-49 age.

xv. Maternal mortality Rate: It is death of women while pregnant or within 42 days of delivery per 1000 live births.

$$\text{MMR} = \frac{\text{No. of mothers dying due to pregnancy, child birth within 42 days delivery}}{\text{No. of Live Births}} \times 1000$$

It is 3.01 at present estimate.

xvi. Perinatal mortality rate: It is calculated by:

$$\text{PMR} = \frac{\text{Late foetal deaths (< 28 weeks gestation (1 week) in 1 year}}{\text{No. of Live Births in one year}} \times 1000$$

It is 33 as per current estimate

xvii. Neonatal mortality rate: It is calculated by:

$$\frac{\text{No. of deaths < 28 days}}{\text{Live births}} \times 1000$$

It is 43 as per current estimate.

xviii. Post Neonatal mortality rate: It is calculated by:

$$\frac{\text{No. of deaths from 28 days to 1 year age}}{\text{Live births}} \times 1000$$

It is estimated to be 23 at present.

xix. Infant mortality rate: It is the ratio of infant deaths registered in one year to the live births of the same year.

$$\text{IMR} = \frac{\text{No. of deaths < 1 year in 1 year}}{\text{Live births}} \times 1000$$

In India it is 58 as per current estimate.

xx. 1 – 4 year mortality rate: It is calculated by:

$$\frac{\text{No. of deaths of 1-4 aged in 1 year}}{\text{1-4 year population}} \times 1000$$

It is estimated to be 5.2% of total deaths.

xxi. Child mortality rate (underfivemortality): It is calculated by:

$$\frac{\text{No. of deaths of < 5 year child in 1 year}}{\text{Live Births}} \times 1000$$

It is estimated to be 17.4 per 1000 under five children (85 per 1000 Live births).

xxii. Child survival index: It is calculated by:

$$\frac{\text{1000—under five mortality rate}}{10} \times 1000$$

Child survival rate is 91.5 as per 2004 estimate.

xxiii. Incidence: It is number of new cases occurring in a defined population during 1 year.

$$\frac{\text{No. of new cases in 1 year}}{\text{Population at risk}} \times 1000$$

xxiv. Prevalence: It refers to the prevailing status at a point of time which includes old and new cases.

Point prevalence is calculated by:

$$\frac{\text{No. of old and new cases in a point of time}}{\text{Population at that time}} \times 100$$

Period prevalence is calculated by:

$$\frac{\text{No. of old and new cases at 1 year}}{\text{Population at risk (MYP)}} \times 100$$

xxv. Sullivan's index: This is expectation of life free of disability. At life expectation of 58 years and disability or sickness period of 7.5 years, Sullivan index is 50.5. It is an advanced indicator available.

xxvi. Health adjusted life expectancy (HALE): It measures healthy life expectancy. It includes time spent in poor health.

xxvii. Disability adjusted life expectancy (DALE): It measures healthy life excluding time spent in poor health.

xxviii. Disability adjusted life year (DALY): It measures burden of disease of a population. One year healthy life lost is equal to 1 DALY.

xxix. Bed occupancy rate and Bed Turn over ratio are utilisation rates which explain the extent of use of health services.

xxx. Per capita income: It is an index of standard of living. According to estimate it is Rs. 23241 at current price.

Source of Statistics

a. Census:

It is a major source of vital events. It is done once in 10 years. First census was in 1881 and latest 13th census was in 2001. Entire population is covered at one time for information on age, sex, marital status, birthplace, religion, literacy, occupation etc. The compiled date is published by census commissioner and Registrar General of India. It is a base line data, helpful for research and Government activity including policy decision.

b. Birth and Death Registration:

It is a reliable source of information. But is still in infancy because of following reasons:

- Lack of completeness
- Lack of accuracy
- Illiterate Primary Reporters
- Revenue and police department transmits the data
- People are not aware of its importance (ignorant)
- Lack of uniformity.

GOI Birth and Death Registration Act for registration of vital events came into effect in 1970.

c. Notification of Diseases:

This is applicable to a list of diseases which help in proper recording, report-ing and surveillance.

d. Hospital Records:

This has been a major source over centuries. Since it is not community based it lacks in power of data.

e. Health Centres:

After district health system, health centres are providing all information which is good source of health statistics.

f. Health Surveys:

It includes General survey and special surveys and sample surveys. They give good data for development of health indicators.

Uses of Statistics

i. It measures the state of health of a community.
ii. It identifies Health problems.
iii. It identifies the health need.
iv. Helps in comparison between:
   a. Past and Present
   b. State to State
   c. Country to Country.

v. Helps in planning and administration of health.
vi. Helps in evaluation of:
   a. Success of nursing care.
   b. Failure of Health programme.
   c. Progress in professional care.
vii. Helps in Research.

NURSING RESEARCH – BASIS

Science and Philosophy

Science is the development of specialty due to keen observation and experiment-ation of man by his knowledge. Direct or indirect methods of demonstration are possible to answer our Biological questions. Documentation of such observation based on scientific approach constitutes science.

Philosophy of science is to apply the knowledge of science for the welfare of mankind, for resource development and for maintenance of positive health.

Source of Human Knowledge

Man has shown adventure in finding an answer for unanswered question since his evolution. For survival of his species "Homo Sipien" he adopted many devices to develop understanding through:

- Observation
- Natural course of events
- Interaction in the community
- Adaptation of education system
- Research.

What is Scientific Method?

Research is the systematic study of one or more problems, usually posed as question that needs answer. Specific approved methods are adopted to study such problems by developing hypothesis and proving such postulated hypothesis. Question taken will have the potential contribution to existing body of knowledge and it should benefit the nursing profession and community.

Research – Definition, Nature, Concept, Scope

Research is a defined as a systematic study of selected problem through specific methods of scientific basis of specified disciplines. It includes experiment, survey, correlation studies with or without Meta analysis and psychometric evaluations. (After knapp 1998)

Nature of research may be observational and hypothesis generation study (descriptive). It may be hypothesis testing study (observational analytical strategy). It may be based on animal and human experiments. Observation as time motion study is also one of the natures of Research called Operational strategy.

Conceptual idea of Research involves a population (group of patients for study), parameters (to describe characteristics of population). Since a representation of population is selected it will be always a "sample" in Research.

Scope of research are multifold, they are:

- Drawing conclusions
- Improving nursing care facility
- Order for new innovations
- Adopting science and technology
- Makes cost benefit
- Bring out cost effective procedures
- Control of health problems
- Prevention of risks.

Characteristics

i. It is attached with significance and relevance.
ii. They are made amenable to scientific study.
iii. Need facility, equipment and resources.
iv. It needs personal interest in researcher.
v. Curiosity leads to research.

Nursing Research – Source, Process, Evaluation

Research in nursing profession is to make judicious decisions in nursing care delivery at individual patient level, at group of patients level and also at large in community who are healthy.

Nursing as a discipline deals with variations of characteristics like cholesterol level, lung function, blood pressure because of pathological variations. This again is determined by biological factors like genetic constitution, age, sex and personality. In majority of cases environmental factors like, life style, stress, strain, diet etc., adds to the process of research.

During the process nurse has to:

- Think scientifically, logically and critically about health problem.
- Assess the available evidence for decision making.
- Be aware of possible risk associated with nursing decisions.
- Identify decisions and conclusions that lack scientific and logical basis.

Evaluation of research is necessary in the following areas of nursing care:

a. Handling of variations in nursing care.
b. Diagnosis of patient's ailments.
c. Diagnosis of community health problem.
d. Predications of likely outcome of an intervention.
e. Selection of appropriate intervention measures.
f. Planning, administration in nursing.
g. Final reports for policy making in nursing profession.

Research Types

There are two types of research available in nursing profession.

Basic Research

This is also called observational research seen as routine research activities.

It may be pure observational type where nursing activities encompass. E.g., breast feeding practices or delivery practices etc.

It may be observational and interview type when response is obtained from respondent and are recorded. Examples are: study of sexual behaviour, community participation in tubectomy camp etc.

It may be observation and analysis where knowledge of analytical epidemiology is used as in Case-Control study or Cohort study.

Applied Research

This is also called explorative research. Main objective is to get new insight or to standardise a procedure. Here, by exploratory applied research nurse can augment her skills or procedures. For example, exploration for a better foetoscope, instrument for a better infusion, a good gadget for an effective first aid etc.

RESEARCH METHODS

There are many methods that are made available as research methods in nursing profession.

Experimental Research Methods

Here researcher is able to modify the risk factors by giving drug, vaccine, nutrient etc. Sometimes changes must have occurred as a coincidence in nature. Experimental research is undertaken with control group or without control group. They are of following types:

i. Randomised controlled trail.
   a. Clinical trail
   b. Field trail
   c. Community study.
ii. Non Randomised trail
   a. Trail without control

b. Natural experiments with or without control

c. Before and after comparison studies.

In clinical study both diseased and healthy are selected. In preventive study only healthy are selected. They may be for treatment, surgery (Therapeutic) protective like : (a) for vaccine or contraceptives (prophylaxis) (b) for side effect of medicaments (safety studies) and can be (c) efficiency studies like copper T efficiency, TBA trained for efficient services etc.

The same is presented in a flow chart: (Fig. 5.25)

Steps taken in clinical trail are:

- Informed consent of participants
- Protocol is drawn
- Reference population is selected
- Study population is selected
- Randomisation done
- Intervention done
- Recorded and followed up
- Data Analysed
- Report prepared.

To overcome Bias, blinding is done which do not allow patient or nurse or data analyst to know about drug or placebo.

Single Blinding	Patient does not know.
Double Blinding	Patient and nurse (Researcher) do not know.
Triple Blinding	patient, nurse and statistician all do not know.

Historical Study

It is retrospective historical study which has already occurred before the start of the study. Here we do not select case or control. Exposed group is selected and studied.

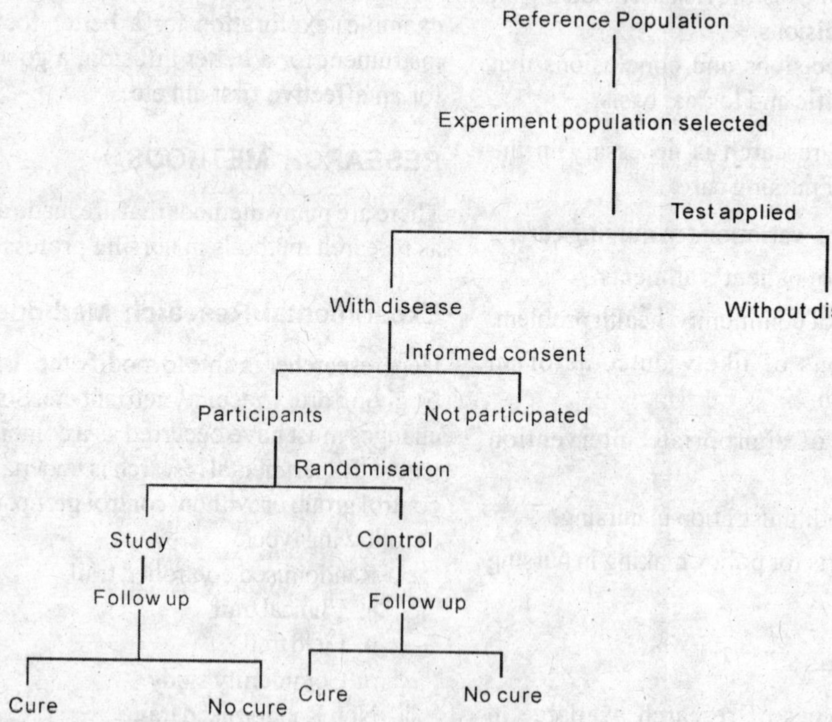

Fig. 5.25: Flow chart of RCT

Cohort Study

It is a prospective study where a Cohort is selected which is a group of people experiencing common characteristics. They can be birth cohort, Marriage cohort, Treated cohort, exposure cohort, Occupational cohort or insured cohort.

Steps in cohort study:

- Identification of reference population
- Selection of study population
- Formulation of cohorts
- Follow up.

Difference between case control study and cohort study:

Table 5.3: Difference between case control and cohort

Case control	*Cohort*
Goes from effect to cause	Cause to effect
Starts with disease	Starts with risk
No risk group	There is a risk group
Cases are selected	Cases are evolved
Odds ratio is available	Relative risk and attributable risk are available
Not expensive	Expensive
Small universe	Large universe
Suitable for rare problem	Not suitable for rare problem
No other information	Yields other information is available
Less attrition	More attrition

Survey

It is a basic tool of research in Health Sciences. There are many types like Impact survey, utilisation survey, Gallup survey, Social survey, Morbidity survey, mortality survey etc., Survey provides the denominator and hence enables comparison. Major uses of survey are:

- To assess magnitude of health problem.
- To guide planning.
- To evaluate National health activities.
- Knowledge, Attitude and Practice can be studied.
- To know the extent of service utilisation.
- Helps to test hypothesis on health related events.

Meticulous planning is needed for a survey. Survey instruments can be Interview, Observation, Questionnaire, schedules, Techniques, investigations.

Field Study

A designed research undertaken at community level constitutes filed study. This can be Rural, Urban, Industrial or Nutritional in nature. It is an active process by a Researcher to visit, observe and collect data at family level or at social unit level. This involves understanding of local customs, culture and traditional value. Field study requires local dialect for information collection.

Case Study

This is extensively used in nursing science and Behavioural science. It involves in-depth study of one or a few cases as representative of a larger number of cases. The subject of investigations may be a few selected characteristics in Individual or family, Case study do not generate information which can be adopted on a wider scale. However "case study" method can be used as an area for testing hypothesis.

Ethical Issues in Nursing Research

Since nursing research involve human population it has to be carefully reviewed at proposal level. Any research on human beings commands certain amount of service benefit may be in the form of cash or kind. So it is advisable to earmark a budget for it.

All examination procedure should be harmless and noninvasive.

Outcome of research must be shared with the community for their welfare.

In interventions, informed consent should be obtained. Confidentiality should be ensured.

Poorer section of society should not be exploited. Special care must be taken to take permission from ethical committees for drug trail, animal experiments and invasive procedures among human subjects.

RESEARCH PROCESS

Overview

It is essential to have overview of the research process from the point view of manpower, money and material. At the beginning feasibility and applicability in nursing set up should be viewed. As far as possible a research should be a need based beneficial proposal where time and money are not wasted.

Steps

Following are the major steps in research process:

i. A good research topic of relevance is selected.
ii. A research problem is selected from the topic. This leads to proper formulation of research hypothesis.
iii. To get a help for further understanding, search for related research work is undertaken.
iv. Objectives research proposal are formulated.
v. Variables that are needed to be measured are clearly spelled out. They are dependent, independent, confounding and background variables.
vi. Strategies are drawn-up for research study. They include descriptive, experimental and operational strategies.
vii. Selection of appropriate sample is done.
viii. Pilot study is undertaken for final preparation of protocol.
ix. Plans for data analysis and interpretation are drawn.

Purpose

The main purpose is to fulfill the objectives of the study and proving the hypothesis by verifications of hypothesis done at protocol.

Review of Literature:

Review of literature is done for information on related aspect of research process.

This helps in:

- Further understanding of research.
- Hin identification of proper and appropriate variables.
- Helps in drawing research hypothesis.
- Helps to design the protocol based on what has been followed earlier.
- Getting familiarity of methods used in the protocol.

The search can be undertaken by:

- Scan of literature, periodicals.
- Discussion with experts.
- Library index search like:
  - International nursing index
  - Excerpta medica
  - Index medicus.
- Computer search like:
  - Medlars
  - Med line
  - Cat Lines.
- Bibliographic.
- Statistical reports.

Research Topic

Research topic must be of current problem oriented. By using outcome of research there must be benefit to patient, family or community (need based study topic). As far as possible the topic should have relevance to the local area or region where it can stand as base line data, for therapy, management or intervention. When information on a particular topic is readily available, it need not be repeated. In case of repetition it can be taken after a lapse of 5 or 10 years for a study on secular changes of characteristics.

Broad area of topic can be study of rare occurrence, of common practical concern, for a need of comparing an alternative treatment modality or for additional information on a given illness.

CONCEPTUAL AND THEORETICAL FRAME WORK

Introduction

Theoretical frame work: Both simple and complex abstracts from a theory are generated imagining expected result of research. This is a developed Theoretical conceptual frame work, containing predicted and speculated elements. Since Theory is symbolic in nature, we may not likely to get all required evidence to prove our speculations. This Theory frame work can be called as "a model".

Theory generates a phenomenon of approach which can lead the way for conducting research in a scientific way.

Accepting a conceived research framework, it is possible to look into do's and don'ts with regard to selection of cases, selection of variables, sample size and even formulating the objectives of relevance.

Operational Deficiencies

- Duration of study may be too long.
- Seasonality (Timing) may not be suitable.
- Accessibility of subjects may be difficult.
- Availability of subjects may be poor.
- Co-operation of other sectors involved may not be there.
- Facility and equipment may be available only after a long time.
- Financial resource may be limited.
- Ethical issue may come in the way of research process.

Variables

Characteristics like sex, presence of illness in an individual, occurrence of birth, death, etc.; are qualitative data. For any characteristics the observation we make is any of the alternative situations for that characteristics. For example male/female, sick/well, survival/dead etc.

When many characteristics are drawn for an individual, classification can be made simultaneously for all these multiple characteristics.

In case of characteristics that are measurable like Hb% age, weight, height, when a character takes any value over a particular range it is called continuous (like plasma protein, age etc.). When a character has only intermitted values over a range they are discrete (like number of diarrhea attack, WBC count etc.).

Hypothesis

Let us study following statements:

"Tropical Oesinophillia is associated with high absolute oesinophillic count".

"Amoxicillin cures pharyngitis to the tune of 100 percent".

"Drug ginger with fatty meal inhibits platelet aggregation".

"Drug consumption and sleep disturbances increases with age".

Above statements are assumptions. They are called hypothesis. Testing the hypothesis involves making assumption about the parameter which can check our assumption.

There are 2 types of research procedures with reference to testing of hypothesis. They are:

- Comparative study on 2 or more population/sample.
- Studying the relationship between 2 or more factors on the population.

In testing hypothesis we have to deal with sampling variation because we make inference on the basis of samples. If the observed sample difference is larger than that which the sampling variation would produce, we can conclude that differences exist in the population.

In the beginning we assume "Null hypothesis" which means that no difference exist between populations.

If an observed value is greater than expected (table) value at a given degree of freedom and at minimum (critical) probability of 0.05 we say significant and say occurrence is not by chance.

Research Design

The validity of research relay upon data analysis, planning and execution of research design. Appropriate design and careful execution are necessary to provide specific answer to hypothesis, which also takes care of complete use of men, material and money used in the research.

Following principles are followed for an effective research design:

i. *Bias:* They are overcome by appropriate sampling techniques and suitable randomising procedures.

ii. *Precision of sensitivity:* This is overcome by collection or data from (as far as possible) a large sample and quality control of instruments that are used in research.

iii. *Use of common research design:* This is necessary to disallow unnecessary and harmful effects of treatment in research activity. Here principle followed are to conduct research on a population which show little variation, study of subgroups for separate studies and evidence based activities are incorporated.

Following simple designs are advocated:

- *Individual comparison:*
  This helps in refinement of experiment on the knowledge of variation on group research. Depending on number of treatment, number of groups is made.
- *Group comparison:*
  Valid conclusion can be drawn by research on group by random allocation of treatment or intervention.
- *Concurrent comparison:*
  Here many groups are simultaneously exposed for specified treatment. Simultaneous trail will reduce the cost of research.

Table 5.4: Allocation pattern in research design

Simple design	
Treatment A	15 Subjects
Treatment B	15 Subjects
Treatment C	15 Subjects
Control	15 Subjects
Total:	60 Subjects
Factorial design	
Treatment A	10 Subjects
Treatment B	10 Subjects
Treatment C	10 Subjects
Treatment A & B	10 Subjects
Treatment B & C	10 Subjects
Control	10 Subjects
Total:	60 Subjects

When 60 subjects are used response of 15 subjects each are available for treatment A, B, C and control. If results are not incoming in the simple design, then Factorial design may help where comparison is possible as under:

- Comparison of A and B
- Comparison of B and C
- Comparison of A and A & B
- Comparison of B and B & C
- Comparison of A and Control
- Comparison of B and Control.

Where again same 60 subjects are sufficient in research design.

iv. Prevalence of event or proportion of event helps in consideration of number of cases to be studied with permissible error of 5%, 10% or at the most maximum of 20% of permissible error rate.

Experimental Design

The experimental design needs the fulfillment of requirement of procedure and good design. A statistician should be contacted before the experiment and not after the experiment. Avoiding post mortem analysis is the best for a good experimental design.

Following principles are followed in a good experimental design:

- Random allocation of individuals.
- No arbitrary correction is allowed.
- Whatever result comes that should be taken.
- Use of control with similar characteristics but without the testing variable.

The controls can be:

Concurrent (Simultaneously used)
Volunteer (not found effective)
Geographical (elsewhere done)
Historical (earlier done).

- Experimental errors should be measured by:

  Randomisation (no over estimation or no under estimation)
  Replication (Repetition).
- Reducing the errors due to working condition.

Common Experimental designs are as under:

- *One way approach*:
  Allotting patients at random to the various treatments.
- *Two way approach*:
  Grouping patients according to known response on them.
- *Latin square approach*:
  E.g.: Treatment can be started by 4 replication to 4 treatments.

A	D	C	B
B	A	D	C
C	B	A	D
D	C	B	A

- *Factorial design*
  When 2 or more factors are under investigation this is found useful.

E.g., of 2 factors at 2 level

	Low Dose	Normal Dose	Total
Old Treatment	15	15	30
New Treatment	15	15	30
	30	30	60

- *Split plot design*:
  This design is used when we need precise information on one factor, on the interaction of this factor on the second factor. Actually precision on second factor is ignored in this study design.
- *Use of analysis of covariance.*

Non Experimental Design

These are observational studies. Depending on risk factor present or not, we get comparative group for observation. Non experimental design has an innate bias. Still it is most feasible and community conducted research design.

Following are types of non-experimental designs:

a. Cross sectional study
b. Prospective study
c. Retrospective study.

Bias in non experimental design is due to case selection type, information collection methods, confounding of variables. This bias of non experimental design can be overcome by:

- Restricting people who are within narrow range to produce confounding.
- Matching the cases for values which influence confounding.
- Sub grouping of study individuals.

- Use of standardised rates.
- Use of Analysis of Covariance for adjustment.

According to Bradford Hill following Criteria can be used to establish casual associations. This is known as Hill's criteria.

1. Study design
2. Strength of association
3. Consistency
4. Correct temporal relationship
5. Dose response relationship
6. Plausibility
7. Specificity
8. Analogy.

SAMPLING

Meaning and Definition

In research it is not possible to study the whole universe which is called population. So we restrict to a sample from that population which is representation of whole population.

Sample is minimum number of objects or individuals for a study which is statistically determined and which represent the population in their characteristics.

What is a Good Sample?

It is a sample size which is sufficient to answer the problem in the research. It depends on the problem to be investigated, precision and resource available.

Sample size determination when prevalence of a disease is known

Prevalence of stroke in a city is 22%. At 10% accuracy what is the sample size of a study on stroke epidemiology.

$$\text{Sample size } n = \frac{4pq}{L_2}$$

where n = sample size

4 = derived from 2 ´ 2 SE (1.96)

p = prevalence of stroke 22%

q = 1-P = 78%

L = 10% of 22 = 2.2 (permissible error)

$$= \frac{4 \times 22 \times 78}{2.22} = \frac{6844}{4.84} = 1418$$

To obtain the estimate of quantitative data like Hb% weight etc.:

What should be the size of sample required to obtain the estimate of weight of infants at 1 year age when 'infant population mean' is 12 kg; SD= 1.5 kg; permissible error at 1%.

$$\text{Sample size} = n = \frac{t^2a \times s^2}{e^2}$$

where t^2a = table value of t at 2SE

s = Sample SD

e = error permissible

e = 1% of 12 = 0.12

$$n = \frac{t^2 \times s^2}{e^2} = \frac{1.96^2 \times 1.5^2}{0.12^2}$$

$$\frac{8.64}{0.0144} = 600$$

When control group is available, sample size will be as under:

Determine sample size for anaemia by Hb% estimation when a pilot study showed the following:

<u>Hb% of 10 patients</u>:

13, 12, 14, 14, 10, 11, 12, 11, 11, 13

Mean = 12.1 SD = 1.37

<u>Hb% of 10 controls</u>

13, 12, 13, 14, 12, 13, 12, 13, 12, 13

Mean = 12.7 SD = 0.67

First we have to find out the pooled SD(S)

$$S = \sqrt{\frac{n_1 s_1^2 + n_2 s_2^2}{n_1 + n_2 - 2}}$$

where S = pooled SD
n_1 = 10 patients
s_1 = 1.37
n_2 = 10 controls
s_2 = 0.67

$$= \sqrt{\frac{\left(10 \times 1.37^2\right) + \left(10 \times 0.67^2\right)}{10 + 10 - 2}} = 1.14$$

$$n = \text{size of sample} = \frac{2t^2 a \times s^2}{(d)^2}$$

where $2t^2a$ = Table value of t = 1.96
S = pooled S.D.
(d) = Minimum difference between case and control

$$= \frac{2 \times 1.96 \times 1.14^2}{0^2} = 10$$

So 10 for study group and 10 for control group.

In case of proportion, at C.I. 95% and range we are satisfied with predicting the event:

HIV/AIDS awareness is 80%. We want to be 95% sure of predicting by studying within 1% either side of the estimated population.

Then sample size will be:

95% of C I cover a distance of ± 1.96 SE under normal curve:

$$\pm 1.96\, \sigma_p = \pm 0.03$$

$$1.96 \sqrt{\frac{0.80 \times 0.20}{n}} = 0.03$$

$$1.96 \sqrt{\frac{0.16}{n}} = 0.03$$

$$1.96 \frac{0.40}{\sqrt{n}} = 0.03$$

$$\frac{0.784}{\sqrt{n}} = 0.03$$

$$0.784 = 0.03\sqrt{n}$$

$$26.13 = \sqrt{n}$$

$$682 = n$$

Types of Sampling

Random

Random Sampling includes:

- Simple random sampling (by Lottery or random numbers).
- Stratified random sampling (sample from each strata).
- Systematic sampling (every 10th case).
- Cluster sampling (selecting natural groups).
- Multi stage sampling (For HIV study 4 stages) is selected (primary), 4 district in 4 states, (secondary), 4 villages in these 4 districts (final).

Non Random

- Area sampling (a non probability sampling).
- Quota sampling (a non probability sampling).
- Incidental sampling (a non probability sampling).
- Purposive sampling (a non probability sampling).

TOOLS FOR DATA COLLECTION

Data collection is a decisive step in research methodology. Hence, proper training of personnel who collect the data is mandatory. Pilot study conducted would have set right the deficiencies in proforma prepared.

There are many methods of data collection in a research design. Following are common and noteworthy as tools for data collection.

Observation

Personal visit and observation by investigator help in observing many details who can detect the salient features of data collection. Qualitative evaluation is better done by the investigator. When more than one observer is involved there is a need for standardisation of evaluation technique.

Interview

Contact is done with individual or case by investigator. He elicits the response from the individual (a respondent). For a sustained prolonged interview, one has to maintain interest. The reaction and attitude of individual can be recorded.

Check List

This is a response sheet where questionnaires are recorded. Schedule or a questionnaire becomes useless if it is inadequately answered. The defect in check list cannot be compensated by any statistical means. Checklist should contain clear and unambiguous questions. As far as possible questions must be self explanatory. Even answers like "not known", others etc., need entry in the check list.

As far as possible the reply is recorded by "a cross" or a "tick" or ringing a category which makes the tabulation also easier.

An assurance to the effect that information collected will be kept confidential makes the respondent free to express his opinion.

Survey

The coverage of survey may include few individuals to whole community, Survey provides denominator which enables comparison. Health, morbidity and utilisation survey are common types of surveys.

Case Study

It is an in-depth analysis of a few cases or subjects. The method entails a comprehensive work up. The data collected will be enormous, when compared to surveys. But case study does not give a denominator and hence cannot be compared.

Sociometry and Sociogram

Sociometry is a technique of deter-mining and identifying good respondents. It also identifies the non cooperative. When such preference or rejection is seen in a society, by prior visit, advanced briefing and motivating for interrogation is advisable.

Sociogram is a map or description which allows the investigator to know the cooperative and non cooperative group. It is a description of social reaction, either by active group or by shy group. Sociogram developed at pilot study needs attention by frequent visits and motivation.

Scaling Methods

There are 4 types of scales that are used by the investigator for data collection. They are:

- Nominal scale (Category or quality described).
- Ordinal scale (Category where distance between category not known).
- Interval scale (accepted physical measurement).
- Ratio scale.

MEASUREMENT AND DATA COLLECTION

Introduction

Data collection is mainly dependant on precision of measures used in the study, how investigation was planned and how executed. Collection of definite answers, venturing for unambiguous reply puts the measurements at valid position.

Item Analysis

Measurement used in data collection is scientific based when it follows set of rules and scientific basis.

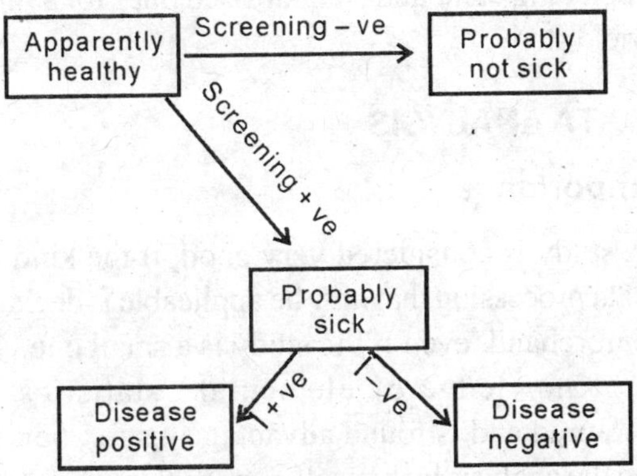

Fig. 5.26: Measure of a screening test

Table 5.5: Difference between screening and diagnostic tests

Screening	*Diagnostic test*
Done on healthy	Done on sick
It is a group test	Done on individual
Accuracy less	Accuracy more
Not for treatment	Basis for treatment
An active process	A passive process
Test is on criteria	On clinical criteria

Reliability

Reliable conclusion is possible by a large universe of study. It is dependent on individual variability and test variation. Common causes of poor reliability are:

- Biological variation
- Technical variation
- Intra and inter observer variation.

Validity

It measures accuracy of a Test. Indicators that are used to measure validity are sensitivity, specificity, positive and negative predictive values.

Extent of disease detection by a Test is sensitiveness or True positiveness.

Extent of normalcy detected by a Test is specificity or true negativeness.

Predictive values are probability of percentage of +ve or –ve result.

Let us put this information in a contingent table:

Test	Disease +	Disease –	
+	a (True +ve)	b	= a+b
–	c	d (True –ve)	= c+d
	a+c	b+d	= a+b+c+d (prevalence)

Example:

Heart attack

ECG	+	–	
+	23(a)	4(b)	27(a+b)
–	7(c)	66(d)	73(c+d)
	30 (a+c)	70 (b+d)	100

Sensitivity (True +ve) $= \frac{23}{30} \times 100 = \frac{a}{a+c} \times 100 = 76.7\%$

Specificity (True –ve) $= \frac{66}{70} \times 100 = \frac{d}{b+d} \times 100 = 94.3\%$

False +ve $= \frac{4}{70} \times 100 = \frac{b}{b+d} \times 100 = 5.7\%$

False –ve $= \frac{7}{30} \times 100 = \frac{c}{a+c} \times 100 = 23.3\%$

Predictive value of +ve

$$= \frac{23}{27} \times 100 = \frac{a}{a+b} \times 100 = 85.2\%$$

Predictive value of –ve

$$= \frac{66}{73} \times 100 = \frac{d}{c+d} \times 100 = 90.4\%$$

Source of Error

There are a few factors in Data collection which cannot be eliminated. They are even controlled by the investigator. They are called experimental error because they are associated with random variation of the experiment. Randomisation and replication make this error less important.

When we draw conclusion we are likely to make 2 types of error viz. Type I error and Type II error. (They are called a and b respectively). Actual situation is tabulated as:

Null Hypothesis

Table 5.6: Type I & II errors

	Rejected	*Not Rejected*
NH (True)	Type I (α)	No error
NH	No error	Type II (β)

It is not possible to reduce them totally. If one is reduced other raises.

Table 5.7: Illustration for understanding errors

	Sulpha Treatment	*Cloxicillin Treatment*	
A.	100 Patients 30% cure	100 Patients 55% cure	
B.	Sulpha Treatment 30 Patients Cloxicillin Treatment 30 patients	Type 1 (α) Used 5%	gives 40% cure
C.	Remaining 60% is type II (β) error.		
D.	If β error is 60% then remaining 40% is nothing but power of test (sensitiveness)		

Pilot Study

This is pre survey check of planning done. Suppose proforma and questionnaire are prepared, they are subjected for a test in the field, by administration. Reliability of questions and response is checked and necessary alteration can be made for the future reliability of the study. Unclear and ambiguous areas are removed replacing clear and standardised ones for a high yield study.

DATA ANALYSIS

Importance

A study is considered very good, if the kind of data processing that may be applicable is decided beforehand, even if the study is a small one.

Knowledge of elementary statistics is required and is found advantageous for, he can do the analysis by himself. Personal involvement of investigator in analysis adds immensely to the reliability and value of Nursing research. If the investigator is amateur, it has to be checked by a senior statistician. Very good nurse and who has shown excellence in nursing care, goes to request the help of statistician to do analysis for her. Association of statistician and senior faculty from the beginning brings best result out of the research. Application of appropriate statistical analysis is the secret of success and efficiency.

Data Processing—Inferential and Computer

Data collected from research always reflect the objectives formulated at the beginning. Analysis of small data may not be a problem if an orderly procedure is followed. In case of large sample where we come across multiplication of factors, planning for an efficient data analysis is required.

There are many constraints in handling large set of data:

- Errors
- Incompleteness
- Inconsistency.

Manual data analysis is cumbersome if the study is of large scale. Coded material, entered in specified manner in columns designed, will help in processing and analysis of data. Individual records and master registers or Master table must be available for a quick reference, whenever it is called for.

Manual Data Analysis

This involves direct handling of records, use of ordinary or edge marking cards, edge punch cards. Cards are cheaper and effecting the correction is easy. Simple tables, cross tables gives us tabulated data which needs description for observation. Observational description requires proportion, ratio and percentages. Further we may have to make a few contingent tables or statistical tables to enable us to apply statistical tests. This becomes inferential because we infer from statistical tests.

Computer Data Analysis

Computer is an electric device to which we can feed and store innumerable size of data and the analysis of such data will be at a very great speed. According to the cost, power and size, they are of following types:

i. Mainframes
ii. Mini computers
iii. Micro computers
   a. Personal type
   b. Compact desk top type.

Magnetic storage units are:

i. Floppy diskette
ii. Hand Disc (Winchester)

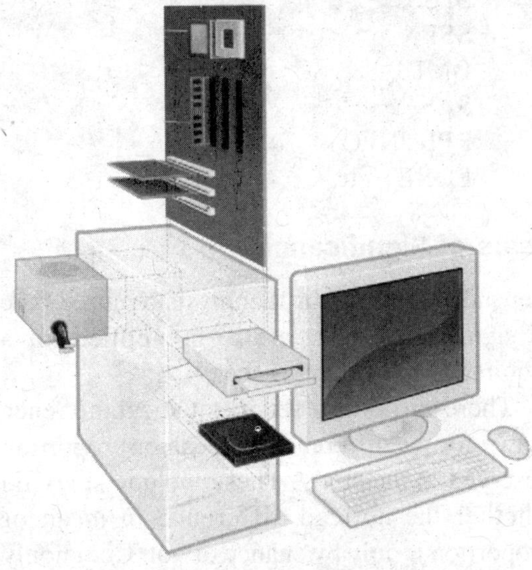

Photo: Parts of computer
(Central processing unit, visual display unit, input and output device)

iii. Cassette tapes
iv. Printing and plotting units

Common Floppy diskettes have following variations:

Sizes – $3^{1/2}$", $5^{1/4}$", 8"
Density – High and low
Capacity – 360 Kb to 1.44 Mb.

Computer languages required for operation are:

COBOL (common business oriented language).

FORTRAN (formula translation).

BASIC (beginners all purpose symbolic instruction code)

PASCAL – C.

Using these languages (software) a programme is prepared (Instructions) for the computer to execute any given job of data analysis.

There are readymade set of instructions (package) for specific statistical analysis, they are:

SPSS
SSP
BMDP
SAS
EPI- INFO
EGRET etc.

Tests of Significance

Depending on statistical analysis required type of significance tests are to be applied for a required statistical inference.

There are definite set of statistical inference drawn for the difference of mean or proportion observed in the study. These include study on whether the noticed difference in mean or proportion is only by chance or not. Commonly this area of significance test includes:

- Difference between Mean of sample and population.
- Difference between 2 sample Means.
- Difference between proportion of sample and population.
- Difference between 2 proportions.

Common significance tests applied are:

1. S.E. of the difference between 2 Means
2. S.E. of the difference between 2 proportions
3. Chi square test
4. t Test
5. Z Test.

Let us compute these five tests of significance by specific illustrations:

Standard Error of the Difference between Two Means:

Following is the data collected during a survey:

	No.	Mean height (inches)	S.D.
Englishmen	6400	67.85	2.56
Australians	1600	68.55	2.52

There is a difference of 0.7 inches in the mean. Is this significant?

$n_1 = 6400 \qquad S.D._1 = 2.56$

$n_2 = 1600 \qquad S.D._2 = 2.52$

$$S.E._{\bar{x}_1-\bar{x}_2} = \sqrt{\frac{SD_1^2}{n_1}+\frac{SD_2^2}{n_2}}$$

$$= \sqrt{\frac{2.56^2}{6400}+\frac{2.52^2}{1600}}$$

$$S.E._{\bar{x}_1-\bar{x}_2} = 0.07066$$

$$\text{Twice the } S.E._{\bar{x}_1-\bar{x}_2} = 0.141322$$

Actual difference 0.7 inches is greater than twice the $S.E._{\bar{x}_1-\bar{x}_2}$ (0.141322); hence significant. It is true that Australians are taller and it is not by chance.

Standard Error of the Difference between Two Proportion S.E.^ P – P

A study on arsenic poisoning was conducted during 2002 (2 year follow up study) where following observation was made.

Arsenic type	*Deaths*	*Survival*	*Total*
Paris green	66	48	114
White arsenic	148	161	309

First let us find % of Survival

In paris green it is 42.1%

In White Arsenic it is 52.1%.

$$S.E._{\hat{p}-p} = \sqrt{\frac{p_1q_1}{n_1}+\frac{p_2q_2}{n_2}}$$

$$= \sqrt{\frac{42.1\times 57.9}{114}+\frac{52.1\times 47.9}{309}}$$

$$= 5.427$$

$$\text{Twice } S.E._{\hat{p}-p} \quad 10.854$$

Observed difference (52.1 – 42.1 = 10) is less than Twice $S.E._{\hat{p}-p}$ (10.854).

Hence not significant and there is no strong evidence of any difference between types of Arsenic in survival rate.

Chi-square Test (x^2)

The ratio of male to female birth in nature is 1:1. One of the survey conducted by III year nursing students in Lucknow, showed the proportion as 52:48 (52 Males are born for every 48 females). Could this difference be due to chance?

Following are the four steps:

i. First: Let us prepare a contingent table:

	Natural	*Lucknow*	*Total*
Male	50	52	102
Female	50	48	98
	100	100	200

ii. Second: Let us find expected value Male birth 102 for 200, for 100 it is 102/200 x 100 = 51 etc.

	Natural	*Lucknow*	*Total*
Male	50(51)	52(51)	102
Female	50(49)	48(49)	98
	100	100	200

iii. Third: Apply X^2 Test by using formula X^2

$$= \frac{\Sigma(O-E)^2}{E}$$

Where 0 = observed value

E = Expected value (calculated)

$$X^2 = \frac{\Sigma(O-E)^2}{E} =$$

$$\frac{(50-51)^2}{51} + \frac{(52-51)^2}{51} + \frac{(50-49)^2}{49} + \frac{(48-49)^2}{49}$$

$$= 0.79 = 0.08$$

iv. Fourth: Find out degree of freedom by (c – 1) (r – 1)
where c = column
r = row
Here (2 – 1) (2 – 1) = 1
D.F. = 1

v. Fift: Find out table value of X^2 for D.F. = 1 at P=0.05
(P = Probability)
This is 3.84

vi. Sixth: Inference drawn. i.e. $x^2_{cal} < x^2_r$ at D.F.1 , P = 0.05
that means x^2 calculated (0.08) is less than x^2 table value, at D.F. = 1 and at P = 0.05.
∴ not significant

Statistical inference: The difference is only by chance.

't' Test

Ten nurses showed I.Q. as under:
70, 120, 110, 111, 88, 83, 95, 98, 107, 100.
At National level average I.Q. of a nurse is 100.
Apply 't' Test to test the significance.

Steps followed are:

i. First: Note that it is to find out that difference between sample mean (10 nurses) which is to be calculated and population mean (100) (it is available) is statistically significant.

ii. Second: It is a small sample, apply t test.

iii. Third: Find out mean and S.D. of 10 values.

x	$(x-\bar{x})$	$(x-\bar{x})^2$
70	– 28.2	795.24
120	21.8	475.24
110	11.8	139.24
111	12.8	163.84
88	– 10.2	104.04
83	– 15.2	231.04
95	– 3.2	10.24
98	– 0.2	0.04
107	8.8	77.44
100	1.8	3.24
982		1999.6

$\bar{x} = 98.2$

Sample S.D. $= \sqrt{\frac{\Sigma(x-\bar{x})^2}{n-1}} = \sqrt{\frac{1999.6}{9}}$

$= 14.91$

iv. Four: Apply t test

$t = t = \frac{\bar{x}-\mu}{s/\sqrt{n}}$ where $\bar{x}$ sample mean (98.2)

μ = population mean (100)

s = sample S.D. (14.91)

n = size sample (10)

$= \frac{98.2-100}{14.91/\sqrt{10}} = \frac{1.8}{4.7136} = 0.3818$

v. Five: Find out D.F by n-1
Here 10 – 1 = 9 ie., D.F. is 9

vi. Six: Find table value for D.F. = 9:P = 0.05.
It is 2.262

$\frac{98.2-100}{14.91/\sqrt{10}}$

Infer: Calculated 't' value (0.3818) is less than table value at DF 9 and P=0.05.

Statistical inference : Accept null hypothesis; Mean difference of 1.8 among 10 nurses is only by chance.

Z Test

Following are the illustrations for z test:

The mean height of 100 nursing staff at Delhi was 150 cms with a S.D. of 10 cms.

The population mean (say all India level study) of nurse population is 154 cms.

Does the sample mean significantly different from 154 cms ?

Apply Z test for the difference between sample mean and population mean.

$Z = \frac{\bar{x}-\mu}{SD/\sqrt{n}}$ where

$\bar{x}$ = mean of sample (150 cms)

μ = population mean (All India) (154 cms)

SD = 10 cms

n = 100 nurses.

$Z = \frac{150-154}{10/\sqrt{100}} = \frac{4}{1} = 4$

Infer: Z calculated is more than 2.54 indicating that it is highly significant.

Statistical inference: The difference is significant. 100 nursing staffs at Delhi have lower heights than All India Value.

Interpretations and Implications in Nursing Research

Statistical inference is not a final diction in nursing care, but it helps in planning, programming, implementing and also evaluating all routine and special nursing care services.

Data analysis gives an inference which suggests the following:

- There is association
- The difference is not significant
- The occurrence is not by chance
- We accept null hypothesis
- We reject null hypothesis
- Can conclude that a given variable is dependent on another
- There is goodness of fit etc.

In nursing profession it is always advisable to draw conclusion at the critical probability of 1 in 20 i.e. at P = 0.05. this has to be considered for a given degree of freedom in most of the occasion.

At higher probability of 1 in 100, 5 in 1000 or 1 in 1000 it is highly or very highly significant. (P = 0.01, P = 0.005, P = 0.001 respectively).

PRESENTATION AND DISSERTATION OF FINDINGS

Need and Importance of Writing

With formulated objective and postulated hypothesis, the nurse investigates and conducts research to arrive at validated hypothesis. When a fruitful observation is arrived and is found useful and beneficial to nursing community, it has to be presented in the form of a report or in the form of a dissertation (as a part of fulfillment of degree). From this the nursing community should get the benefit and research result should be a guide in nursing care, nursing management or nursing technique. The presentation made should be comprehensive in nature and a nurse should take care of the guidelines given for the scientific presentation or for submission of a dissertation.

This amounts to publication of results of research. The publication can be in the form of project, thesis, study, case study, research, clinical trail or a dissertation.

All nursing council and affiliated universities that embodies nursing colleges and nursing schools define the presentation or dissertation as under:

Definition and Components

"It is a formal, often lengthy treatise or a disclosure especially the one which is written by a nursing student at a course, degree or P.G. course."

The components of presentation or dissertation are as under:

Title.
Introduction with Aims and objectives.
Review of Literature.
Material and methods.
Results and observations.
Discussion.
Summary.
References.

Title

- Short, informative and concise.
- No abbreviations allowed.
- It may contain place, duration and type of study.

Introduction

- It should state as to why the topic is selected.
- It should state the purpose.
- It should give specific objectives.
- It should not exceed 500 words.

Review of Literature

- Give pertinent references.
- Critical approach to early works.
- Appropriate description must follow.
- No conclusions on other's work.

Material and Methods

- Outlines the scientific approach.

- Sampling, selection criteria and collection procedure and investigations should come.
- If any unusual method or technique, it can be taken to appendix.

Results/Observation

- Should follow order of objectives.
- Stratification is done by tabular and graphical presentation.
- Should have statistical measure.

Discussion

- Interpret the result of the present study.
- If disagrees with other studies what could be the reason for.
- Arrive at generalization from findings.
- Spurious correlations are avoided.
- Should make a note of limitations of the study.
- It can profound the future work establishment, from the present study.
- Comparative statement of present study and earlier studies make better presentation.

Note: A few advocate observation and discussion to be put together.

Summary and Conclusion

- Avoid all experimental details.
- Should be schematic presentation of a problem, outcome and result.
- Major conclusions are imperative.

References

- Always expected in Harvard style i.e. arranged alphabetically.
- It can also be in Vancouver style (the list is at the order of appearance in the text).
- Scientific nursing article commands Vancouver style.
- Nursing dissertation commands Harvard style.

Examples of references

1. Text book:
   Single author:
   Prabhakara G.N. Textbook of Community Health for Nurses, Peepee Pub. 2003, 670 pp.
   Two authors:
   Both names to be written here.
   Three authors:
   Prabhakara G.N. *et al.* etc., are written here.
2. Newspaper article:
   Editorial in "Deccan Herald" July 19, 2003.
3. Unpublished material:
   Prabhakara G.N. – Medical internship, a review, Medical education cell, JIPMER, Pondicherry, 1974 pp 73 (Mimeographed).
4. Journal:
   Prabhakara G.N. "Infant feeding patterns in slums of Bangalore" 1987 Ind paed, 24: 10 : pp 895-898.

A Model of Bibliography

A study of Medico Social profile of under five children suffering from diarrhoeal diseases by Dr. Mahenderkar. A.G. *et al.* at Pune (1991) showed that incidence of diarrhoea was more in low socio-economic group, and is inversely proportional to the literacy status of mother. Fifty percent of mothers had no knowledge of O R T therapy.

Appendix

This includes any of the following:

- A map of study area.
- Details about an experiment or procedure.
- A score system.
- Clinical photo of cases.
- Master table of the study.
- Schedule/proforma of the study.
- Standard criteria used etc.

Critique and Application in Nursing

Nursing care approach has brought out voluminous documents, Journals, Books, Reports, inferences from seminar, symposia and workshop. Reading these updates the knowledge. At the same time critical evaluation of Journal, report etc. is needed to be made in the form of Journal club or presentation of articles.

Evaluation of report or a Journal should critically review objectives, research methodology, statistical inference and conclusions.

This allows student nurse to develop an insight of Recent nursing development under the guidance of a Nursing Tutor.

FURTHER REFERENCES

1. Prabhakara G.N. "Biostatistics" (Jaypee).
2. W.H.O. – Teaching Health Statistics.
3. Simpson – Basic Statistics (Oxford I B H).
4. Woods Catasaro – Nursing Research (C V Mosby).
5. Prabhakara G.N. – Short Text Book of P.G. Orientation Coarse (Jaypee).
6. Prabhakara, G.N. – Short Text Book of Professional Medical Ethics (Paras).
7. Prabhakara, G.N. – "Essential Medical Education" (Mehta).
8. Prabhakara, G.N. – "Policies and Programmes of Health in India" (Jaypee).
9. Prabhakara G.N. – "Trends, Issues and Management in Nursing" (Peepee).

6

Demography and Family Planning

DEMOGRAPHY

Importance

Community health nursing or public health nursing is directly connected with people. Public health is related to population change, size of family, type of family, composition of family, morbidity and mortality of the family and hence public health nursing serves population to meet the health needs which might have been met or unmet. Moreover population is influenced by marriages, migrations and social mobility apart from births and deaths which are occurring as a natural process.

Terminologies

Demography

Demography is the study of human population with respect to size, type, composition, pattern and distribution.

Population Dynamics

Population dynamics is the study of mode of change of population and the factors responsible for such changes.

Social Mobility

Social mobility is movement of people with the purpose of family settlement, occupational placement and temporary stay on account of religious, philanthropic and national purpose.

Marriage

The term marriage can well be defined as the socially acceptable bondage in the process of family formation.

Fertility

Fertility is the child bearing process in the reproductive age group.

Demographic Gap

Demographic gap is the difference between births and deaths. It helps to know the rapid growth of population.

Malthusian Theory of Population Explosion

This theory postulates that over population is controlled by natural calamities like volcano, earthquake, floods, epidemics, etc. Though it is not a scientific version it can only be an antithesis of population.

Improvident Maternity

Improvident maternity is said to occur to a woman when the childbirth occurring to that woman who has already given birth to three children of whom one is alive. It is 42.8% in India.

Population Education

Population education is a health education programme which provides for a study of population situation in the community, country and world with the purpose of developing rational and responsible attitude among present generation towards family planning behaviour.

Demographic Cycle

With change of time, population change occurs which are noted is 5 cycles. They are:

- High stationary
- Early expanding
- Late expanding
- Low stationary
- Declining.

They are depicted in the Figure 6.1.

Major Sources of Demographic Data

There are many sources of data for demography and they are ongoing over many centuries. But, of late, importance is given through legislation (like Registration of Birth and Death Act) and a national commitment of Census. Four major sources are to be noted. They are:

- Registration of births, deaths, marriages and migration.
- Census.
- Hospital records, health centre records.
- Notification of diseases.

Effects of Over Population

Impact of overpopulation on the society is many. Major effects noticeable are hindrance to national development, unemployment, illiteracy, poor housing, non availability of health care facility, poor environmental sanitation and fast development of slums and shanty towns with its consequences.

Fertility

Fertility is child bearing among women of 15-45 age group. Uninterrupted marriage life, without

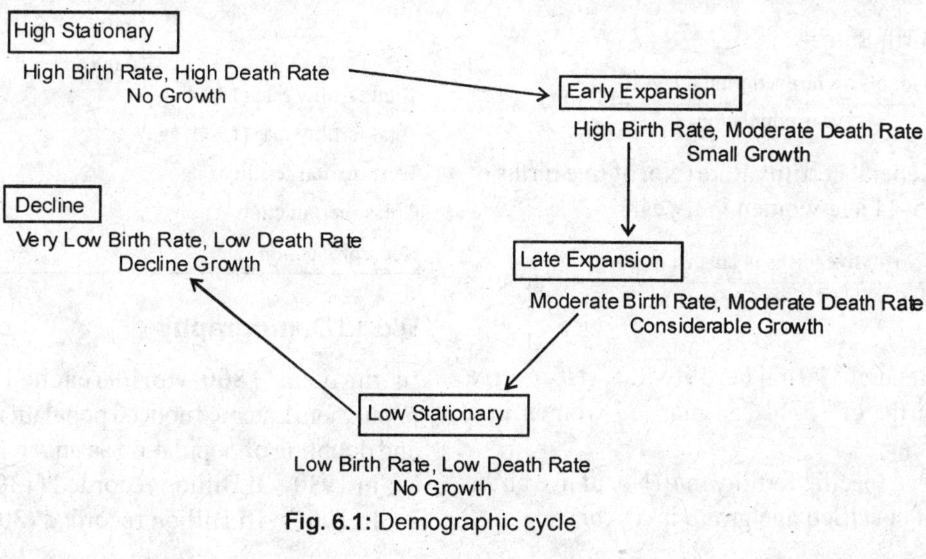

Fig. 6.1: Demographic cycle

protection, can allow 8-10 children is the fertility status. Factors which influence fertility are:

i. Age at marriage—on an average age at married in India is 21.1 years among girls.
ii. Married life—longer married life has high fertility rates.
iii. Spacing—postponement of pregnancies.
iv. Literacy—Illiteracy is associated with high fertility.
v. Income—Higher income (per capita income) show low fertility.
vi. Religion and caste—studies from International Institute for Population science, Mumbai has shown its observation as under:

Religion/Caste	*Fertility Rate*
Hindu	2.78
Muslim	3.59
Christian	2.44
Upper Caste	2.10
Lower Caste	3.90

vii. Nutrition—It indirectly influence fertility.
viii. Acceptance of family planning—This has determined the fertility rate.

Fertility Indicators

1. Birth Rate =

$$\frac{\text{No. of live births during the year}}{\text{Mid year population}} \times 1000$$

2. General Fertility Rate (No. of live births of 15-44 age women in a year)

$$\text{GFR} = \frac{\text{No. of live births in an area in a year}}{\text{15-44 age population}} \times 1000$$

3. General Marital Fertility Rate (No. of live births of 15-44 age married women in a year).
4. Age specific fertility rate (No. of live births of specified age group in a year).
5. Age specific marital fertility rate (No. of live births of 15-44 age married women in a year).
6. Total fertility rate (Average no. of live births of women during 15-44 age).
7. Total marital fertility rate (Average no. of live births of married women during her 15-44 age).
8. Gross reproduction Rate: It is No. of girls born to women in her 15-44 age.
9. Net Reproduction Rate: It is the number of daughters which a new born girl will bear.
10. Child women ratio, pregnancy rate, abortion rate and marriage rate are other fertility indicators.

Present fertility indicators are given in table (Estimates).

Table 6.1: Fertility indicators

Birth rate = 24.1		
General Fertility Rate = 95.3		
General marital fertility rate = 132.6		
Age specific fertility rate =		
15-19 years –	0.046	
20-24 years –	0.214	
25-29 years –	0.171	
30-34 years –	0.090	
35-39 years –	0.044	
40-44 years –	0.016	
45-49 years –	0.006	
Total fertility rate (15-44 age)		3.29
Total fertility rate (15-49 age)		3.32
Total marital fertility rate		4.7
Gross reproduction rate		1.4
Net reproduction rate		1.46

World Demography

In the year 1800 world reached 1 billion population. Later we noticed population explosion and doubling of population as under:

In 1930 – II Billion recorded (130 years)
In 1960 – III Billion recorded (30 years)

In 1974 – IV Billion recorded (15 years)
In 1987 – V Billion recorded (12 years)
In 1999 – VI Billion recorded (12 years)

Now, annual growth rate of the world is 14 percent. China and India are among most populous countries. Present demographic picture of the world are:

Population	- 6313,000,000
Annual Growth Rate	- 1.1 %
Birth Rate	- 21 per 1000 MYP
Death Rate	- 9 per 1000 MYP
Current growth	- 176 per minute (92,543,000 per year)

India—Demography

India reached 1 billion population on 11-05-2000. India thus has 2.4 % of land area and 16.87 % of world population. As per census report, post independent India population is as under (First census was in 1881):

1951	–	361,088,090
1961	–	439,234,771
1971	–	548,159,652
1981	–	683,329,097
1991	–	846,302,688
2001	–	1027,051,247 (Total 35 states/UT[5])

The total population of India as at 0.00 hours on 1.3.2001 stood at 1,027,015,247 persons. With this India become only the second country in the world after China to cross 1 billion mark. It is expected to reach 1.53 billion by 2050. The population of India rose by 21.34 % between 1991 and 2001. The sex ratio (female to male) in 2001 is 933 and 986 as per 2003 estimate. The literacy rate is reckoned at 65.38%.

Rural urban proportion of India is as under:

	Population	*Percentage*
Rural	741,660,293	72.2
Urban	285,354,954	27.8
Total	1,027,015,247	(100.0)

Male and female proportion of India is as follows:

	Population	*Percentage*
Male	531,277,078	51.7
Female	495,738,169	48.3
Total	1,027,015,247	(100.0)

Dependency ratio (above 65 years and below 15 years) is 55.5% (8.3% and 47.2% for 65 + and below 15 respectively).

Density of population in India as per 2001 is 324 persons per square kilometre area. The estimate for 2004 is 363 persons per square kilometre area.

Average family size is 3.0 members per family. Literate is 65.38% (male = 63.9% and female = 66.9%)and life expectancy is 62.10 for males and 64.00 for females. India has 3 mega cities (10 million population) viz., Mumbai, Kolkata and Delhi.

Proportion of population by age and sex are as follows:

Age	*Male*	*Female*
0-4	11.3	10.8
5-14	21.6	21.0
15-44	47.7	48.6
45-64	15.0	14.3
65 +	4.4	5.3
	(100.0)	(100.0)

The age structure of a population is best represented as age pyramid. The age pyramid of India has broad base and a tapering top. In developed countries it (pyramid) shows bulge in the middle and a narrow base.

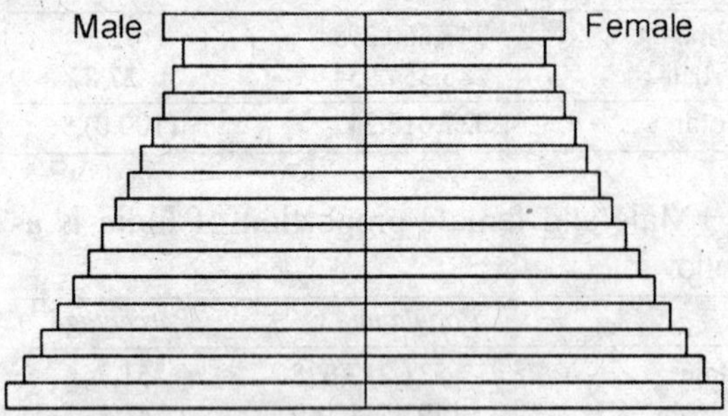

Fig. 6.2: Age pyramid of developing countries

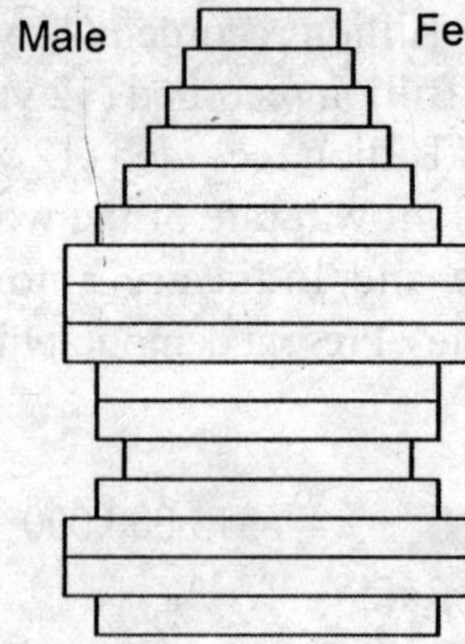

Fig. 6.3: Age pyramid of developed country

National Population Policy

To achieve National Demographic goals India developed National population policy in 1976, modified in 1977 and restructured in 2000. The National Population Policy of 2000 has laid emphasis on women's education, child survival, unmet needs of family planning, coverage of under-served population, adolescent health and education and participation of men in Planned Parenthood. Following are the demographic goals of NPP by 2010:

1. Service, supply and infrastructure for unmet needs of RCH.
2. Free and compulsory education up to 14 years of age and school drop-out reduced to below 20%.
3. IMR to 30 per 1000 live births.
4. MMR to 1 per 1000 live births.
5. 100% coverage of UIP.
6. Age at marriage for girls 18 years.
7. 100% deliveries by trained persons.
8. Cafeteria approach of family planning methods.
9. Registration of vital events 100%.
10. Integrated approach for RTI and STD.
11. Control of communicable disease by priority.
12. Integration and availability of Indian system of medicine for RCH care and home visiting.
13. Total fertility rate is brought to replacement level by 2010 by promoting small family norm.
14. F.P. is made as family welfare and as a people centred programme.

New Concepts with New Terms for Population Health

Global Burden of Disease (GBD)

It is a project to estimate health gaps for a comprehensive set of disease and injury causes, and for major risk factors or in the populations of the world using or all available mortality and health data and methods to ensure internal consistency and comparability of estimates. To measure health gaps DALY (Disability Adjusted Life Year) is used.

Health Adjusted Life Expectancy (HALE)

Any number of summary measures which use explicit weights to combine health expectancies for a set of discrete health state into a single indicator estimating the expectation of equivalent years of good health. It is also called healthy life expectancy.

International Statistical Classification of Diseases and Related Health Problems (ICD)

It is classification of diseases and other causes of mortality that was entrusted to the WHO in 1948, along with the constitutional mandate to have it periodically revised as necessary. The current 10th revision was issued in 1992 and come to effect on 1.1.93. The ICD is a member of the WHO family of International classifications.

International Classification of Functioning, Disability and Health (ICF)

It is an international classification published by WHO in 2001 as endorsed by the 54th world health assembly in resolution 54.21. As a revision of the ICIDH, the ICF is a member of the WHO family of International classifications.

International Classification of Impairment Disabilities and Handicaps (ICIDH)

A classification published by WHO for trail purpose in 1980 in accordance with the 1975 International Revision Conference and world health assembly resolution WHA 29.35 of 1976. It has now been superseded by the ICF.

Life Expectancy (LE)

It is a generic term summary measures of population mortality that estimate the expectation of year of life lived, called period life expectancy.

Period Life Expectancy

It is summary measures of population mortality that calculates the expectation of year of life lived in a fictitious birth cohort assuming that each age the cohort experience the specific mortality rates, observed in the real population during a specified time period.

Summary Measures of Population Health (SMPH)

They are indicators that summarise the health of a population into a single number. SMPH combine information about mortality and population health states. They may summarise either average health level or inequality for a population.

Sullivan's Method

It is a method of calculating health expectancies using data on current prevalence of health states in a population.

Years of Healthy Life (YHL)

It is a form of DFLE based on two questions collected in USA National Health Interview survey, which are concerned with activity limitations and perceived general health.

Years Lived with Disability (YLD)

It is the component of the DALY that measures the lost years of healthy life through living in states of less than full health.

Years of Life Lost (YLL)

It is the component of the DALY that measures the year lost through premature mortality.

Effective Components of Population Growth

Main components which effectively influence population growth are birth rate, death rate and growth rate. In spite of all efforts, birth and death rates remain high and population health has to be drawn towards this angle. Common causes of high birth rate in India are: (a) Marriages are done as universal phenomena. (b) Early marriages where about 50 to 56% are married before attaining age of 20 years. (c) Illiteracy and low standard of living influence high birth rate. (d) Custom dictating that all women should marry and all men must have a son influence high fertility, and (e) Awareness of small family norm is very less. Measures to overcome these factors are discussed under concerned chapter.

Present century response of low death rate can be attributed to (a) Large scale epidemics and great famine, are news of the past. (b) Death causing diseases are either controlled or prevented. (c) Accessible and affordable health care. (d) Impact of National Health programmes, and (e) Socioeconomic and health development activities.

Effort to reduce death rate still further is a hard task because it involves environmental manipulations and human nutrition.

Growth rate used to be steadily 2.0 percent and has come down to 1.7% in 2003 (estimate).

Current goal of these effective components of population growth by 2007 is as under:

Birth rate	–	21 per 1000 MYP
Death rate	–	9 per 1000 MYP
Growth rate	–	1.2 percent
Growth stabilisation	–	up to 2050

Population Dynamics in Nursing

There is a close interaction between population dynamics and medicine. The practice of nursing service administration and the management of health development require an understanding of the current size and composition of the population and the determinants of changes in these characteristics. Nursing planners must also be able to describe such changes quantitatively.

Population statistics has made the task possible in population size determination. The increase in population may be any of the following ways:

1. Natural increase
2. Arithmetic progression
3. Geometric progression

Following is the illustration that how population can be estimated by above methods:

Illustration:

i. 1991 population of a town = 65,000
ii. 2001 population of that town = 78,000
iii. Births from 1.1.91 to 30.6.95 = 14,000
iv. Deaths from 1.1.91 to 30.6.95 = 7800
v. Immigration from 1.1.91 to 30.6.95 = 3,100.
vi. Emigration from 1.1.91 to 30.6.95 = 375.

* Now we need to calculate population of 1995 (mid year population).

A. Midyear population of 1995 by National increase method:

= census + (births – deaths) + Immigration – Emigration)

= 78,000 + (14,000 – 7,800) + (3100 –375)

= 78,000 + 6200 + 2725

= 86,925.

B. Midyear population of 1995 by Arithmetic progression method:

$$\text{Where: } P_2 + \frac{P_2 - P_1}{n} \times d$$

P = Population to be calculated
P_1 = Population in 1991
P_2 = Population in 2001
d = Duration after 1991
n = Census period = 10 years

$$= 78{,}000 + \frac{13000}{10} \times 4½$$

= 83,850

C. Midyear population of 1995 by Geometric progression method:

$$P_n = P_o\left(1 + \frac{r}{100}\right)^n$$

Where:

Pn = Population to be calculated on 1.7.95.

Po = 78,000 (1991)

r = Rate of growth

$$= \frac{13{,}000}{65{,}000} \times 100 = 2\%$$

$$P_n = 78{,}000\left(1 + \frac{2}{100}\right)^{4.5}$$

= log 7800 + [(4.5) × log 1.02]

= 4.8921 + (4.5) (0.0086)

$= 4.8921 + 0.0387$

$= 4.9309$

By antilog conversion of 4.9309 we get,

$P_n = 85{,}270$

Demography and Genetics in Nursing

This aspect is the behaviour of genes in a given population. The study of genes in population rather than in individuals is the province of that branch of human genetics known as "population genetics". Let us take tallness of nurse population. There can be 3 possibilities.

Very tall = AA
Moderate = Aa
Short = aa

If A = Tall, a = short, Total must be 100 say p + q = 100 percent.

i.e., proportion of tallness + proportional shortness = 1

In above proportion, the sperms and eggs will contain then in same proportion and with random making (say marriage and off spring) the various gametic combinations can be:

$p^2 + 2pq + q^2$

i.e. AA + 2Aa + aa

Hardy and Weinberg postulated that population is static and not gene pool which is influenced by many factors. They pronounced (Hardy-Weinberg law) that "the relative frequencies of each gene allele tend to remain constant from generation to generation in the absence of external forces".

Estimated spontaneous mutation rate per million genes per generation for some of the traits are given in Table 6.2:

Table 6.2 : Gene mutation rate in population

Trait		*Mutation Rate*
Autosomal dominant disease		
• Retinoblastoma	–	20
• Polyposis coli	–	20
• Chorea	–	5
Autosomal recessive disease		
• Albinism	–	28
• Total colour blindness	–	28
• Phenylketonuria	–	25
Sex linked recessive disease		
• Haemophilia	–	30

Because of improved medical and nursing care we are prolonging the life of many individuals, who otherwise would have died before reaching child bearing age. So 'bad' genes in population cannot be eliminated. The only solution which a demographer can give is that affected persons might be persuaded not to have children. Legislative sterilisation is not universally accepted but voluntary motivation of not to have children can be made acceptable.

FAMILY PLANNING

Importance

Reproductive and sexual health care including family planning is a key intervention for improving the health of women and children along with considering human right. Beijing platform for action has aptly said.

"Reproductive rights embrace certain human rights that are already recognised in national laws, international human rights documents and other relevant consensus documents. These rights rest on the recognition of the basic right of all couples and individuals to decide freely and responsibly the number and spacing and timing of their children and to have the information and means to do so, and the right to attain the highest standard of sexual and reproductive health."

The benefits of family planning can be tabulated as under (Table 6.3):

Terminology Used

Family Planning: Family planning refers to practice that help individuals or couples to attain certain objectives like:

a. To avoid unwanted births.
b. To bring about wanted births.
c. To regulate the interval between pregnancies.
d. To control the time at which births occur in relation to the ages of the parents.
e. To determine the number of children in the family.

Small Family norm: "A concept to stabilise the country with 2 children per family which help to achieve NRR 1 and made acceptable into the lifestyle of people."

Spacing: "Postponing succeeding pregnancy to maintain 3 to 4 years difference between 2 children."

Eligible Couple and Target Couple: The eligible couple rate is 150 per 1000 population in India. Eligible couple register is basic document in public health nursing. The priority group in target couple is eligible couple which can be differentiated by Table 6.4:

Unmet Need for FP: There is a gap between women's reproductive intension and their contraceptive behaviour. And it is a KAP gap (Knowledge attitude and practice). When married women prefer to avoid pregnancy but nevertheless not using method are attended on priority base. This unmet need is estimated to be 25 percent among eligible women.

Table 6.4: Difference between target couple and eligible couple

Target couple	*Eligible couple*
Age group of 15-45 years	Following are deducted from target couple • Primary sterility • Secondary sterility • Early menopause

Couple Protection Rate: It is an indicator of the prevalence of contraceptive practice in the community. It is the percentage of eligible couples effectively protected against childbirth by approved methods of family planning. By 60% of CPR we can achieve N.R.R. of 1.0.

Incentive and Disincentives in Family Planning:

These are measures to encourage couples to practice family planning as a strategy.

Table 6.5: Incentive and disincentive in family planning

Incentive	*Disincentive*
• Tubectomy 200.00	Improvident maternity
• Laparoscopy 145.00	No housing loan
• Vasectomy 180.00	No subsidised medical treatment
• Motivation of tubectomy 10.00	
• Motivation of vasectomy 40.00	
• One special increment	
• 14 days leave (women)	
• 7 days leave (men)	
• Green card to individual acceptances (for special attention)	

Table 6.3: Benefits of family planning

Women	*Children*	*Men*	*Families*	*Nation*
• Protect from unwanted pregnancies • Saved from unsafe abortions • Are health benefits	• Save life of children	• Better life in family	• Family well being	• National Development • Economic improvement

Scope

F.P. is not just birth control. It includes many more family welfare activities. Hence family planning is called Family Welfare Planning. They are:

- Spacing of pregnancy
- Advice and treatment of sterility
- Infertility treatment
- Education for planned parenthood
- Sex education
- Screening of cancer cervix
- Genetic counselling
- Preparation for pregnancy and delivery
- Marriage counselling
- Adoption services.

Health Aspect of F.P.

a. *Women Health:* By not allowing unwanted pregnancy, limiting the number of children to two, and timing of pregnancy for above 20 years to 35 years we can bring down maternal mortality and morbidity.

b. *Foetal Health:* Timing of pregnancy can avoid congenital anomalies. The quality of health of foetus is better if proper planning of the family is done.

c. *Infant and Child Health:* Family size and spacing of pregnancy has an impact on infant and child health. Growth and development is good with small family norm.

Organisation of F.P. Services

Health and family welfare are essential component and is primary responsibility of Government for its delivery to the community. There is an organised set up for the F.W. programme in India.

Family planning organisations in India is sideline of health services and it is accounted from central government to village. This is depicted in Figure 6.4.

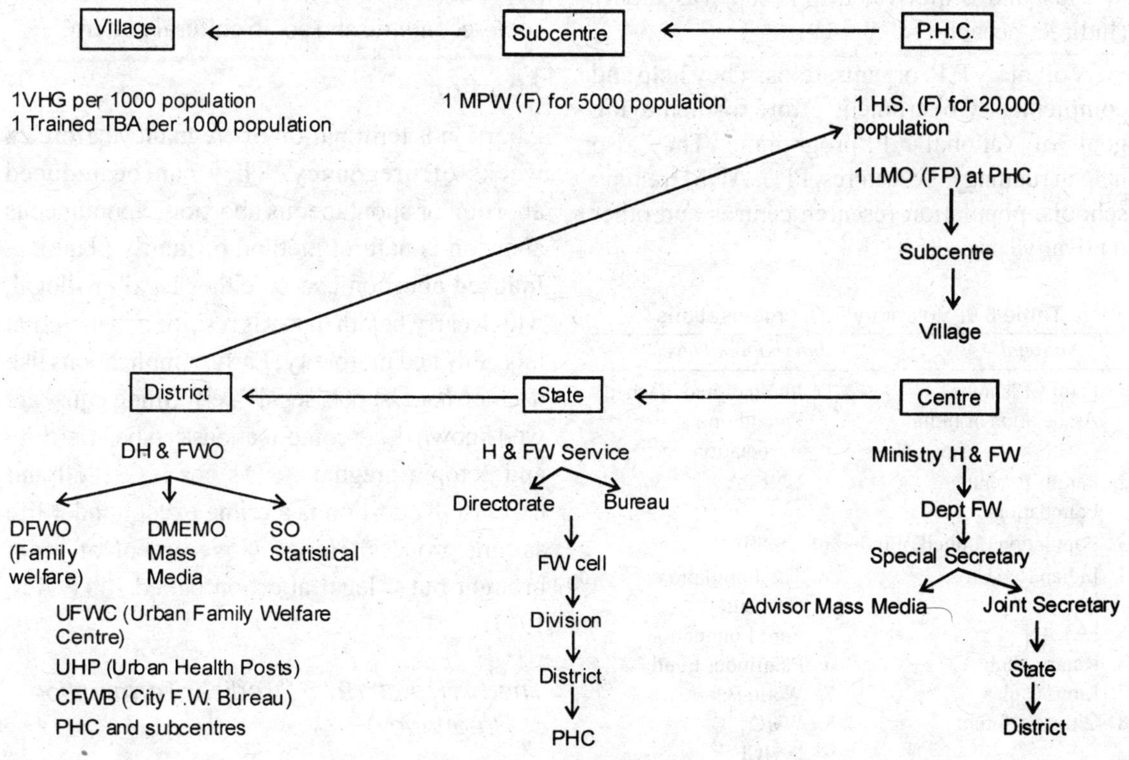

Fig 6.4: Organisation of family planning in India

Post Partum Programme (PPPC)

In the year 1969 All India hospital post partum programme was introduced. Since women who have recently delivered can be easily motivated and that they are available at hospital during lying - in period, PPC has gained impetus as hospital based maternity - centered family planning approach. PPC is in OBG department of a medical college or in OBG unit of a District hospital and coordinated by a programme officer. It helps in the following:

Women are motivated to accept F.P. before discharge (Direct acceptors – Immediate).

Woman is motivated to accept F.P. after discharge before 42 days after delivery (Direct acceptance – delayed).

Women are motivated to accept F.P. after 42 days after delivery (Indirect acceptor).

Husband is motivated to accept vasectomy (Indirect acceptor).

Voluntary F.P. organisations: They help and complement Government effort for achieving goals of National F.P. programme. They also help in running F.W. centres, PPC, ANM training schools, population research centres and other innovative projects.

Table 6.6: Voluntary F.P. organisations

National level	*International level*
1. Family Planning Association of India	1. International Planned Parenthood Association
2. Family Planning Foundation	2. UNFPA
3. Population Council of India	3. USAID
4. Indian Red Cross	4. The Population Council
5. I.M.A.	5. Ford Foundation
6. Rotary Club	6. Pathfinder Fund
7. Lions Club	7. World Bank
8. Citizen's forum	8. WHO
	9. UNICEF

Social Aspect of F.P.

Traditional beliefs like God gives children; A son is for sending parents to heavenly abode; children are wealth; children are future care takers; sterile women is not socially accepted etc., are having negative effect in contraceptive use by couples. Though awareness of F.P. is by over 60% of married couple, people are not generally favouring F.P. because of social aspect of F.P. associated with deep rooted religious beliefs, attitudes and practices.

Rapidly growing population is eroding the Government effort and finance towards providing basic necessities like food, shelter, clothing, education and medical care. It is having a negative impact on socio economic growth in the country. This aspect of socio-economic impact needs to be disciplined under changing socio-economic and socio cultural pattern.

Abortion

Abortion is termination of pregnancy before 28 weeks of pregnancy. They can be induced abortion or spontaneous abortion. Spontaneous abortion is natural method of family planning. Induced abortion can be either legal or illegal, which carry health hazards resulting in maternal mortality and morbidity. Early complications like haemorrhage, shock, sepsis, performing injury are well known. Late complications can be infertility and ectopic pregnancy. As per IPC 1860 and CCP 1898 abortion is a crime except under life saving process. Hence Government of India brought out a legal abortion called MTP Act, 1971.

The MTP Act 1971 (Medical Termination of Pregnancy)

This lays down the conditions, persons to perform and place to perform for MTP.

Indications:

Medical – When pregnancy cause injury or death to mother.

Eugenic – When abnormal growth is established.

Humanitarian – When rape has caused pregnancy.

Socioeconomic – When socioeconomic cause can lead to death or injury to mother.

Failure of contraceptive – Failed F.P. methods causing pregnancy.

Written consent of guardian when pregnant woman is lunatic or minor is a requirement.

Person to Perform MTP

By RMP if below 12 weeks, who has experience in OBG.

By 2 RMP opinion if above 12 weeks who have experience in OBG.

Place to Perform MTP

It must be in a hospital, health centre or any approved place.

Following Amendments are done in 1975 in MTP:

i. DH and FWO can certify a doctor to conduct MTP.
ii. An RMP who conducts 25 MTP in a hospital is permitted to conduct MTP.
iii. Experience in OBG means.
   - 6 months house surgeoncy in OBG.
   - PG in OBG.
   - RMP of before 1971 needs 3 year OBG practice.
   - RMP of after 1971 needs 1 year OBG practice.
iv. DH and FWO can certify place of conducting MTP.

Thus MTP is a safe, legal abortion made universally available for family planning in the country.

Family Planning

Fertility Awareness Based Methods (FABM)

Fertility awareness means that a women learns how to tell 'when the fertile time of her menstruation starts and ends'. This helps a woman to know when she could become pregnant. The couple avoids pregnancy by changing their sexual behaviour during fertile days.

i. *Abstain from vaginal intercourse:* Avoiding vaginal sex completely during fertile time. This is called periodic abstinence and natural F.P. method.
ii. *Use of withdrawal (coitus interruptus)*: The male withdraws before ejaculation and avoids semen deposit into vagina. There are other sexual contacts without vaginal intercourse as per studies conducted in sex behaviour in communities.

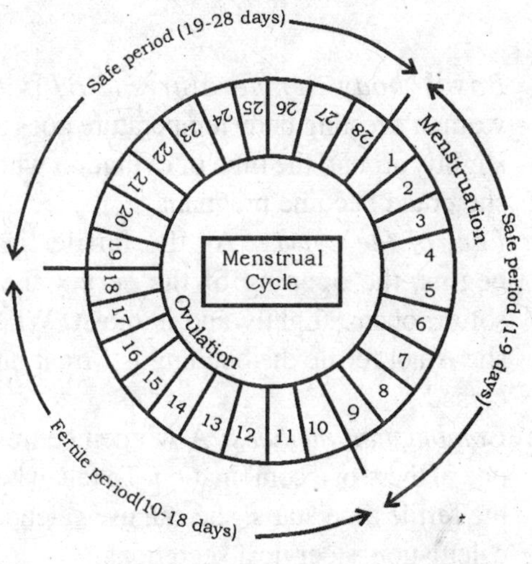

Fig. 6.5: Fertile period in menstrual cycle

iii. *Calendar calculation:* A women can count calendar days to identify the start and end of the fertile time. The number of days depends on the length of previous menses.

iv. *Cervical secretions:* When a woman sees or feels cervical secretions, she may be fertile. This is to be differentiated with just a sense of vaginal wetness.

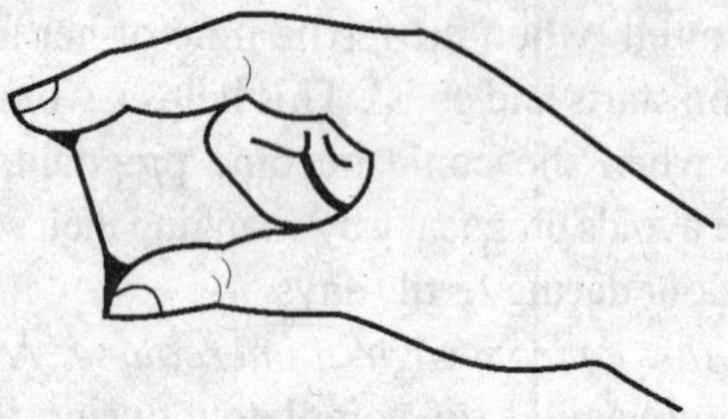

Fig. 6.6A: Cervical secretion +ve

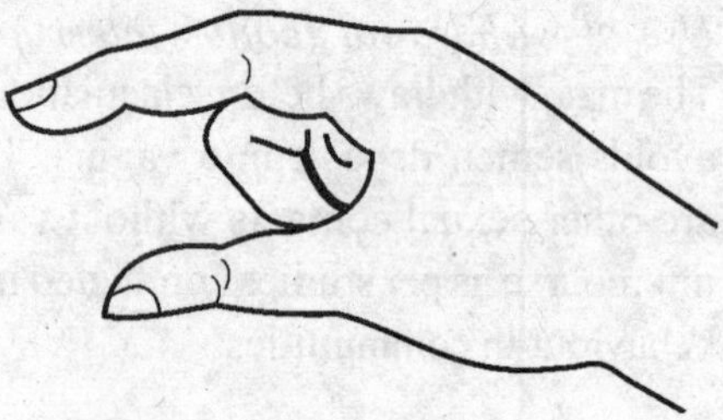

Fig. 6.6B: Cervical secretion –ve

v. *Basal body temperature (BBT):* A women's resting body temperature goes up slightly around the time of ovulation when she could become pregnant.

vi. *Feel of the cervix:* As the fertile time begins, the opening of the cervix feels softer, opens slightly and is moist. When she is not fertile the opening is firmer and closed.

vii. *Combination methods:* A women can use one of these or a combination. To tell, when the fertile time starts, she can use calendar calculation + cervical secretions.

When the fertile time ends, she can use BBT + Cervical secretion + Calendar calculation.

Lactational Amenorrhoea Method (LAM)

A women uses lactational amenorrhoea method (breast feeding) when:

- Her baby gets little or no other food or drink except breast milk, and she breast feeds often, both day and night.
- Her menstrual periods have not returned.
- Her baby is less than 6 months old.

LAM is effective for up to 6 months after childbirth.

LAM protects the milk supply by avoiding pregnancy.

The women should be planning to start another F.P. method.

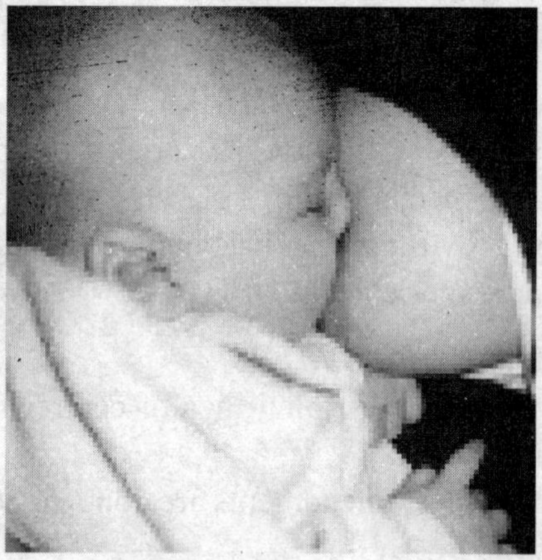

Photo: L.A.M. for F.P.

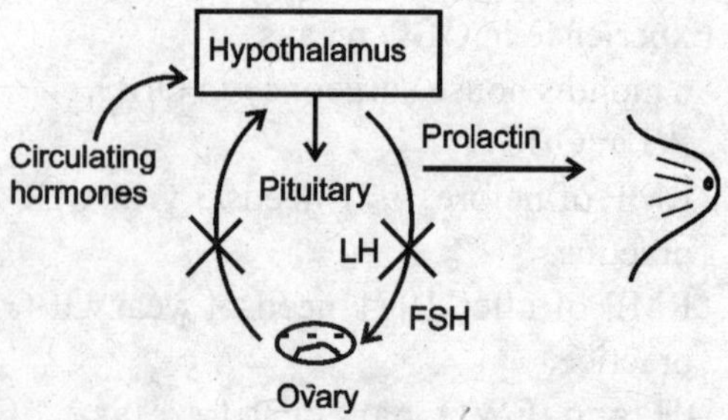

Fig. 6.7: Breastfeeding as F.P. method

During lactation, circulating hormones, particularly progesterone gives hypo-thalamus a signal that there is no need of L.H. (Leutinising Hormone) and F.S.H. (Follicle Stimulating Hormone) and thus ovulation is prevented. As long as continuous breast feeding is there, the cycle is expected, but not 100 % sure. Once menstruation occurs LAM cannot be considered as a contraceptive device.

Vaginal Methods

Vaginal methods are contraceptives that a woman places in her vagina shortly before sex. Common vaginal methods are:

Spermicides:
They include foaming tablets or suppositories, melting suppositories, foam, melting film, jelly and cream. The active ingredient is a surface acting agent which attaches to sperm and inhabit their oxygen intake.

Diaphragm:
It is a soft rubber cup that covers the cervix. It should be used with spermicidal jelly or cream. Checking proper placement of a diaphragm is very important (Fig. 6.10).

Cervical Cap:
It is similar to diaphragm but smaller, but not widely available in developing countries.

Vaginal Sponge:
It is available by trade mark 'Today', made of polyurethane foam sponge with nonoxynol-9 as spermicide. But failure rate is high with vaginal sponge.

Intra Uterine Device (IUD)

An I.U.D. usually small, flexible plastic frame. It has copper wire or copper sleeves on it. (Exception - Lippes Loop). It is inserted into women's uterus through her vagina.

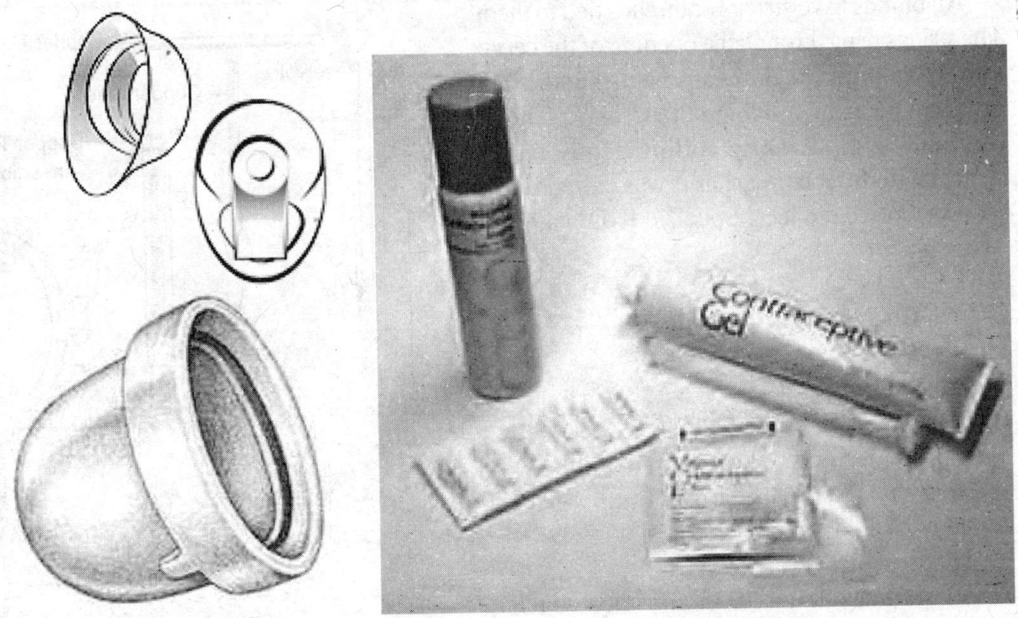

Cervical Caps

Spermicides

Fig. 6.8: Vaginal methods of F.P.

Checking Proper Placement of a New Diaphragm or Cervical Cap

An experienced user of diaphragm or cap or else a specifically trained provider must show a new user how to place the device within the vagina. She should allow the woman to practice privately, and then she should check placement.

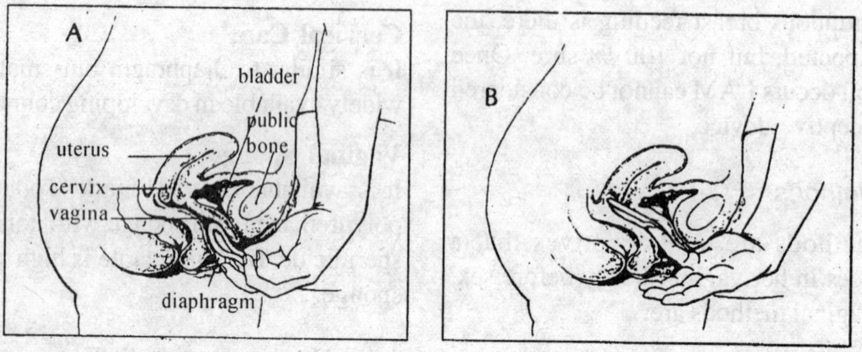

To insert a diaphragm, a woman squeezes its sides together and pushes it into her vagina as far as it will go (A). Then with her finger she checks that the diaphragm fits snugly behind the pubic bone and covers the cervix (B).

Fig. 6.9: Checking proper placement of diaphragm or cervical cap

All brands have strings or threads tied to them. The strings hang through the opening of the cervix into the vagina. The user can check that the IUD is still in place by touching the strings. A nurse can remove the IUD by pulling gently on the strings with forceps. Earlier it was called IUCD (contraceptive device). Specific IUD's are:

Copper T
T Cu - 380 A
M L Cu 375 (multiload)
Nova T
Progestasert
LNG - 20

Lippes loop is no longer used in India.

Most commonly used I.U.D.'s are T Cu 380 A and MLcu - 375.

Types of IUD are:

i. First generation IUD (nonmedicated IUD).
ii. Second generation IUD (copper containing).
iii. Third generation IUD (Hormone releasing).

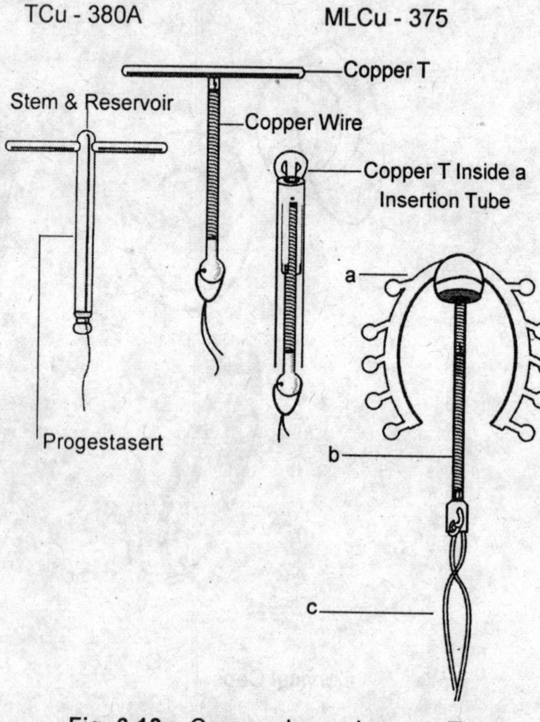

Fig. 6.10 : Commonly used copper T and multiload MLcu – 375

There are many advantages of copper T. They are:

a. Low expulsion rate
b. Low side effects
c. Easy to insert
d. Better tolerated
e. High protection rate and
f. Useful as post coital contraceptive.

Mechanism of Action:
It brings out cellular and biomedical changes in the endometrium and uterine fluids which impair the viability of gamete.

Table 6.7: Effectiveness of IUD

	Pregnancy rate	*Expulsion rate*
Copper T	0.9 per 100 women after 12 months of IUD use.	8.0 per 100 women after 12 months of IUD use.
Multiload 375	0.1 women after 12 months of IUD use.	2.1 women after 12 months of IUD use.

Contraindications:

1. Acute pelvic infection
2. Chronic pelvic infection
3. Menorrhoegia

Before putting IUD, one has to exclude the following:

Pregnancy
Anaemia due to iron deficiency
Anaemia due to hook worm
Large fibroid

Side effects of IUD and their management:

Table 6.8: Management of IUD side effects

Side Effects	*Management*
Increase in menstruation	Watch for anaemia
Uterine cramp	Exclude other causes
Extrusion	Check threads frequently
Pregnancy	Always remove IUD
Anxiety	Support and reassure

Most ideal time for IUD insertion is during menstruation or within 10 days of the beginning of a menstrual period. Post puerperal insertion has several advantages. Follow up of IUD cases are required and nursing staff should encourage this.

Condom

A condom is a sheath or covering made fit over man's penis. They are known by many trade names. Most condoms are made of thin latex rubber. Some are coated with a dry lubricant or with spermicide. Different size, shapes, colour and texture are made available in some places.

Nirodh is available in 3 brands:

a. Dry *nirodh.*
b. Delux *nirodh* (lubricated).
c. Super delux *nirodh* (thin and lubricated).

Its use has shown pregnancy rate 2-3 per 100 women year. It is a common barrier method of contraceptive used in F.P. programme.

Sterilisation

Tubectomy:
Female sterilisation provides permanent contraception for women who will not want more children. It is a safe and simple surgical procedure. It can usually be done with just local anaesthesia and light sedation. Proper infection prevention procedures are required. The common approaches are mini-laparotomy and laparoscopy. They are also called V.S.C. (Voluntary Surgical Contraception), T.L. (Tubal Ligation), Minilap, etc.

Laparoscopy:
Sterilisation is done by using laparoscope. Abdomen is inflated with nitrous oxide tubes. When tubes are accessible, clips are put and tubes are occluded. It has to be done only in 2nd month after delivery. Post operative observation is for 48 hours. Multi purpose worker (Female)

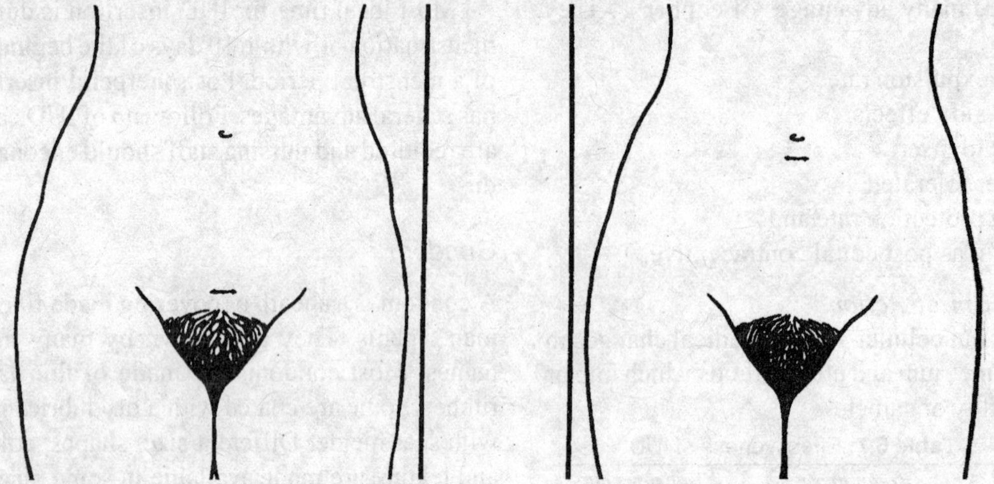

Minilaparotomy for female sterilization invovles a small incision just above the pubic hair.

Laparoscopy for female sterilization usually involves 1 small incision just below the naval.

Fig. 6.11: (A) Minilaparotomy incision (B) Laparoscopy incision

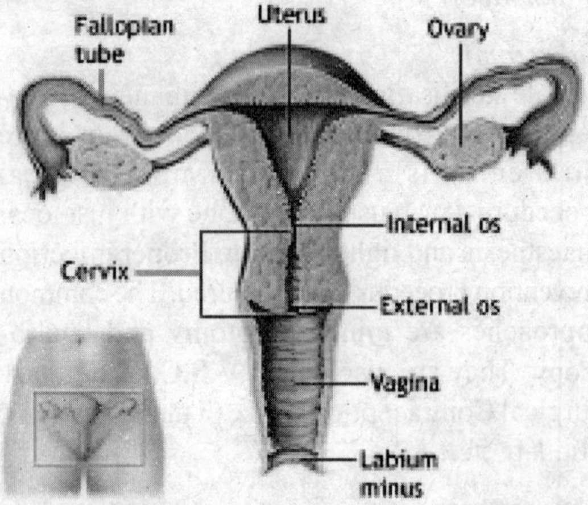

Fig. 6.12: Diagrammatically shown tubes blocked

and health supervisor will pay home visiting on 10th day and 12th month after operation. Least complications are recorded in the hospital practice.

Minilap Operation:

With a small incision under local anaesthesia, tube is identified, ligated and sterilised. This is also called as Pomeroy technique. Because of safety, efficiency and ease, it is used in tubectomy camps. It is suitable for post partum tubal sterilisation.

Vasectomy:

Vasectomy provides permanent contraception for men who decide they will not want more children. It is safe, simple, quick surgical procedure. It can be done in a clinic, a camp with proper infection prevention procedures. Guidance and counselling at nursing care require telling that it is not castration and it does not affect testicles or it does not affect sexual ability.

New, No-scalpel Vasectomy

The differences noticed from convent-ional procedure are:

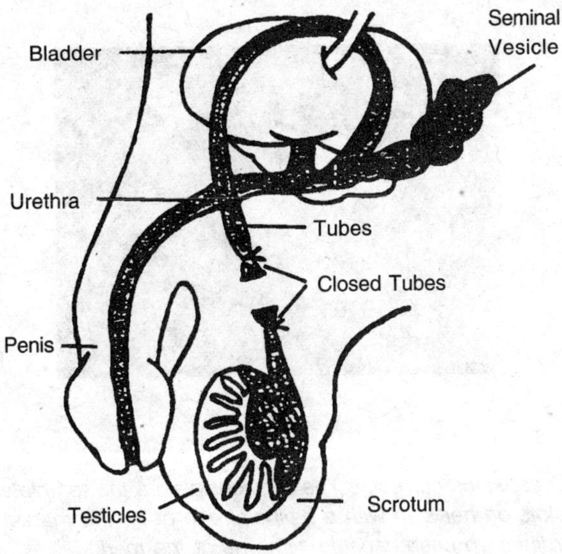

Fig. 6.13: Closed tubes in vasectomy

a. Use of a small puncture (instead of 2" incision) in the scrotum.
b. Special anaesthesia technique needs only 1 needle puncture instead of 2 or more.

Advantages are:

a. Less pain
b. Less bruising
c. Short recovery time
d. Less operating time.

Main advice given after vasectomy is that usually until 30 ejaculations, the persons will have the chance of impregnating his partner. Vasectomy does not alter sperm production or hormone output. It is simpler, faster and less expensive sterilisation method.

Side effects noticed after vasectomy are:

a. Sperm granules.
b. Spontaneous recanalisation.
c. Rise in circulating antibodies against ones own sperm as an autoimmune response is seen.
d. Anxiety and psychological depression.

Implants

They are sub dermal implants for long term contraception. Commonly used Norplant is a set of 6 small plastic capsules.

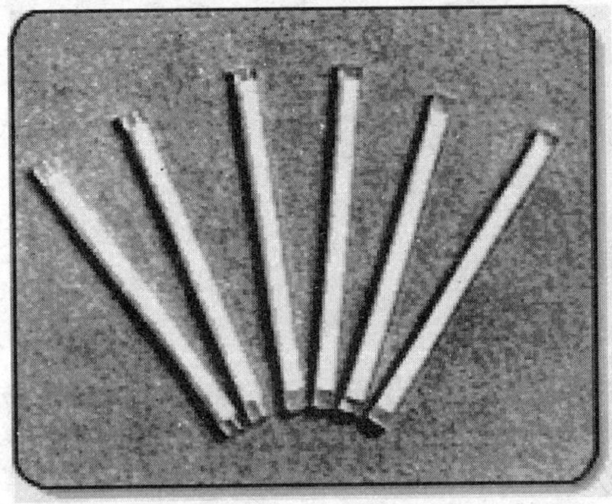

Fig. 6.14: Norplant

Each is about the size of a small matchstick. The capsules are placed under the skin of a women's upper arm. They contain progestin similar to a natural hormone that woman's body makes. It is released slowly from all 6 capsules. Thus the capsules supply a steady, very low dose. It does not contain oestrogen (Figs. 6.15 and 6.16).

It provides 5 years of contraception, and is reversible with removal.

Injectable Hormones

Women who use this method receive injections to prevent pregnancy. Common preparations are:

DMPA (Depot Medroxy Progesterone acetate).

NET – EN (Norethisterone enantate).

Common type of injectable is RMPA given every three months. It contains progesterone similar to the natural hormone that a woman's body makes. The hormone is released slowly into

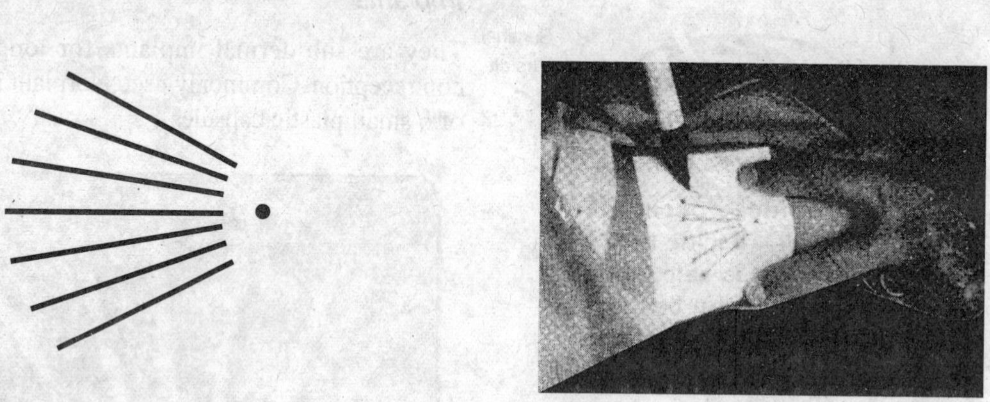

The template (left) can help providers position Norplant capsules correctly. The provider places the template against a woman's arm and marks the ends of the 6 slots on her skin with a ballpoint pen or similar marker (see photo). When inserting the capsules, the provider lines up each capsule with one of the marks.

Fig. 6.15: Marking the slots on the skin

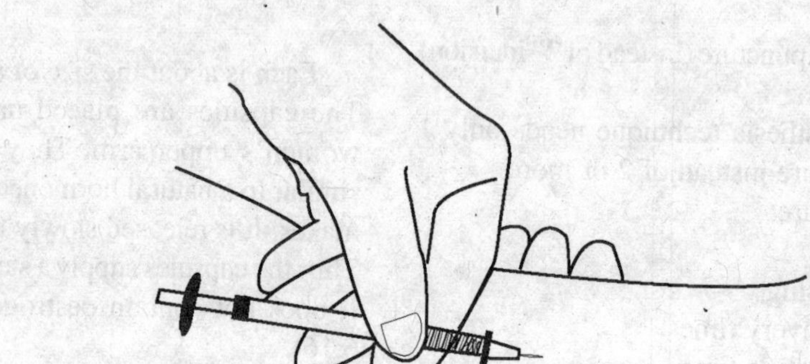

Using proper infection-prevention procedures, the provider inserts each Norplant *capsule just under the skin of a woman's upper arm.*

Fig. 6.16: Inserting norplant

the blood stream. (Trade names: Depot Provera, Depot Megestron) NET–EN is given every 2 months.

(a)

(b)

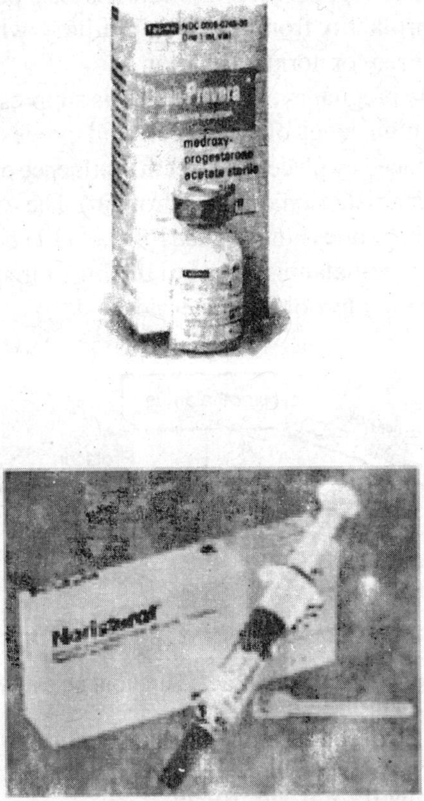

Fig. 6.17: Injectable material

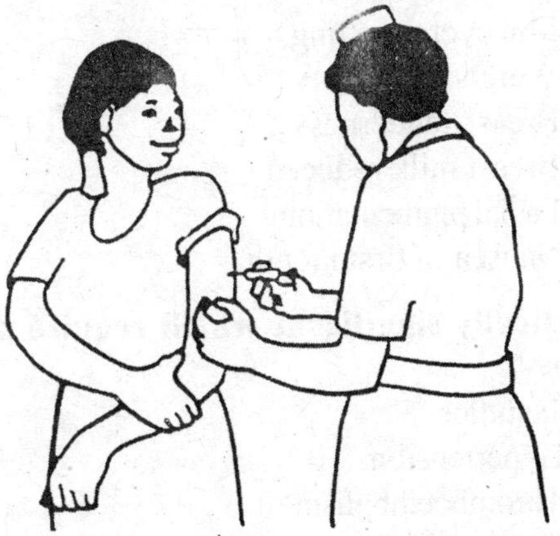

Fig. 6.18: Administration

Mode of Action: The suppression of ovulation through feedback mechanism.

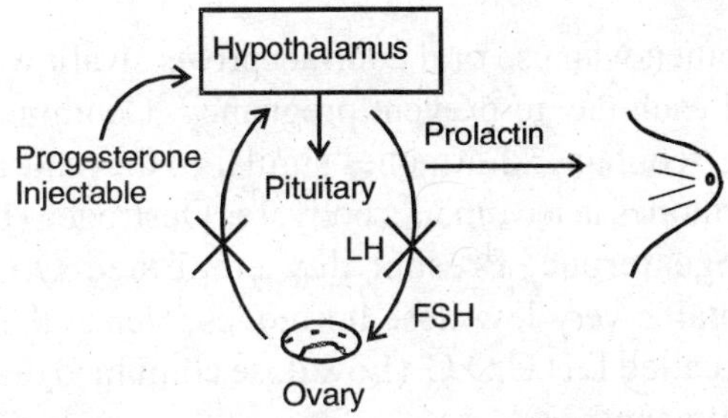

Fig. 6.19: Altered hormonal cycle by injectables

Injectables do not affect breast milk

Contraindications:

- Hypertension
- Diabetes
- Large fibroid.

Side Effects:

- Irregular bleeding
- Amenorrhoea
- Delayed return of ovulation
- Hypertension
- Changes in carbohydrate metabolism.

Injectables are given during first 5 days of menstrual cycle deep IM to gluteus maximus. Post injection massage is disallowed.

Oral Contraceptives

They are effective contraceptives when properly used, which have nearing to 100% effectiveness. Oestrogen and progesterone by gonads are called physiological steroids. Synthetic oestrogens are ethinyl oestradiol and mestraol. Synthetic progesterones are norethisterone lynestrenol and levonor-gestrel. They are grouped under 5 heads:

1. Combined (oestrogen progesterone pill).
2. Progesterone only pill (POP).
3. Post coital pill.

4. Long acting pill.
5. Male pill.

Combined Pill

Women who use oral contraceptives swallow a pill each day to prevent pregnancy. Combined O.C. contains 2 hormones similar to the natural hormones in a woman's body. (a) Oestrogen (b) Progesterone. Present day combined O.C. contains very low dose hormones. Hence they are called L.D.C.O.C. (Low dose combined oral contraceptives).

There are 2 types of pill pockets. Some contain 28. These contain 21 active pills which contain hormones, followed by 7 reminder pills of a different colour that do not contain hormones. Other type contains only 21 active pills.

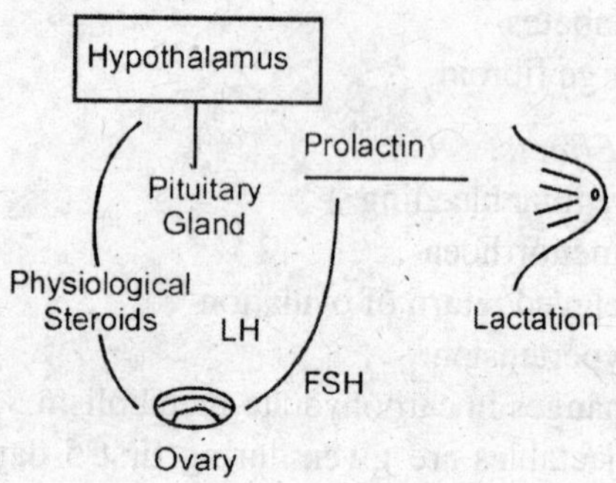

Fig. 6.20: Cyclical interaction by hypothalamus, pituitary and ovary, in normal menses

The hypothalamus controls ovarian activity. It senses the amount of circulating oestrogen and progesterone and when the level drops, Gonadotrophin releasing factors are produced, which enable the anterior pituitary to produce the gonadotrophins FSH (Follicle stimulating Hormone) and LH (Luteinising Hormone). The FSH stimulates development of ovarian follicle and the LH is concerned with the rupture of the follicle at the time of ovulation. Oestrogen is produced while the follicle is developing and it is at its peak at the time of ovulation and progesterone is produced from the corpus Luteum after ovulation.

The hypothalamus also controls the production of prolactin from anterior pituitary which is required for normal lactation.

In pregnancy, menstruation is suppressed by the high level of oestrogen and progesterone produced by placenta under the influence of HCG (Human Chorionic Gonadotrophin). The Anterior pituitary does not produce FSH and LH because the hypothalamus reacts to the high circulating levels of physiological steroids.

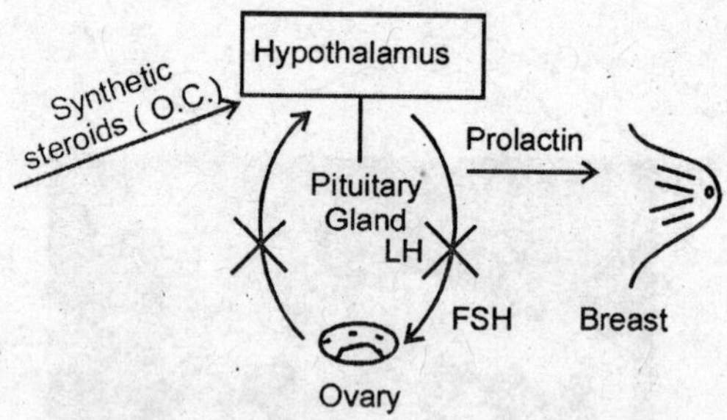

Fig. 6.21: How O.C. act in preventing ovulation

Reaction and Effects of Combined Pill:

Medically not significant:

- Decreased menstrual loss
- Amenorrhoea
- Mid cycle spotting
- Weight change
- Breast tenderness
- Breast milk reduced
- Facial pigmentation
- Nausea in first month.

Medically significant which require attention:

- Jaundice
- Hypertension
- Thromboembolism
- Glycosuria
- Severe headache

- Chronic cervical erosion
- Monilial vaginitis
- Fibroid enlargement.

Contraindications for Combined Pill:

Table 6.9: Complication of combined pill

Absolute contraindication	*Careful supervision*
Acute liver disease	Renal or cardiac disease
History of	
Thromboembolism	Diabetes
Cancer breast	Hypertension
Lactation	Sickle cell anaemia
Prediabetes	Major surgery

Government of India has commercialised 2 types of combined oral contraceptives. They are:

1. Mala N (Free supply through health and nursing care)
   Norgestrol 0.3 mg
   Ethinil oestradiol 0.03 mg
2. Mala D (21 active 7 brown piacebo) (Under social marketing at low cost)
   Norgestrol 0.3 mg
   Ethinil oestradiol 0.03 mg

Progestogen Only Pill (POP)

Women who use progestogen only pill, swallow a pill every day to prevent pregnancy. Progestogen – only pill contain very small

- ***Missed 1 pill?*** Take 1 now. Take the rest as usual.
- ***Missed 2 or more in a row? Which ones***? (See below)

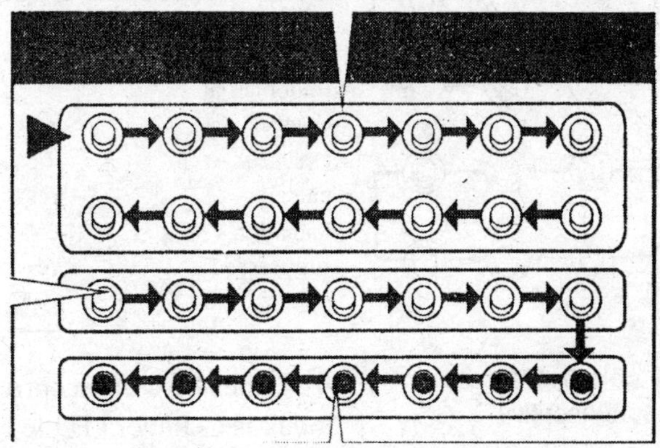

Fig. 6.22: Action for missed pills

amounts of only progestin (1/10th of dose of combined pill). They are best for breastfeeding women. They do not reduce milk production.

Contraindications:

There are no contraindications to POP:

Side effect of POP:

Irregular bleeding at first
Amenorrhoea later
Increased pregnancy risk

It is suitable for women who are:

Lactating
Sub fertile
Spacing of children

POP to be taken everyday. It is best to take at the same time each day. Taking pill more than a few hours late increase the risk of pregnancy and missing 2 or more greatly increases the risk.

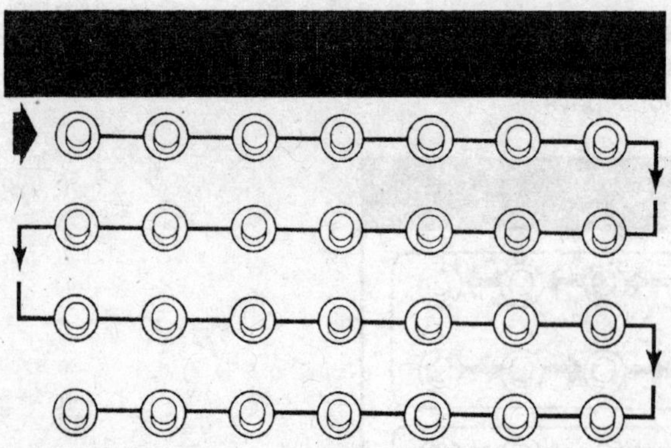

28 or 35 pills of the same colour: These are progestin-only oral contraceptive

Fig. 6.23: POP pill

After 1 pack, one should take first pill from next pack on the very next day. All pills are active, hormonal and there is no wait between packs.

Post Coital Contraceptive

They are recommended within 48 hours of unprotected intercourse.

a. IUD Copper-T is inserted if acceptable.
b. Double the dose of standard combined pill. i.e., 2 o.c. immediately followed by another 2 pill 12 hours later.
c. As emergency contraception 4 tablets of pills containing 30 mg oestrogen, at one time itself.

Long Acting Once a Month Pill

Quinestrol + progestogen are advocated but are associated with high failure rate.

Male Pill

A derivative of cotton seed oil "gossypol" for 6 months orally has produced azoospermic in men. It is not in routine clinical use.

Comparative merits of 3 common hormonal contraceptives:

Table 6.10: Merits of hormonal contraceptives

Effects	*Combined pill*	*POP pill*	*Injectable*
Ovulation suppressed	Yes	No	Yes
Endometrial changes	Yes	Yes	Yes
Cervical mucous	Yes	Yes	Yes
Lactation suppressed	Yes	No	No
Pregnancy	0.5%	2-10%	1.0%

Order of contraceptive effectiveness as on today is as under (Table 6.11):

Vaccines for Birth Control

Only known vaccine known by clinical trail is "hcG vaccine", i.e. beta sub unit of human chorionic gonadotrophin, which blocks continuation of implanted ovum. Booster dose at 12th

Table 6.11: Order of OC effectiveness

Order	*Method*
1.	Sterilisation
2.	Combined pill
3.	Injectable hormone
4.	I.U.D.
5.	P.O.P.
6.	Sheath or diaphragm
7.	Spermicide or withdrawal

month is recommended. Birth control vaccine is only an academic interest and not in clinical practice.

National Family Planning Programme (NFPP)

In 1952 India launched FP programme. The approach is "Extension education approach" for motivating people to accept small family norm. Since 1965 to 1970 IUD (Lippes loop) made the score in F.P. programme. Later Copper-T has been used under National F.P. programme. In 1966 Ministry of health got bifurcated to health and F.P. wings. The infrastructure of F.P. was strengthened. In every 5 years plan, top priority is being given to F.P.

PPC in 1970 and MTP in 1971 were added as additional forces in Family Planning. National population policy gave vivid picture for action in 1976.

In 1977 F.P. was renamed as FWP since it involved family welfare activities.

Primary health care approach, HFA approach, long term demographic goal of NRR 1 by 2007 which imply 2 child family norm, goal of BR 21, goal of DR 9 and CPR of 60% are strategic phenomena under NFPP in India.

Seventh five year plan incorporated UIP, ORT (under CSSM) under F.W. planning.

Since 1997 we have unified R.C.H. integrated with Eighth five year plan for need based, client oriented service.

In the year 2000, Government of India reinforced the comprehensive National Population Policy.

Financial allocation to FWP is better reviewed by following table:

Table 6.12: Financial allocation to family welfare programme

Year	*Expenditure*
First 5 year plan	0.65 crore
Fifth 5 year plan	285.6 crore
Tenth 5 year plan	58920.3 crore

National F.P. programme is evaluated from time to time through evaluation of:

- Need
- Plan
- Performance
- Effects
- Impact.

FURTHER REFERENCES

1. Census of India 2001–Provisional data, Government of India.
2. Population reports – The John Hopkins University, Baltimore.
3. National Population Policy, 2000, G.O.I., New Delhi.
4. All India Hospitals (PPC) F.P. programme – G.O.I.
5. Alan Emery – Elements of Medical Genetics (Churchill Livingstone).
6. WHO – Improving access to quality care in F.P.
7. WHO – Population Information programme. John Hopkins Baltimore. (The Essentials of Contraceptive Technology).
8. Prabhakara G.N. "Policies and Programmes of Health in India 2004 (Jaypee).
9. Government of India, DGHS, Health Information 2003, New Delhi.

7

Concept of Health, Disease and Prevention

World Health assembly has the main target of governments for "the attainment of all citizens of the world of a level of health that will permit them to lead a socially and economically productive life."

Health is a necessity for overall socio-economic development of a nation.

HEALTH

Health implies a sufficient reserve of strength of physical action, strength of agility and strength of endurance and mental poise to meet the demands of daily life. It is characterised by: (a) Sense of well being, (b) Ability to work efficiently and with enthusiasm, (c) Cheerfulness, (d) Self confidence, (e) Self control, (f) Absence of illness, (g) Conduct better in the society, (h) Good mental attitude, (i) Absence of anxiety, (j) Day's fatigue disappear with undisturbed sleep. The ancient Indians used to attribute health to absence of illness and well balanced body and mind.

Health, now, is considered as a fundamental right of man, which is to be attained by improved quality of life.

Changing Concepts of Health

i. *Biomedical Theory:* It is based on germ theory of disease but has overlooked other aspects.
ii. *Ecological Theory:* According to this, illness is caused by maladjustment of environment.
iii. *Psychosocial Theory*: It relates the illness to psychosocial aspect of disease occurrence in man.
iv. *Holistic Theory:* This theory compromises by consolidating Biomedical, Ecological and psychosocial theories encompassing all sectors to illness causation.

WHO Definition of Health

"Health is a state of complete physical, mental and social well being and not merely an absence of disease or infirmity."

This also emphasized the quality of human organism expressing the adequate functioning of the organism in given conditions, genetic and environmental.

Beyond 2000 has added one more aspect to extend the definition of health viz.;

"To lead a socially and economically productive life."

'Health' now, has new philosophy which include (a) Human right (b) Productive life (c) Intersectoral (d) Integral part of development (e) Quality of life (f) Involve responsibility (g) Social investment; and (h) Wide social goal.

Health Dimensions

i. *Physical:* At individual level it covers complexion, good flesh, normal skin, good appetite and coordinated movements. At community level crude death rates and life expectancy are used to measure physical dimensions.
ii. *Mental:* No internal conflicts, well adjusted, has self esteem, has self control.
iii. *Social:* Harmony in life and good social interaction.
iv. *Spiritual:* Meaningful and purposive life, integrity, principles.
v. *Emotion:* Feelings.
vi. *Vocational:* Physical work for satisfaction
vii. *Others:* Philosophy, culture, socio-economic, nutrition, educational dimensions.

Positive Health

Maintaining perfect functioning of the body by improving the quality of life is suggestive of positive health. Each country, each nation, each state, each family and each individual set their own standard for defining health. This varying concept has given a new idea of relative concept of health.

Concept of Well Being

This concept is given with the background of quality of life which denotes the level of living.

U.N. document has used the term level of living, which includes health, food, education, occupation, working condition, housing, social security, clothing, recreation, leisure and human rights. Corresponding to this WHO has given new term "Standard of living" by defining it as "Income, occupation, standard of housing, sanitation and nutrition, the level of provision of health, educational, recreational and other services may all be used individually as measure of socio-economic status and collectively as standard of living index."

According to WHO quality of life is defined as "the condition of life resulting from the combination of the effects of the complete range of factors such as those determining health, happiness (including comfort in the physical environmental and a satisfying occupation), education, social and intellectual attainments, freedom of action, justice and freedom of expressions."

Index of Quality of Life

i. PQLI (physical quality of life index): It considers IMR, life expectancy and literacy which varies from 0 to 100.
ii. HDI (Human Development Index): It considers life expectation, literacy and income, which varies from 0 to 1.

Current HDI estimate for India is 0.6 based on current life expectancy.

Health Spectrum

At a given point of time we come across all categories of people in varying state of health. It can be represented as under:

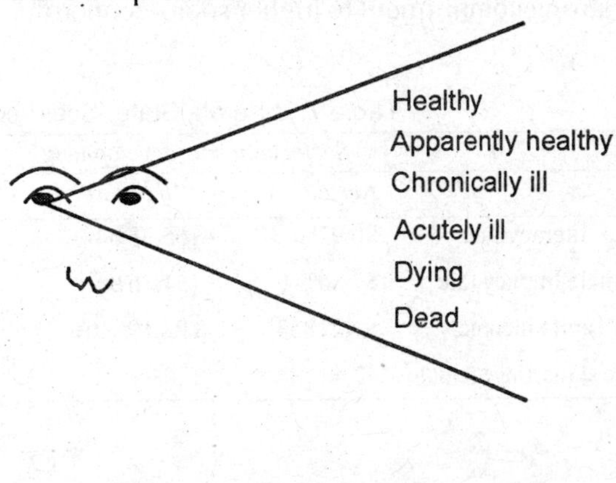

Determinants of Health

i. Human trait which is genetically determined.
ii. Lifestyle which is socioculturally determined.
iii. Surrounding which is man's environment.
iv. Income, education and occupation, which is socio-economic condition.
v. Availability and accessibility of health services.
vi. Demographic character of population like very young, very old etc.

Ecology of Health

Ecology is a science of mutual relation-ship between living being and its surroundings, Ecosystem is being altered by urbanization, industrialization, deforestation, dams etc. Resurgence of diseases and occurrence of new problems are examples of change in ecosystem.

Health and Development

As a right to protection of health, responsibility of health has come to one and all for a fruitful development. Health responsibility lies on the following:

- On each individual.
- On every community.
- On every state and it is global.

Socio-economic development of a nation determines the health status of the community. A strong commitment to higher socio-economic development has yielded a real positive development in health status in case of Kerala State. It can be represented under following indicators (Table 7.1):

Health development can be measured by developing health indicators, which may be grouped as under:

i. *Mortality:* Crude Death, Life expectation IMR, MMR etc.
ii. *Morbidity:* Incidence, Prevalence, hospital stay etc.
iii. *Disability*: Expectation of life free of disability (Sullivan's index). Health adjusted life expectancy (HALE), disability adjusted life year (DALY) etc.
iv. *Nutrition:* LBW, weight, height etc.
v. *Health care delivery:* Doctor Nurse Ratio.
vi. *Utilisation:* Fully immunised children.
vii. *Psychosocial:* Suicide, homicide
viii. *Environment:* Protected water supply, Air pollution.
ix. *Socioeconomic:* Per capita income.
x. *Health policy:* Amount spent on water supply.
xi. *Quality life:* HDI, PQLI.
xii. *Miscellaneous:* Social security, welfare schemes.

Health Status in Developing Countries

With the comparison of developed countries, health status of developing country like India needs stabilization and further development. table 7.2 gives a comparative picture:

Table 7.1: Kerala State: Socio-economic and health development

	Socioeconomic development			*Health Development*	
	Kerala	*(All India)*		*Kerala*	*(All India)*
Gen. literacy rate	90.92%	(65.38%)	IMR	12.0	(58.0)
Female literacy rate	87.86%	(54.16%)	CDR	6.1	(7.5)
Per capita income	Rs.21853	(Rs.19040)	G.R.	0.9	(1.93)
Age at marriage female	22.4	(20.1)	Life Expect	66.5	(61.5)

Table 7.2: Health profile comparison between India and U.K.

Health Profile	*India*	*U.K.*
Disease pattern	Infections	Cancer and Metabolic
Socioeconomic Character	Rural	Urban
	Joint family	Single
	Agriculture	Industry
	Per capita income	
	Low	High
	Literacy rate	
	Low	High
	Standard of living	
	Low	High
	Medical care	
	Low	High
Demographic Character	More young population	Older Population
	More paediatric problem	Geriatric
	High birth rate	Low birth rate
	High death rate	Low death rate
	High growth rate	Low growth rate
	High IMR	Low IMR

Recent Area of Interest in Health

Health care, Nursing care are services rendered to individual, families and community by health professionals.

Health System relates to management sectors involving service givers.

Levels of Health Care are:

Primary – Care at first contact.

Secondary – District hospitals, Community health centres

Tertiary – Super specialty care.

Health Team: Each member in a professional group has specific and recognised function in the team. It is a group of persons who share a common goal and common objectives which are determined by the needs of the community.

Health for All: It is an attainment of a level of health that will permit them to lead to a socially and economically productive life.

Primary Health Care: It is "Essential health care based on practical, scientifically sound and socially acceptable methods and technology made universally accessible to individuals and families in the community through their full participation and at a cost that the community and the country can afford to maintain at every stage of their development in the spirit of self determination."

DISEASE

It is condition of body, organ or tissue in which functions are disrupted or deranged.

Causation of Disease

i. *Germ Theory:* Body dysfunction by pathogens.
ii. *Epidemiological Triad*: Apart from pathogen, host character and environment also are considered. It can be represented as a triangle.

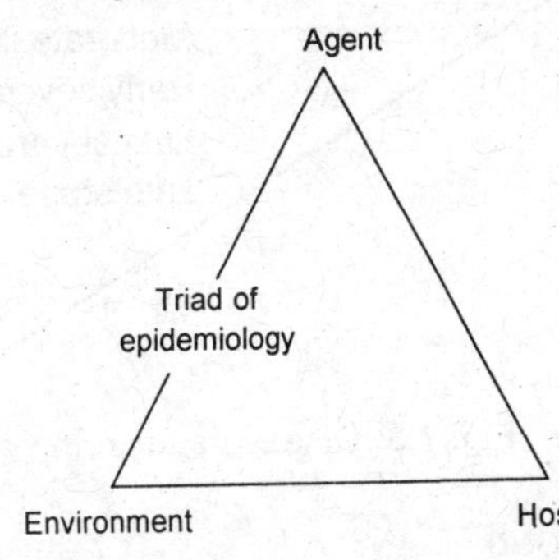

Fig. 7.1: Epidemiological triad

iii. *Multifactorial:* It was described by Pettenkofer whose idea gave rise to multiple aetiology like social, economical, cultural, genetic, psychological and biological.

Recent Area of Interest

Iceberg of Disease

Like an iceberg, presymptomatic and what health professional cannot see is exceedingly high. This phenomenon is called Iceberg of disease.

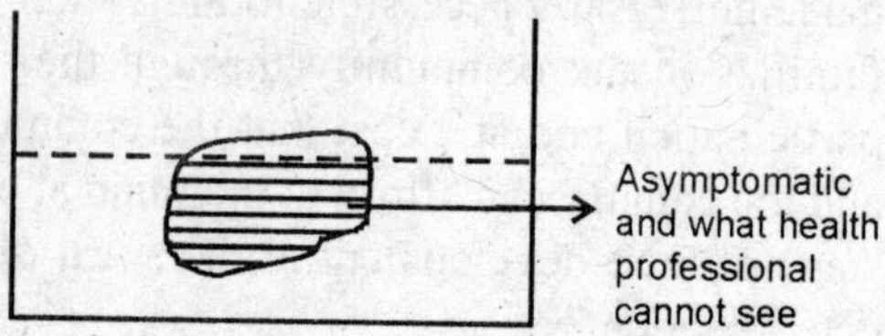

Fig. 7.2: Iceberg of disease

Disease Spectrum

Similar to light spectrum the disease gives the picture of disease at a given point of time in the community.

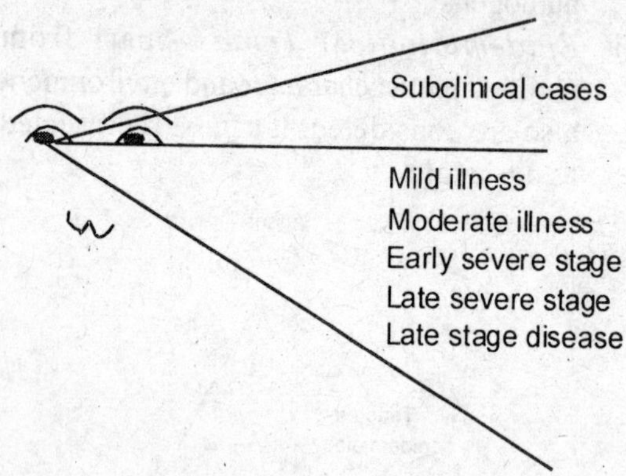

Fig. 7.3: Disease spectrum

Risk Group

There are some biological, physical and sociocultural situations that defines risk group. They become target group for risk approach. E.g.; risk mothers, at risk infants etc.

Risk Factors

For many non communicable diseases, where agent is not specific, the aetiology is discussed under risk factors. For example:

Table 7.3: Example of risk factors

Cancer	– Smoking, irradiation, alcohol
Diabetes	– Obesity
Traffic accident	– Seat belt, helmet, alcohol
Atherosclerosis	– Elevated serum cholesterol

Natural History of Disease (NHD)

Each disease has its own unique natural history, in the absence of intervention. Knowledge of NHD of a disease is helpful in intervention therapy. The events of NHD can be outlined as under (Fig. 7.4):

In pre disease state interaction among agent, host and environment occurs which bring agent and host together to produce disease. This provokes a stimulus to bring about changes in human body.

In disease state we notice tissue changes and physiological changes and agent gets established and multiples. Depending on host reaction and body immunity, illness advances or recovery occurs. If disease advances it manifests as disability, defect and chronic state. Later Fatal stage may culminate in death.

Primary prevention in prepathogenic period, Secondary and Tertiary prevention in pathogenic period is marked in Fig. 7.4.

CONTROL

Control is operational procedures aimed at reducing the incidence of disease. When a stage

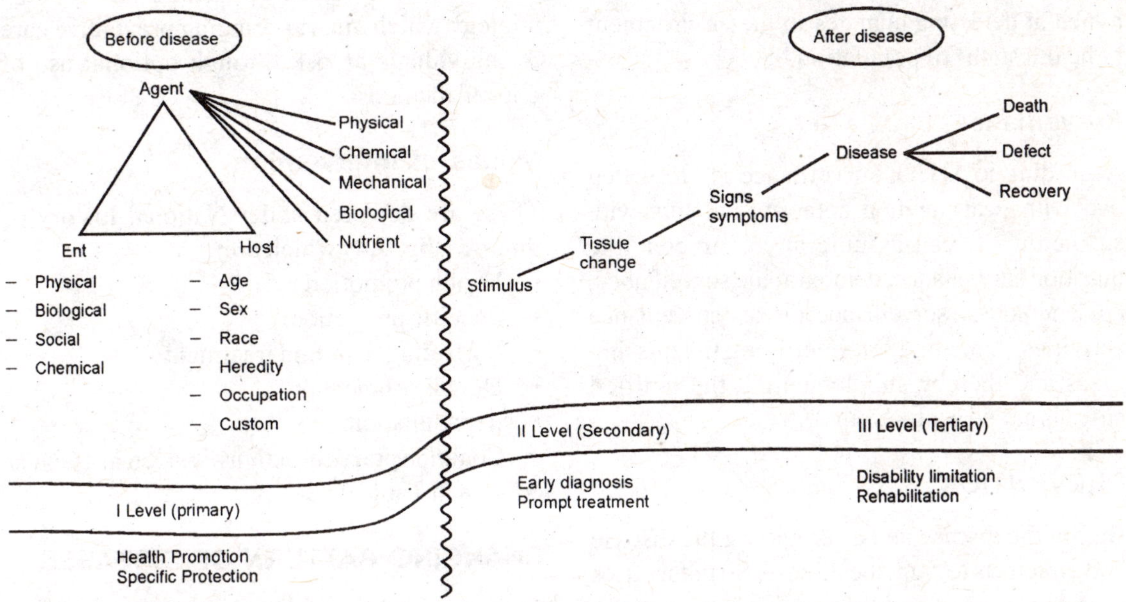

Fig. 7.4: N.H.D.

Table 7.4 : Difference between control and eradication

	Control	*Eradication*
Definition	To reduce incidence to acceptance level e.g.; cholera control	Total extirpation of disease agent e.g.; Polio eradication
Objective	To reduce mortality and morbidity (no more a public Health problem)	To uproot the disease
Area of operation	In high incidence area	Total coverage
Duration of operation	Indefinite	Time limited
Economic aspect	Recurring	Cheap
Case finding Confirmation Epidemiological Investigation	Not important	Very important

of control has come, the disease can be eliminated by eradication. The difference between control and eradication is tabulated as Table 7.4:

Monitoring

According to Last, monitoring is "the performance and analysis of routine measurement aimed at detecting changes in the environment or health status of population".

Surveillance

According to WHO, surveillance is "to watch over with great attention, authority and often with suspicion". It can assume any character like nutrition surveillance, demographic surveillance, epidemiological surveillance, disease surveillance activities. A method for identifying the missing cases and thereby supplementing the notified cases is called sentinel surveillance.

PREVENTION

Before the disease and after getting the disease body interacts to fight the disease. So nature tries to preserve and restore the health when impaired. With advance in science and technology man wants to utilize the knowledge of advancement in preventive and curative medicine to promote health. These formulations are seen with the process of prevention.

Levels of prevention are:

- Primordial
  Prevention of development of disease by not changing to harmful life style.
- Primary
  Action taken before disease to remove possibility of getting it.
- Secondary
  Action which halts the progress of disease.
- Tertiary
  Action taken to reduce disability.

WHO has recently recommended 2 approaches under primary prevention (first level of prevention); one is population strategy, which is directed at the whole population irrespective of individual risk level. Here population strategy is directed towards socioeconomic, behavioural and lifestyle changes. The other is high risk strategy which aims at bringing preventive care to individuals at risk through optional use of clinical methods.

Modes of Intervention

These are depicted under National history of disease (Fig. 7.4) which are:

- Health promotion
- Specific protection
- Early diagnosis and treatment
- Disability limitation
- Rehabilitation.

Common practical activity is given in a tabular column in Table 7.5.

CHANGING PATTERN OF DISEASES

As part of health development changing pattern of disease is noticed in developed countries. Infectious diseases are extinct and now leading causes of death are cancer, heart diseases, accident, stroke and metabolic disorders. Silent epidemic of Alzheimer's disease is progressively seen in U.S.A.

In developing countries infections are still the main cause of high mortality.

Above picture emphasises the need for planning in advance the approaches in future health planning and management.

POPULATION MEDICINE

Population medicine is a common ground for a concern to promote health and to prevent diseases. This area considers population medicine which includes Hygiene, Public Health, Preventive Medicine, Community Health, Social Medicine and Community Medicine.

Hygiene

It is the science of health and embraces all factors which contribute to healthful living.

Table 7.5: Examples of intervention therapy in prevention

Primary		*Secondary*	*Tertiary*	
Health promotion	*Specific protection*	*Early diagnosis and treatment*	*Disability limitation*	*Rehabilitation*
* Health education	* Immunisation	* TB patient	* Physiotherapy polio case	* Artificial limb to limbless
* Life style change	* IFA prophylaxis	* Leprosy case	* IV fluid to severe dehydration	* Gardener job to leprosy cured.
* Use protected water	* Chemoprophylaxis	* Hypertension case	* Bed rest, sedation to IHD	* Family restoration of TB cured
* Mosquito control	* Seat belt, helmet	* Cancer cervix case	* IV therapy in severe malaria	* Brill schooling to blind
* Food fortification	* Food safety	* Severe malnutrition	* IV therapy in meningitis	* Reconstructive surgery to leprosy patient

Public Health

The organised application of local, state, national and International resources to achieve health for all, i.e. real public health.

As early as 1952, World Health Organisation has adopted Winslow's definition of Public Health which is as under:

> "The science and art of preventing disease, prolonging life and promoting health and efficiency through organized community efforts for the sanitation of the environment, the control of communicable infections, the education of the individual in personal hygiene, the organization of medical and nursing services for early diagnosis and preventive treatment of disease and the development of social machinery to ensure for every individual a standard of living adequate for the maintenance of health, so organizing these benefits as to enable every citizen to realize his birthright of health and longevity."

Preventive Medicine

It is a branch of medicine based on aetiology as applied to healthy people. It is timely application of all means to promote the health of people.

Community Health

It is "all the personal health and environmental services in any human community, irrespective of whether such services were public or private ones". Earlier hygiene moulded to sanitation which got changed to preventive and social medicine. The same area is now "Community Health". This was called community medicine till today.

Social Medicine

It is the study of man as a social being in his total environment.

Community Medicine

It is the successor of public health, preventive medicine, preventive and social medicine. In community medicine we come across measures like community diagnosis and community treatment.

I.C.D. CLASSIFICATION OF DISEASES

It is a system of classification needed to group diseases for an ultimate uniform classification. WHO has brought out ICD 10th with 3 volumes which give detailed report of classification.

It is arranged into 21 major chapters (I to XXI). For e.g. XI: is disease of digestive system.

Each major chapter has 3 character categories to cover its content. For e.g. XI: Diseases of digestive system has (K00 – K93).

Most of 3 character category is subdivided by means of 4th numeric character after a decimal point, allowing up to 10 sub categories. When 3 categories are subdivided 'X' is used for data processing.

For example

Chapter XXI is Factors influencing health status and contact with health service. It has ZOO-Z99 sub category. Further sub-categories can be seen.

For example

High Risk Sexual Behaviour

Z 72.5 (z 72 is from XXI) 0.5 is sub category.

I.C.D. helps in health management and facilitates research and help in international comparison.

FURTHER REFERENCES

1. Leavel and Clark—Preventive medicine for the doctor in his community (McGraw Hill).
2. Prabhakara G.N.– Short Textbook of PSM (Jaypee).

8

Environment and Health

Environmental Health is the science of safe guarding health in broader sense includes;

'Water, Air, Soil, Housing, Waste, Radiation, Plant life, Animal Life, Bacteria, Virus, Insects, Rodents, Animals, Human customs, Culture, Habits, Income, Occupation, Religion and such many more things'

Environmental Pollution has been a constant threat to mankind.Human activities, urbanization and industrialization are blamed for the poor environmental hygiene.

IMPORTANCE

Physical development, health and survival are influenced by physical,chemical, social, spiritual and Biological environments. Man lives in this group of Environment where he adjusts and readjusts to the surroundings.Control of these environments which exercises deleterious effects on health, constitutes environmental health.

Much of ill health in India is due to poor environmental health in terms of unprotected water, air pollution, soil pollution, poor housing, vectors around us and social interactions interwoven. High Death rate and high morbidity rate are due to poor environmental sanitation, which needs improvement in the battle of prevention of diseases and promotion of community health.

United Nations conference on the Human environment focused worldwide attention on the environmental hazards that threaten human beings. At present WHO and UNO have taken up the task of wide range survey of environmental hazards to human health.

Sanitation is equally a forceful word in environmental health which is defined as the Science of Safeguarding Health. According to the National Sanitation Foundation of USA "Sanitation is way of life It is the quality of living that is expressed in the clean home, the clean farm, the clean business, the clean neighborhood and the clean community. It comes from people,it is nourished by knowledge, grows as an obligation and an ideal in human relations."

The first global conference on health promotion"Supportive environments for Health" called upon the people in all parts of the world to engage actively in making environments more supportive to health. This clear picture of Environment and Health is expressed by the world commission on environment and development in its report "Our Common Future" which provides a new understanding of the imperative need of sustainable development.

TYPES OF ENVIRONMENT

i. Physical environment include Housing, Human congregation, Meteorology, Air, ventilation, Noise, Lighting, Radiation, Water, Solid Waste and Liquid Waste.
ii. Chemical environment include organic and inorganic chemicals that exist in human placement and human occupations.
iii. Social environment include ways of living, religion, caste, customs, culture, attitude, beliefs, moves, education, occupation and standard of living.
iv. Spiritual environment include integrity, principles, ethics, purpose of life and commitment to some higher being.
v. Biological environment include Bacteria, virus, rickettsiae, fungi, helminths, protozoa, insects, rodents and other animals.

Biological environment is detailed under communicable diseases, social and spiritual environment is detailed under sociology and psychology and chemical environment is detailed under human occupations. In the present chapter all physical and materialistic surroundings are highlighted.

Physical Environment

Housing

House refers to a physical structure where unit of society the family lives, but the concept is slowly changing to "Human settlement" which allow the extended outlook of a house, where people live, interact and pursue their goals, WHO has coined the word residential environment which is used by man for his activity and desired devices for his family well being.

Healthful Housing:

American Public Health Association has given basic principles of healthful housing. On similar lines WHO has given following Healthful Housing criteria:

- It gives physical protection and shelter.
- Adequate provision for cooking, eating, washing and excretory functions.
- It prevents spread of infections and communicable diseases.
- Protects from noise.
- Protects from atmospheric pollutions.
- Housing material is free from toxic and harmful chemicals.
- Encourage personality development.
- Promote mental health.
- To attain social goals like:
  - Family life
  - Access to community facility
  - Social participation
  - Economic stability.

Need of Housing:

i. Physical needs like air, temperature, lighting, rest, recreation.
ii. Physiological needs like privacy, family life.
iii. Health needs like water, sanitary latrine, balanced diet, protection from insects and animals.
iv. Protective needs like accidents, fire, electricity etc.

Housing Standards:

Environmental Hygiene committee of Government of India has given some minimum housing standards that are to be maintained by building regulations through Municipality, Corporation, Town planning and urban development authorities.

Bathing Facility: House should have adequate bathing facility.

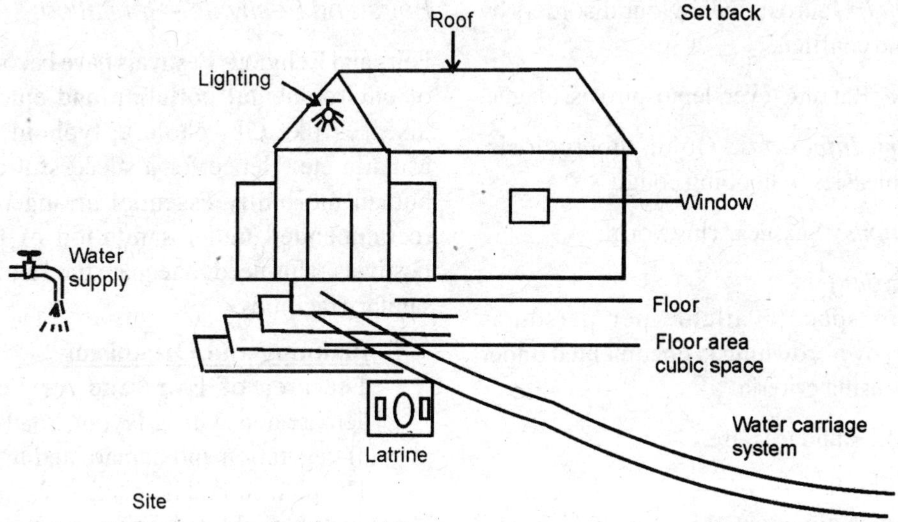

Fig. 8.1: Minimum housing standards

Cubic Space: It should be 500 cubic feet per person.

Floor: Pucca floor, no crack and damp proof.

Floor Area: 100 square foot per person.

Garbage Disposal: Daily removal by sanitary method for proper disposal.

Kitchen: Adequate provision for separate and sanitary area for food preparation.

Lighting: It is expected to have a D.F. (day light factor) of 1.0 or above 1.0.

Privy: Sanitary RCA latrine and water carriage system is a must under criteria of healthful housing.

Roof: It should be more than 10 feet.

Rooms: According to family size and needed privacy, number of rooms are suggested.

Refuse Disposal: Daily disposal and transport for sanitary disposal is advocated.

Site of the House – In an elevated place, in a residential area of a town and subsoil water must be below 10 feet.

Set Back: The built up area is restricted to 2/3rd of site. Wind direction and ventilation are considered.

Walls: Strong and weather resistant.

Windows: Window area shall be 1/5th of floor area.

Water Supply: Safe and wholesome water supply is guaranteed.

Washing: Should have provision for washing facility

In case of rural housing criteria, additional considerations are suggested and recommended. They are:

- Cattle shed 25 feet away.
- Manure pit at the back yard or side yard

Housing Related Diseases:

Accidents: Home accidents like fire, electrocution, fall, and fracture.

Arthropod Borne: Vector borne diseases by mosquito, housefly.

Psychosocial: Neurosis, behaviour disorders by isolation and conflicts.

Rat Menace: Rat bite fever, leptospirosis, plague.

Respiratory Infections: Cold, tuberculosis, influenza, measles, whooping cough.

Skin Infections: Scabies, ringworm.

Over Crowding

If the floor space available per person is inadequate, overcrowding is documented under healthful housing criteria.

Accepted standards are:

- 70-90 esq. – for 1 person.
- Infant is not counted.
- Child 1–10 year is ½ people.
- 2 persons above 9 years not husband wife of opposite sex are not obliged to sleep in the same room.

Current Status

Housing is viewed as an important component of national economy. In Five Year Plans assistance to disadvantaged groups (single women, widows, physically handicaps, SC/ST, Rural etc.) are undertaken. House site and construction assistance are part of Minimum Needs Programme.

Absolute homeless families are in Lakhs in India. Urban housing crisis is increasing due to hiked inflation. Slum and shanty town has no healthful and housing conditions. N.B.O. (National Buildings Organisation) HUDCO (Housing and Urban Development Corporation) and HHF (Hindustan Housing Factory) are functioning to achieve goals of healthful housing to the community, under IAY(*Indira Awas Yojana*) house with 1 room, 1 kitchen, and RCA latrine, a bath and a smokeless *chullah* are being constructed which also give employment opportunity to rural youth.

Fairs and Festivals– Sanitation:

Fairs and Religious Festivals have become source of environmental pollution and epidemics of diseases like GE, cholera, typhoid, Dengue, Malaria etc. Hence for a successful control of human morbidity essential arrangements are recommended under sanitation of Fairs and Festivals. This needs adequate fund and adequate sanitary facilities.

i. **Planning and Organising**:
The area of Fairs and /or Festival is demarcated with a layout, roads, cleared of vegetation and demarcated into blocks. The plan should help a fact sheet which is made available to visiting pilgrims or people.

ii. **Accommodation**:
Organisers, police personal, Health authorities and visiting people should have required accommodation. It should have sanitary conveniences. Room accommodation should be 10 feet height and 10% of floor area with window. Pits, pools etc., are smoothened to avoid future breeding places.

iii. **Health Facility**:
The area should be under supervision of a health officer and assisted by required Health Assistants. Facility for routine treatment, first aid and an ambulance are prime requisites. Treatment facility for burns and accidents is facilitated.

iv. **Water Supply**:
Adequate safe and wholesome water supply arrangement is looked into through feasible methods like:

- Filtered, Chlorinated water from water works
- Deep Tube wells
- Piped water connection

v. **Conservancy:**

Sweeping of roads, residential blocks are got done by whole time conservancy staff. They are also delegated the duties of cleaning of Latrine, Urinals.

One sanitary worker for 2000 expected pilgrims or people is the standards aimed at. Dust bins at reachable to collect dust, their removal by trucks are to be arranged. Latrine for males and females are to be planned separately. Trench latrine is ideal which is to cater as under:

- 1 day fair—2 seat per 1000 people.
- More than 1 day – 1 seat per 100 people.

Adequate urinals are to be provided in Fairs. A pit 4 feet square, 5 feet depth is filled with broken bricks. At corner of pit kerosene tin filled with saw dust and bottom perforated is placed.

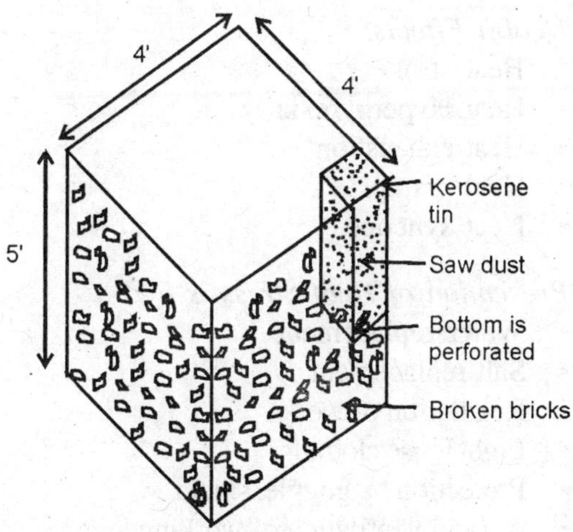

Fig. 8.2: Urinals for fairs

Satisfactory arrangement for refuse disposal is expected.

vi. **Food Hygiene:**

Supervision of food sale is exercised. Glass cover to cut fruits, sweets and eatables is enforced to avoid fly nuisance, care of food handlers and hygiene of food catering area are also enforced.

vii. **Immunisation:**

This depends on the place of fair or festival. Depending on its geographic location, vaccination for cholera, typhoid, and meningitis are advocated. Pilgrims are expected to get vaccinated before specified days and before coming to *Mela*, as specified by corporation health authorities. In some of the international congregation, certification of vaccination is mandatory.

viii. **Health Inspection Check Post:**

Health staffs are posted in check post to keep surveillance on patients with infections disease, who are not allowed to Fairs and festival, to avoid spread of diseases.

ix. **Vigilance on Social Problems:**

Personnel from police and volunteers are drawn to check *goondaism*, theft, public unrest, prostitution, alcoholism and drug abuse.

Meteorological Environment

These are physical surroundings that comprise of:

a. Temperature
b. Humidity
c. Atmospheric pressure
d. Rainfall
e. Wind
f. Clouds, these are summated to represent Meteorology or weather forecasting for the given geographical area.

Temperature

Atmosphere temperature is variable during the day, during the season and at given latitude. It is higher at ground level and goes on reducing as we move up to higher attitude. Thermometers are used to measure atmospheric temperature.

Mercury thermometers are used to record maximum temperature, because of its great expansible character. Ether is used to record lower temperature because of its great condensation power.

Dry Bulb Thermometer

This is Commonly used to record air temperature.

Wet Bulb Thermometer

When bulb of thermometer is kept wet by a muslin cloth, it shows air temperature depending on the dryness of air.

Maximum Thermometer

It is a mercury thermometer.

Minimum Thermometer

It is an alcohol thermometer.

Six's Maximum and Minimum Thermometer

It is a combination of maximum and minimum thermometers which are used in Indian Meteorological observations.

Globe Thermometer

Bulb of thermometer is painted with matt black paint which absorbs radiant heat and air temperature.

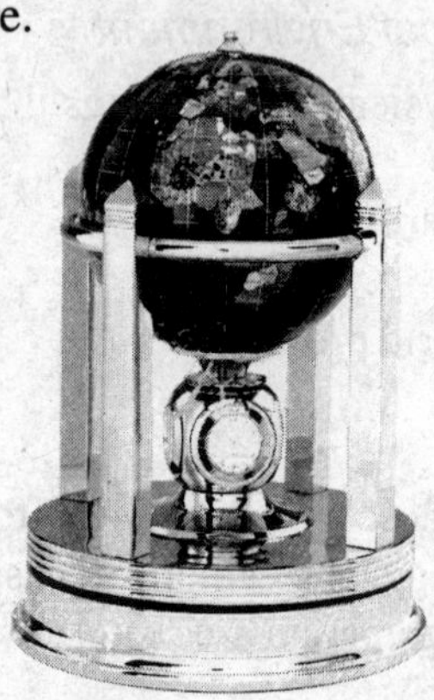

Fig. 8.3: Globe thermometer

Kata Thermometer

It is used to find out cooling power of the air (Fig. 8.4).

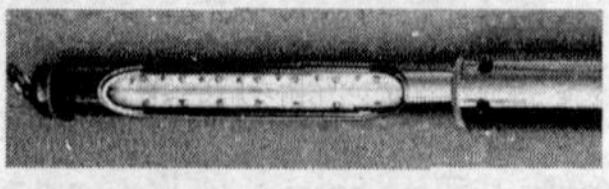

Fig. 8.4: Kata thermometer

Cooling power of the air is expressed as millicalories per square cm per second.

Indices of Comfort in Kata Thermometer:

Dry Kata 6 and above	Indicate Thermal comfort
Wet Kata 20 and above	

Types of Kata are:

a. Standard Kata – range 100-95^{0}F (Red)
b. High temperature Kata – 130-125^{0}F (Dark blue)
c. Extra high temperature – 150 -145^{0}F (Magenta)

Common heat stress indices are available like (a) Equatorial comfort index. (b) Heat stress index. (c) Predicted four hour sweat rate.

Heat stress index up to 10 is tolerable and heat strain starts with 10 and 40 HSI, is sever heat strain.

Health Effects:

- Heat stroke
- Heat Hyperpyrexia
- Heat exhaustion
- Heat cramps
- Heat syncope.

Prevention of Heat Stress is by:

- Water replacement
- Salt replacement
- Regulation of work
- Light loose clothing
- Protection by goggle, shield
- Air and ventilation of working area.

Effect of lower temperature:

- Numbness
- Loss of sensation
- Muscular weakness
- Immersion foot (Trench foot)
- Frostbite.

Above cold stress can be prevented by protection and using warm water.

Global Warming

Emission of green house gases to atmosphere mainly CO_2 can bring about rise in global surface temperature, rise in sea level and extreme climatic events like cyclone, heat wave and draught. This affects global ecosystem.

Humidity

Humidity is expressed in terms of the water content in air (Aqueous Tension). Air temperature determines humidity. We notice dew collection when air temperature is very low. If it is measured in percentage it is called Relative humidity. If humidity is expressed in actual by weight for a given value it is Absolute humidity. Below 30% of relative humidity and above 65% of relative humidity is not comfortable. Low humidity cause dryness of nasal mucosa and cause ENT problems.

To measure humidity following instruments are used:

i. Hygrometer (Dry and wet bulb thermometer).
ii. Sling Psychrometer (Dry and wet bulb with rotation facility).
iii. Assmann Psychrometer.

In case of hydrometer, it directly measures air temperature. Air is allowed by force due to rotation, at recording, in case of sling Psychrometer. In Assmann Psychrometer, fan air at 5 meters per second is allowed to bulbs for recording. The readings of dry and wet bulbs are referred in Psychrometric chart (Nonogram) to get the following:

- Air temperature
- Relative humidity
- Wind speed
- Absolute humidity.

Rain Fall

Water precipitated from atmosphere is rain water. Depending on level of precipitation the water may be in the form of snow, hail, dew or frost. Rain fall is measured by "Rain gauge". Rainfall of 8 mm in a day or 41 mm in a month is unit of expression with the measure by Symons Rain gauge.

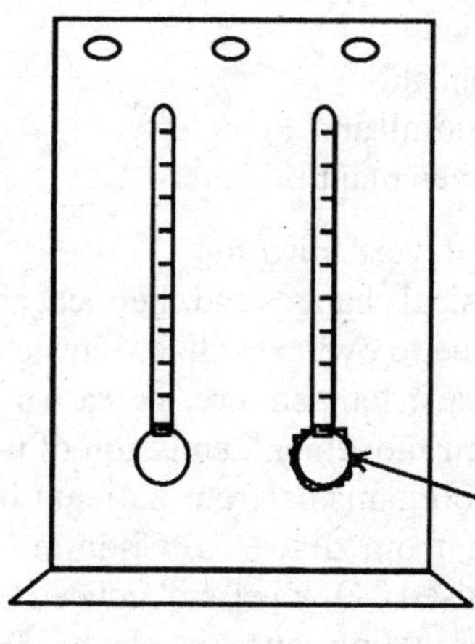

Fig. 8.5: Dry and wet bulb thermometer

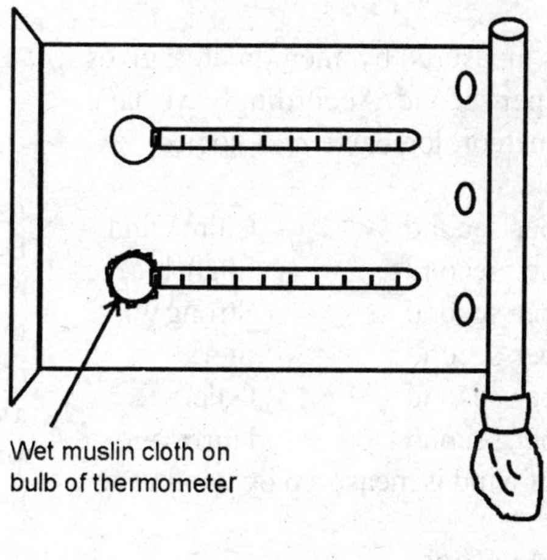

Fig. 8.6: Sling thermometer

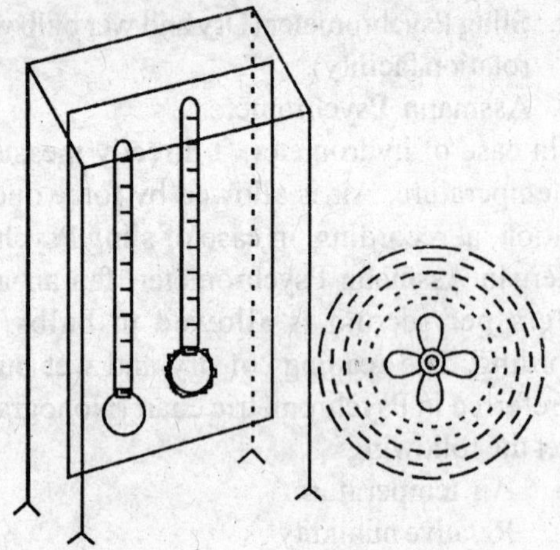

Fig. 8.7: Assmann psychrometer

Wind Velocity:

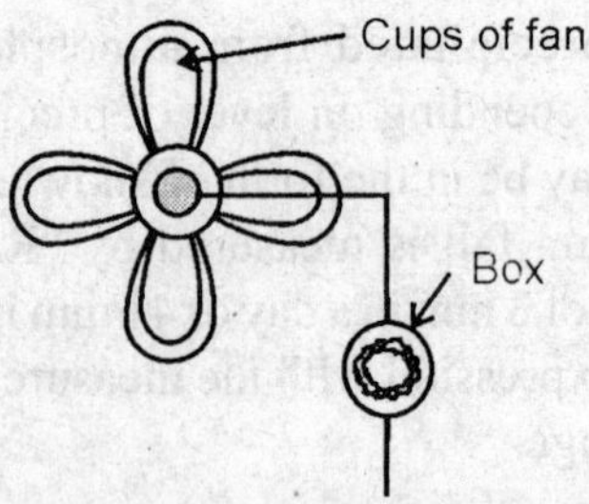

Fig. 8.8: Anemometer

Air velocity is measured by anemometer, gives the unit metre per second. Accordingly we have the following meteorological terminologies.

0.5 meter per second	– Calm wind
3.3 meter per second	– Slight breeze
10.0 meter per second	– Strong wind
15-20 meter per second	– Storm
25-30 meter per second	– Gale
30-50 meter per second	– Hurricane

Direction of wind is measured by wind vane.

Clouds and Weather

It gives sequence of weather in a geographical locality. Common man uses the word bad weather, good weather by these observations. Satellite installation by Government of India has given highly sensitive and accurate idea of weather and values for weather forecasting.

Air and Ventilation

Air

Biosphere has life only by the presence of air which supply oxygen, cools the body, gives stimulus to special sense. Polluted air can cause high morbidity and mortality.

Composition of air:

1. Nitrogen 78.1 %
2. Oxygen 20.93 %
3. CO_2 0.03 %
4. Other gases
5. Water vapour
6. Ammonia traces
7. Suspended matter

Air gets polluted very easily by:

a. Traffic, Trade
b. Organic matter decomposition
c. Combustion of oil, gas, coal
d. Human and animal respiration

Nature simultaneously disallows air pollution through

a. Wind
b. Sunlight
c. Rainfall and
d. Green plant life.

Effect of Overcrowding:

Both physical changes and chemical changes are noticed due to overcrowding. Physical changes include rise in temperature, increase in humidity, reduced air movement, emission of body odors and microorganisms from patients if they are suffering from diseases. Chemical changes include raised CO_2 level and reduced O_2 content.

Overcrowding causes headache, drowsiness, inability to concentrate. Discomfort in overcrowding is due to physical changes and not because of chemical changes.

Measurement of Thermal Comfort:

i. Cooling power of the air by Kata thermometer.
ii. Corrected effective temperature (CET) which combines Air temperature, Humidity and air movement and radiant heat. Globe Thermometer is used in recording Air temperature.
iii. Predicted Four hour sweat rate (P_4SR).

It is called McArdle's maximum allowable sweat rate which is 3 for an upper limit of comfort zone.

Table 8.1: Comfort zone

	CET	*P_4SR*
Comfortable	77-80°F	
Comfort zone	–	1–3 litres
Hot, uncomfortable	81-82°F	–
Just tolerable	–	3-4.5 litre
Intolerable	86°F	4.5 + litres

Air Pollution: Air is said to be polluted if substance of human and animal activity is raised and that can cause human ill health. Air can get polluted by:

a. Motor vehicles which emit hydrocarbons, CO, Lead, Nitrogen Oxide and particulate matter.
b. Industry emits smoke, SO_2, Nitrogen Oxide and fly ash.
c. Domestic combustions of coal, wood etc.
d. Others like nuclear energy, pesticide spray etc.

Man is in direct effect of 10 kms of atmosphere and not above that from earth surface. Rise in Atmospheric temperature make pollutions to diffuse vertically. If cooling of lower layer has occurred then vertical air diffusion is not possible allowing pollutants to get trapped at lower level as smog. This is called temperature inversion. Important pollutants are CO, CO_2, H_2S, SO_2, SO_3, NO_2, organic compounds, metals, radio active compounds and photo chemical oxidants.

Table 8.2: Indoor air pollutants

Possible source	*Pollutant*
Smoking	Tobacco particle
Combustion	CO, CO_2
Coal	SO_2
Resin products	Benzene
Fire proofing	Asbestos
Appliances	Mineral fibre

Hazards of Air Pollution:

i. Respiratory tract irritation
ii. Impaired lung function
iii. Lung cancer
iv. Cough, ARI
v. Asthma
vi. Hindrance in neuropsychological development.

Control of Air Pollution:

a. By air monitoring for SO_2, Smoke index, and dust measurement.
b. Follow up of criteria and guidelines for maximum permissible allowance for individual substances.
c. Monitoring of air pollution through data base in selected cities.
d. Containment of harmful substances.
e. Discarding and replacing old technology process with new safe process.
f. Vegetation and development of green belt.
g. Acts and Amendments to enforce clear air.
h. Development of network of Laboratories.
i. Air disinfection by ventilation, ultra-violet radiation and allowing clean air by triethyelene glucol vapour.

Table 8.3: Maximum upper limit of chemicals in air

Substance	*Maximum limit*	*Averaging time*
CO	30 mg/m^3	1 hour
H_2S	150 microgram/m^3	24 hours
Lead	0.5-1.0 microgram/m^3	1 year
NO_2	150 microgram/m^3	24 hours
SO_2	350 microgram/m^3	1 hour

Ventilation

Ventilation is a process of controlling air quality in terms of temperature, humidity and purity, Minimum fresh air supply to man is 300 to 3000 cubic feet per hour per person. Air is allowed to have recommended cooling power of the air. Optimum floor space is suggested to 50-100 square feet.

Types of Ventilation

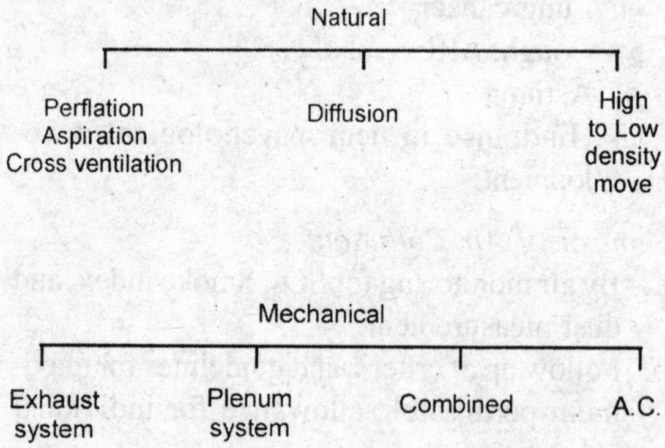

Fig. 8.9: Types of ventilation

Natural Ventilation:

A: Wind movement in a chamber is called perflation. When there is obstruction, it is aspirated. Windows or doors when facing each other cross ventilation is produced.

B: When a small space is provided air is diffused slowly.

C: Temperature difference outside and inside make air movement possible.

Mechanical Ventilation:

A: Exhaust an takes the air out and is called exhaust system.

B: Centrifugal Fans blow air inside and is called plenum system.

C: A combination of exhaust and plenum system is used.

D: Air conditioning in O.T., hospital, ICU, ICCU, IPCU is very helpful. The air is filtered and saturated with water vapour. The excess moisture is removed and the air is heated to desired temperature. Care is taken to see that outside and inside temperature is maintained to below 20'F.

Noise

Noise is defined as unwanted sound i.e. wrong sound, in wrong place at wrong time. Modern life is associated with noise pollution. Major source comes from automobile, factory, industry, airway, roadway, television and sound systems.

Table 8.4: Acceptable noise level

Home	40 dBA
Office	45 dBA
Industry	60 dBA
Classroom	40 dBA
Hospital ward	20 dBA

Table 8.5: Noise level in decibels

Whispering	10 dB
Talking	60 dB
Speech	80 dB
Radio music	85 dB
Shouting	80 dB
Crying	80 dB
Road roller	120 dB
Plane takes off	150 dB

Above 90dB and 4000Hz, whistling and buzzing in ears occur. Temporary or permanent hearing losses are affected based on noise level and duration of exposure. Sleeplessness, psychosis, neurosis and fatigue are common due to noise pollution.

Suggested Measures to Control Noise Pollution:

i. Town planning
ii. Vehicle and traffic control
iii. Noise proof constructions

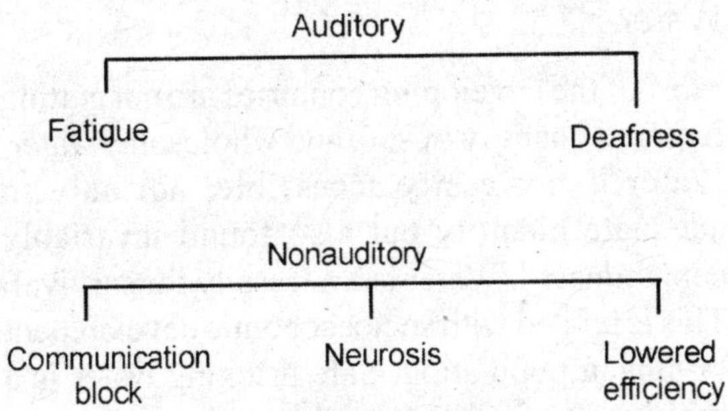

Fig. 8.10: Effects of noise

iv. Source reduction in industry
v. Ear plug and Ear muff use
vi. Legal regulations
vii. Public awareness on noise pollution.

Lighting

Lighting is an essential part for good vision, efficiency physiological functions and vitamin D supply. Brightness of light is measured by candle power whereas amount of light reaching surface is measured by foot candle.

D.F. (Day Light Factor):

$$D.F. = \frac{\text{Indoor illumination}}{\text{Outdoor illumination}} \times 100$$

Day light Factor is a ratio between instantaneous illumination indoors and simultaneously occurring illumination outdoors. Living room should have 8% D.F. and kitchen 10%. Since artificial lighting is to be depended, systems of artificial lighting like Direct, indirect, semi direct, semi-indirect and direct-indirect have came up in daily life. Light from above and from left is ideal for reading and studying, lighting standards are laid down for each visual activity. Avoiding glare, an illumination of above 30 times the requirement is rule of thumb for visual task.

Radiation

Men are continuously exposed to radiation through cosmic rays, U.V. rays, X-rays, α rays, β rays and γ rays, both natural way and man made exposures. Further over the past 25 years, therapeutic procedures have been developed in the field of Radiology, based on (mainly) angiographic techniques. Diagnostic procedures involving injection of contrast media comes under the heading of invasive diagnostic radiology. Interventional radiology on the other hand comprises procedures with a predominantly therapeutic objective. Here from Nursing care point of view it takes care of informed consent and the level of acceptable risk for diagnosis.

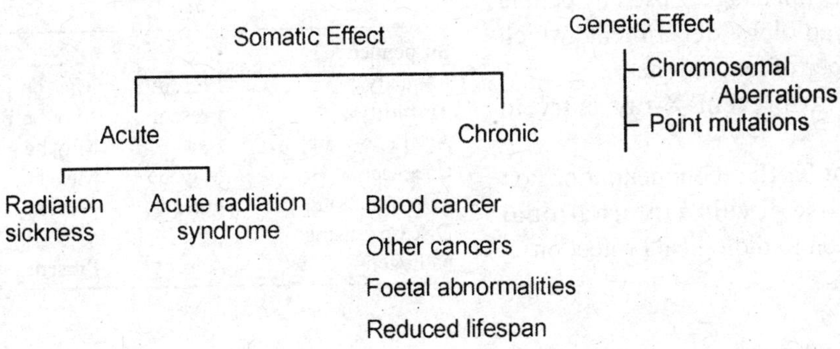

Fig. 8.11: Biological effects of radiation

Natural Radiation:

From outer space cosmic rays are emitted. In soil and rock radioactive elements like thorium, uranium, radium are present, even human body does contain minute quantity of isotopes of K_{40}, Sr_{90} and C_{14}.

Man-made Radiation:

X-ray is the greatest source used in hospital practice. Nuclear explosions release energy and ionising radiation. T.V., Luminous watches etc., also contribute to our exposure. Ionising radiation is one where radiation penetrates the tissue and gets deposited in tissues.

Effects of Radiation:

Since man is exposed to radiation during diagnosis and for intervention, the scope has widened to cover fluoroscopy, ultrasound, computerized tomography (CT scan) and Magnetic resonance imaging (M.R. scan). The Biological effects of radiation is classified as in Figure 8.11.

Radiation Protection:

i. Pregnant women are not exposed to radiation unnecessarily.
ii. Leakage of X-ray machines and defective machines are avoided and discarded.
iii. All working in X-ray unit, isotope unit, cobalt therapy unit, luminous parts industry and atomic energy are subjected for periodic check-up.
iv. Dosimeter or film badge is used by people working in radiology department, which checks the dose of ionization.
v. Lead apron to prevent X-ray entry to workers body.
vi. Adaptation of ICRP recommendations on radiation dose levels (International Commission on Radiological Protection).

Water

Most of the developing countries are not getting required quantity of safe and wholesome water. Water is not easily accessible, not only in adequate quantity but also found invariably contaminated. Water is a necessity for survival. This is related with socioeconomic development of human population. Safe drinking water is a basic need of primary health care which is the key to attain health for all. There is considerable improvement in urban water supply in late 2000, but rural India has not attained the requisite provision of protected water for the community. Now Government of India has included water as a component in RCH, Nutrition programme and health awareness programme.

Safe and Wholesome Water:

The criteria for safe and wholesome water are:

i. It should be potable.
ii. It should meet aesthetic value by colour, taste, turbidity.
iii. It should be free from harmful chemical substances.
iv. It should be free from pathogens.

Difference between polluted and contaminated water:

Table 8.6: Difference between polluted and contaminated water

	Polluted water	*Contaminated water*
Suspended impurity	Present	May be present
Turbidity	Present	May be present
Aesthetic view	Bad	May be good
Chemical contamination	May be present	May be present
Disease causing pathogens	Absent	Present

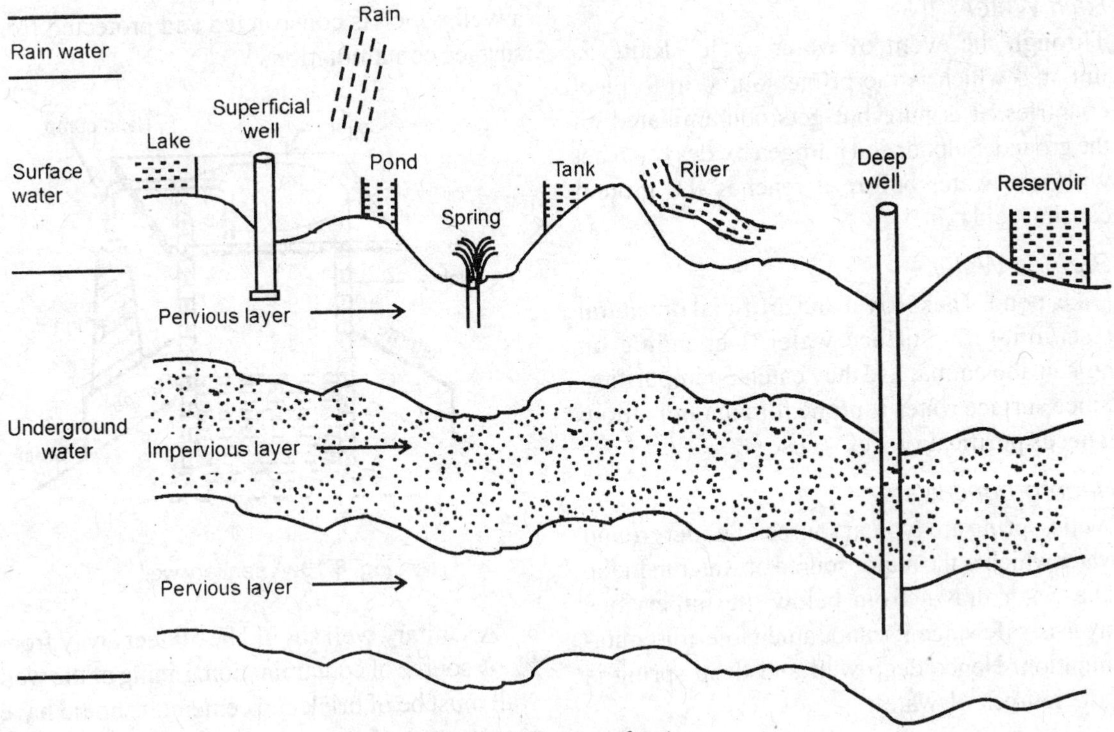

Fig. 8.12: Source of water

Uses of Water

Table 8.7: Uses of water

Domestic	*Public*	*Industry*	*Agriculture*
Drinking	Swimming pool	Raw material	Irrigation
Cooking	Fountain	Process material	Farming
Washing	Ponds	Cooling material	Plantation
Bathing	Fire force		Cash crops
Ablution	Public park		Food crops
Gardening			
Power	*Carriage system*		
Hydropower	Solid waste		
Steam power	Liquid waste		
Sullage	Sewage		

Rain Water

Through the event of water cycle" Rain" is initiated which is the prime source in tropical countries. It is pure but gets contaminated on the ground. Sulphur and nitrogen oxides can react with rain water before it reaches the ground causing acid rain.

Surface Water

Lake, pond, Tank, River and artificial or natural reservoir form surface water. Depending on human and animal use they catch up impurities. Since surface water is prone for contamination, it needs purification before use.

Underground Water

Wells, spring are typical source of underground water which is the major source of water in India. The water drawn from below the impervious layer is safe since it is not amenable for contamination. Hence deep well and deep spring is safe sources of water.

Types of Wells

i. *Shallow well:* It taps water from above the impervious layer, soft often grossly contaminated and not long lasting.
ii. *Deep well:* It taps water from below the impervious layer, hard, bacteriologically pure and provides constant supply.
iii. *Katcha well:* They are dug wells dries early, gets easily contaminated.
iv. *Pucca well:* They are dug wells dries early, do not get easily contaminated.
v. *Step well:* Steps provided well where people can enter and collect water. It is the cause of Guinea worm infection.
vi. *Artesian well:* It is a kind of deep wells, where water is jet out by subsoil pressure.
vii. *Tube well:* They are driven well and are called sanitary wells.

Sanitary Well

From public health point of view sanitary well is a well which is constructed and protected from surface contamination.

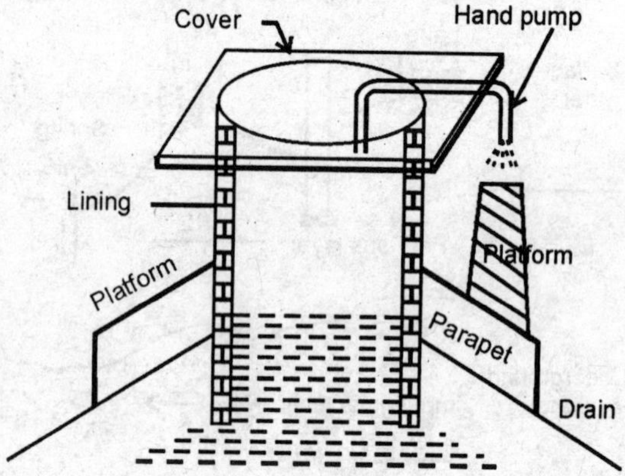

Fig. 8.13: A sanitary well

A sanitary well should be 50 feet away from likely source of contamination. Lining of the well wall must be of brick and cement. It should have a parapet wall and a platform round the well. Drain is provided which drains beyond the zone of influence. Well is covered and a pump set is fixed.

Water Pollution

The impurities derived from atmosphere, catchment area and soil, pollutes a given source of water. Industry and urbanization worsens the pollution. Sullage, sewage, industry waste and agricultural wastes dominate in water pollution. Cross connection and leakage also cause water pollution.

Water pollution is indicated by:

i. Suspended solids
ii. B.O.D.
iii. C.O.D.
iv. Nitrogen
v. Dissolved oxygen

Water Pollution Law: To control water pollution a comprehensive legislation, the

Water (Prevention and Control of Pollution) Act 1974 is available with Water Boards.

Water Borne Diseases:

Bacterial	– Typhoid, Paratyphoid, Dysentery, Infantile Diarrhoea, Cholera
Viral	– Hepatitis A, Poliomyelitis, Infantile Rota Virus Infection
Protozoal	– Amoebiasis, Giardiasis
Helminthic	– Roundworm, Threadworm
Leptospiral	– Weil's disease
Others	– Schistosomiasis Guineaworm infection Fish tapeworm

To control water pollution Parliament has passed "Prevention and Control of Pollution Act, 1974".

Purification of Water

Domestic Scale

Boiling for 10 minutes and keeping in the same vessel.

Bleaching powder commercially available contains 33% of available chlorine. In case of stabilized bleaching powder it is about 70% of available chlorine.

Chlorine Tablet – 0.5 Grams of one tablet is sufficient for 20 litres of water.

Iodine – It is only for emergency disinfection.

$KMnO_4$ – Though it is good, not accepted from aesthetic point of view.

Filters: Candle filters are commercially produced. In this contaminated water is allowed to filter slowly through a porous ceramic material. This cannot filter virus. Types of filters available are Pasteur Chamberland Filter, Berkefeld Filter and Katadyn Filter.

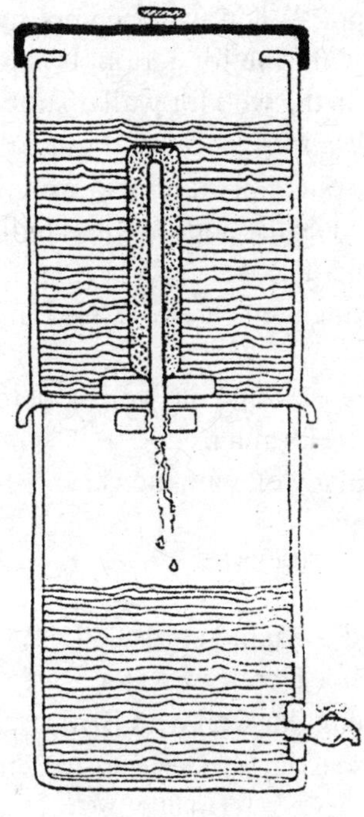

Fig. 8.14: Candle filter

Double Pot Method:

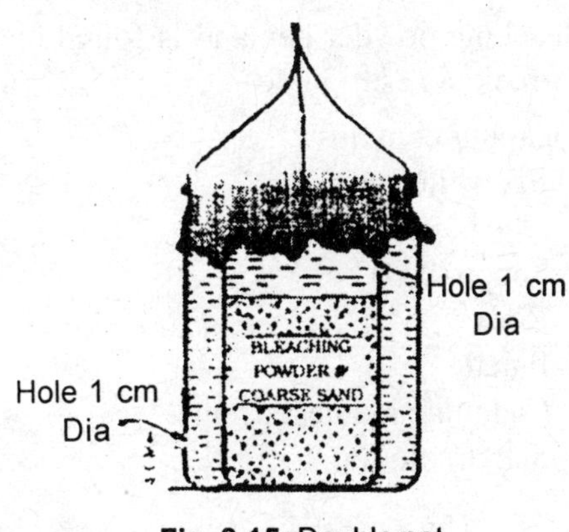

Fig. 8.15: Double pot

Double pot is a product of NEERI, Nagpur. There are 2 pots one placed inside the other. Inner pot has hole in upper portion and in outer pot the hole is 4 cm above the bottom. Mixture of 1:2 bleaching powder and coarse sand is kept in inside pot. When water enters there is slow release of chlorine for action. It is lowered and immersed in the well for well disinfection.

Well Disinfection: Subsoil water through well is a major source of water and well disinfection is to be periodically done in Rural India to prevent water borne disease.

Following steps are followed in well disinfection:

a. Volume of water in well is determined by following formula.

   i. Circular well with metric values:

$$\text{Volume of water (Litres)} = \frac{3.14 \times d^2 \times h}{4} \times 1000$$

when d = Diameter of well
h = Depth of water

   ii. Rectangular well with British value:
   Volume (Gallons) = Length × Breadth × 6.25 × Depth of water

   iii. Circular well with British values.
   Volume (Gallons)= $D^2 \times W \times 5$ = gallons
   Where D = Diameter of well
   W = Depth of water

b. Bleaching powder demand is found out by Horrock's Test.

   Apparatus contains:
   - Six white cups
   - One black cup
   - Scoop (2 G)
   - Rods
   - Pipette
   - Cadmium iodide reagent
   - Starch solution.

   Procedure:
   Sample of water to be tested is taken in 6 white cups mark. They are numbered 1 to 6. Standard solution of bleaching powder is prepared in black cup by taking 1 scoop bleaching powder. This standard solution is taken in a pipette and added 1 drop to first, 2 drops to second till 6 drops to 6th cup. They are allowed for 30 minutes as contact period by constant stirring. After 30 minutes 3 drops cadmium iodide and 1 ml starch solution are added and observed for colour change. From inference bleaching powder demand is calculated (e.g. if 3rd cup onwards blue colour appeared, then 3 × 2=6G. of bleaching powder is needed for 100 gallons of water. (*Note:* If there is no change, experiment is repeated with 6 to 12 drops of standard solution).

c. Required quantity of bleaching powder is taken in a bucket, prepared as paste in the beginning and later to a homogenous solution.
d. Supernatant solution of (c) is taken in a bucket and mixed to well water by constant jerky movement (in the evening).
e. Allowed over night for action.
f. Next morning well water is tested for residual chlorine which should be at least 0.5 PPM (1 PPM after 1 hour contact period is ideal) by orthotolidine test.

Large Scale

In a water reservoir procedure followed are (i) Storage (ii) Filtration and chlorination.

Storage: 24 hours storage help in settling of suspended impurities, oxidation by anabolic bacteria can occur and sunlight may help in certain disinfection.

Filtration: It can be either slow sand Filtration or Rapid sand filtration. In case of more suspended solid content and high turbidity of source of water, pre-filtration with gravel or other course material before sand filtration is an effective means of preventing the rapid blocking of the sand filters (Fig. 8.16). Raw water is passed vertically or horizontally through different compartments and collected in outlet chamber. If vertical flow is chosen, either up flow or down flow is possible, but up flow filters are easier to clean and thus more likely to operate effectively.

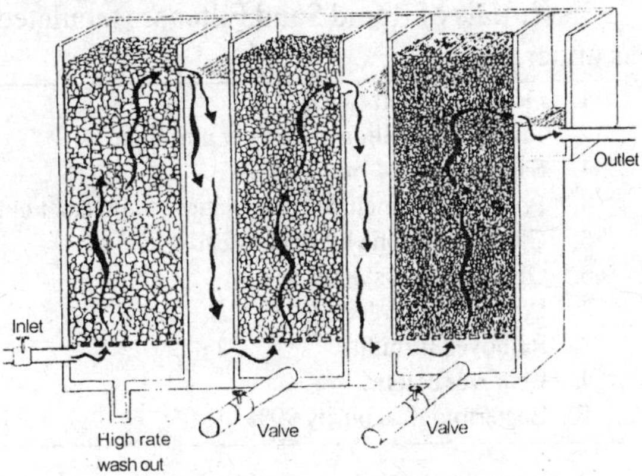

Fig. 8.16: Vertical upflow gravel prefilter

Slow Sand Filtration:

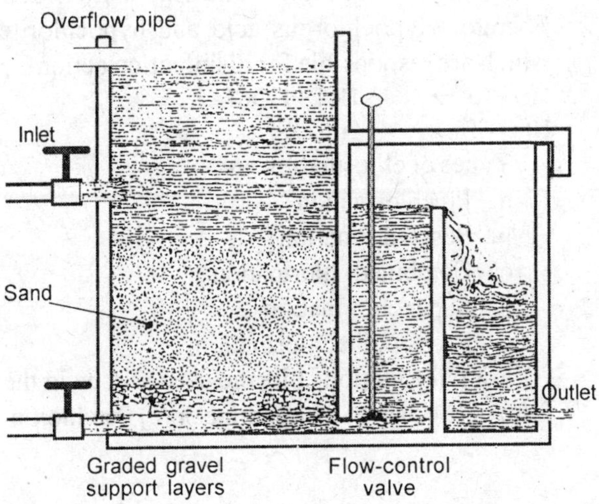

Fig. 8.17: Slow sand filter

Slow sand filtration improves physical, chemical and microbiological quality of water. It is reliable and less expensive and is therefore particularly useful in small community water supplies. The Biological layer (it is also called vital layer or Zoogleal layer or schmutzdecke) is made of algae, plankton diatoms and bacteria which are responsible for removal of organic matter and oxidize ammoniacal nitrogen.

Essentials of slow sand filtration are tabulated as under:

Table 8.8: Essentials of slow sand filter

1.	Occupies large area
2.	Rate of filtration is 3 million gallons per acre per day
3.	Effective sand size is 0.3 mm.
4.	Pre-filtration is plain sedimentation
5.	Washing of bed is by scraping
6.	Operation is not skilled work
7.	Loss of head allowed 4 feet
8.	Turbidity is removed
9.	Colour is removed.
10.	100 percent bacterial purity (99.9%)

Elements of slow sand filtration are outlined in Figure 6.18:

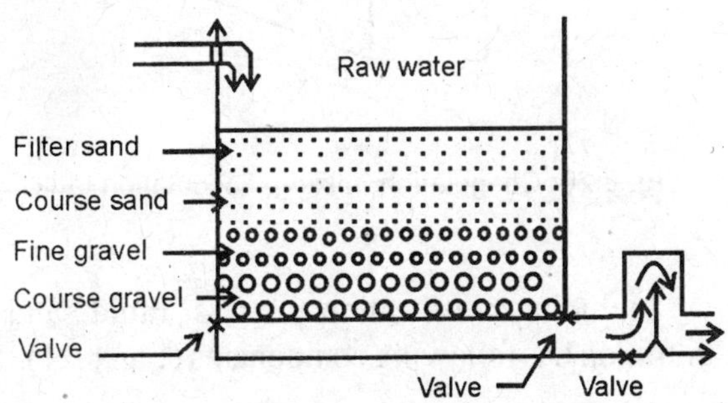

Fig. 8.18: Element of slow sand filter

Loss of head is, resistance offered by sand, in due course of time of filtration, which needs periodic cleaning.

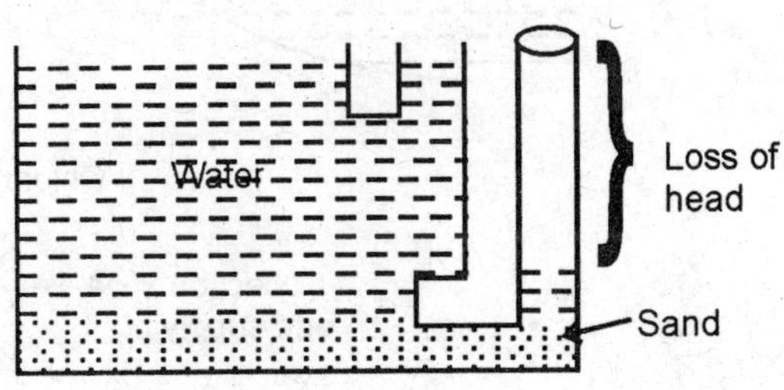

Fig. 8.19: Loss of head

Rapid Sand Filtration:

There are two types of Rapid Filters. Paterson Filter acts on the gravity and cand's filter acts on the pressure. Before filtration or prefiltration, coagulation is allowed in rapid filtration which takes off suspended impurities.

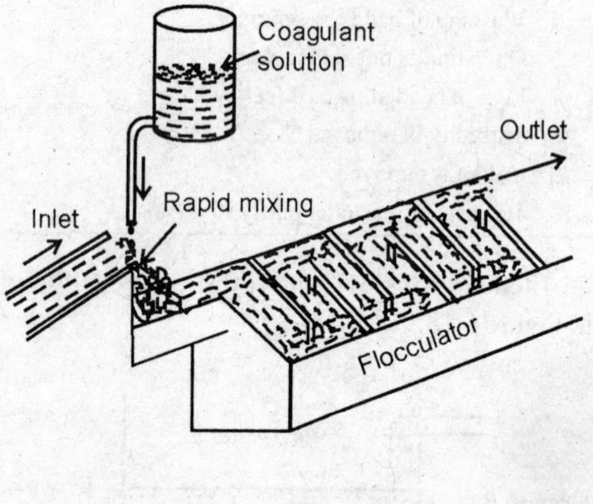

Fig. 8.20: Coagulation, mixing, flocculation tank

Including prefiltration process, rapid sand filtration has following components (Fig. 8.21).

Essentials of Rapid Sand Filter are tabulated as under:

1. Occupies small space.
2. Filters 200 million gallon per unit filter.
3. Sand size is 0.4 mm.
4. Pre-filtration includes coagulation, sedimentation.
5. Cleaning is done by Back wash.
6. Operation is a skilled one.
7. Loss of head 6 feet.
8. Removes turbidity.
9. Removes colour.
10. Bacteriological purity 99%

(ii) Chlorination:

Chlorine is used in water purification as a supplement to sand filtration. It kills bacteria, Oxidises minerals, reduces bad odor and prevent green algae-formation. Chlorine with water liberates Hypochlorous acid and hypochlorite which are responsible for disinfection action.

HO + Cl → HCl + HOCl

$H^2 O Cl^2$ → H + OCl

Types of chlorination are:

a. Prechlorination
b. Post chlorination
c. Combined chlorination
d. Super chlorination
e. Break point chlorination

For chlorination chlorine used will be in the form of (a) Gas (b) Chloramine or (c) Perchloron.

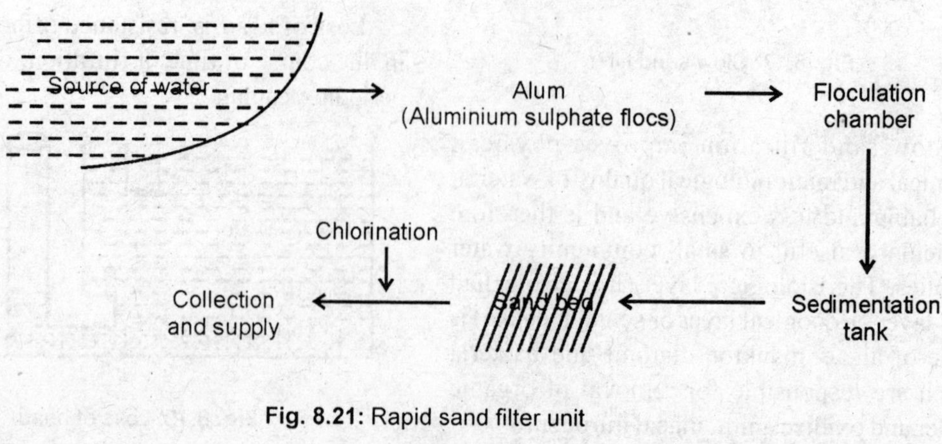

Fig. 8.21: Rapid sand filter unit

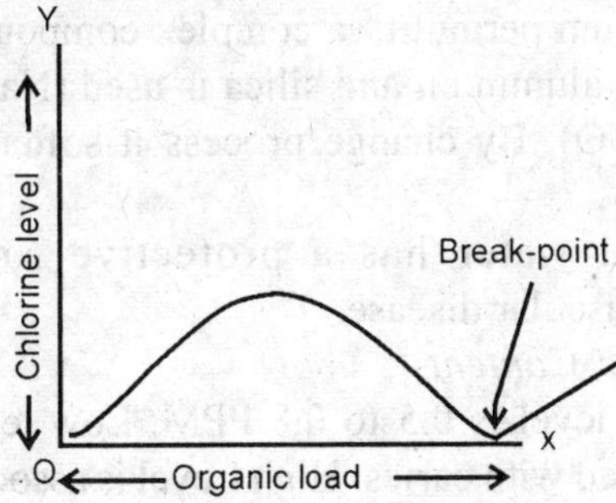

Fig. 8.22: Break point chlorination

Figure illustrates that chlorine added kills bacteria and oxidize organic material. A point where no bacteria, no organic matter and no chlorination are traceable is called Breakpoint (a misnomer) after which free chlorine starts appearing in water.

Principles of Chlorination:

1. Water must be clean and not turbid.
2. Chlorine demand is found out.
3. Contact period of 1 hour is allowed (minimum 30 minutes).
4. Residual chlorine of 0.5 mg/litre after 1 hour contact period is allowed.

Guidelines for Drinking Water Quality:

I. *Acceptability*
 a. Physical
  i. Should not be turbid
  ii. Should not have colour
  iii. No bad smell or taste
  iv. Should be cool.
 b. *Inorganic*
  i. Chloride less than 600 PPM
  ii. Hardness below 500PPM
  iii. Ammonia below 0.2 PPM
  iv. pH between 6.5 – 8.5
  v. H_2S below 0.05 PPM
  vi. Iron below 0.3 PPM
  vi. Sodium below 200PPM
  viii. Sulphate below 250PPM
  ix. TDS (Total dissolved solid) below 600 PPM
  vii. Zinc below 0.1 PPM
  xi. Manganese below 0.1 PPM
  x. Dissolved O_2 (level for not to cause bad odour)
  xi. Copper below 1 PPM
  xii. Aluminium below 0.2 PPM.

II. *Microbiological:*
 a. Coliform organisms are tested by Multiple tube method. They should be less than 10 MPN (Most Probable Number) per 100 ml.

Table 8.9: Minimum samples for water test

Population	*No. of monthly sample*
< 5000	1
5000-100,000	1 per 5000 population
>100,000	1 per 10,000 population + 10 additional sample

Bacteriological standards laid down are:

- In 95% sample no coliform should be seen
- No E.coli in any sample in 100 ml
- MPN (Coliform) should be below 10/100 ml
- Should not be positive in two consecutive samples

 b. Virologically it must be pure
 c. Biologically no organism should be present.

III. *Chemical Aspect:*
 Following upper limit are fixed for criteria under potable water (all ppm):

Arsenic	0.005
Cadmium	0.003
Chromium	0.05
Cyanide	0.07
Fluoride	1.5
Lead	0.01
Mercury	0.001
Nitrate (No_3)	50

Nitrite (No_2)	Zero
Benzene	10

IV. *Radiological Aspect:*

α Radioactivity below 0.1 Bq/L

β Radioactivity below 1.0 Bq/L.

Surveillance of water supply to the community should have following measures:

i. Check at new source of water
ii. Water source is protected
iii. Sanitary survey carried out
iv. Sampling done properly as per specifications
v. Bacteriological surveillance includes:
   a. PCT (Presumptive coliform test)
   b. Detection of faecal contamination
   c. Colony count
   d. Biological examination
vi. Chemical surveillance is done.

Hardness of Water

Temporary hardness is due to bicarbonates and permanent hardness is due to sulphates and chlorides. Soft water has less than 1 mEq/ Litre of hardness whereas very hard water has over 6 mEq /Litre of hardness. Hardness cause:

a. More soap usage
b. Scaling of boilers
c. Fabrics do not last longer
d. Not suitable for industries.

Removal of hardness is as under:

i. Boiling (for temporary hardness):
   $Ca(HCO_3)_2 \rightarrow CaCO_3 + H_2O + CO_2$
ii. Addition of lime (for temporary hardness):
   $Ca\ (OH)_2 + Ca(HCO_3) \rightarrow 2\ CACO_3 + 2\ H_2O$
iii. Addition of sodium carbonate (for both temporary and permanent hardness):
iv. $Na_2CO_3 + Ca(HCO_3)_2 \rightarrow 2\ NaHCO_3 + CaCO_3$
v. $CaSO_4 + Na_2CO_3 \rightarrow CaCO_3 + Na_2SO_4$
iv. Base exchange process:

Sodium permutit, a complex compound of sodium, aluminum and silica is used ($Na_2\ Al_2\ Si_2O\ H_2O$). By change process it softens the water.

Hard water has a protective role in cardiovascular disease.

Fluorine Content:

Normal level is 0.5 to 0.8 PPM. Low level is associated with caries. High Level is associated with fluorosis.

Swimming Pool Sanitation

Health hazards associated with swimming pool are:

- Fungal infection of skin
- Warts
- Eye, Ear, Nose, Throat infection
- Respiratory infection
- Intestinal infection
- Accidents.

Preventive Measures:

i. Rules and regulation for personal hygiene is formed.
ii. Everyday 15% of water is replaced.
iii. Chlorination and maintenance of Residual chlorine 1 PPM is advocated.

Health Education

It includes convincing felt need of protected water and for giving up unhygienic practices.

National Water Supply and Sanitation Programme

It was started in 1954. In 1972 it envisaged Accelerated Rural Water Supply Programme. Government identified problem villages (no water within distance of 1.6 km and at depth of 15 meters) for assistance. A norm of water supply of 40 litres per head per day and one hand pump for every 250 population was planned. Current status is that 85% of population are getting safe water supply.

A community level participatory programme called *Swajaldhara* was launched in 2002. *Swajaldhara I* at *Panchayat* level and *Swajaldhara II* at district level help to manage water supply and sanitation including conservation measures.

Waste Disposal

Health hazards due to improper disposal of waste are known and its need is to be understood by nursing professionals. They are called upon to give advice on some occasion.

Solid Waste

This depends on life style, living standard, urbanization and industrialisation. Per head solid waste produced on an average works out to be 1.0 to 2.0 kg per day. Vector borne diseases will increase with the accumulation of solid waste material. Sanitary disposal of waste is a must for positive health. Following sequence follows which can lead to diseases if dumping is done:

- Ferments and decomposes
- Fly breeding
- Vector borne disease occur
- Water pollution
- Soil pollution
- Aesthetic point of view.

Terms used:

Garbage – Fruit and vegetable waste
Rubbish – Paper, plastic, wood, metal, old container, glass pieces, bricks, pipes, sludge and solid of domestic waste
Ash – Burnt material in powder form
Storage – by waste bin, plastic bin etc.
Collection – House to house collection by cart, truck, corporation van etc.

Sanitary Methods of Disposal

a. *Urban Area:*

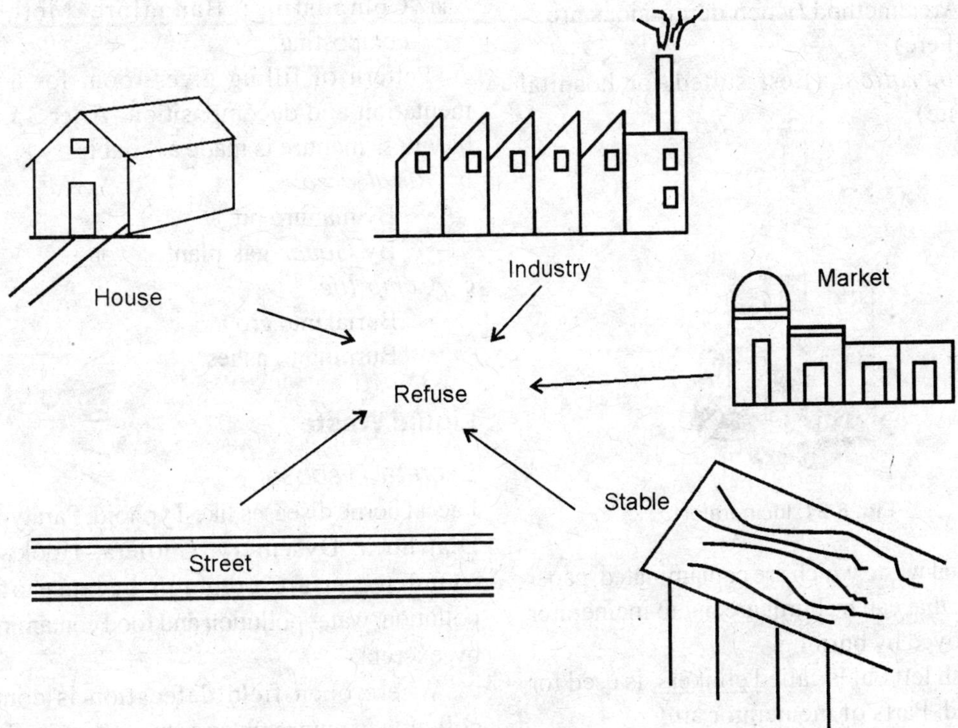

Fig. 8.23: Sources of refuse

i. Controlled tipping on sanitary landfill

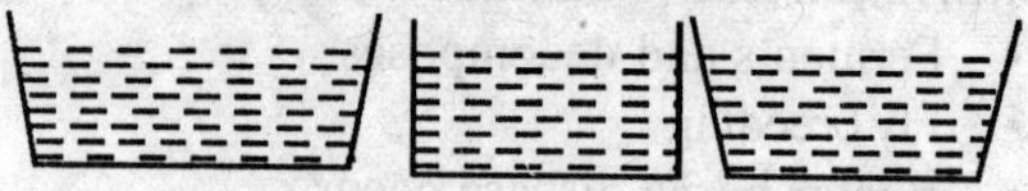

(Raised temperature at 60°C kills pathogens)

- Trench method (when land is available)

1 acre per 10,000 population is sufficient.

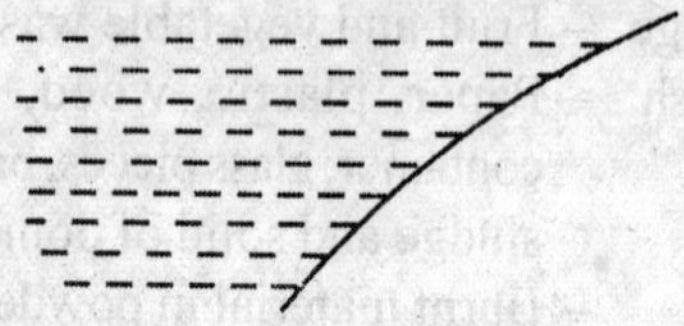

Trench at 9 meter width and 3 meter height works out better.

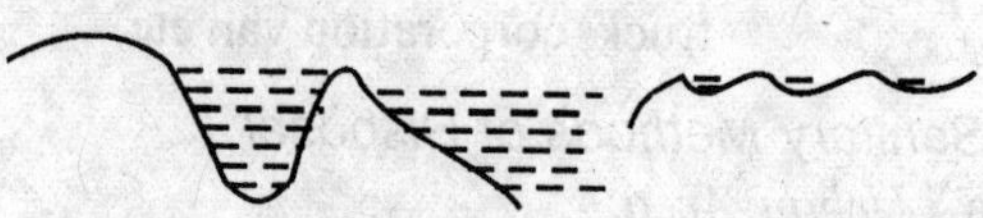

- Ramp method (when slope is there)
- Area method (when depressions are there)

ii. *Incineration:* (Best suited for hospital waste)

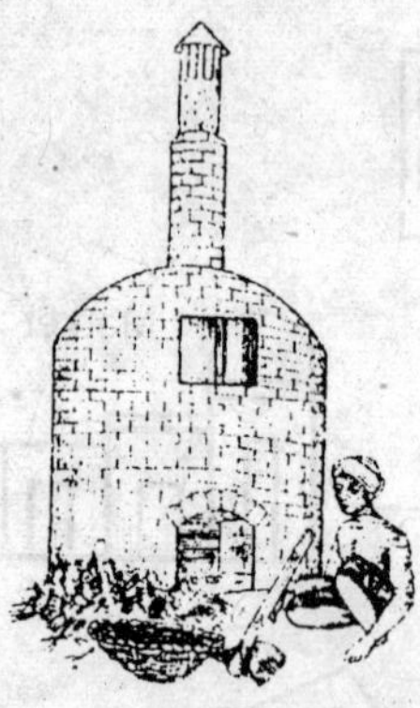

Fig. 8.24: Incinerator

Hospital waste which are contaminated, paper and waste that can be burnt are put to incinerator and destroyed by burning.

The ash left out is called <u>clinkers</u>, is used for metal road. Parts of incinerator are:

- Furnace built fire proof
- Platform for tipping refuse
- Stoker for raking refuse to fire
- Baffle plate to drive fumes to chimney.

Common pattern of incinerators are:

- Double cell meldrum type.
- Single cell horsfall destructor type.

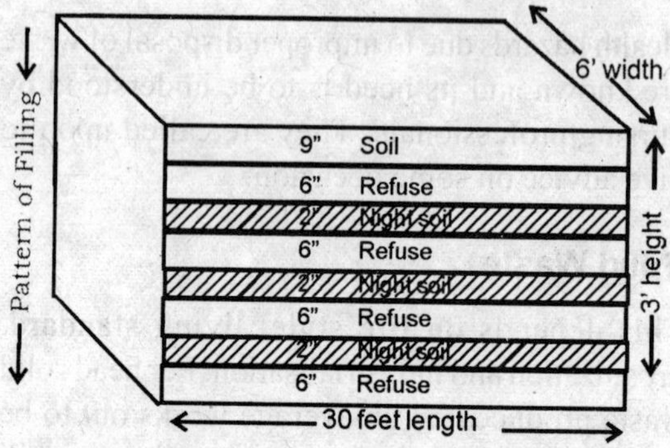

Fig. 8.25: Dimensions of excavation, pattern of filling in Bangalore method of composting

iii. Composting: Bangalore Method of composting.

Pattern of filling gives room for hot fermentation and decomposition. After 3 months harmless manure is made available:

b. *Rural area:*
   - By manure pit
   - By *Gobar* gas plant.

c. *Camp life:*
   - Burial into ground.
   - Burning to ashes.

Liquid Waste

Excreta Disposal

Faecal borne diseases like Typhoid, Paratyphoid, Diarrhoea, Dysentery, Cholera, Hookworm, round worm are common because of soil pollution, water pollution and food contamination by excreta.

Where open field defecation is common pollution of environment is the outcome, Enteric fever and hookworm anaemia is highest in their prevalence.

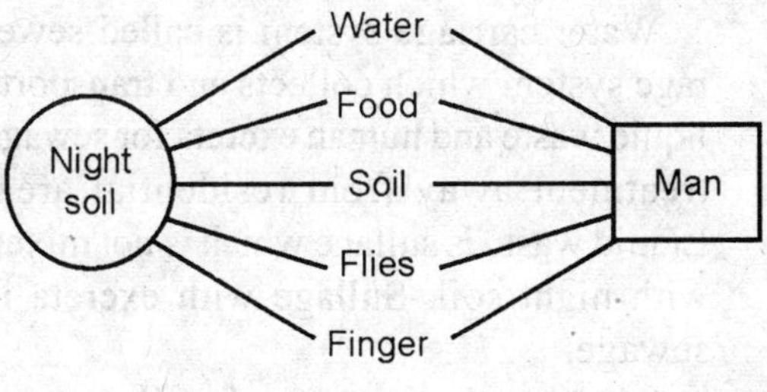

Fig. 8.26: Faecal borne disease transmission

i. *Bore hole latrine:*

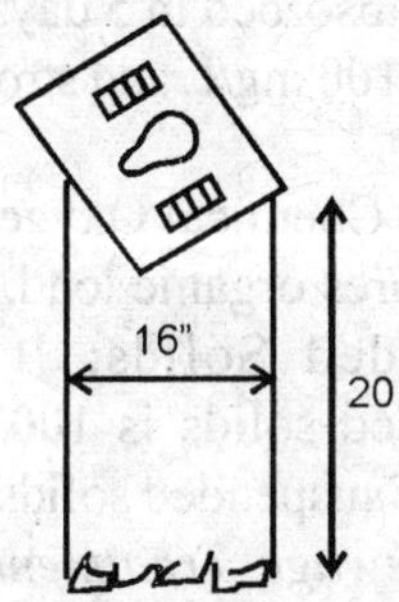

Fig. 8.27: Bore hole latrine

ii. *Dug well latrine:*

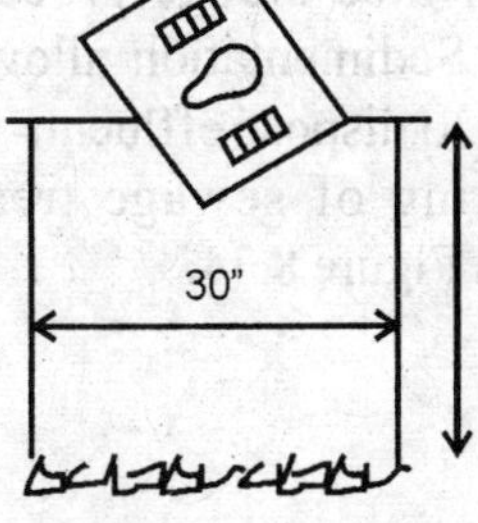

Fig. 8.28: Dug well latrine

iii. *R.C.A. latrine (Research-cum-action):*

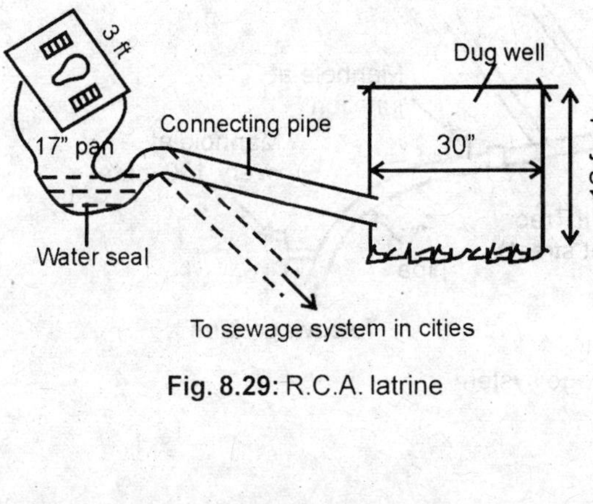

Fig. 8.29: R.C.A. latrine

iv. *Sulabha shouchalaya*:
It is found by *sulabha* organisation of Dr. Bindeshwar Pathak to provide clean toilet facility to public on small payment. Amount collected is used for maintenance of *sulabha souchalaya.*
This is an improved version of RCA latrine at low cost is a model. Construction and maintenance through charging Rs. 1.00 for the users has maintained it to be a sanitary latrine. It is very useful in slums and is adapted in many pars of India as sanitary facility to the country.

v. *Septic tank:*

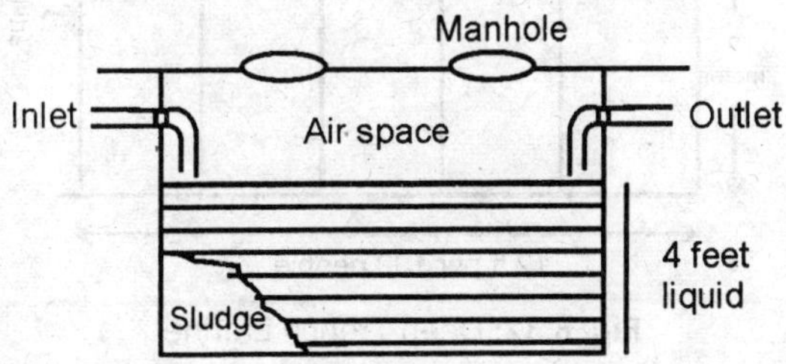

Fig. 8.30: Septic tank

Latrine is connected to septic tank when there is no sewerage system. Capacity is 500 gallons. Retention period is 24 hours. Sludge undergoes anaerobic digestion, scum undergoes aerobic digestion. It is the best economical and commonly used sanitary method of disposal of sewage.

vi. *Aqua privy:*
This is also same as septic tank but on a smaller scale. One cubic meter size is sufficient for a family of 4 members for 5 years.

For camp life

- Shallow trench latrine for short duration camp (Fig. 8.31).
- Deep trench latrine for long duration camp (Fig. 8.32).

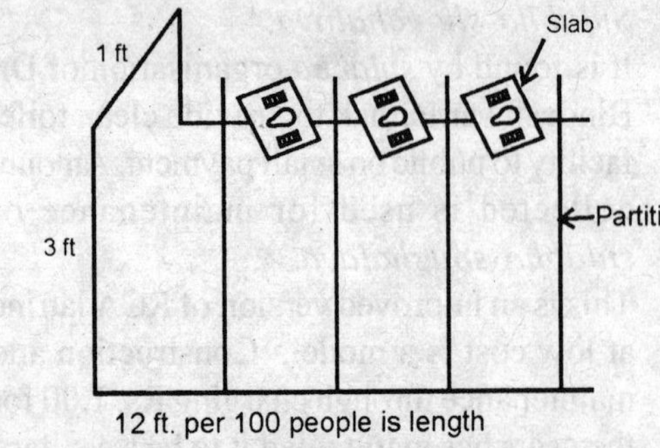

Fig. 8.31: Shallow trench latrine

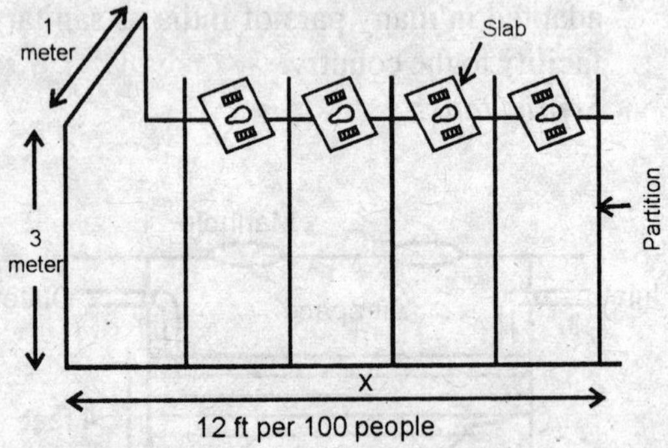

Fig. 8.32: Deep Trench Latrine

When Sewerage System is Available

i. *Water Carriage System:*

Water carriage system is called sewerage system which collects and transports liquid waste and human excreta for sewage treatment away from residential area. Liquid waste is sullage which is not mixed with night soil. Sullage with excreta is sewage.

Sanitary indicators of sullage and sewage:

i. B.O.D. (Biological Oxygen Demand): It is O_2 absorbed in 5 days at 20°C. it is weak at 100 mg/L and strong at 300 mg/L.
ii. C.O.D. (Chemical Oxygen Demand): It measures organic load.
iii. Suspended Solids: It is weak if suspended solids is 100 mg/L and is strong if suspended solids is 500 mg/L

ii. *Modern Sewage Treatment:*

Liquid waste from sewerage is screened and sedimented. Later it is subjected for aerobic oxidation either by Trickling Filter or by Activated sludge process. Later, secondary Sedimentation allows to treat sludge and to dispose effluent.

The working of sewage treatment is depicted in Figure 8.34.

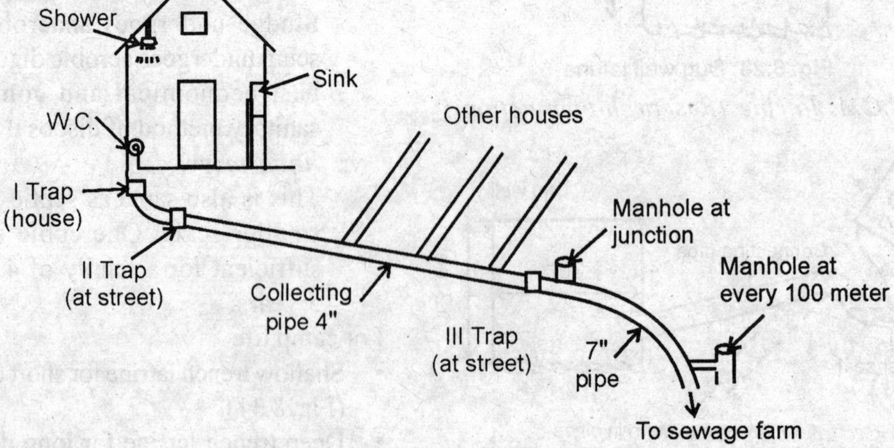

Fig . 8.33: Water carriage system

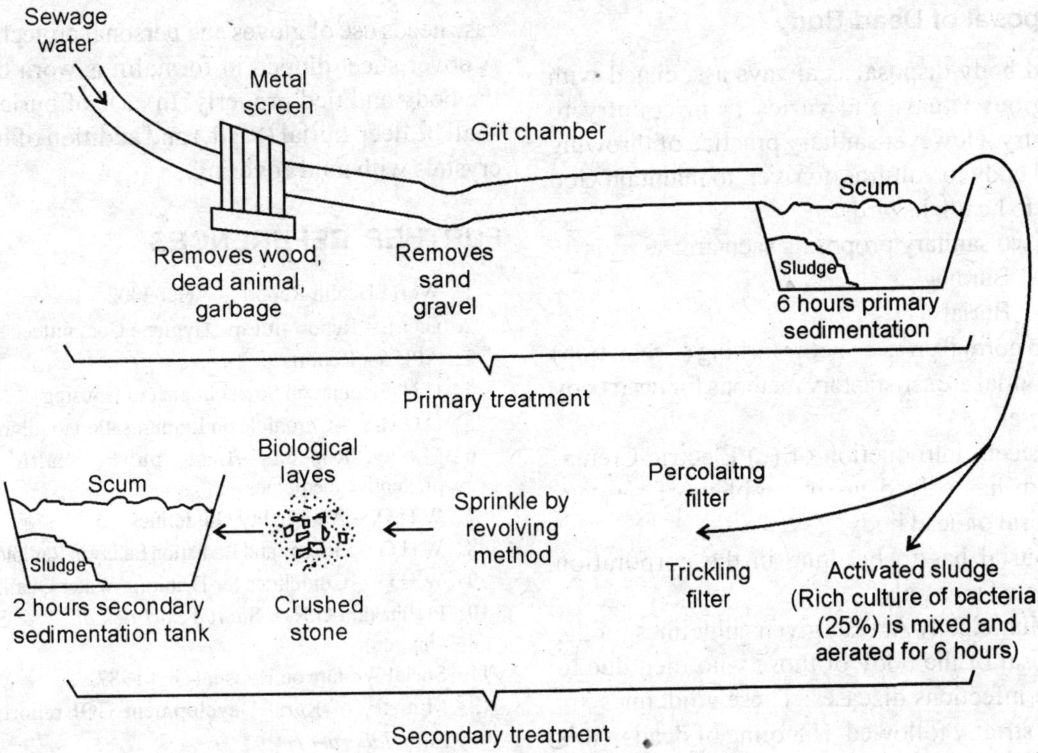

Fig. 8.34: Modern sewage treatment

iii. *Oxidation Pond:*

This is an open pool containing liquid waste and sewage which undergoes both aerobic digestion and anaerobic digestion which take place at the outskirt of a town. In Bhilai first experiment of oxidation pond by public engineers was successful for a population of 1 lakh.

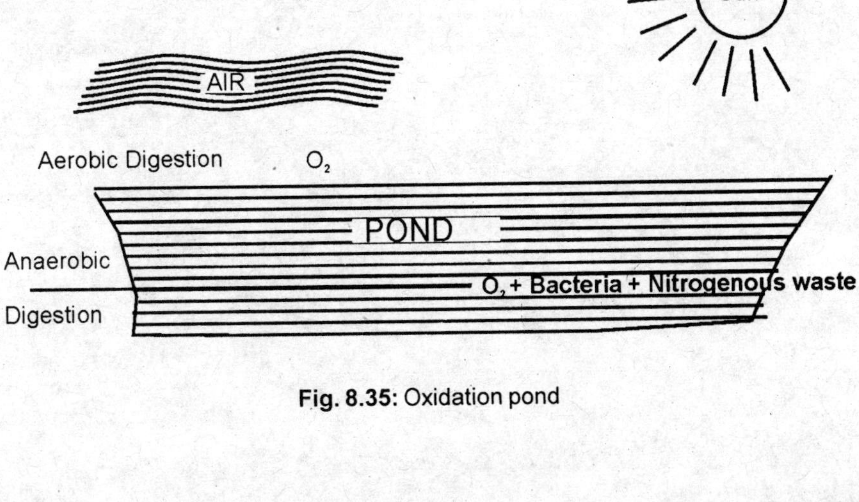

Fig. 8.35: Oxidation pond

Disposal of Dead Body

Dead body disposal is always associated with religious rituals and varies from country to country. However sanitary practice of throwing dead body to vultures, to river, to maintain God lead to health hazards.

Two sanitary proposals seen are:

a. Burning

b. Burial.

In normal process both Burning (Cremation) and Burial are satisfactory methods for dead body disposal.

Recent introduction of (c) Electric Crematorium has solved urban problem of sanitary disposal of dead body.

Burial has to be done in the corporation allocated area only.

Municipally Act has given guidelines for the disposal of the body of those who died due to acute infections diseases. These guidelines are to be strictly followed. Handling of dead in this case needs use of gloves and personal protection. A cover sheet dipped in formalin is worn over the body and tied properly. In case of burial, it shall be deep burial (> 3ft.) and addition of lime crystals with mud covering.

FURTHER REFERENCES

1. World Health Report – WHO 2002.
2. G.O.I. – Report of Env. Hygiene Committee.
3. APHA– Reports.
4. U.N. Seminar on Social Impact of Housing.
5. D.G.H.S. – Chronicle on Immunisation to pilgrims
6. Maxcy, Rosenau—Last—public health and preventive medicine.
7. W.H.O. – Air Quality Guidelines.
8. W.H.O. – Efficacy and Radiation Safety in Radiology.
9. W.H.O. – Guidelines for Drinking Water Quality.
10. Prabhakara G.N. – Short Text Book of P & S M (Jaypee).
11. Social Welfare on Housing GOI 1987.
12. Ministry of Rural Development GOI report on *Swajaldhara.*

9

Medical Entomology

IMPORTANCE

Insects, arachnids, crustaceans and other arthropods cause pathological conditions in man, which are known from the time of Old Testament (Exodus 8:24) which described grievous swarm of flies and in sixth century when *Sushruta* recorded filaria infection. The science is directly concerned with the biology and control of offending arthropods and with the recognition of the damage they cause. All of them are related to individual health as well as group health. The field of entomology made a good appearance after 1910. Greatest entomological discoveries on record are:

- Plague
- Malaria
- Yellow fever
- Typhus.

Experiencing disease, human death and search for survival gave great impetus to the subject and we started to know about vectors on these lines – How they live? How they carry disease? How they are classified? What is the biology? and How they may be destroyed?

In 1874 Othmar Zeidler synthesized DDT in Germany and its value was shown by Paul Muller in 1939 in Switzerland.

Scope

The subject helps us to understand morphology, life cycle, bionomics, disease transmitted and control measures. Both medical and public health importance are proved beyond doubt.

HEALTH PROBLEM

In day to day patient care and nursing care we come across umpteen number of vector borne (arthropod borne) diseases. Malaria, Filaria, Brain Fever, Dengue Fever, Typhoid, Diarrhoea, Typhus, Plague, Monkey Fever, Scabies and Guineaworm infection are very common diseases in Nursing care services. All the vectors are (colloquially) called "Insects" whose population in 1 square mile is equal to human population in the world. This identifies the area of importance around us. Millions of people are getting diseases through the bite of insects. Severe malaria is causing deaths; filaria and Brain fever is incapacitating people. Trachoma is causing preventable blindness.

CLASSIFICATION

Group	*Example*	*Characters*
1. Crustaceans	Cyclops	Head Thorax joined, 5 pair legs 2 pair antennae, No wings, Live in water
2. Arachnida	Ticks Mites	No body division 4 pair legs, No Antennae, No Wings, Live on Land
3. Insecta	Mosquito Flies Lice Flea	Head, Thorax, abdomen are seen, 3 pair legs, Antennae 1 pair, some have wings, Live on land

MODE OF TRANSMISSION

Direct Contact

Transfer of arthropod from man to man occurs. For example in scabies and pediculosis disease occurs with 2 living factors. Man and arthropod (itch mite or head louse).

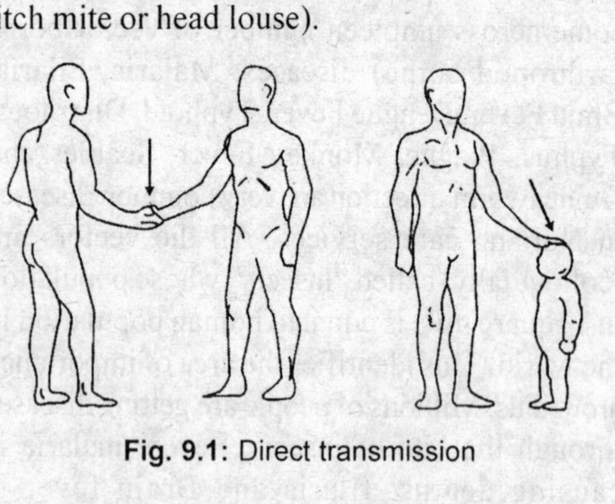

Fig. 9.1: Direct transmission

Mechanical

Mechanically parasite is transferred by arthropod to a man. Examples are diarrhoea, dysentery, typhoid, food poisoning and Trachoma. Here, disease occurs with 3 living factors viz. Man, Arthropod (House Fly) and Parasite.

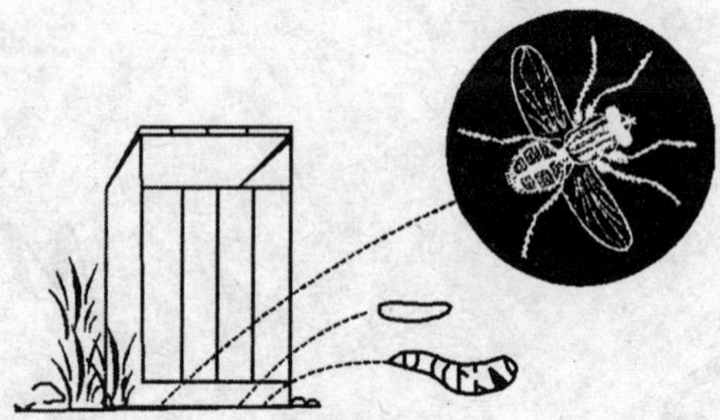

Fig. 9.2: Mechanical transmission

Biological Transmission

They are of 3 types:

i. Propagative, e.g. plague bacteria multiplies in rat flea.
ii. Cyclopropagative, e.g. malaria parasite multiplies and undergoes cyclical change in mosquito.
iii. Cyclodevelopment, e.g. filaria parasite undergoes cyclical changes in mosquito, e.g. guinea worm undergoes cyclical changes in cyclops.

Parasite is transmitted from man to man by arthropod (Mosquito bite). Examples are:

Mosquito bite	:	Malaria, yellow fever, Dengue fever, filaria
Louse bite	:	Epidemic typhus, relapsing fever
Fly bite	:	Leishmaniasis, sleeping sickness, river blindness.

Here 3 living factor play in transmission process viz, Man, vector (Mosquito, Louse etc.) and Parasite.

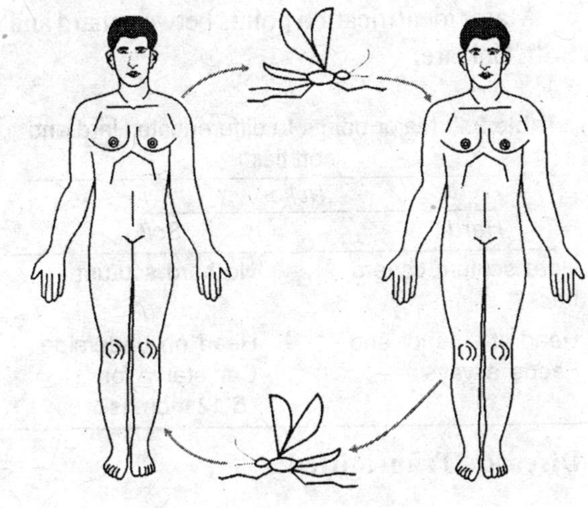

Fig. 9.3: Biological transmission

Suppose an animal reservoir play its role in transmission, biological transmission of parasite to man by arthropod (flea etc.) from animal reservoir (rat) occurs. Here 4 living factors play their role viz Man, Vector (Flea etc.) Parasite (plague bacilli etc.) and animal reservoir (rat etc.)
Examples: Plague – Rat Flea – Rat – Man
K.F.D. – Tick – Monkey – Man

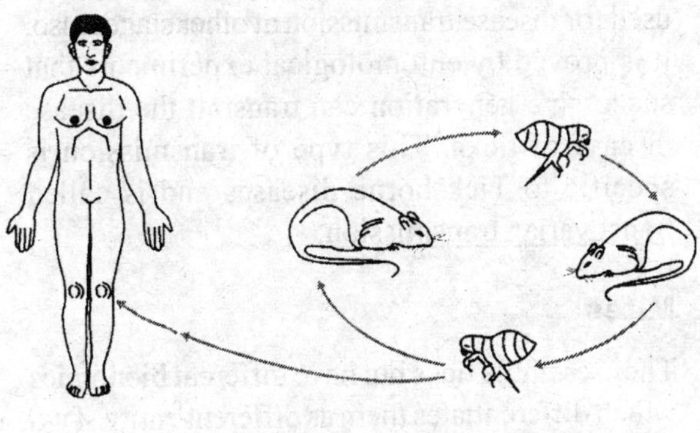

Fig. 9.4: Biological transmission where animal reservoir is seen

ARTHROPOD BORNE DISEASES

Common diseases are tabulated under transmitted or causing vector:

Table 9.1: Arthropod borne diseases

Vector	*Disease*
Cyclops	Guinea worm
Hard tick	Typhus, viral encephalitis, K.F.D.
Soft tick	Relapsing fever
Mite	Typhus
Itch mite	Scabies
Mosquito	Malaria, filaria, J.E., dengue, yellow fever
House fly	Typhoid, cholera, G.E. trachoma
Sand fly	Kalaazar, Sand fly fever
Tsetse fly	Sleeping sickness
Lice	Typhus, relapsing fever
Flea	Plague
Black fly	River blindness

VECTORS OF PUBLIC HEALTH IMPORTANCE

Cyclops

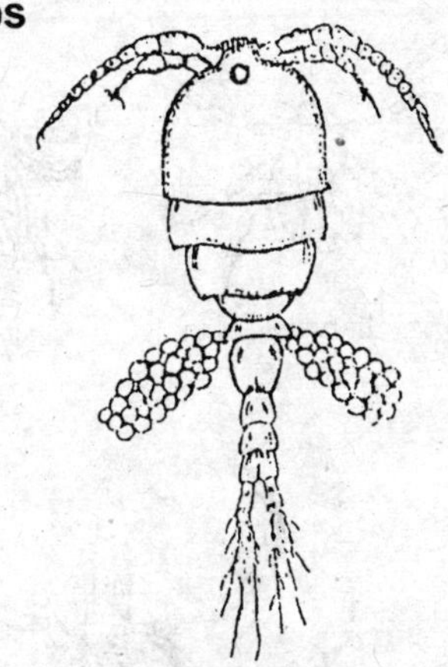

Fig. 9.5: Cyclops

Cyclops is a tiny vector of the size of a pin head. It is pear shape, body is semitransparent and the tail is forked; Pigmented eye, 5 pair legs and 2 pair antennae are present.

Diseases transmitted – Guinea worm infection (D. medinensis and Fish tape worm (D. latum) infection.

Control Measures

Physical methods:

- Straining with muslin cloth
- Boiling the water

Chemical methods:

- Bleaching powder to water (5 PPM)
- Lime (4 grams per 5 litres)
- Abate (1 PPM)

Biological method:

- Barbel fish will eat cyclops
- Gambusia fish will eat cyclops

Social method:

- Abolition of steep wells and introduce pipe water supply.

Ticks

They are of 2 kinds (a) Hard Tick (b) Soft Tick. They are oval shape, 4 pair legs, no antennae. Males are smaller. Soft tick can withstand starvation. Life cycle passes through stages of

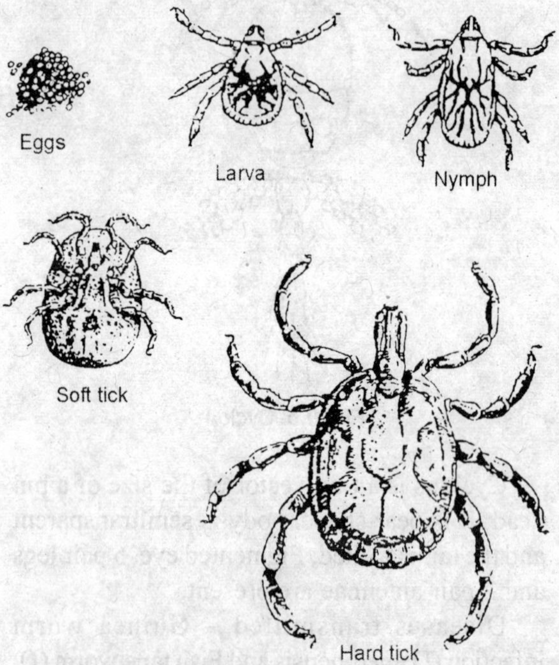

Fig. 9.6: Life cycle and morphology of ticks

Major identification points between hard and Soft Tick are:

Table 9.2: Major points to differentiate Hard and soft tick

Ticks	
Hard	*Soft*
Hard scutum covers back	No hard scutum
Head at anterior end	Head on underside
Feeds always	Can starve for 6-12 months

Diseases Transmitted:

Table 9.3: Tick borne disease

Hard Tick	*Soft Tick*
Tick Typhus	Relapsing Fever
K.F.D.	

<u>Special note on Transmission of Tick Borne Disease</u>:

Ticks suck blood and cause anaemia. They secrete a neurotoxin at bite causing local neurotoxic effect. Larva stage and nymph stage can also bite and transmit disease. Hence <u>transtagial</u> is used for disease transmission at other stages also. It is proved by entomological experiments that successive generation can transmit the disease in case of ticks. This type of transmission is specific to Tick borne diseases and is called <u>transovarian transmission</u>.

Mites

They resemble ticks but have different bionomics which differentiates them as different entity. Two forms are medically important. They are:

a. Trombiculid mite and
b. Itch mite.

Mites are spider like in their appearance. They pass through stages of egg, larva, nymph and adult. Life cycle takes about 6 weeks and life span is observed to be 6 months (Fig. 9.7).

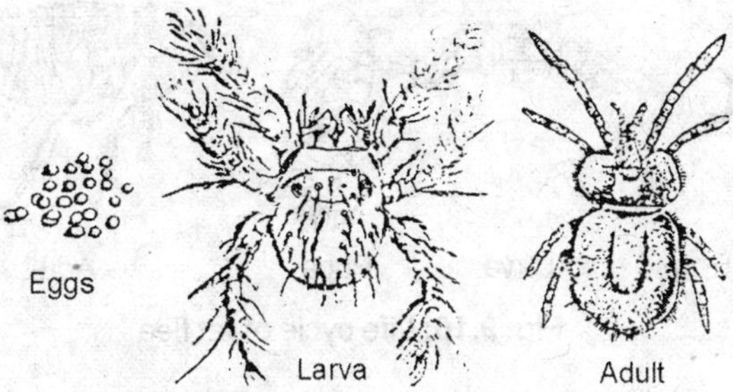

Fig. 9.7: Cycle of mite

Disease transmitted by trombiculid mite is scrub typhus.

Control measures for Ticks and mites are the same. They include:

- DDT, Lindane or Malathion at 1 pound per acre as insecticide.
- Insecticide dust on pet dogs which harbour ticks and mites.
- Abolition of crevices in residential area reduces the vector density.
- Repellents are used by workers who are exposed in areas where ticks and mites are prevailing.

Sarcoptes Scabiei (Itch Mite) (Scabies)

Scabies is one of the oldest known diseases of poor sanitation. Small globular arthropod is just visible to naked eye. Female mite burrows to epidermis, breeds in epidermis and cause intense itching; hence the name itch mite.

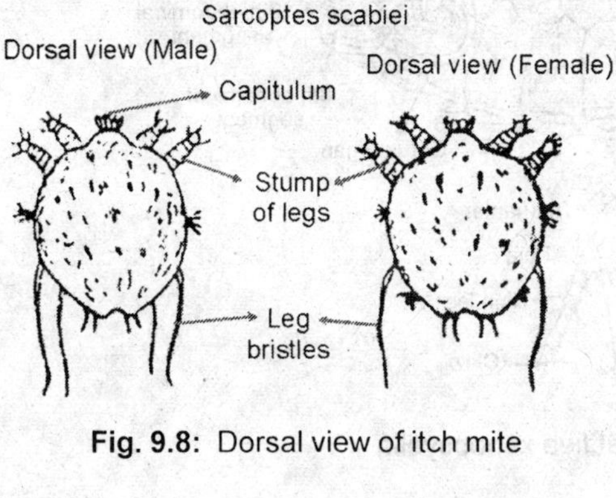

Fig. 9.8: Dorsal view of itch mite

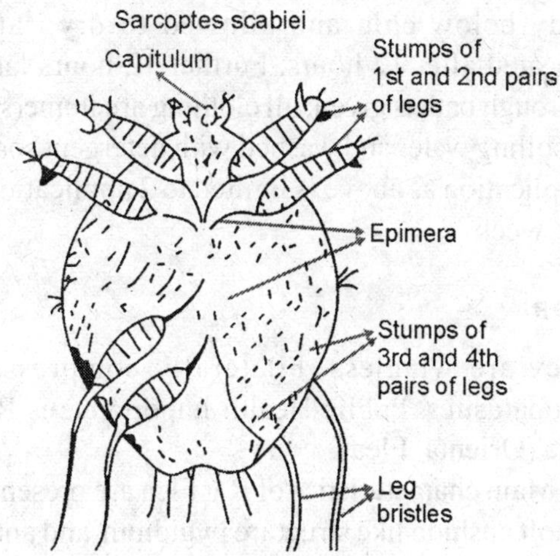

Fig. 9.9: Ventral view of itch mite

Female itch mite is differentiated when skin scrape of scabies patient is examined under microscope. It is bigger than male and has long tubular suckers in all 4 pairs of legs. Close contact and contaminated clothes spread scabies from person to person. Hands, Wrist, Elbow are common sites of scabies. Infected scabies draws patient to the hospital care than non infected scabies case. Itching, poor sanitation, secondary infection leading to pustule, other members of family are seen afflicted, are diagnostic of scabies.

Scabies Control

- All family members of family are given treatment simultaneously.
- 1.0% Lindane in any vegetable oil is a good sarcopticide, applied twice a week till cure.
- 5.0% Tetmosol application thrice a day till cure.
- 10.0% Sulphur ointment daily for 4 days is best and economical.

Specific Treatment and Nursing Care with Benzyl Benzoate (25.0%):

25% Benzyl benzoate is applied to all parts of

body below chin and allowed to dry; later repeated after 12 hours. Further 12 hours later thorough bath is given; all clothing are immersed in boiling water and washed with detergent soap. Application as above is limited to 2 applications per week.

Flea

They are wingless, bilaterally compressed ectoparasites. Public Health importance is Rat Flea (Oriental Flea).

Main characteristics of Rat Flea are presence of soft cushion like structure pygidium and ante-pygidial bristle (Fig. 9.11). Sex is differentiated by the fact that female is bigger and possesses spermatheca which is roughly shaped a (in astia) b (in braziliences) c (in cheopis).

Other types of flea are:

Human flea	–	Pulex irritants
Dog flea	–	Ptenocephalus canis
Cat flea	–	Ptenocephalus felix
Sand flea	–	Tunga penetrans

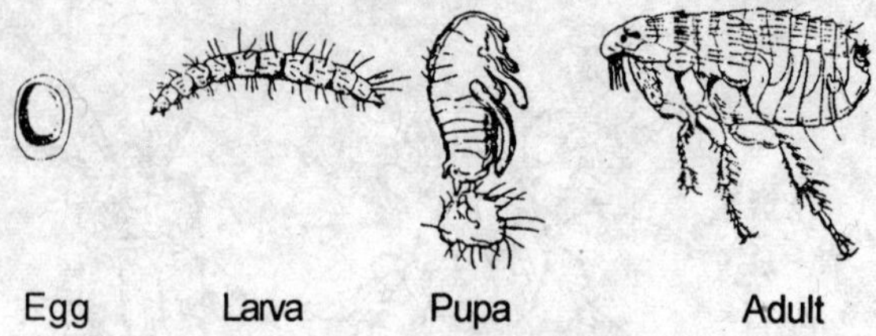

Fig. 9.10: Life cycle of rat flea

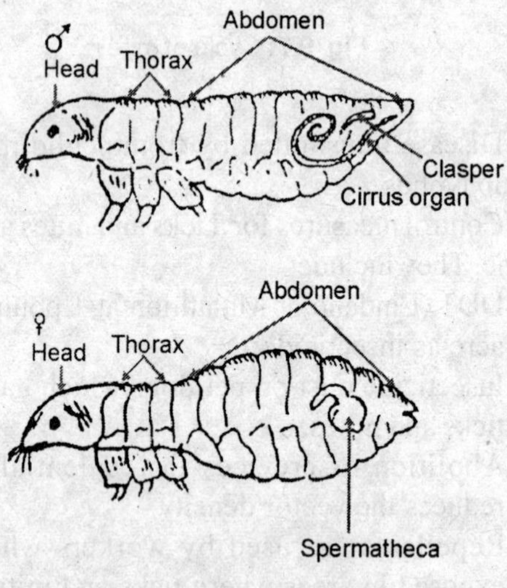

Fig. 9.12: Differentiation of sex in rat flea

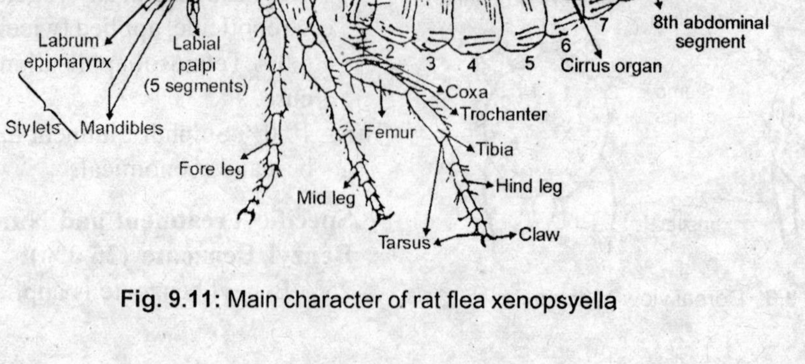

Fig. 9.11: Main character of rat flea xenopsyella

The body is divisible into head, thorax and abdomen. Life cycle passes through egg, larva, pupa and adult. Life cycle takes about 20 days to complete. Life span is about 40 days in tropical area. Infected Flea may have blocked or partially blocked ventriculus and they are dangerous in spreading plague bacilli.

Disease Transmitted:

- Plague
- Endemic typhus.

During entomological survey, following Flea indices are used:

1. General Flea index (No. of flea per rat)
2. Specific Flea index (No. of any one species per rat)
3. Percentage incidence (percentage of each species per rat)
4. Rodent infestation rate.

Control Measures:

1. Carbaryl or diazinon 2%
2. Malathion 5%
3. Rat Burrow closure with concrete
4. Use of Repellent (Diethyltoluamide)
5. Rat control measures.

Lice

They are small wingless ectoparasite of man which are dorsoventrally compressed. Head louse (pediculus capitis) and Body louse (pediculus corporis) are similar in their morphology. Pubic louse (phthirus pubis) is crab like which is not known to transmit any disease.

Morphologically body is divisible into head, thorax and abdomen. It passes through stages of egg, nymph and adult. Adult lives for about 2 months. It is transmitted from person to person by direct contact, and indirectly through cloth, bed, comb, brush etc.

Diseases transmitted by head or body louse are:

- Epidemic typhus
- Relapsing fever
- Trench fever
- Dermatitis.

Pubic louse in pubic area and in perineal region is a nuisance. Their presence is suggestive of poor personal hygiene.

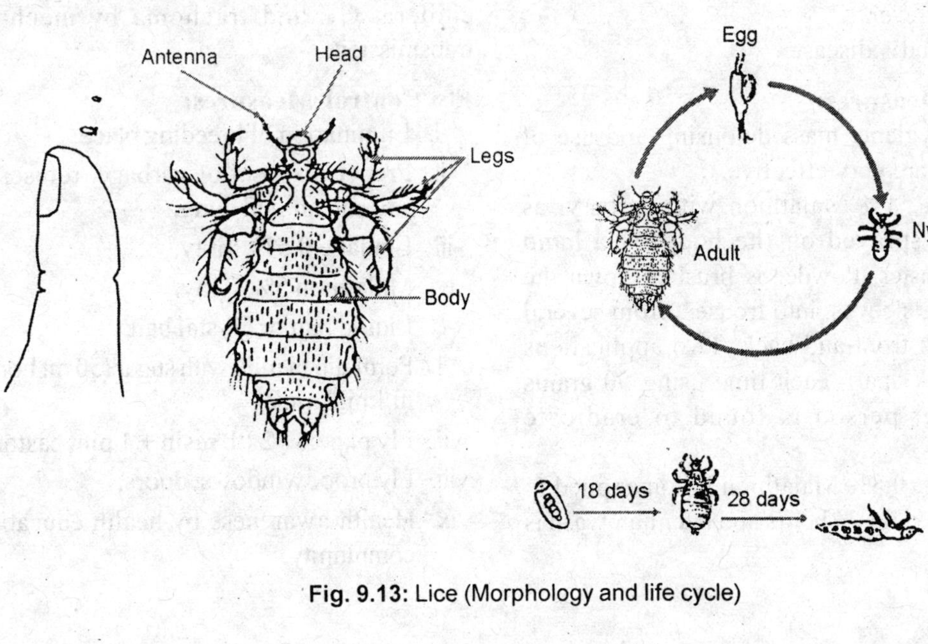

Fig. 9.13: Lice (Morphology and life cycle)

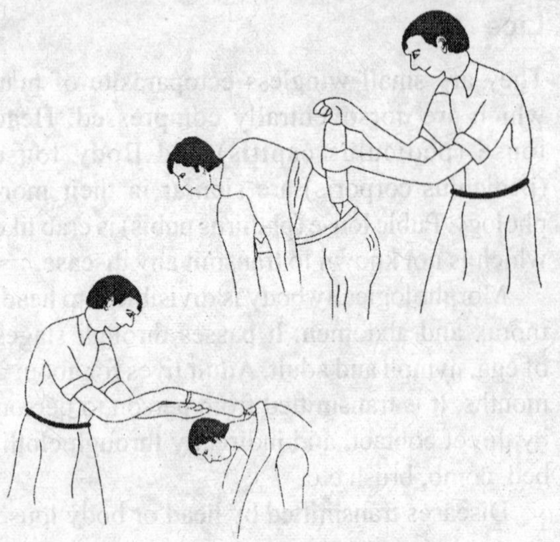

Fig. 9.14: Delousing method

Species:

- Pediculus humanus capitis (Head louse)
- Pediculus humanus corporis (Body louse)
- Phthirus pubis (Pubic louse)

Diseases transmitted by Head and Body louse:

- Epidemic typhus
- Relapsing fever
- Trench fever
- Vagabond's disease

Control Measures:

Personal hygiene, mass delousing and use of insecticide are very effective.

Body Louse: 1% Malathion with carbaryl as powder is sprayed on the body by a hand operated duster. Powder is brushed down the neck, up the sleeves, into trousers from several angles, both front and back. Two applications with 1 week apart, each time using 50 grams powder per person is found to eradicate pediculosis.

Head Louse: 0.5% Malathion lotion applied to head, allowed for 24 hours and later hair wash is given.

Flies

Flies are most common and most abundant insects found in human surroundings.

House Fly

They are nonbiting common house fly called Musca domestica. Their density is an index of poor sanitation.

It has head, thorax and abdomen, a pair of antennae, a pair of eyes, a proboscis, a pair of wings and 3 pair of legs.

Life cycle passes through stages of egg, Larva (maggot), pupa and adult. Life cycle is about a week to 10 days and life span is about 15 days

Larva infestation in wound, lesions or post injury, post operative, advanced cancer phase are great nursing care problem known as Myiasis. Daily application of irritant to remove maggots and cleaning is a cumbersome process in regular nursing care. Fly control and good sanitation and not allowing their lying eggs on wounds are both cost benefit and effective (Fig. 9.15).

They are vectors for typhoid, diarrhoea, cholera, GE and trachoma by mechanical transmission.

Fly Control Measures:

i. Elimination of breeding place.
ii. Proper disposal of garbage, refuse, night soil and animal dung.
iii. Lindane 0.5% spray.
iv. Malathion 5% spray.
v. Liquid bait or crystal bait.
vi. Formalin in milk with sugar (50 ml Formalin in 1 pint milk).
vii. Fly papers (2 Lb resin + 1 pint castor-oil).
viii. Fly proof windows, doors.
ix. Health awareness by health education of community.

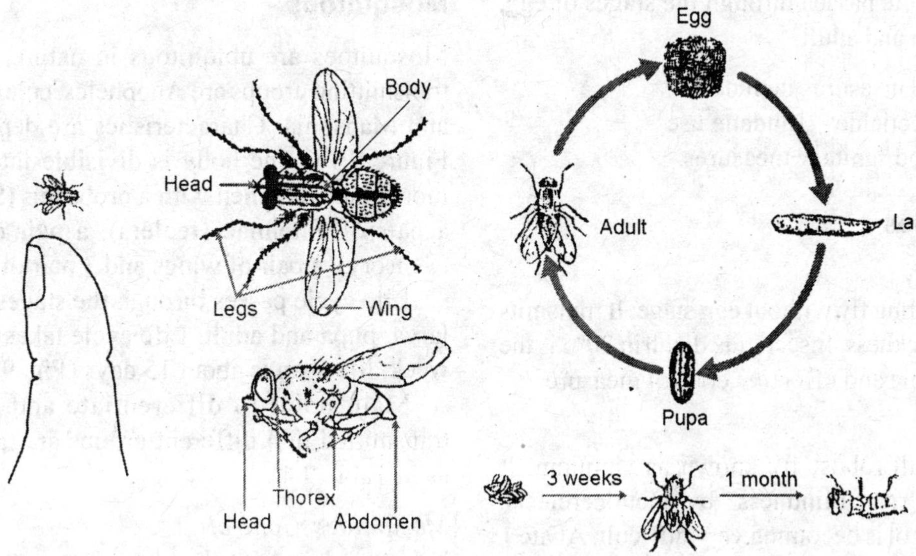

Fig. 9.15: Life cycle of house fly

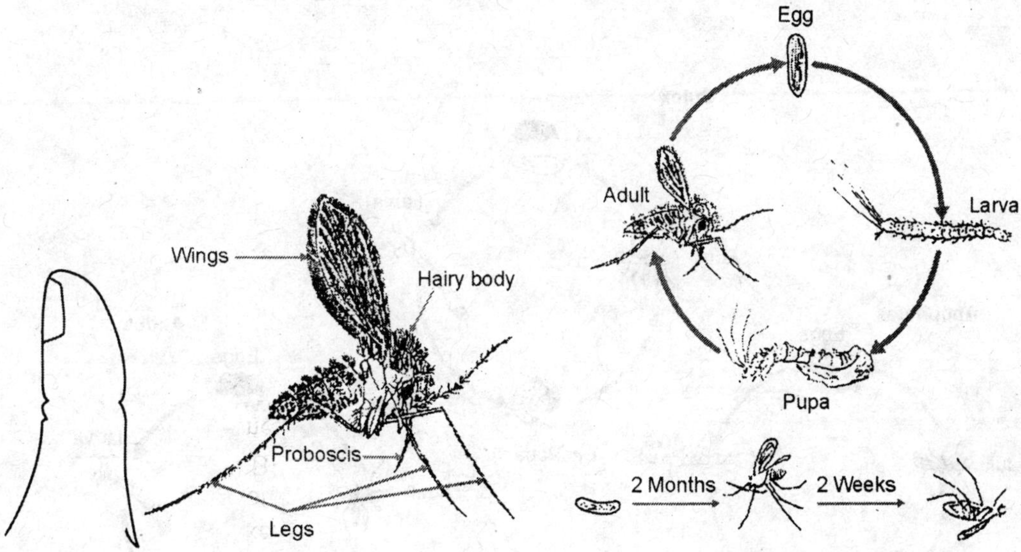

Fig. 9.16: Adult sand fly and life cycle

Sand Fly

They are smaller but visible by disproportionate legs. They are important vectors of Kalaazar, Oriental sore and sand fly fever.

They are differentiated from mosquitoes by:

- Smaller size than mosquito.
- Upright, lanceolate hairy wings.
- Long, slender out of proportion legs.

Life cycle passes through the stages of egg, larva, pupa and adult.

Control measures include:

- Insecticide – Lindane use
- Good sanitary measures.

Other Flies

Tsetse Fly

This is a biting fly without egg stage. It transmits sleeping sickness. Insecticide dieldrin 20% is the only feasible and effective control measure.

Black Fly

It is a small robust fly known as simulum. It transmits "river blindness" by onchocerciasis. Adult control is becoming very difficult. Abate 1 PPM for 10 minutes is found an effective control measure.

Mosquitoes

Mosquitoes are ubiquitous in nature, disease transmitting groups are Anopheles, culex, Aedes and Mansonia. Characteristics are depicted in Figure 9.18. The body is divisible into Head, thorax and abdomen with a proboscis (Sucker), a pair of antennae (feelers), a pair of palpi (Sensory), a pair of wings and 3 pair of legs.

Life cycle passes through the stages of egg, larva, pupa and adult. Life cycle takes about 1 week; life span is about 15 days (Fig. 9.17).

Main point to differentiate and disease transmitted in 4 different groups are tabulated as in Table 9.4.

Mosquitoes Control:

Integrated approach where more than one method is used for best result. Common measures are enumerated as under:

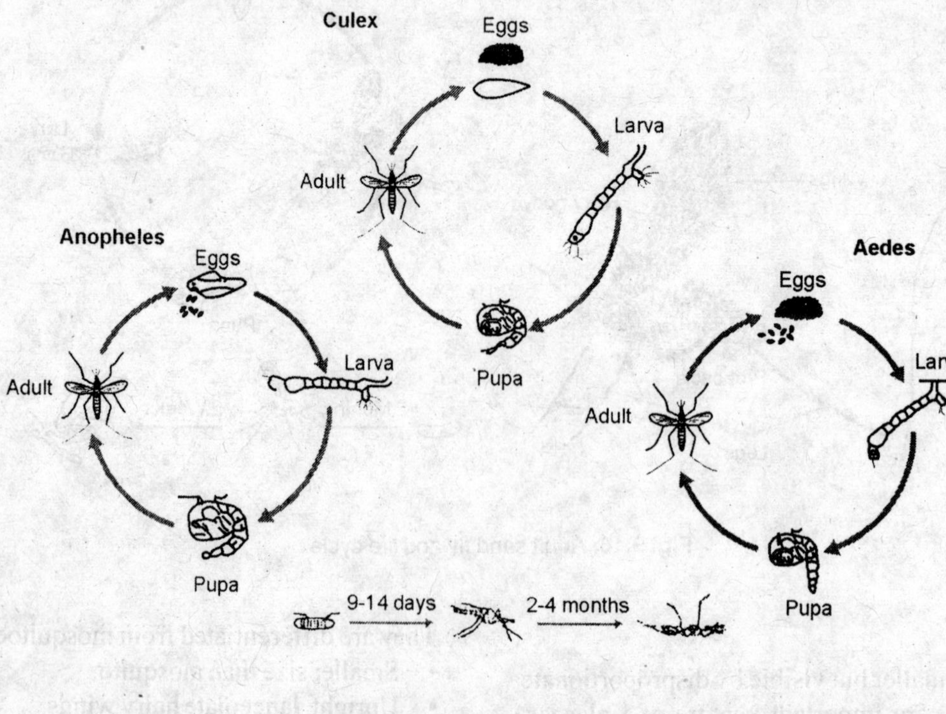

Fig. 9.17: Life cycle of mosquitoes

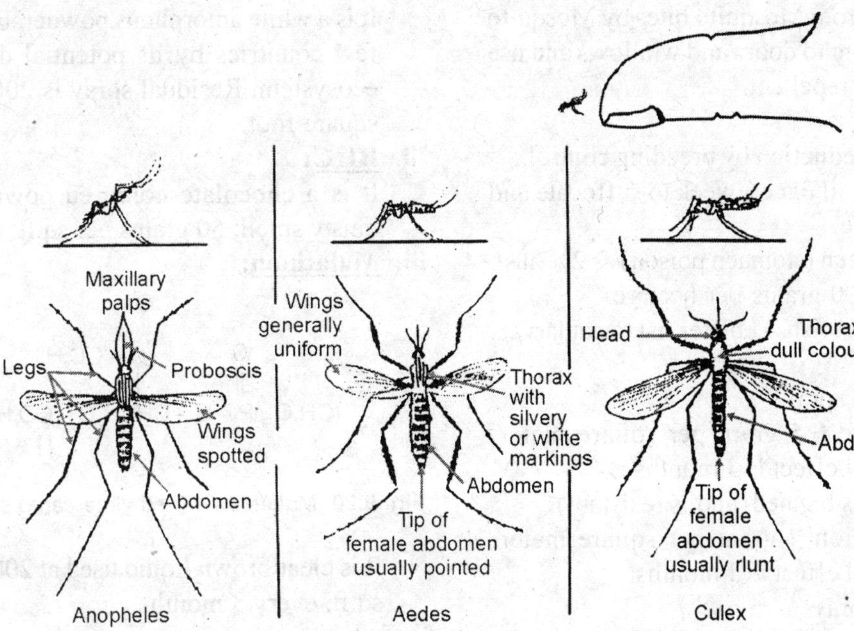

Fig. 9.18: Characteristics of different mosquitoes

Table 9.4: Differentiation and disease (mosquitoes)

	Anopheles	*Culex*	*Aedes*	*Mansonia*
Egg	Single, boat shape	Cluster, oval shape	Cluster, oval shape	Cluster, oval shape
Larva	Floats parellel Siphon tube absent Palmate hairs present	Float perpendicular Siphon tube present Palmate hairs absent	Float perpendicular Siphon tube present Palmate hairs absent	Float perpendicular Siphon tube present Palmate hairs absent
	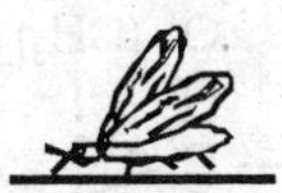	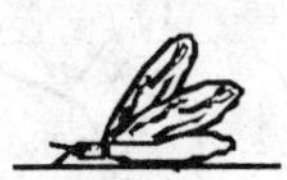	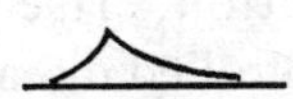	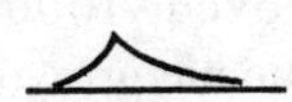
Adult Resting	No hunchback at rest	Hunch back at rest	Hunch back at rest	Hunch back at rest
	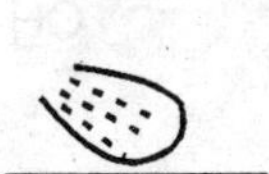	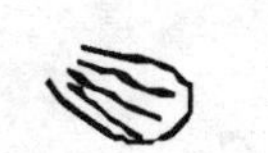		
Wing	Spotted wing	No spotted	No spotted	No spotted
	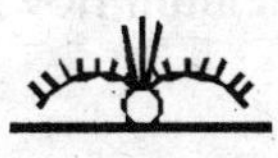	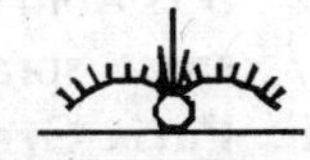	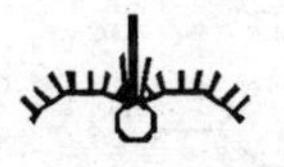	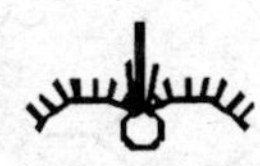
Mouth part	Long palpi female	Short palpi female	Short palpi female	Short palpi female
Disease	Malaria	Urban filaria J.E.	Dengue	Rural filaria

1. Protection from Mosquito bites by Mosquito net, screening to doors and windows and use of mosquito repellent.
2. For Larva
   a. Source reduction by breeding control.
   b. Mineral oil once a week to suffocate and kill larvae.
   c. Paris green (stomach poison) as 2% dust.
   d. Abate 100 grams per hectare.
   e. Gambusia fish, Lebister fist to eat larvae.
3. For Adult
   a. Residual spray
      i. Lindane 0.5 gram per square meter; residual effect is 3 months.
      (DDT is banned, and is resistant)
      ii. Malathion 2 gram per square meter; residual effect is 3 months
   b. Space spray
      Pyrethrum 1.02 gram per 1000 c.ft.
   c. Fogging by fenitrothion.
   d. Releasing sterile male to atmosphere is still at research phase and feasibility not sound.

INSECTICIDE

Control of insects which transmits diseases is done by insecticides. This area is an achievement of public health during 20th century. It has lead to improved food production, rise in socioeconomic growth and controlled diseases that used to cause deaths in human beings.

They are classified in figure 9.22 (see next page).

Some Common Insecticides

i. DDT

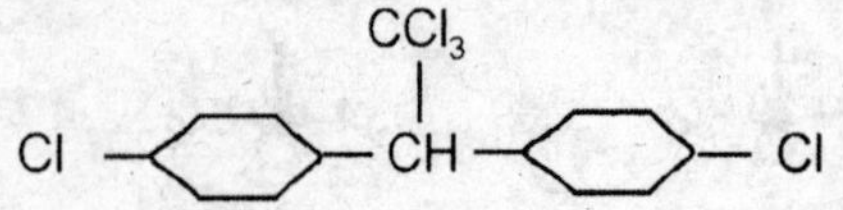

Fig. 9.19: Dichloro diphenyl trichloro ethane

It is a white amorphous powder, banned in few countries by its potential danger to ecosystem. Residual spray is 200 mg per square foot.

ii. BHC:

It is a chocolate coloured powder with musty smell; 50 grams per sq.ft. is used.

iii. Malathion:

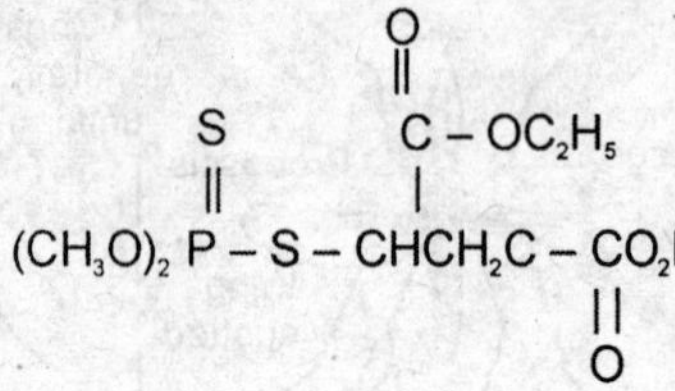

Fig. 9.20: Malathion – Diethylmercapto succinate

It is clear brown liquid used at 200 mg per sq.ft. every 3 months.

iv. Abate:

It is brown viscous liquid used at 1 PPM as larvicide.

v. Fenthion:

It is brown liquid with garlic smell; used at 100 mg per sq.ft. as larvicide.

vi. Dichlorovos:

It is used in aircraft disinfection.

vii. Pyrethrum:

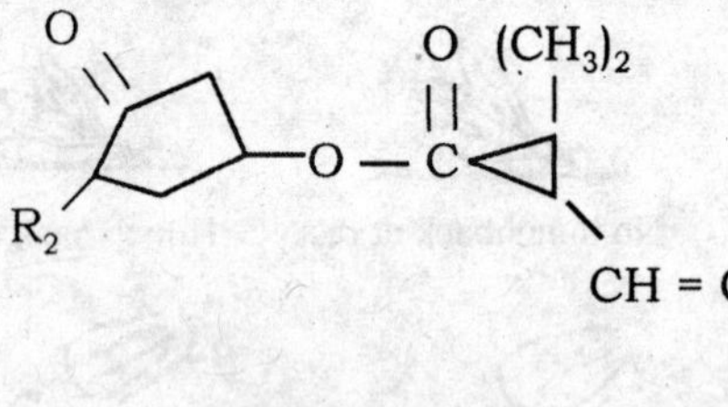

Fig. 9.21: Pyrethrum

It is from chrysanthemum flower used as space spray.

viii. Paris Green

It is copper aceto arsenite, a green powder, used at 2% dust spray for larvicide.

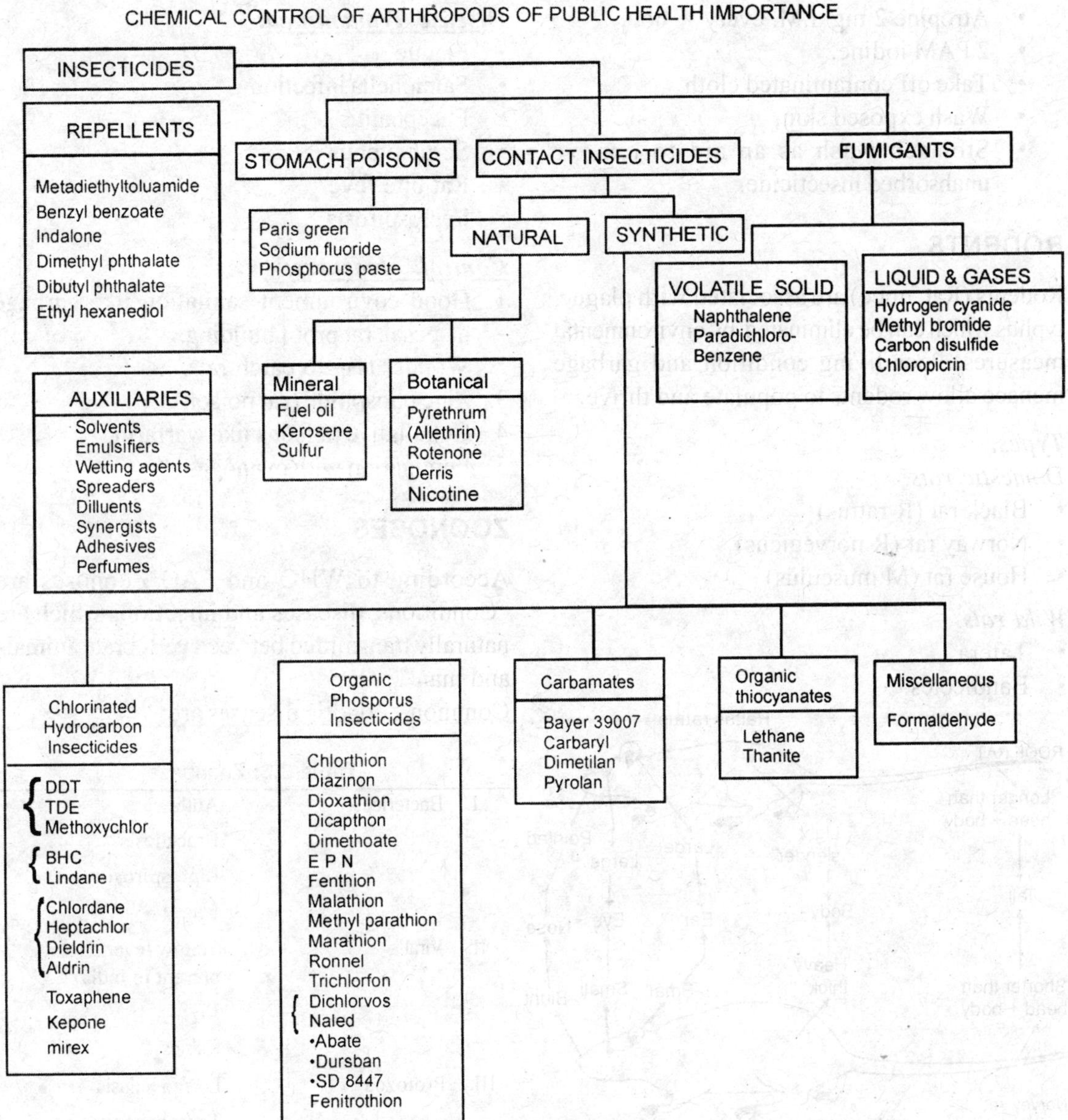

Fig. 9.22: Insecticides

Insecticide Resistance

"It is the development of an ability in strain of insects to tolerate doses of toxicants which would prove lethal to the majority of individuals in normal population of the same species". The knowledge of insecticide resistance helps in selection of proper insecticide in vector control.

Toxicity

Headache, giddiness, apprehension, restlessness, cold sweating, salivation, uncontrolled urination and defecation, loosing consciousness, ataxia and respiratory paralysis are the manifestation of toxicity. Tick-20 poisoning is common in hospital emergency. The treatment includes:

- Atropine 2 mg I.M. every ½ hour.
- 2 PAM iodine.
- Take off contaminated cloth.
- Wash exposed skin.
- Stomach wash as an aid to remove unabsorbed insecticide.

RODENTS

Rodents (Rat, mice) are associated with plague, typhus which can be eliminated by environmental measures. Poor living condition and garbage menace allow rodents to populate and thrive.

Types:

Domestic rats:

- Black rat (R rattus)
- Norway rat (R norvegicus)
- House rat (M musculus)

Wild rats:

- Tatera
- Bandicotes.

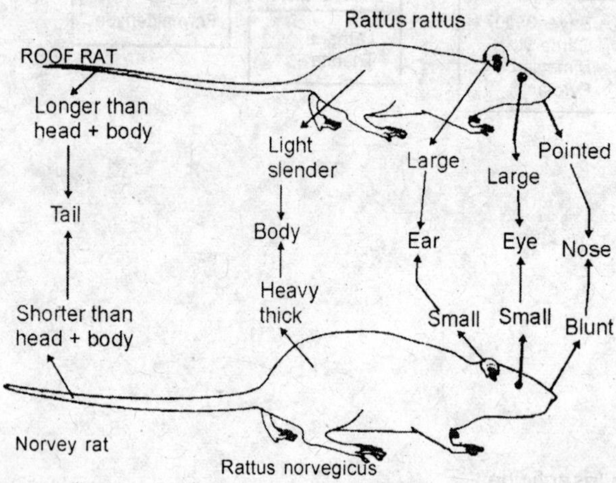

Fig. 9.23: Black rat and Norvey rat

Table 9.5: Character differences

R. rattus	*R.norvegicus*
Slender body	Heavy body
Long nose	Blunt nose
Long Tail	Short tail
Large eye and ear	Small eye and ear.

Disease Transmitted:

- Plague
- Salmonella infection
- Encephalitis
- Scrub typhus
- Rat bite fever
- Leptospirosis.

Control Measures:

1. Good environment sanitation like garbage disposal, rat proof building.
2. Wonder trap to catch rats.
3. Zinc phosphide (rat poison).
4. Cumulative poisons like warfarin.
5. Fumigation with cyanogas.

ZOONOSES

According to WHO and FAO Zoonoses are "Conditions, diseases and infections which are naturally transmitted between vertebrate animals and man".

Common Zoonotic diseases are:

Table 9.6: Zoonoses

I.	Bacterial	–	Anthrax
		–	Brucellosis
		–	Liptospirosis
		–	Plague
II.	Viral	–	Yellow fever (Not present in India)
		–	J.E
		–	Rabies
III.	Protozoa	–	Leishmaniasis
		–	Trypanosomiasis
IV.	Helminthic	–	Schistosomiasis
		–	Echinococcosis
		–	Taeniasis
		–	Trichinellosis

Components of Control of Zoonoses:

i. Diagnosis and treatment in animals.
ii. Sanitation of wool, hide, horn and fats.

iii. Protection of man from animal bites.

iv. International, national and state programme implementations like:
- UNEP (United Nations Env. Programme)
- MAB (Man and Biosphere Programme)
- EHCP (Environmental Health Criteria Programme).

FURTHER REFERENCES

1. Herm's Medical Entomology (MacMillan).
2. WHO – Control of arthropods of P.H. Importance.
3. Ratnaswamy—Medical Entomology (S. Viswanathan).
4. Prabhakara G.N.—Short Textbook of P. & SM (Jaypee).
5. CFTRI – Pesticide residues in foods and their safety limits.

10

Nutrition in Nursing Care and Therapeutic Diets

IMPORTANCE

The pattern of infection, disability, growth and development depends on nutritional status of an individual. It is also influenced by women's educational status, changes in agricultural practice and provision of hygienic food. Malnutrition in Measles, whooping cough and other infections is known to cause serious complications in children. Diet and hygiene determine child's mortality. Knowledge of infection (Germ Theory) helped in understanding the relevance of proper food hygiene. Discovery of vitamins, their benefits to growth and health have reemphasised the importance of diet for the health of an individual. It was for the first time, Head of NIN Hyderabad in 1920; Dr. Mc Carrison found that rat fed by Indian traditional diet showed good growth than rat fed by European diet. This unravelled the knowledge "Protective factor" of vitamins. However early study goes to 1750 when scurvy was treated by lime juice.

Presently nutrition has proved to be associated with socioeconomic development of a nation. Infection, immunity, fertility, Maternal Health, child health and health of sick all depend on nourishment they get. We have nutritional indicators to monitor community nutritional status.

Definition

Nutrition is a science of food and nutrients and their relation to human health.

Nutrient is specific dietary constituent.

Dietetics is the practical application of principles of nutrition.

Diet is the food article in consumable form.

Therapeutic Diet is modification of diet for therapeutic purpose.

Nutritional Epidemiology is epidemiological assessment of nutritional status of communities which include:

- Nutritional survey
- Diet survey
- Nutritional surveillance
- Growth monitoring
- Nutritional rehabilitation
- Nutritional intervention.

Food

Foods are grouped under following category for feasible explanation and comparison.

1. Cereals and millets
2. Pulses (legumes)

3. Vegetables
4. Nuts and oil seeds
5. Fruits
6. Animal foods
7. Fats and oils
8. Sugar and *Jaggery*
9. Condiments and spices
10. Miscellaneous foods.

Major Food Sources of Nutrients are tabulated below:

Table 10.1: Source of food for nutrients

Nutrient	*Food*
Energy	Cereals, pulses, roots, tubers, fats, oils, sugar, *Jaggery.*
Protein	Milk, Egg, Fish, Meat, Liver, Pulses, Nuts, Oilseeds.
Fat	Butter, Ghee, Vegetable Oils, Hydrogenated fats, nuts and oilseeds.
Carbohydrate	Cereals, pulses, sugar, *Jaggery*, Roots, tubers.
Fibre	Green leafy vegetables, Fruits, Unrefined cereals, pulses, legumes.
Calcium	Milk, Milk products, *Ragi*, Green leafy vegetables.
Iron	Liver, green leafy vegetables, rice flakes, whole wheat flour, *ragi*, pulses.
Vitamin A	Fish, Liver oil, Butter, Ghee, Milk, Carrot, Green leafy vegetables, papaya, mango.
B complex	Milk, Egg, Liver, Home-pound rice, Whole Wheat, Whole gram, pulses, green leafy vegetables, nuts, oil seeds.
Vitamin C	Gooseberry, Lime, orange, guava, tomato, lettuce, sprouted gram.
Vitamin D	Milk, Sunlight.

Nutritive Value of Food

Very often we need the availability of proximate principles and available calories in food/food raw materials. They can be tabulated for every 100 grams by their weight as under:

Nutritional Profile of Food

Each food has its own profile. This knowledge is important for formulating diet composition and supplementation.

i. *Cereals:* They form bulk of diet. It is deficient in Lysine (Limiting Aminoacid). Milling of rice takes off nutritive element. Parboiled rice has good high Vitamin B quantity. Parboiling (Partial cooking in steam) is a method of preserving nutrient. Paddy is soaked in hot water at 70° for 3 hours; drying and steaming follows; later dried and milled (CFTRI Process). Protein content of wheat is 16%.
ii. *Millet:* Smaller grains *jowar, bajra, ragi* are examples. In *Jowar* limiting amino acid are lysine and threonine. *Ragi* is rich in calcium.
iii. *Pulses:* All pulses have 20% protein except soyabean which has 40%. Germinated pulses have higher content of vitamins. *Kesaridhal* is associated with Lathyrism.
iv. *Vegetables:* They are grouped under greens, roots, tubers and other vegetables. They yield low calorie, form bulky food; but provide vitamins and minerals.
v. *Nuts, Oilseeds:* Nuts contribute minerals, essential fatty acids. Acceptable balance foods are MPF, *Balahar,* and Malt food.
vi. *Fruits:* They are protective foods. Since they are eaten raw they provide good amount of vitamins and minerals.
vii. *Animal Food:* They provide high quality protein. Reference proteins are milk and egg which are nearly perfect food.
    a. **Milk:** Casein is the chief protein. Buffalo milk contains high fat content (8.8%). Skimming removes fat. Toning means 1 part water 1 part natural milk and 1/8 part skim milk powder. Vegetable milk is prepared from groundnut, soyabean etc.

Table 10.2: Nutritive Value of Common Foods

Foodstuff	*Protein*	*Fat*	*Carbohydrate*	*Calories*
Cereal	9.9	2.3	71.0	344
Bread	7.8	0.7	51.9	245
Salt biscuit	6.6	32.4	54.6	534
Sweet biscuit	6.4	15.2	71.9	450
Pulses	22.6	2.0	58.4	342
Green leafy vegetables	3.8	0.6	6.0	45
Roots, tubers	1.2	0.2	16.0	70
Other vegetables	2.2	0.3	6.3	36
Nuts, oilseed	15.2	46.6	20.4	578
Condiment, spice	9.8	6.6	40.6	261
Fruit	1.1	0.4	7.6	79
Meat	21.0	4.9	0.8	131
Egg	13.3	13.3	0.0	173
Milk	3.6	5.8	4.7	85
Curd	3.1	4.0	3.0	60
Butter	0.0	81.0	0.0	729
Ghee	0.0	100.0	0.0	900
Oil	0.0	100.0	0.0	900
Sugar	0.1	0.0	99.4	398
Honey	0.3	0.0	79.5	319
Jaggery	0.4	0.1	95.0	383
Sago	0.2	0.2	87.1	351

b. **Egg:** About 60 gram egg has 6G. Protein, 6G. Fat, 30 mg calcium, 1.5 mg iron and provide 70 calories. Boiled eggs are nutritionally superior (Boiling destroys *avidin* a vitamin preventing factor). Cholesterol content of egg is related to CHD.

c. **Fish:** It is food of good biological value and a food with balanced amino acids. They are richest source of Vitamin A. Sea fish is rich in iodine.

d. **Meat:** Flesh of cattle, sheep and goat are commonly used. They give 20% protein. They are source of Zinc and Vitamin B.

viii. **Fat, Oil:** They are source of energy and Vitamin A, D, coconut and palm contain polysaturated fatty acids. Hydrogenated fat is called *vanaspati.*

ix. *Sugar, Jaggery:* They are source of natural sugars.

x. *Condiment, Spice:* Mustard, ginger, garlic, cardamom, *Hing*, Clove and Pepper are examples. They stimulate appetite and increase palatability.

xi. *Miscellaneous:* Coffee, Tea, Cocoa, aerated waters, alcohol, i.e. beverages are examples.

PROXIMATE PRINCIPLES

Protein

They are nitrogenous compounds. They form 20% of body weight in adult. Dietary proteins provide essential amino acids viz., leucine, isoleucine, lysine, methionine, Phenylalamine, Threonine, Valine, Tryptophan and histadine. They help in new tissue formation. Biologically complete protein is one which contains all essential amino acids.

Functions
- Repair of tissues
- Maintain osmotic pressure
- Antibodies produced.

Sources
Animal source: Milk, meat, egg, fish etc.
Plant source: Pulses, Oilseeds.

Evaluation
By NPU (Net protein utilisation).

Requirement
1 G. per kg body weight.

Fat

They are of 3 types; simple, compound and derived. Lauric, palmitic and stearic acid form saturated fatty acids. Examples are ghee, butter, milk, cheese, eggs, meat and fish.

Oleic acid, linoleic acid form unsaturated fatty acids; unsaturated fatty acids are found in vegetable oils. Examples are groundnut oil, mustard oil, sesame oil, coconut oil.

Research has shown that Essential Fatty Acids reduce serum cholesterol and LDL.

Polysaturated fatty acids are precursors of prostaglandins that are called as 'local hormones' are known to play role in physiological functions.

Trans Fatty Acids
They are geometrical isomers of Cis unsaturated fatty acids due to partial hydrogenation. In commercial sector the process of increasing shelf value has created the development of Trans Fatty Acids. Two problems with this are elevating LDL and decreasing HDL which increases coronary heart disease risk. Chips, crackers, whipped toppings, packaged cookies, candy, packaged doughnuts, pies, cakes deep fried fast foods, cake mixes, energy bars are main sources of trans fatty acids.

Sources
- Animal source like ghee, butter, cheese, egg etc.
- Vegetable source like (oilseeds) groundnut and coconut etc.

Functions
- Yield calorie
- Support body viscera
- Act as local hormones

Visible and Invisible Fats
Major intake is from invisible fat and their measurement is difficult.

Hydrogenation
It is a process of converting oil to Semisolid form in presence of a catalyst.

Refining
Process of removing rancid material oil.

Health Effect
- Obesity
- Thick skin, other changes of skin
- Heart disease
- Cancer of some organs.

Requirement
15-20% of total calories. (Indian diet provide 30-40% total calories).

Carbohydrate

- Starch sugar, cellulose are forms of carbohydrate.
- Requirement – 60 to 70% of total calories.

VITAMINS

They are essential nutrients made up of organic compounds. Their deficiency leads to various disorders.

Water Soluble Vitamins

i. *Thiamine:* It is called vitamin B_1 and helps in utilisation of carbohydrate.

Source: Cereal, wheat, pulses, nuts, fish.
Loss: By Milling, prevention by parboiling.
Deficiency: Dry beriberi, wet beriberi and infantile beriberi.
R.D.A.: 0.5 mg/1000 calories.

ii. *Riboflavin:* It is vitamin B_2 helps in cellular oxidation.
Source: Milk, egg, liver, green leafy vegetables.
Deficiency: Angular stomatitis, glossitis.
Requirement: 0.6 mg/1000 calories.

iii. *Niacin:* It helps in metabolism of proximate principles.
Source: Liver, meat, fish, groundnut.
Deficiency: Pellagra.
Prevention: By supplementation.
Requirement: 6.6 mg/1000 calories

iv. *Pyridoxine:* It is called B_6
Source: Milk, liver, meat, egg yolk, fish, legumes.
Deficiency: Peripheral neuritis.
Requirement: 2 mg per day.

v. *Pantothenic acid:* It helps in adrenal gland function and in synthesis of corticosteroids. Requirement is 10 mg per day.

vi. *Folic acid:* This helps in synthesis of nucleic acids.
Source: Liver, meat, egg, milk, fruit and leafy vegetables.
Deficiency: Megaloblastic anaemia, glossitis.
Requirement: 100 micrograms per day.

vii. *Vitamin B_{12}:* This helps in synthesis of DNA, along with folic acid.
Source: Liver, meat, egg, milk, cheese.
Deficiency: Megaloblastic anaemia.
Requirement: 1 microgram per day.

viii. *Vitamin C*: It is called ascorbic acid. It is needed for collagen formation.
Source: Fresh fruits and green leafy vegetables.
Deficiency: Scurvy.
Requirement: 40 mg per day

Fat Soluble Vitamins

i. *Vitamin A:* It is required for vision, for glandular and epithelial tissue functioning, for skeletal growth, as facilitator.
Source: Animal source: liver, egg, butter, fish, meat.
Plant source: Spinach, amaranth, green leafy vegetables, papaya, mango, pumpkin
Fortified foods: Vanaspathi, margarine, milk.
Deficiency: Night blindness, Bitot's spots, dryness and eye softening.
Correction: Early deficiency is corrected by 2,00,000 IU of vitamin A orally on 2 successive days.
For community based intervention 2,00,000 IU orally once in 6 months to preschool children.
Requirement is 600 mcg retinol or 2600 mcg β carotene.
Criteria for Eye Problem in Community: Eye problem is said to exist if prevalence in population at risk 6 months to 6 years is:

1 %	Night blindness
0.5%	Bitot's spot
0.01%	Corneal xerosis
0.05%	Corneal ulcer
5.0%	Serum retinol level below 10 micrograms per dl.

Requirement: Adult requires 600 μg of retinol.
Hypervitaminosis: It is associated with Vitamin A.

ii. *Vitamin D:* It helps in calcium and phosphorous absorption, stimulates bone formation and permit normal growth of tissues.
Source: Sunlight, liver, egg, butter, fish.
Deficiency: Rickets, osteomalaca.
Requirement: 2.5 micrograms per day.

iii. *Vitamin E:* It is called tocopherol.
Source: Cottonseed, Sunflower seed, egg yolk, butter.
Deficiency: Not specific.

iv. *Vitamin K:* It stimulates the production and release of coagulation factors.
Source: Green leafy vegetables, fruits, milk
Deficiency: Bleeding tendency.
Requirement: 0.03 mg/kg per day.

MINERALS

Minerals are chemical elements that are required for growth, repair and regulation of body functions.

Major Minerals

Calcium: It helps in formation of bones, teeth, helps in muscular contraction, in coagulation of blood.
Source: Milk, milk products, *ragi, sitaphal.*
Deficiency: Not demonstrated.
Requirement: 500 mg per day.

Other Major Minerals

Phosphorous, sodium, potassium and magnesium

Trace Elements

They are chemical elements that are required by the body in small quantities.

i. *Iodine:* It is required for the synthesis of Thyroid hormones.
Source: Sea foods, cod liver oil, milk, meat and some vegetables. Cabbage and cauliflower interfere with iodine utilisation and hence are called goitrogens.
Deficiency: Hypothyroidism, growth retardation, abortion, stillbirth, cretinism, deafmutism.
Requirement: 150 microgram per day.

ii. *Iron:* This is present in human body both in circulating form and in storage form.
Functions: Formation of haemoglobin, Brain Development and function, Temperature regulation, muscular activity.
Source: Liver, meat, fish, cereal, green leafy vegetables, legume, nuts, *jaggery,* dried fruits.
Iron has vital importance during pregnancy, Lactation and young children.
Deficiency: Anaemia.
Requirement: 30 mg dietary iron (0.9 mg absorbable form).

iii. *Fluorine:* It is essential for bone and teeth function.
Source: Water, sea foods, tea, cheese.
Deficiency: Dental fluorosis, skeletal fluorosis.
Requirement: 0.5-0.8 mg per litre in drinking water.

iv. Other trace elements are: zinc, copper, cobalt, chromium, selenium and molybdenum.

Anti Oxidants

During normal physiological function, certain food substances that decrease the adverse effects of reactive oxygen species and reactive nitrogen species are called antioxidants. Rise in free radicals are produced by faulty diet, carcinogen exposure, sunlight, toxic drugs, over exercise, high animal diet, nicotine, chemicals, infections, vasoconstrictions, radiation, excess heat and excess cold.

For chemical stability electrons from other molecules are required. Vitamin A, C, E and Trace elements act as antioxidants by donating an electron. Plant source form antioxidants and examples are:

Carrots
Palak
Sweet potato
Turnip
Watermelon

Cabbage
Pumpkin
Lettuce
Green pepper
Tomato
Banana
Plums
Peaches
Amla, lemon
Pineapple
Orange
Watermelon
Guava
Vegetable oil.

CALORIE

It is the prime requisite of the body for effective growth and development. It is expressed by calories (in terms of kilo calorie). For international comparison calorie is replaced by Joule. For purpose of conversion 1 calorie (Kcal) = 4184 Joule. The energy available by proximate principle is as under:

Protein	4 calories (17 Joule) per gram
Fat	9 calories (37 Joule) per gram
Carbohydrate	4 calories (17 Joule) per gram

In view of the currently recommend adult body weight, the reference man and reference women are redefined as under:

Reference Man

He is between 20-39 years age weight 60 kg, is free from disease and physically fit for active work. On each working day he is employed for 8 hours in occupation that usually involves moderate activity. While not at work he spends 8 hours in bed, 4-6 hours sitting and moving about, and 2 hours walking and in active recreation or household duties.

Reference Woman

She is between 20-39 years age healthy, weight 50 kg. She may be engaged for 8 hours in general household work, in light industry or in any other moderately active work. Apart from 8 hours in bed, she spends 4-6 hours sitting or moving around in light activity, and 2 hours walking or active recreation or household chores.

Caloric Requirement

For B.M.R. – 1 calorie per hour per kg.
For daily activity – additional.
For occupation – additional.

Energy Requirement of Reference Person

Sex	*Body weight*	*Activity*		
		Sedentary	*Moderate*	*Heavy*
Male	60 kg	2425	2875	3800
Female	50 kg	1875	2225	2925

BALANCED DIET

Balanced diet is an accepted means to safeguard population from nutritional deficiencies. It is defined as a diet containing required proximate principles, calorie, vitamins, minerals and trace elements that can meet the requirement for healthy life. This also allows provision of extra nutrients for given situations like pregnancy, lactation and sickness. In constructing the balanced diet following guidelines are used as base line (adult):

Protein	–	1 G per kg body weight
Fat	–	15-20% of total calories
Carbohydrate	–	50-60% of total calories
Iron	–	28 mg
Retinol	–	600 mg (2400 Im)
Thiamine	–	1.2 mg
Riboflavin	–	1.4 mg
Nicotinic acid	–	16 mg
Pyridoxine	–	2.0 mg
Vitamin C	–	40 mg
Folic acid	–	100 micrograms
Vitamin B_{12}	–	1 microgram

Following tables give balanced diet for given specific situations:

Adult Man

Table 10.3: Balanced diet for adult man

Items (Grams)	*Sedentary*	*Moderate work*	*Heavy work*
Cereals	460	520	670
Pulses	40	50	60
Leafy vegetables	40	40	40
Other vegetables	60	70	80
Roots and tubers	50	60	80
Milk	150	200	250
Oil and fat	40	45	65
Sugar or *jaggery*	30	35	55

Adult Woman

Table 10.4 : Balanced diet for adult woman

Item(Grams)	*Sedentary*	*Moderate work*	*Heavy work*
Cereals	410	440	575
Pulses	40	45	50
Leafy vegetables	100	100	50
Other vegetables	40	40	100
Roots and tubers	50	50	60
Milk	100	150	200
Oil and fat	20	25	40
Sugar or *jaggery*	20	20	40

Children

Table 10.5 : Balanced diet for children

Item(Grams)	*1-3 years*	*4-6 years*
Cereals	175	270
Pulses	35	35
Leafy vegetables	40	50
Other vegetables	20	30
Roots and tubers	10	20
Milk	300	250
Oil and fat	15	25
Sugar or *jaggery*	30	40

Adolescence

Table 10.6: Balanced diet for adolescence

Item (Grams)	*Boys 10-12 years*	*Girls 10-12 years*
Cereals	420	380
Pulses	45	45
Leafy vegetables	50	50
Other vegetables	50	50
Roots and tubers	30	30
Milk	250	250
Oil and fat	40	35
Sugar or *jaggery*	45	45

Allowance During Pregnancy

Table 10.7: Additional allowance during pregnancy

Cereals	35 grams	Yield 293 calories
Pulses	15 grams	
Milk	100 grams	
Sugar	10 grams	

Allowance During Lactation

Table 10.8: Additional allowance during Lactation

Cereals	60 grams	Yield 521 calories
Pulses	30 grams	
Milk	100 grams	
Fat	10 grams	
Sugar	10 grams	

Balanced diet for elderly people above 65 years.

Table 10.9: Balanced diet for elderly

	Woman > 65 years	*Man > 65 years*
Cereals	225	350
Pulses	40	50
Vegetables	150	200
Green leafy vegetables	50	50
Roots and tubers	100	100
Fruits	200	200
Milk, milk products	300	300
Sugar	20	20
Fats and oils	20	25

PRUDENT DIET

This is the diet developed by National Nutrition and Food Policy to achieve highest level of health. It is called prudent diet if following criteria are adopted in a diet:

a. Fat intake below 20-30% of total calories
b. Saturated Fat below 10% of total calories
c. Carbohydrate should contain high fibre
d. Fats, alcohol restricted
e. Salt below 5 grams per day
f. Protein below 15-20% of daily intake
g. Junk foods avoided (Ketchup, cola).

NUTRITION AND HEALTH

There are many health problems which are due to nutritional deficiency, adulteration or harmful excesses. Major concerns are detailed below;

P.E.M.

This is commonly seen during infancy. It affects growth, development and mental outlook of a child. *Kwashiorkar* and *Marasmus* are two clinical types of P.E.M. Among preschool children, it is 2 percent. Among malnourished, 20% are severely malnourished (Grade III and IV) and remaining are mild and moderate (Grade I and II).

Earlier it was called PCM (Protein calorie Malnutrition) because of concept of protein gap. Now since energy gap is there, the cause is taken over to food gap in causation of PEM.

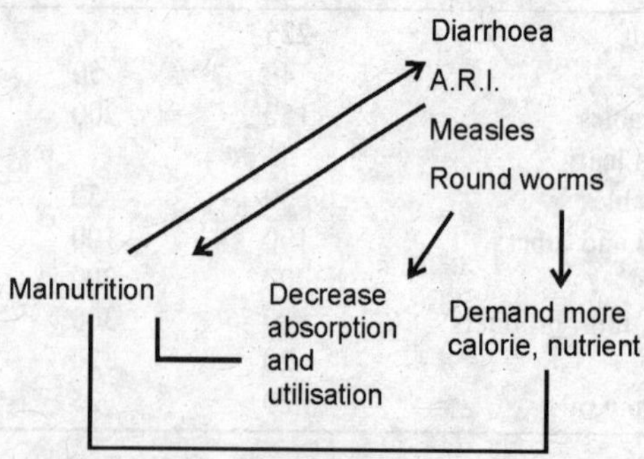

Fig. 10.1: Vicious cycle of infection and malnutrition

Figure 10.1 demonstrates the vicious cycle of infection and malnutrition.

Other Environment causes are:

- Poor R.C.H.
- Failure of Lactation
- No exclusive breast feeding
- Child rearing practice
- Weaning practice
- Overcrowding in the family.

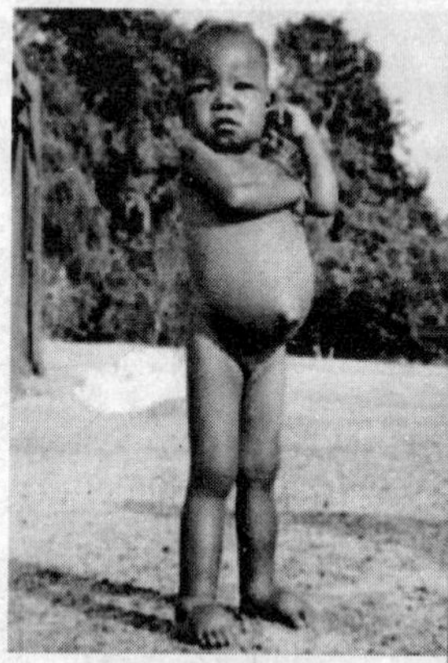

Photo: Kwashiorkor

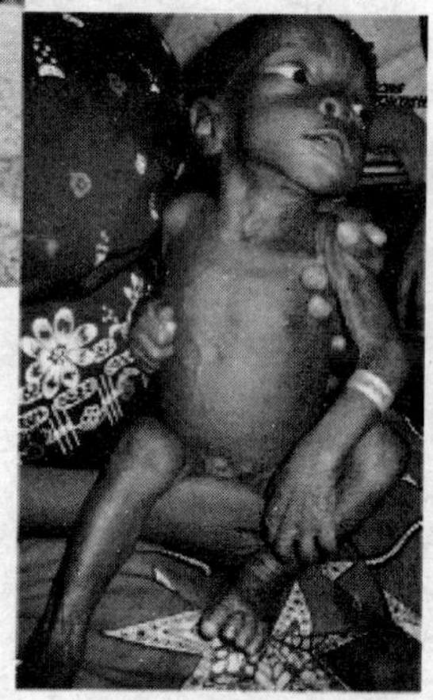

Photo: Marasmus

Difference Between *Kwashiorkar and Marasmus*:

Table 10.10: Difference between kwashiorkar and marasmus

	Kwashiorkar	*Marasmus*
Muscle wasting	Not obvious	Obvious
Fat wasting	Not obvious	Obvious
Oedema	Present	Absent
Weight/ Height ratio	Low	Very low
Mental change	Irritable	Quiet
Appetite	Poor	Good
Diarrhoea	Present	Present

Contd.

Contd.

Skin change	Flaky paint dermatosis	Nil
Hair change	Silky, pluckable	Nil
Liver change	Enlarged	Nil
Serum albumin	Low	Normal
Plasma aminoacid ratio	Raised	Normal

Types of P.E.M.

According to Gomez the degree of P.E.M is classified in terms of weight retardation as under, by a coefficient value.

$$\text{Weight in \%} = \frac{\text{Weight of child}}{\text{weight of normal for same age}} \times 100$$

Below 60%	=	III degree
60–74%	=	II degree
75–89%	=	I degree
90+	=	Normal

All anthropometric values like weight, height, chest circumference, head circumference and mid upper arm circumference are used to classify P.E.M. (Malnutrition) into following categories:

Normal

I Degree Malnutrition } Mild
II Degree Malnutrition }

III Degree Malnutrition } Severe
IV Degree Malnutrition }

Planning above grouping is of practical help for supplementary nutrition to mild type and therapeutic nutrition (Double the dose of supplementary nutrition) to severe degree.

Ecology of Malnutrition (P.E.M.)

According to Jelliffe it is man made and related to environmental factors which are preventable in nature. They are:

a. *Conditioning influences:* Measles, Diarrhoea, Helminthic infestation, Malaria, Tuberculosis.
b. *Cultural influences:* Food habit, religious taboos, food fads, child rearing practices.
c. *Socio-economic influences:* Poverty, low income, illiteracy, overcrowding.
d. *Food production:* Reduced food production, maldistribution, spoiling due to improper storage.
e. Accessibility of health services.

Role of Protein Assessment in P.E.M.

The Quality protein (Reference protein) is a determining force in the causation of PEM. It is the product of digestibility coefficient and biological value divided by 100. It indirectly shows the ratio of Nitrogen retained to nitrogen intake.

If a food has low NPU, the protein requirement is high and accordingly the quantity of food also to be increased.

Prevention of P.E.M.

It needs multidimensional activities which can be tabulated in Table 10.11.

L.B.W. (Low Birth Weight)

It is defined as birth weight of newborn below 2500 grams. Its prevalence is 28-30% in Developing countries. Main cause has been growth retardation due to poor socioeconomic conditions. In India the national goal to achieve 10% by 2010 is aggregated in the National Health Policy.

According to gestational age LBW can be grouped under 3 categories:

- Pre Term (less than 259 days)
- Term (259 to 293 days)
- Post Term (294 days above).

Table 10.11: Prevention of P.E.M.

Primary prevention		*Secondary prevention*		*Tertiary prevention*
Health Promotion	Specific Protection	Early diagnosis Prompt treatment	Disability Limitation	Rehabilitation
MCH nutrition Supplementation	High protein rich diet	Nutrition Surveillance	Hospital Treatment	
Exclusive Breastfeeding	Immunisation	Diagnosis of P.E.M.	Case follow up	Nutrition Rehabilitation
Nutrition Education Family Planning	Food Fortification	Supplementary Nutrition Therapeutic Nutrition Deworming		

Three main causes that need attention to overcome L.B.W. are:

- Malnutrition
- Infection
- Unregulated Fertility

Preventive Measures:

- Identification of risk cases and attending to Medical and Nursing care.
- Dietary improvement of pregnant women.
- Control of Maternal infections.
- Control of PET, Toxaemia, Diabetes, Hypertension.
- Family planning.
- Improvement of socioeconomic condition.

Treatment of L.B.W.:

Here, there is a great role of Nursing care which includes:

- Incubatory care for regulation of Temperature, humidity, oxygen supply.
- Nasal feeding since baby cannot suck properly.
- Antibiotic to prevent neonatal infection.

Neonatal Intensive Care Unit (NICU): The role of Nursing care is at most important in a NICU for the prevention of neonatal death by attending to intervention of the following conditions:

- Lung collapse (atelectasis).
- Malformation (Where paediatric surgery are suggested).
- Pulmonary haemorrhage.
- Birth trauma leading to brain haemorrhage.
- Pneumonia.

Vitamin A Deficiency

Vitamin A deficiency is one of the causes of preventable blindness in India. Young children are susceptible for xerophtalmia. This is associated with Faulty feeding practice and ignorance. South India show higher incidence of Vitamin A deficiency than North India.

Prevention and control is done under three strategies (Vitamin A Therapy):

1. *Long Term Strategy:* Nutrition education, Treatment of infections, immunisation, and periodic massive dose (2 *lakh* unit) of retinol in oil every 6 months.
ii. *Medium Term Strategy:* Fortification of foods with vitamin A (*Dalda*, sugar, Tea, Margarine, skimmed Milk).
iii. *Short Term Strategy:* (Oral dose of Retinol palmitate)

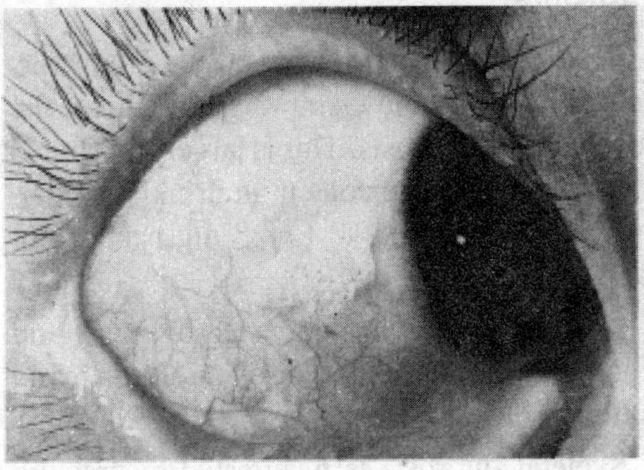

Photo: Bitot's spot (foamy)

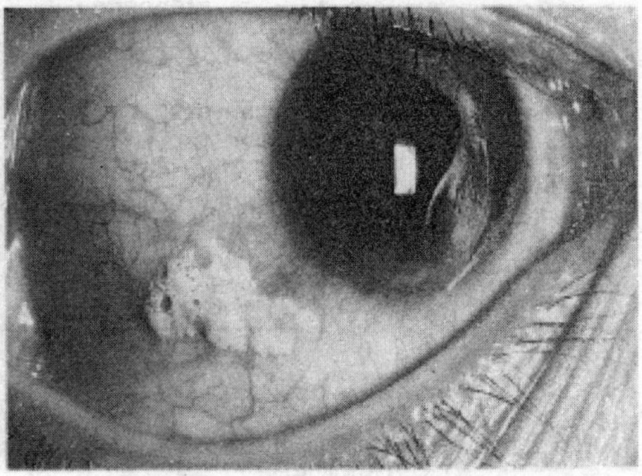

Photo: Bitot's spot (cheesy)

To pregnant – 2.75 mg per day
To lactating – 11 mg once a week
Newborn – 27.5 mg at birth
Infants – 110 mg once in 6 months
Young children – 55 mg once in 6 months.

Anaemia

Anaemia is a condition in which haemoglobin content of blood is lower than normal as a result of deficiency. Very commonly iron deficiency is the cause of anaemia.

Table 10.12: Hb% in anaemia diagnosis

W.H.O. Criteria for anaemia	
Adult male	13 G%
Adult female	12 G%
Pregnancy	11 G%
Children upto 6 years	11 G%
Children above 6 years	12 G%

Cause:

Inadequate intake
Poor bioavailability of dietary iron
Loss by haemorrhage.

Effect:

Maternal mortality
Foetal mortality
Abortion
P.P.H.
L.B.W.

Prevention of Anaemia:

i. In severe anaemia (8 G%) blood transfusion.
ii. In mild and moderate anaemia.
   - I.F.A. 60 mg Iron, 0.5 mg Folic acid daily to mothers till Hb% is corrected.
   - I.F.A. 60 mg Iron, 0.5 mg Folic acid daily for 3 months to pregnant woman.
   - I.F.A. 20 mg Iron, 0.1 mg Folic acid daily to children till Hb% is corrected.

Other measures

- Fortification of salt with iron.

Iodine Deficiency

Iodine deficiency is increasingly becoming public health problem since it is giving wide spectrum of disorders. They can be enumerated as (Fig. 10.2).

Goitre and cretinism are greatly associated with Iodine deficiency. "Himalaya goitre belt" is biggest goitre belt in the world.

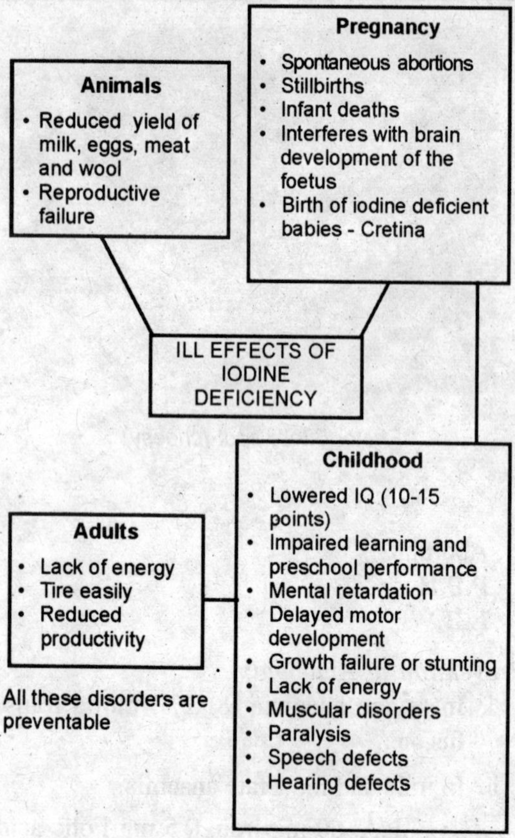

Fig. 10.2: Ill effects of Iodine deficiency

Epidemiological studies have shown the following observations:

- 140 million people are living in endemic area.
- In endemic belt, goitre is nearly 36% in prevalence.
- In endemic belt, 15% are neonatal hypothyroidism.

Control Programme:

- Iodised salt (15 PPM I_2 at consumer level).
- Iodine monitoring and surveillance.
- Manpower engaging in health care work is trained on goitre control.
- Health education.

Fluorosis

In India common occurrence of Dental fluorosis, skeletal fluorosis and Genu valgum indicate the prevalence of fluorosis. This is largely attributed to excessive fluorine content in drinking water. The normal range is 0.3 to 0.8 mg per litre of water.

Dental fluorosis is manifested by white and yellow patches on teeth, corrosion in teeth and mottling of teeth.

Skeletal fluorosis is manifested by fracture and indisposition to move which cripples the individual.

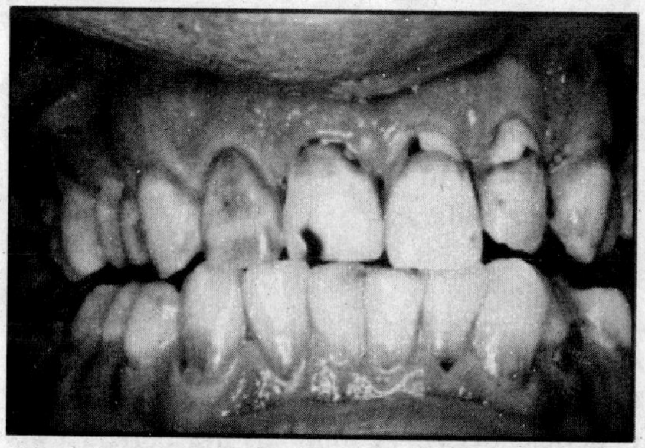

Fig. 10.3: Dental fluorosis

Recent studies have shown that *Jowar* eating area has higher retention of ingested fluoride leading to Genu Valgum.

Control Measures:

- Changing the water source.
- Chemical Treatment by *Nalagonda* Technique (Fig. 10.5).

Lathyrism

It is called Neurolathyrism, a paralytic disease caused by consuming contaminated non edible pulse " *Lathyrus Sativus*" (*Kesridhal*). It is high in middle part of India when compared to

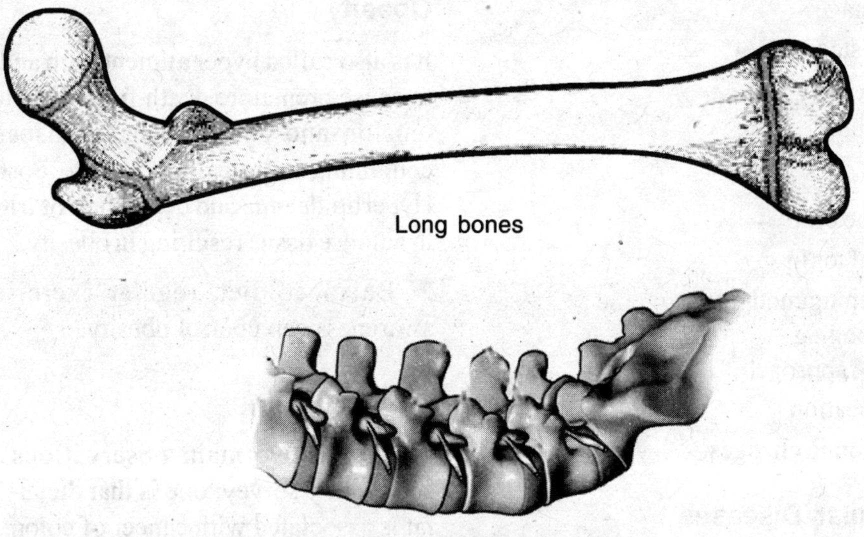

Fig. 10.4: Skeletal fluorosis

peripheral states of the country. The toxin identified is BOAA (Beta oxalyl amino alanine) which produce neuroparalysis. Clinically it shows following stages:

- Latent stage

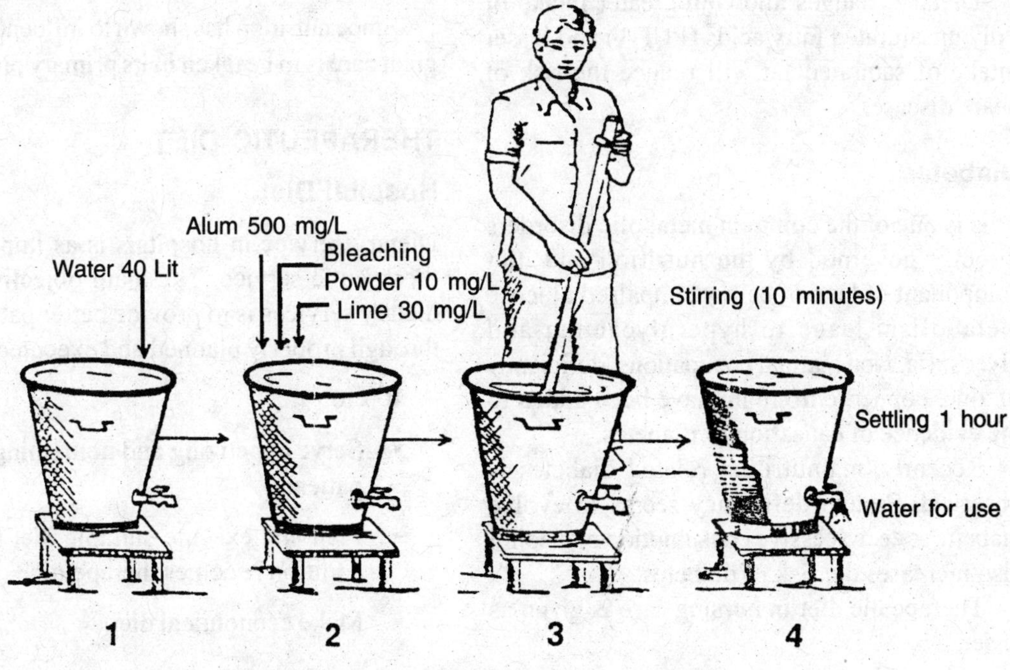

Fig. 10.5: Nalgonda technique (Defluoridation)

- No stick stage
- One stick stage
- Two stick stage
- Crawler stage.

Control Measures:

- Banning the crop
- Removal of toxin
  - By steeping method
  - By parboiling
  - Genetic approach
- Health education
- Socioeconomic changes.

Cardiovascular Diseases

Nutrition is associated with coronary heart disease. There are supported studies that have shown that elevated blood level of cholesterol and elevated blood level of Low density lipoprotein (LDU) result in the development of atherosclerosis.

Dietary changes allowing greater intake of Poly unsaturated fatty acids (PUFA) and lesser intake of saturated fat will reduce the risk of heart diseases.

Diabetes

This is one of the common metabolic disorders directly governed by the nutrition and diet component of human beings. Impaired glucose metabolism leads to hyperglycaemia and glycosuria. Non manual occupations, deficiency of zinc, copper, chromium have been added to the evidence of causation of diabetes.

Recently, malnutrition related diabetes is observed. Protein deficiency seems to evolve diabetic state. Excessive consumption of alcohol also increases the risk of diabetes.

Therapeutic diet in nursing care is given as under:

Obesity

It is also called hyper alimentation and is known to cause premature death from diabetes, hypertension and coronary heart diseases. Diet containing more calorie lead to Post Prandial Hyperlipidaemia and deposition of triglycerides in adipose tissue resulting in obesity.

Balanced diet, regular exercise, health awareness can control obesity.

Cancer

There are two main observations noted in community survey: one is that dietary intake of fat is associated with cancer of colon, the other is high consumption of fat (per capita consumption of fat) is associated with breast cancer.

Aflatoxin, saccharin and a few food additives and food contaminants are blamed to be carcinogenic.

Since nutrition has shown to influence cancer, great care is to be taken in its primary prevention.

THERAPEUTIC DIET

Hospital Diet

Dietary service in hospitals is as important as therapeutic service. The main objective of the dietary services is to provide better patient-care through properly planned and executed diets.

It is to:

- Serve appetizing and nourishing meal to patients.
- Plan and execute suitable diet which in addition becomes therapeutic.
- Make economical diet.

Following are Common Hospital Diets:

Normal Full Diet (All in grams except otherwise mentioned)

Item	*Veg*	*Nonveg*
Cereal	350	350
Bread	50	50
Pulses	50	25
Milk/curd	550 ml	300 ml
Greens	300	300
Potato	100	100
Butter	10	10
Oil	20	30
Sugar	50	50
Fruit	150	150
Meat/Fish/Chicken	—	100
Or		
Egg	—	Two
Tea or coffee	7/15	7/15
Salt	10	10
Condiments	15	15
Yield:		
Calorie	2500	2500
Protein	75	80
Fat	60	70
CHO	420	400

Full Liquid Diet (All Acute Illness)

Item	*Amount (g.)*
Milk	1 Litre
Bread	100
Butter	20
Egg	One
Greens (for soup)	150
Potato	100
Sugar	50
Fruit	150
Tea/Coffee	7/15
Salt	10
Provide:	
Calorie	1500
Protein	45
Fat	60
CHO	190

Liquid diet for Fever, Diarrhoea, Post Operative, Diabetes, Jejunostomy, Ca-Oesophagus, Anorexia nervosa, Cannot chew, Severe burns, Gastric surgery

Item	*Quantity (g.)*
Cow's milk	500 ml
Sugar	100
Orange juice	250 ml (six)
Dhal for soup / Cereal Kanji	25
Tea/Coffee	7/15
Provide:	
Calorie	1000
Protein	20
Fat	20
CHO	180
Sodium	285 mg

Obesity Diet

Item	*Quantity (g.)*
Skimmed milk	500 ml
Bread	25
Cereal	100
Curds	200
Channa	50
Dhal	25
Greens	500
Oil	10
Tea/Coffee	7/15
Salt	10
Condiment	15
Fruit	2 portions
Provide:	
Calorie	1200
Protein	47 G
Fat	30 G
CHO	183 G

Foods to avoid:

Whole milk, cream, butter, oil, ghee, fried food, honey, sugar, sweets, ovaltine, horlicks, cocoa, cheese, banana, mangoes, grape, jam, *arvi*, potato, soda, alcohol, dried fruits and nuts.

Foods allowed liberally:
All vegetables, lime juice, clear soup, pepper water, skimmed milk and all fruits.

Low Cholesterol Diet for Coronary Heart Disease, Atherosclerosis, Hypercholestraemia

Item	*Quantity (g.)*
Skimmed milk	600 ml
Bread	25
Cereal	100
Curds	300
Channa	50
Dal	25
Veg	400
Fruit	150
Honey	20
Sugar	10
Oil	10
Tea/Coffee	7/15
Provide:	
Calories	1200
Protein	54 G
Fat	13 G
CHO	214 G

Peptic Ulcer Diet

Item	*Quantity (g.)*
Milk	1.5 litre
Egg	1
Cream	25
Sugar	50
(1 Egg can replace 100 ml milk)	
Provide:	
Calorie	1375
Protein	54 G
Fat	76 G
CHO	115 G

Bland Diet for Gastric Ulcer, Gastritis, Diarrhoea, Haemorrhoids

Item	*Quantity (g.)*
Milk	1 litre
Crestless white bread	50
Butter	25
Egg	1
Or	
Channa	25
Or Chicken / Fish	100
Rice	150
Dhal	25
Cooked veg.	200
Potato	50
Banana	1
Sugar	50
Tea / Coffee	7/15
Yield:	
Calorie	2075
Protein	58 G
Fat	68 G
CHO	305 G

Guidelines In Diabetic Diet

Free foods: Leafy veg, tomato, cucumber, radish, lime, clear soup, black coffee/Tea, butter milk, sour chutney, pickle, pepper, *jeera* water, *Jamun* fruit.

Foods to avoid: Potato, yam, *arvi*, mango, grape, banana, alcohol, wine.

Foods prohibited: Glucose, sugar, honey, all sweets.

Food equivalents:

50 G rice=any one		
	Bread	75G.
	Wheat Porridge	50 G.
	Dosa	2
	Idli	2
	Potato	150 G
	Biscuit	4

1 portion fruit 10 grams CHO = Anyone	=	100 grams of Apple, Guava, Green Mango, Orange, *Musambi*, Plum, Papaya, Pear, Peach, *Leechies*, Pomegranate, 150 grams of grape, yellow melon 300 grams of Watermelon 50 grams of Banana, Grape, Mango

Protein Free and Sodium Free Diet for Hepatic Coma, Acute Anuria

Sago Kanji

a.	Sago	50 ml
	Water	500 ml
	Sugar	50
b.	Lemon	10 ml
c.	Orange	200 ml
d.	Glucose	100
	Water	500 ml
e.	Tea/Coffee	7/15

Feeds once in 2 hour provide.

Calorie	–	900
Protein	–	2 G.
Fat	–	1 G.
CHO	–	215 G.
Sodium	–	Nil

High Protein Diet for Liver Cirrhosis

Item	*Quantity (gms)*
Skimmed milk	1 litre
Channa	100
Curds	200
Rice	300
Dal	50
Veg	200
Potato	100
Salt free butter	10
Sugar	100

Provide:		
Calorie	–	2500
Protein	–	100 G
Fat	–	40 G
CHO	–	430 G
Sodium	–	730 mg

Gluten Free Diet for Celiac Disease

Foods allowed : Rice, Corn flour, Soya products, Lean meat, fish, egg, milk, Milk product, Sugar, honey, All veg, fruit, Butter, Ghee, Oil

Foods prohibited: Wheat products-*atta, sooji, Maida*, biscuit, bread, *ragi*, oat, rye.

Low Purine Diet for Gout

Item		*Quantity (g.)*
Milk		200 ml
Bread (white)		50
Butter		10
Channa		50
Curds		200
Rice		150
Oil		10
Greens		300
Fruit		2 portion
Salt		10
Sugar		25
Tea/Coffee		7/15
Yield :		
Calorie	–	1600
Protein	–	40 G
Fat	–	45 G
CHO	–	240 G

Dietary Recommendation in Renal Calculi

If stone is uric acid, urate–Eliminate

Meat, meat product, shellfish, dhal, wholegrain cereal, oat meal, dried pea, bean, spinach. (Give alkaline ash and neutral).

If stone is oxalate, eliminate

Green plantain, spinach, *arvi* (colocasia root), Sweet potato, beet, currants, figs, almond, cashew nut, grape.

If stone is Phosphate – Carbonate

Give acid ash diet.

High ash foods are:

Wholegrain cereal, meat, fish, egg, nut.

High alkaline foods are:

Dhal, greens, roots, milk, milk product, fruit, coconut.

Neutral foods are:

Tea, coffee, sugar, butter, oil.

NUTRITIONAL ASSESSMENT

It is a community health device to assess individual and group nutritional status by available field methods. This gives the prevalence and distribution of nutritional problem in a community.

Clinical Examination

It is clinical assessment of nutritional deficiencies. ICMR has formulated a schematic proforma for this type of clinical assessment, which is as under:

CLINICAL

1. General: Normal Built/Thin built/ Sickly
2. Hair: Normal/dull and dry/dys-pigmented/thin and sparse/ easily pluckable /flag sign
3. Face: Diffuse depigmentation/naso-labial dyssebacea/moon face
4. Eyes: Conjunctiva—normal / dry on exposure for ½ min /dry and wrinkled / Bitot's spots / brown pigmentation /angular conjunctivitis /pale conjunctiva
   Cornea—normal / dry /hazy or opaque
5. Lips: Normal/angular stomatitis/ cheilosis
6. Tongue: Normal / pale and flabby /red and raw / fissured / geographic
7. Teeth : mottled enamel/ caries /attrition
8. Gums: Normal / bleeding
9. Glands: Thyroid enlargement / parotid enlargement
10. Skin: Normal/dry and scaly/ follicular hyperkeratosis
11. Nails: Koilonychia
12. Oedema: In dependent parts
13. Rachitic changes: Knock-knees or bow legs / epiphyseal enlargement/beading of the ribs/pigeon chest
14. Internal system : Hepatomegaly / psychomotor change/mental confusion/ sensory loss / motor weakness/ loss of position sense / loss of vibration sense / loss of ankle and knee jerks / calf tenderness/ cardiac enlargement/ tachycardia.

ANTHROPOMETRIC

Weight (kg):

Head circumference (cm):

Height (cm):

Chest circumference (cm):

Mid-upper-arm circumference (cm):

Skinfold :

Anthropometry

This is measurement of following on individuals:

- Height
- Weight
- Skinfold

} Adult

- Head circumference
- Chest circumference
- Mid upper arm circumference

} Paediatric

Laboratory Assessment

They are:

Hb % (Anaemia)
Stool exam (worms)
Urine exam (Diabetes)
Serum level for metabolites
(Serum retinol, folate).

Assessment of Functional Indices

- Capillary fragility (Vitamin C)
- Cutaneous hypersensitivity (Zinc)
- Prothrombin Time (Vitamin K)
- Sperm count (Zinc)
- EEG (Nerve function)
- Vaso pressor response (Vitamin C).

Diet Survey

By enquiry and data collection on personal visit, information on food consumption is done in the following ways:

- Weighment of raw food.
- Weighment of cooked food.
- Oral questionnaire.
- Stock inventory.

Minimum of 7 days or 3 days data gives average value for:

i. Per capita consumption of calories.
ii. Per capita consumption of nutrient.

Other Methods

They are morbidity data, mortality data, data on ecology and health education services.

NUTRITIONAL SURVEILLANCE

It is defined as keeping a watch over nutrition of a community to take decision on required improvement for better nutrition. It helps in long term planning, management, evaluation and to get over nutrition crisis.

Difference Between Nutritional Surveillance and Growth Monitoring:

Table 10.13: Difference between surveillance and monitoring

Nutritional surveillance	*Growth monitoring*
Detect under-nutrition by diagnosis	Preserve normal growth by health education
A sample study	All 0-6 age children
By trained worker	By educating mothers
Precise instrument used	Simple instrument used
Referral to hospital	Referral to P.H.C.

Following indicators are used in nutrition surveillance:

- Birth weight
- Proportion of breast feed
- Proportion of weaned feed
- Height for age
- Weight for age
- Weight for height
- Clinical signs.

The above indicators are used in nutrition surveillance. Each state has a unit to monitor this surveillance called state level National Nutrition Monitoring Bureau.

SOCIAL NUTRITION

Food and nutrition is part of civilization which endorse the security and safety of a society and when it comes to individual it endorses survival.

Social interaction influence under-nutrition, over-nutrition, imbalance and specific nutritional deficiency.

Food habit, custom, belief and tradition make people to develop an attitude which determines the nutritional status of a community. Psychological aspect of love, affection, social prestige is shown through food. Family passion like rice eaters, wheat eaters shapes dietary habits, Foods which are avoided, tabulated below, depict food fad which can influence nutritional status.

Table 10.14: Foods avoided under the pretext of hot, cold and other beliefs

Pregnancy	*Lactation*	*Children*	*Elderly*	*Sick*
Papaya	Dhal	Sugar	Rice	Solid food
Carrot	Greens	Banana	Oil	Rice
Leafy vegetables	Rice, fruits	Curds	Spices	
Iron	Banana	Cucumber	Meat	

Cooking practices like direct cooking, boiling, frying, pressure cooking influence the content of nutrient of the diet.

Alcoholism in a society also influences nutrition in a negative way.

FOOD HYGIENE

With the understanding of germ theory, protection of food from contamination by pathogens resulted in an awareness of food hygiene. It is the status of how food in its different placement is maintained. Production, handling, distribution and serving apart from storage decide the quality of food. Bacterial toxin and bacterial contamination hall mark the illness due to food borne diseases.

Food borne disease is an illness either by toxins or pathogens caused by their entry to body through food. This has become a major relevance in the days of mass catering era. They are classified as under:

A. *Toxins:*
   a. *Natural Toxin:* Lathyrism, endemic ascitis.
   b. *Produced Toxin:* Botulism, Staphylococcal.
   c. *Chemical Toxin:* Mercury, Lead, DDT.

B. *Infections:*
   a. *Bacterial:* Typhoid, Paratyphoid, Botulism, Diarrhoea, Infantile diarrhoea.
   b. *Viral:* Hepatitis, GE.
   c. *Parasite:* Tapeworm, Round worm, Amoebiasis, Thread worm.

Milk Hygiene

Next to water, milk is a major vehicle of transmission of diseases. Main diseases which are transmitted through milk are:

- Tuberculosis
- Brucellosis
- Anthrax
- Leptospirosis
- Typhoid
- Para cholera.

It is possible to maintain milk hygiene in the prevention of milk borne diseases. They are:

- Measures on positive health of cows and buffalos.
- Dairy sanitation.
- Pasteurisation.

Methods of Pasteurisation are:

i. HTST method (High Temperature and short time method) where milk is rapidly heated to 72°C, held for 15 seconds and rapidly cooled to 4°C.
ii. Holder (Vat) Method where milk is kept at 66°C for 30 minutes and then quickly cooled to 5°C.
iii. UHT (Ultra High Temperature) method where milk is rapidly heated in 2 stages, first heated to 125°C, cooled rapidly to room temperature followed by heating to 125°C under pressure. In both stage heating is for 10 seconds. Rapid cooling to room temperature and bottling is followed.

To test the effect of pasteurisation Methylene Blue reduction test is done; when methylene blue is added to 10 ml milk and kept at 37^0C and observed for disappearance of blue colour. Quick disappearance is an index of poor pasteurisation.

Meat Hygiene

Animal food which is also an important part of diet can cause disease like tape worm infestation (Beef tapeworm, pork tapeworm), Bacterial infection (anthrax, actinomycosis, tuberculosis) and food poisoning.

Procedures that are followed in meat hygiene are:

- Veterinary examination of animals brought to slaughter house.
- Slaughter house sanitation.

Fish Hygiene

Traditionally stiffness, bright red gills and clear permanent eyes are known to exhibit good eatable fish.

After death autolysis by bacteria causes concern and should be taken care of in avoiding hepatitis, Para cholera and fish tape worm infestation. Of late tinned fish are being adjudged best if they posses following criteria:

- No rusting
- No leakage
- No evidence of tampering
- No bloom out phenomenon at opening.

Egg Hygiene

Eggs are sterile inside and are bound to get contaminated by soil, faecal matter in the environment. Bacteria including Typhoid organism can penetrate a cracked shell which can cause food poisoning.

Inspection and good preservation technique help in overcoming disease by poor egg hygiene.

Fruits and Vegetables

Sanitation of fruit and vegetables is a challenge to modern society.

Disposal of garbage is public health problem in market place, particularly so in corporation areas, since garbage is a source of transmission of Amoebiasis and worm infestation. Since fruits and vegetables are eaten raw, it poses problem with poor food sanitation.

For an effective hygiene of fruits and vegetables, action on following is relevant.

- Proper sanitation in handling of fresh fruits and vegetables.
- Washing fresh fruits/vegetables especially leafy vegetables with potassium permanganate solution.
- Proper disposal of garbage.
- Proper storage methods of perishables.

FOOD TOXINS

Food toxins are common causes of food poisoning. Epidemics of Gastro enteritis are traced, most often, to food toxins. Common toxins are described below.

Epidemic Dropsy

Outbreaks of epidemic dropsy with the manifestation of non inflammatory bilateral swelling of legs, diarrhoea, cardiac failure and death, and even glaucoma used to occur and the cause was discovered in 1926 when it was attributed to contamination of mustard oil with argemone oil. In 1941 "*Sanguinarine*" the toxin was identified for causing dropsy. Contamination was by ignorance (accidental) and also for commerce (deliberate).

Toxin prevention is possible by avoiding seed contamination and enforcement of PFA Act.

Aflatoxin

It is fungal toxin by *Aspergillus flavus* which infest food grains particularly ground nut. Many deaths have occurred because of liver failure. Among children, the clinical condition is described under "Indian childhood cirrhosis".

Prevention of toxin is possible by health education for not consuming the contaminated food grain. One has to ensure proper storage after drying. If moisture content is maintained below 10 percent, toxin formation is prevented totally.

Ergot

Ergot is a Field fungus known as *Claviceps fusiformis*, which grows as black mass. Consumption of ergot causes ergotism.

Nausea, vomiting, giddiness, drowsiness, cramps of limbs, gangrene of limbs are usual manifestation of ergotism.

Control is possible by health education and removal of infested grains by hand-picking. Infested grains can be removed by floating in 20% salt water.

Neurolathyrism

Contamination of edible Dhal with nonedible harmful dhal viz. *Kesaridhal* (Lathyrus sativus) which produce a neurotoxin BOAA (Beta oxalyl Amino Alanine). Neuroparalysis starts with difficult gait to crawling. The clinical stages are described according to ambulatory condition of the patient.

- Latent stage
- No stick stage
- One stick stage
- Two stick stage
- Crawler stage.

Prevention is possible by banning the crop, parboiling, health education and genetic approach.

Endemic Ascites

Millet (Panicum miliare = *Gondhli)* is contaminated with crotalaria seeds (*Jhunjhunia)* which contain hepatotoxin called pyrrolizidine alkaloid. Ascites and jaundice are common clinical manifestations.

Prevention is by health education and deweeding crotalaria plants.

Fusarium Toxin

Sorghum and rice gets infested with Fusarium fungi. G.I. manifestation is common. Control of grain contamination and disallowing the use of contaminated grains prevent toxic effect.

FOOD ADDITIVES

Many chemicals used as additives to increase shelf life of food, improve taste, to change the texture, to give a colour, are called food additives. All junk foods like (Biscuit, cake, confectionery, jam, jelly, coke, ketchup) contain food additives. Food additives are not nutritious, and are added intentionally.

Indiscriminate use of additive pose health problems, Contaminants incidental through packing, insecticides and environmental conditions also pose a threat to public health.

Permitted Food Additives are:

- Colouring agents (Saffron, turmeric)
- Flavouring agents (Vanilla)
- Sweetening agent (Saccharine)
- Preservative agent (Sorbic acid, acetic acid).

These additives are controlled by G.O.I. through:

- F.P.O. (Fruit Products Order).
- P.F.A. Act (Prevention of Food Adulterations Act).
- B.I.S. (Bureau of Indian Standards).

FOOD FORTIFICATION

Reinforcement of nutrients with additional supplies to prevent deficiency is called food fortification.

This is mainly to improve the quality of diet of a community.

Examples:

Fluoridation of water

Iodization of salt

Vitamin A and D to *vanaspathi*

Vitamin A and D to milk

Salt with Iodine and Iron.

Food fortification is a long term nutritional measure in the control of nutritional health problem.

FOOD ENRICHMENT

This process is the restoration of nutrient value of a food to its normal level. It is not a feasible process that can be adopted for a community nutrition programme. Mainly because of its temporary addition which can wean off again, enrichment is possible at the distribution level.

Example of vegetable oil when looses its vitamin content, enrichment with vitamin A and D is done at the source of distribution.

FOOD ADULTERATION

Food adulteration causes concern because it allows the food to loose its quality and at the same time, it may be injurious to health.

Common types of adulteration are noted in the Table 10.15:

Table 10.15 : Common food adulterants

Food		Adulterant
Asfoetida *(Hing)*	-	Resin, gum, grit
Butter	-	Starch, animal fat
Black pepper	-	Papaya seed
Cereals	-	Soapstone bits
Chilli powder	-	Brick powder
Coffee powder	-	Chicory, tamarind husk
Dhal	-	*Kesaridhal*
Dhania powder	-	Cow dung powder
Ghee	-	*Vanaspathi*
Haldi	-	Lead chromate powder
Ice cream	-	Starch, cellulose
Milk	-	Water, starch
Mustard seed	-	Argemone seed

Common Food Standards:

i. The *Agmark* standard (By Directorate of Marketing and Inspection).
ii. ISI Mark (By Bureau of Indian Standards).
iii. PFA Standards (By Central Committee for Food Standards).
iv. Codex Alimentarius (By Commission from FAO/WHO).

P.F.A. Act 1954

To ensure pure food and to avoid deceptive trade practices; prevention of Food Adulteration Act was enacted in 1954. Recently in 1986 it was amended for the third time giving it a more coverage. Food adulteration is punishable by life imprisonment and or fine. Food Laboratories help in final decision in this regard.

NATIONAL NUTRITIONAL PROGRAMMES

In the early part of post Independence due to high prevalence of malnutrition, Govt. of India launched several nutritional programmes. Early emphasis has been on increased food production and supplementary feeding to the vulnerable groups. The aim of all nutrition programmes is to provide additional nutrients to target groups to fill the gap between intake and requirement.

These can be described under following heads:

For Overall Nutritional Status

A.N.P.

Applied Nutrition Programme was introduced in 1960 to make people conscious of their nutritional needs and to increase production of foods for required consumption. Evaluation showed no desired awareness could be generated in the public. The community kitchen and school garden could not function properly. The programme lacked effective supervision and has become defunct.

S.N.P.

Major beneficiaries of special nutrition programme which was started in 1970 were preschool children, pregnant women and lactating mothers. This provided supplementary nutrition, supply of vitamin A solution and IFA tablets. The aim was for:

- 300 calories and 12 grams protein for a child.
- 600 calories and 20 grams protein for women and is for 300 days a year.

Because of lack of infrastructure it is not efficiently functioning.

Balwadi Nutrition Programme

This was started in 1970 for 3-6 aged children in rural areas, under social welfare department. This provided preprimary education along with providing 300 calories and 10 grams protein per day.

Mid Day Meal Programme

Mid Day Meal Programme (Centre):
It was launched in 1961 throughout the country, to improve children school attendance. The meal as a supplement supplying 1/3 of total calorie and half of protein need with local preparation and as low cost meal is an added attraction to school children. A model meal is to contain the following:

Cereal / millet	–	75 Grams
Pulses	–	30 Grams
Oil	–	8 Grams
Leafy vegetable	–	30 Grams
Non leafy vegetable	–	30 Grams

Now mid day meal programme is a part of Minimum Needs programme.

Mid Day Meal Programme (States):
Few states have taken up their own state level budgetary schemes to provide Mid day school Meal. Major examples are, Chief Minister's Noon Meal Programme" in *Tamil Nadu*, Chief Minister's Mid day school Meal "*Akshara Dasoha*" and "*Anna Dasoha*" in Karnataka.

Specific Disease Prevention Programmes

Vitamin A Prophylaxis Programme

This was started in 1970, by administering massive single dose of all preparation of Vitamin A (2 lakh I.U.) orally to all preschool children every 6 months through health workers.

Prophylaxis Against Nutritional Anaemia

It was started under the name National Nutritional Anaemia prophylaxis programme (NNAPP) with an objective of assessment, treatment, prophylaxis and monitoring anaemia among mothers. Distribution of IFA Tablets to Mothers and Children (1-12 years) was taken up through RCH centres, PHC's and ICDS *Anganwadies.*

Control of Iodine Deficiency Disorders

Started in 1962, Widened to national network, mounted in 1986 to replace plain edible salt by iodised salt in a phased manner. This is helping a lot in bringing down Iodine Deficiency Disorders. The programme is called NIDDCP (National Iodine Deficiency Disorders Control Programme).

Other Indirect Programmes

I.C.D.S.

Integrated child development service programme started in 1975 to help ICDS beneficiaries namely 0-6 age children, pregnant, lactating and women of reproductive age group. Supplementary nutrition and Therapeutic nutrition are being carried out at *Anganwadi l*evel which is evaluated by growth monitoring.

I.P.P.

India population project is an indirect nutritional programme through Family Welfare Schemes in selected places.

FURTHER REFERENCES

1. JS Garow WPT James A Ralph–Human Nutrition and Diseases (Churchill Livingstone).
2. ICMR—Nutrient requirement and R.D.A. for Indians.
3. NIN—Menu Low Cost Balanced diet S. India.
4. NIN—Menu Low Cost Balanced diet N. India.
5. NIN—Dietary Tips for the elderly.
6. Shanti Ghosh—Nutrition and Child care (JP).
7. WHO—Preventing controlling Iron deficiency.
8. WHO—Vitamin A deficiency and ill consequences
9. General Nursing and Midwifery 1986.
10. Ordinances of University of Health Sciences in Nursing.
11. Prabhakara, G.N.—Lecture notes to ICDS Medical Officers, COPOS (Mimeographed).
12. Prabhakara, G.N.—Policies and Programmes of Health in India (JP) 2004.
13. Rivers et al Brit Med Jour 37 (1) 1981.
14. WHO document 2004.
15. Health series from Voluntary Health Association.

11

Reproductive and Child Health (RCH)

INTRODUCTION

Pregnant women, lactating mothers and children below 14 years have been the vulnerable group in a community. Their health indicates and determines the community health. Total women population of India as per 2001 census is 495, 738, and 169 which constitute 48.27 % of the total population. Among this 15-45 year age group women constitute 22% of total population. 45 to 49 year age group women constitute 1.67 % of total population. Thus total of women15-49 age group form 23.67 % of total population. Children below 14 years form 42 % of the total population, thereby together (women 15-49 age + children below 14 years) constitute 65.67% of total population. This highlights the magnitude of mother and child health problems which the country has to encounter.

Mothers and children are special risk group. In developing countries mortality and morbidity in these sector are high, calling for a national level measures. Since MCH coverage can cover health of the nation, special health services under R.C.H. is formulated which are for the benefit of child survival and safe motherhood in the community.

Union Ministry announced the allocation of 40,000 *crores* on the II phase of RCH called R.C.H II with a goal of reducing MMR. This Phase II programme started on 1st April 2005. It also announced establishment of 3000 centres for the prevention of parent to child transmission of HIV; establishment of 380 centres where pregnant women are given ART

DEFINITION

Under RCH programme, Govt. of India, Ministry of Health and Family Welfare has defined the term as under:

"People have the ability to reproduce and regulate fertility. Women are able to go through pregnancy, child birth safely; the outcome of pregnancies is successful in terms of maternal and infant survival and well being. And couples are able to have sexual relations free from fear of pregnancy and of contracting disease."

CONCEPT OF RCH

It is an integrated approach of service which provides health services to young women and young children through family welfare programmes like UIP, ORT, CSSM, ARI control, emergency and essential obstetric care, MTP services, RTI and STD control, essential new born care and vitamin A prophylaxis.

RCH PACKAGE

As mentioned under concept of RCH, the components under RCH are depicted in Figure 11.1:

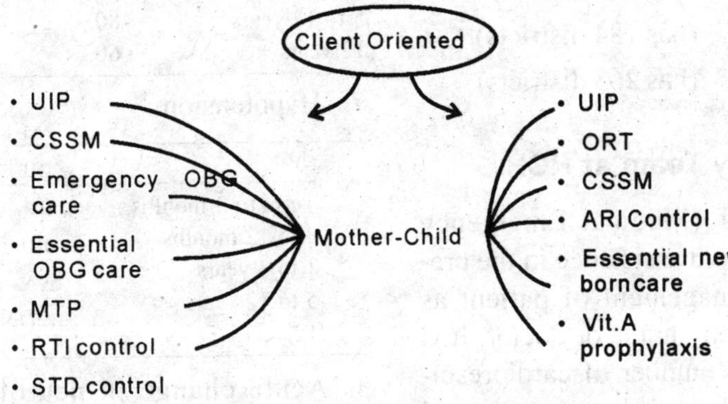

Fig. 11.1: RCH package

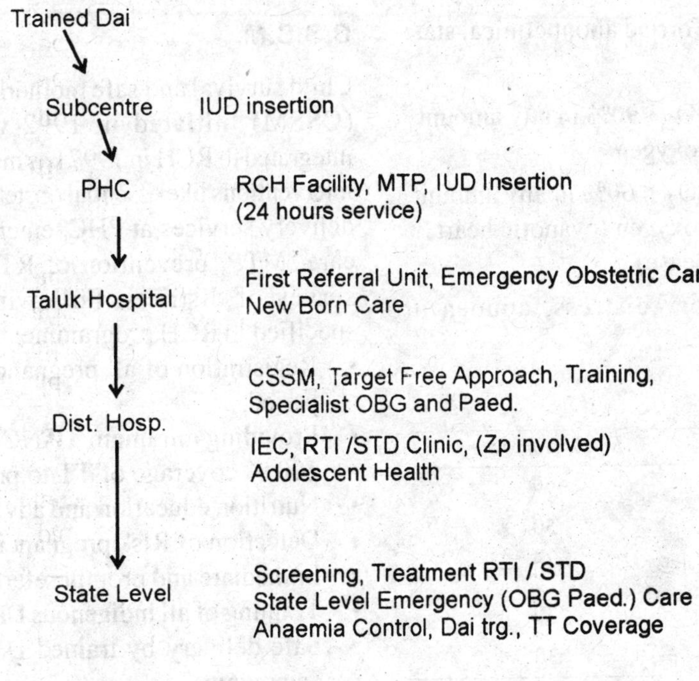

Fig. 11.2: Planned RCH care in H and FW services

RCH DIFFERENTIAL APPROACH

Based on crude birth rate and female literacy rate, districts are grouped under 3 categories for RCH programme initiation.

A Category – (has 58 districts)
B Category – (has 184 districts)
C Category – (has 265 districts)

Medical Emergency Team at RCH

The purpose of MET (Medical Emergency Team) is to provide rapid assistance in the pre-arrest emergency management of patient as deemed necessary by any nurse or doctor. It is hoped to decrease the number of cardiorespiratory arrests in wards and departments and reduce the number of unplanned admissions to ICU.

Criteria for Activation of Medical Emergency Team:

1. Nurse or doctor worried about clinical state
2. Airway threat
3. Hypoxaemia SpO_2 <90% in any amount of oxygen
   SpO_2 < 60% in any amount of oxygen (cyanotic heart disease)
4. Severe respiratory distress, apnoea or cyanosis
5. Tachypnoea

Age	*Respiratory rate*
Term to 3 months	>60
4 to 12 months	>50
1 to 4 years	>40
5 to 12 years	>30
12 years and above	>30

6. Tachycardia or Bradycardia

Age	*Heart rate too slow*	*Heart rate too fast*
Term to 3 months	<100	>180
4 to 12 months	<100	>180
1 to 4 years	<90	>160
5 to 12 years	<80	>140
12 years +	<60	>130

7. Hypotension

Age	*B.P.*
Term to 3 months	<50
4 to 12 months	<60
1 to 4 years	<70
5 to 12 years	<80
12 years +	<90

8. Acute change in neurological status or convulsion.
9. Cardiac or respiratory arrest.

The nurse is expected to notify the treating team and the MET service if a child fulfils any of above criteria.

C.S.S.M.

Child survival and safe motherhood programme (CSSM) initiated in 1992 which later got integrated to RCH in 1997 has major public health interventions like essential obstetric care, 24 hours delivery services at PHC, emergency obstetric care, MTP, prevention of RTI and STD and survey of districts. Following services are specified in RCH programme:

- Registration of all pregnancies, at the early period.
- Providing minimum 3 ANC check ups.
- 100 % coverage of TT to pregnant women.
- Nutrition education and advice.
- Detection of Risk pregnancies.
- Immediate and prompt referral of risk cases.
- Training of all indigenous Dais.
- Safe delivery by trained Dai, MPW in the community.

- Advice on birth spacing.
- Provision of institutional deliveries.

Delivery Service at PHC

To promote and provide institutional deliveries, 24 hours delivery facility at PHC and provision for additional honorarium to attending staff are provided at primary health centre.

M.T.P. (Medical Termination of Pregnancy)

On indication like unintended and unwanted pregnancies, when women accept MTP, it is allowed and conducted at PHC on fixed dates. Manpower training and provision of MTP equipment are attended under the scheme. This is mainly to reduce morbidity and mortality due to unsafe abortions.

Control of RTI / STD

With the collaboration of NACO (National AIDS Control Organisation) which provides assistance to set up clinics, a link with HIV/AIDS control is an ongoing programme. Training of manpower and supply of drug kit are attended under the scheme. This scheme provides provision of contract technician (two) to each district.

U.I.P.

This was earlier a part of CSSM and is now under RCH. Since 1997, provides immunisation against 6 preventable diseases. Supply of DPT, DT, OPV, measles, BCG and cold chain establishment and additional items supporting UIP.

Drug and Equipment Kits

Drug kit and equipment kit to sub centre, PHC under RCH activities are given in appendix.

O.R.T. Therapy

Under the RCH programme ORS packets are supplied to the states. Along with drug kit, every year 300 packets per year, in 2 lots are supplied by the Central Government. Rational use of drug, nutritional care and preventive ORT are motivated to reduce child mortality.

A.R.I. Control

Acute Respiratory Infections are to be prevented to prevent deaths due to pneumonia. Training health workers on recognition and management is undertaken. Through drug kit cotrimoxazole is supplied under the scheme.

Vitamin A Prophylaxis

Five doses of vitamin A to all children below the age of 3 years, is provided each with specified dose.

9 months	–	I dose 1 lakh units
18 months	–	II dose 2 lakh units
24 months	–	III dose 2 lakh units
30 months	–	IV dose 2 lakh units
36 months	–	V dose 2 lakh units

Anaemia Control in Children

Nurse will identify anaemia in children and give 100 tablets for 100 days and such each tablet shall contain 20 mg of elemental iron and 0.1 mg of folic acid. Since 74% of children below 3 years age have anaemia current programme guideline instructs for the provision of iron tablets.

Emergency Obstetric Care

Many deliveries are home deliveries and if they are associated with complications, maternal morbidity and mortality rate will go up. Thousands of referral units are identified under RCH programme. They are strengthened with emergency obstetric kit, equipment kit and skilled health professional. Involvement of NGO for decentralising activities is another novel idea under RCH scheme.

Essential Obstetric Care

This refers to basic maternity service to all pregnant women in the country. This ensures the following:

- Registration of pregnancy at 16 weeks
- 3 ANC check ups by (ANM) MPW
- Safe delivery (Home or Health Centre)
- 3 PNC check ups.

This component is greatly intended at Home visiting and hence a specific criteria of domiciliary care.

Essential New Born Care

This component reduces the perinatal and neonatal mortality in the community. Services extended under following areas:

- Resuscitation of new born with birth asphyxia
- Prevention of hypothermia
- Prevention of infection
- Exclusive breast feeding
- Referral of sick newborn
- Care of LBW babies.

Other Initiatives of RCH Activity

a. RCH camps with obstetricians and paediatricians for specialist's service to remote and outreach areas.
b. RCH outreach activity to cover UIP and MCH services to remote areas.
c. Neonatal care unit establishment at district level hospitals.
d. ICMR model home based neonatal care unit to provide neonatal care at grassroots level.
e. Priority service to high mortality districts by focused interventions. It is called BDCS (Border District Cluster Strategy). This priority also includes integrated management of childhood illness (IMCI).
f. Introduction of Hepatitis B vaccination project in selected districts.

EAG (Empowered Action Group) of Health and F.W. Service, Govt. of India:
This scheme gives priority to UP, Bihar, MP, Rajastan, Orissa, Chhattisgarh, Jharkhand and Uttaranchal.

As per Govt. of India report based on district survey till the end of 1999 has given key indicators.

R.C.H. KEY INDICATORS

a. Currently married women
   Percent married females to total females in the age
   10-14 years – 4.5 %
   15-19 years – 35.3 %
   20-24 years – 81.8 %
   15-44 years – 79.5 %
b. Mean age at marriage – 19.5 years
c. No. of children per married women aged 45-49 years
   - Ever born – 4.3
   - Surviving – 3.7
d. Currently married women with any ANC - 67.2 %. (Any one or two of ANC check up, TT, IFA)
e. Currently married women with full ANC – 14.8 % (all had 3 ANC check up + TT + 100 IFA / Tablets)
f. Institutional delivery - 40.5 %
g. Safe delivery (by trained) - 47.6 %
h. Women with pregnancy complications – 34.8 %
   Swelling hand, feet
   Visual disturbance
   Bleeding
   Convulsions

Weak or no foetal movement
Abnormal presentation.

i. Delivery complications - 36.4%
   Premature labour
   Obstructed labour
   Prolonged labour
j. Post delivery complications - 42.0%
   High Fever
   Lower abdominal pain
   Foul smelling vaginal discharge
   Excessive bleeding
   Dizziness
   Severe Headache
k. Currently married women 15-44 age with symptoms of RTI/STD – 28.8%
l. Currently married women 15-44 age who are aware of AIDS – 41.1%
m. Males aged 20-54 years with symptoms of RTI/STD – 12.7%
n. Males aged 20-54 years who are aware of AIDS – 57.4%

District based rapid household survey by Government of India has given following results 2004 All India Survey:

Mean age at marriage	19.5 years
Birth order 3 and above	42%
Min 3 ANC check ups	50.1%
Complete ante natal care	16%
Couple protection rate	45.7%
Hospital deliveries	40.5%
Fully immunised	47.6%

MATERNITY CYCLE

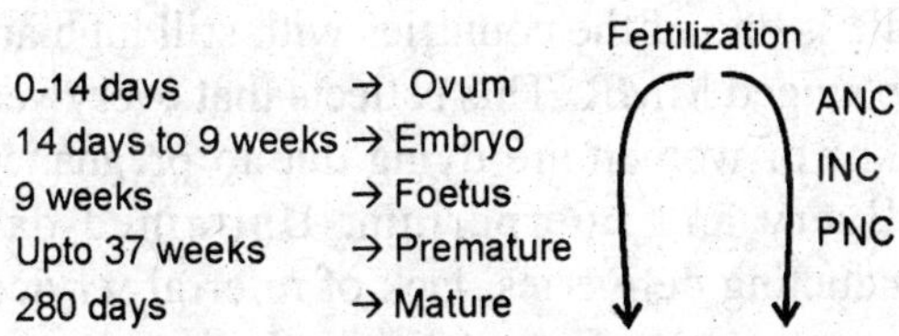

Fig. 11.3: Maternity cycle

Study of maternity cycle is important in understanding physiological basis of pregnancy, delivery and lactation. These periods influence the health of mother and child. Any pathology leads to maternal and infant morbidity and mortality.

R.C.H. PROBLEMS

Malnutrition

Pregnant woman, lactating mothers and children are affected by malnutrition in developing countries. They cause LBW, Anaemia, Toxaemia, PPH. Intrauterine period influence foetal growth and weaning period influence childhood malnutrition. Direct interventions like supplementation, indirect interventions like environmental sanitation prove effective anchor in the prevention of malnutrition.

Infection

Foetal growth retardation, puerperal sepsis and LBW are due to maternal infections. Women infected with Toxoplasma and cytomegalo virus are increasing. On the other hand, diarrhoea, ARI and skin infections of infants are seen to a great extent. Malaria and tuberculosis are serious infection of childhood. Programmes under RCH are aimed at the prevention of those infections.

Uncontrolled Reproduction

Repeated child births have seen their association with anaemia, abortion, LBW and APH. There is need for small family norm to safeguard mother and child health. High birth rate is associated with high IMR and under five death rate (Table 11.1) as per observations by UNICEF and UNDP:

INDICATORS OF R.C.H. CARE

Growth and development of child indicates the care given to a mother during her reproductive

Table 11.1: BR, IMR and UFMR in developed and developing countries

	Developed countries	*Developing countries*
Birth rate / 1000 population	11	24
IMR/1000 LB	7	58
Under five MR/1000 LB	6	85

age. Similarly illness of mothers and children reflex RCH status. But of late mortality rates are indicating the extent of RCH care in the community. These indicators are highlighted below:

M.M.R. (Maternal Mortality Rate)

ICD grouping has brought out the following categories of maternal deaths due to (1) Obstetric complications and (2) Non obstetric complications. The first category includes complications of pregnancy, labour and puerperium. The second category includes previous existing diseases like cardiovascular, renal and other organ disorders.

Pregnancy related death is sometimes used to denote the death of woman while pregnant or within 42 days of termination of pregnancy irrespective of cause of death.

It is also suggested that mother dying from direct obstetric of non-obstetrics causes more than 42 days after termination of pregnancy but before completion of 1 year from delivery may be considered as later maternal death.

WHO has defined MMR as "the death of woman while pregnant or within 42 days of termination of pregnancy irrespective of duration and site of pregnancy from any cause related to or aggravated by the pregnancy or its management but not from accidental or incidental causes."

$$MMR = \frac{\text{Female Death due to complications of pregnancy, childbirth or within 42 days of delivery from puerperal causes in an area during a year}}{\text{Total live births in that area for a year}} \times 1000$$

World Picture:

Table 11.2: IMR per 1000 live births

USA	0.17/1000
UK	0.13/1000
Thailand	0.44/1000
Bangladesh	3.8/1000
India	4.0/1000

Infection and bleeding are common causes of maternal mortality. While hepatitis, heart disorders and endocrine causes are more in developed countries, in developing countries the causes are mostly infection, anaemia, jaundice and malaria.

Table 11.3: Global causes of maternal deaths

Bleeding	25.0 %
Infections	15.0 %
Toxaemia	12.0 %
Unsafe abortion	13.0 %
Obstructed labour	8.0 %
Anaemia, malaria, heart disease etc.	20.0 %
Ectopic, embolism etc.	7.0 %

Other influencing causes of maternal mortality have been:

- Women's age
- Birth interval
- Parity
- Socioeconomic status
- Cultural practices
- Nutritional status
- Environmental sanitation.

Indian Picture:

India is one of the countries with still high and unchanged MMR. This reflects that every year Lakhs of women are dying due to pregnancy, delivery and puerperium. Untrained dais conducting deliveries, lack of referral services are contributory factors. Within India each state shows variable rates with respect to MMR (Table 11.4).

Table 11.4: MMR in different states in India

State	MMR
Gujarat	1.6/1000
Karnataka	1.89/1000
W.B.	1.4/1000
Orissa	2.9/1000
M.P.	4.7/1000
Rajasthan	5.6/1000
U.P.	7.0/1000

Common Causes:

Table 11.5: Causes of MMR in India

Haemorrhage	38 %
Sepsis	11 %
Obstructed labour	5 %
High B.P.	5%
Abortion	8 %
Toxaemia	8 %
Others	25 %

Causes of MMR in India are:

Obstetric cause: Haemorrhage, infection, unsafe abortion

Nonobstetric cause: Anaemia, renal disease, hepatic diseases

Social causes: Age at childbirth, parity, malnutrition, poor transport, social custom.

Prevention of Maternal Mortality:

Tackling obstetric, nonobstretric and social causes reduces the M.M.R.

R.C.H. programme detailed earlier with its components like early registration, anaemia correction, essential obstetric care, emergency obstetric care and preventing complications have an impact on M.M.R.

Foetal Deaths

This is a crude indicator of RCH. No reliable information is available and if available they are usually after 28 weeks of gestation. Hence foetal deaths are redefined under still births.

Still Birth Rate

It is death of foetus weighing 1000 grams or more occurring during one year in every 1000 total births.

Still Birth Rate

$$= \frac{\text{Foetal deaths weighing above 1000 grams, at birth}}{\text{Total LB + Still Births weighing above 1000 g at birth}} \times 1000$$

Present estimate of still birth rate in India is 9, urban areas showing around 8.

Perinatal Mortality Rate

This includes still births and early neonatal deaths.

Perinatal Mortality Rate

$$= \frac{\text{Late foetal and early neonatal deaths weighing above 1000 grams, at birth}}{\text{Total LB above 1000 g, at birth}} \times 1000$$

Perinatal mortality rate is a significant yardstick of measuring obstetric and paediatric care in a country. It is now 33 as per estimate.

Table 11.6: Perinatal mortality rates

Japan	5/1000
U.S.A.	10/1000
Thailand	20/1000
India	33/1000

Following risk groups are identified in influencing high perinatal mortality. They are:

- Elderly mothers
- Young mother
- Parity 5 and above
- Heavy smoking
- Severe anaemia
- Multiple pregnancy.

Causes of perinatal mortality can be grouped under 3 categories:

1. *Antenatal causes:* Maternal diseases, pelvic diseases, birth defects of repro-

ductive organs, Rh incompatibility, Toxaemia of pregnancy, APH.

2. *Intranatal causes:* Birth injury, Asphyxia, obstetric complications.
3. *Postnatal causes:* Premature baby, respiratory distress syndrome, congenital anomalies.

Preventive Steps

Tackling above 3 causes at appropriate time and existing RCH programme include catering TT, IFA, essential obstetric care, emergency obstetric care, safe delivery practice, essential new born care.

Neonatal Mortality Rate

Deaths of newborn occurring from birth till 28 days after birth are called neonatal mortality. It is calculated by:

Neonatal Mortality Rate

$$= \frac{\text{No. of deaths of newborn before28 days after birth in a year}}{\text{Total LB in that year}} \times 1000$$

Neonatal mortality reflects endogenous factors like LBW, birth injury, etc., which affect new born. It is directly related to gestational age and birth weight. In India 60 % of infant deaths are occurring before 28 days after birth of new born babies. It is approximately estimated at present as 37 per 1000 live births (Urban) and 41 in Rural.

Post Neonatal Mortality Rate

It is the ratio of post neonatal deaths in a given year to the total number of live births in the same year. It is calculated by:

Post Neonatal Mortality Rate

$$= \frac{\text{No. of deaths of children between 28 days to 1 year in a year}}{\text{Total LB in that year}} \times 1000$$

This mortality is influenced by exogenous factors like diarrhoea, ARI, malnutrition. Large family and high birth order are found significantly related to this mortality. It is estimated to be, at present, 23 per 1000 live birth.

Infant Mortality Rate (IMR)

It is the ratio of infant deaths registered in a given year to the total number of live births of the same year. It is calculated by:

$$\text{I.M.R.} = \frac{\text{No. of deaths of children below 1 year of age in a year}}{\text{Total LB in that year}} \times 1000$$

It is one of the most important and sensitive indicator of RCH. It is a unique rate because it covers a large 1 year age population, when they suffer from disease or condition which are specific to that age and intervention brings out remarkable decline of IMR.

Table 11.7: IMR in developed and developing countries

Developed countries		*Developing countries (per 1000 live births)*	
Japan	3	Bangladesh	56
USA	7	India	58

I.M.R. of India is estimated, at present, at 58 per 1000 live births. Most of urban studies have shown a declined rate of IMR when compared to rural areas.

I.M.R. is greatly related and influenced by female literacy rate and birth rate. Statistical significant relation (r) is established by taking values of 15 states (Table 11.8).

State	Female literacy Rate	Birth Rate	IMR
A.P.	50.17	20.4	59
Assam	56.30	26.3	66
Bihar	33.57	30.7	61
Gujarat	58.60	24.6	53
Karnataka	57.45	21.8	49
Kerala	87.86	16.7	12
M.P.	50.28	30.2	79
Maharastra	67.51	19.9	36
Orissa	50.97	23.0	77
Haryana	56.31	26.3	61
Punjab	63.65	20.6	45
Rajasthan	44.34	30.3	67
T.N.	64.55	18.3	41
U.P.	42.98	31.3	72
W.B.	60.22	20.3	40
	(1)	(2)	(3)

Causes of I.M.R.:

i. Neonatal causes:
- L.B.W.
- Birth injury
- Birth defect
- Rh incompatibility
- Diarrhoea
- A.R.I.
- N.N.T.

ii. Post neonatal causes:
- Diarrhoea
- A.R.I.
- Malnutrition
- Birth defects
- Other infections

Table 11.8 : I.M.R., female literacy, birth rate of selected states (correlation established)

	$r_{\text{Female Literacy Rate : Birth Rate}}$ i.e., $r_{1:2}$	$r_{\text{Female Literacy Rate : IMR}}$ $r_{1:3}$
n= shift S-sum 3	15	15
Σ_x = shift S-sum 2	845.39	845.39
Σ_x^2 = shift S-sum 1	49838.02	49838.02
Σ_y =shift S-sum → 2	360.7	818
Σ_y^2 = shift S-sum → 1	9007.49	49078
Σ_{xy} = shift S-sum →3	19626.09	43482.47
$\bar{X}$ = shift S-var 1	56.35	56.35
$\bar{Y}$ = shift S-var → 1	24.046	54.53
r	$r_{1:2}$ = - 0.821373271 - 0.8214	$r_{1:3}$ = - 0.836780125 - 0.8368
Statistical inference	Higher the Female Literacy Rate lower the Birth Rate. **Found statistically significant correlation between female literacy rate and Birth Rate.**	Higher the Female Literacy Rate lowers the IMR **Found statistically significant correlation between female literacy rate and .IMR.**

I.M.R. is influenced by following factors:

Table 11.9: Factors influencing I.M.R.

Biological	*Economical*	*Sociocultural*
Birth weight	Income of family	Early marriage
Mother's age	Standard of living	Sex of child
Birth order	Purchasing power of family	Breast feeding
Multiple pregnancy	Affordability	Planned motherhood
Family size High fertility	Possessions	Mother's education Broken family Unwed mother Overcrowding

Foetal and infantile mortality are defined as above (Fig. 11.4):

Prevention of I.M.R.

i. Good Antenatal care
ii. U.I.P.
iii. Exclusive breast feeding
iv. Growth monitoring
v. Small family norm
vi. Good sanitation
vii. Essential obstetric care
viii. Essential paediatric care
ix. Female literacy
x. Socio-economic development.

Child Death Rate

It is calculated by:

$$\text{Child death rate} = \frac{\text{No. of deaths of children 1 - 4 age in a year}}{\text{Total No. of children 1 - 4 age (MYP)}} \times 1000$$

Child death rate reflects environmental conditions and sociocultural conditions of the family. A child has high risk of dying at 2nd year of life.

It is estimated, at present, at 17.4 (Urban 10.2%) percent of total deaths.

Common causes of child death rate in India are:

- Diarrhoea
- A.R.I.
- Malnutrition
- Other infectious diseases
- Accidents.

Prevention of 1-4 year mortality lies on the specific control measures against causes mentioned above.

Child Mortality Rate (Under 5 Mortality)

It is the annual number of deaths of children under 5 years expressed as a rate per 1000 live births.

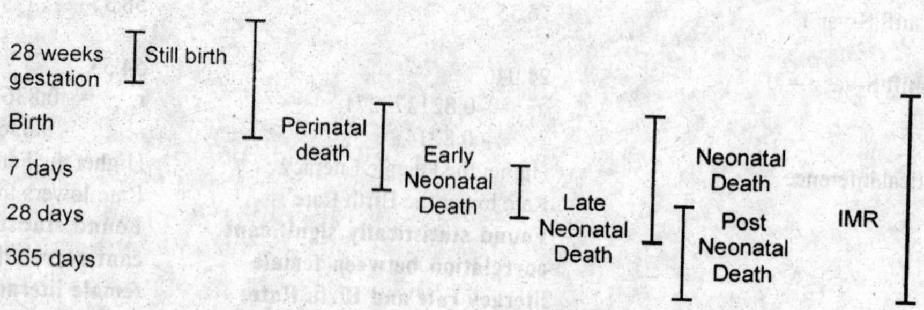

Fig. 11.4: Notation of foetal and infantile mortality

$$\text{C.M.R.} = \frac{\text{No. of deaths of children below 5 years in a year}}{\text{No. of LB in that year}} \times 1000$$

Table 11.10: C.M.R. of selected countries

(per 1000 LB)

Country		C.M.R.
Japan	–	4
U.S.A.	–	8
Sri Lanka	–	14
Thailand	–	21
India	–	85
Pakistan	–	101

Causes of Child Mortality Rate:

- A.R.I.
- Neonatal infections
- Diarrhoea
- Measles, malaria
- Malnutrition
- Accidents.

Note:

C.M.R. estimate, at present, is at

85/1000 live births

OR

17.4/1000 under five years population

Prevention is action on noted causes and control of influencing factors.

Child Survival Index

It is calculated by:

$$\text{C.S.I.} = \frac{(1000\text{–Child mortality rate}}{10}$$

$$= \frac{(1000) - 85}{10} = 91.5$$

Note the calculation:

85 – Child mortality rate

85 – Die out of 1000

Remaining is 1000 – 85 = 915

For 1000 .... 915 survive

For 100 .... $\frac{915}{1000} \times 100 = 91.5$

IMNCI (Integrated management of neonatal and childhood illness

Common childhood illnesses are diarrhoea, acute respiratory infection, measles and malnutrition. They overlap each other. Hence to look beyond treatment of a single illness, IMNCI a cost effective preventive and promotive step is launched by Government of India.

Following steps in the integrated case management process are suggested:

Danger signs are checked
(Convulsion, unconsciousness, not taking feed, vomiting)
↓
Main symptoms are assesses
(Cough, difficulty breathing, diarrhoea, fever, ear problems)
↓
Assess nutrition, assess immunisation, assess feeding problems
↓
Check other problems
↓
Classify into **Red** (urgent referral),
Yellow (treatment at OPD)
and **Green** (home management)

Vandemataram Scheme:

Vandemataram logo is given to voluntary doctors who volunteer for RCH work. Patients are also given *Vandemataram* cards to go these doctors who attend IFA tablet distribution, oral contraceptives distribution, TT injections etc., and further referral from *Vandemataram* doctors are also made available.

Janani Suraksha Yojana:

It is 100% centrally scheme under national rural health mission where cash assistance with institutional care during antenatal, during delivery and during post partum care is given. This can help to reduce MMR, IMR through encouraging delivery at health institutions and focusing at institutional care among women in below poverty line families.

SOCIAL WELFARE PROGRAMMES FOR R.C.H.

They are grouped under 3 heads:
1. Programmes for women
2. Programmes for children
3. Combined programmes.

I.C.D.S. (Integrated Child Development Services)

In pursuance of the National policy for children, I.C.D.S. scheme was initiated in 1975. It is an integrated package of:
a. Supplementary nutrition
b. Immunisation
c. Health check up
d. Medical referral service
e. Nutrition education
f. Health education, and
g. Non-informal education of 0–6 children (See Figure 11.5 on the next page).

Administration of I.C.D.S.

Under Ministry of Social and Women Welfare, Integrated Child Development service is being undertaken through state directorate. There are urban, rural and tribal blocks which are administered by CDPO; under CDPO 4 *Mukhya sevikas* each controlling 20–25 *Anganwadies* acts as mentor to AWWs. Each *anganwadi* has an AWW who is a community woman who helps in AW functionaries. 1978 and 1982 surveys gave good results which allowed great expansions. At present there are 5691 ICDS projects operating. Of late Adolescent Girl scheme was sanctioned to 507 blocks as a special intervention to 11–18 year age girls. Some blocks were sponsored by NGOs and few others were sponsored by World Bank.

Recently we have proposal for:
a. Universalisation of I.C.D.S. scheme
b. Setting up of community nutrition centres and
c. Sanction of *Indira Mahila Yojana* are under consideration.

I.C.D.S. coverage is considered good based on the fact that:
a. There is reduction in severe malnutrition among children.
b. Birth weight is gained among beneficiaries.
c. Good immunisation coverage.
d. Reduced I.M.R., and
e. Reduced child mortality rate in the area under ICDS coverage.

Objectives of I.C.D.S.

a. To improve the nutritional and health status of children in the age group 0–6 years.
b. To lay the foundations for psychological, physical and social development of the child.
c. To reduce mortality and morbidity, malnutrition and school dropout.
d. To achieve an effective coordination of policy and implementation among the various departments working for the promotion of child development, and
e. To enhance the capability of the mother and nutritional needs of the child through proper nutrition and health education.

Package of services in I.C.D.S.

Pregnant women	Health check up TT Supplementary nutrition Nutrition Education Health Education
Lactating mothers	Health check up Supplementary nutrition

Contd.

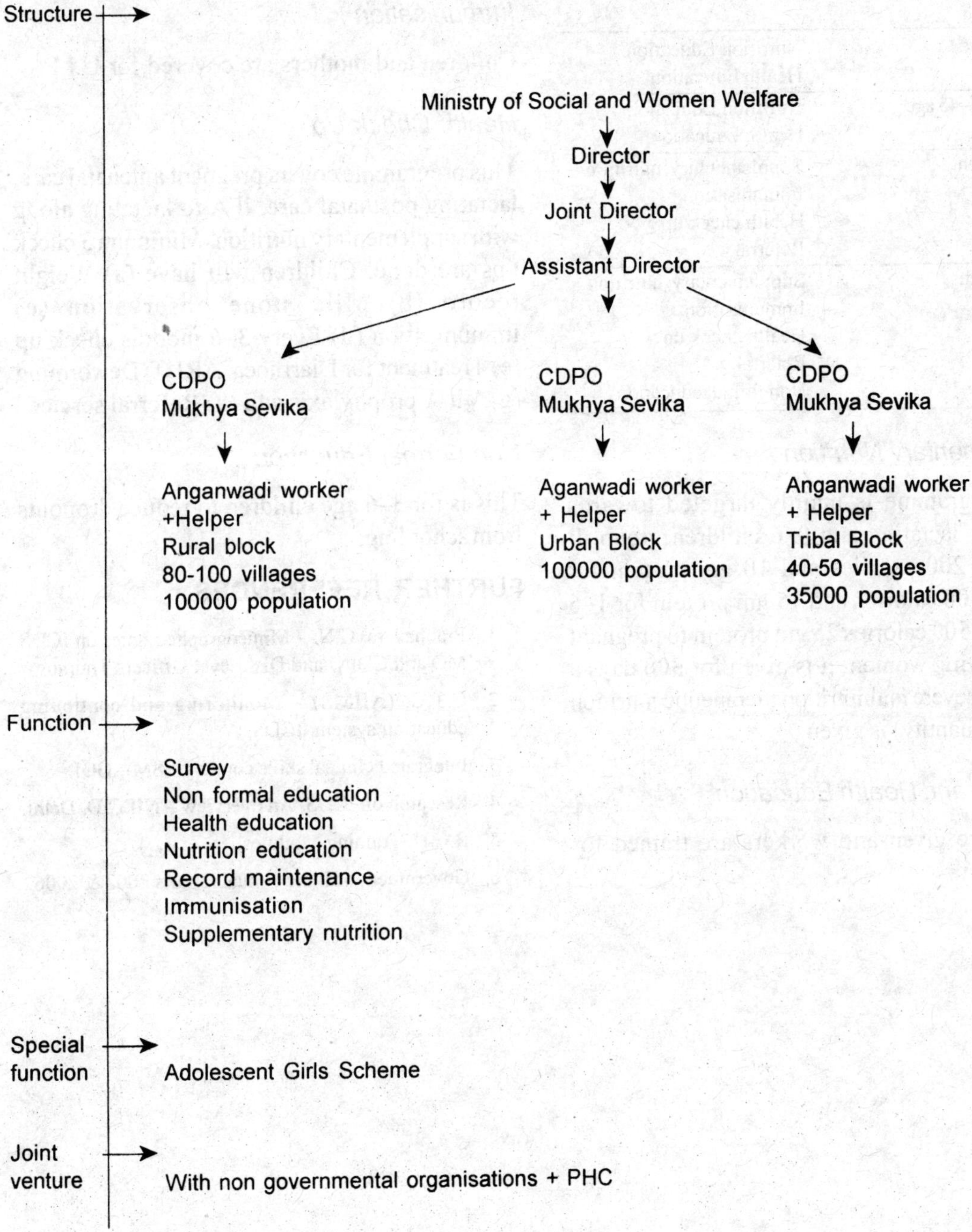

Fig. 11.5: Administration of integrated child development service scheme in India

Contd.

	Nutrition Education Health Education
Women 15–45 age	Nutrition Education Health Education
0–3 children	Supplementary nutrition Immunisation Health check up Referral
3–6 children	Supplementary nutrition Immunisation Health check up Referral Non formal education

Supplementary Nutrition

This programme is mainly targeted towards pregnant, lactating and 0–6 children group. It provides 200 calories and 10 gm protein for infants; 300 calories and 15 gm protein for 1–6 children; 500 calories 25 gm protein to pregnant and lactating women. It is given for 300 days a year. For severe malnutrition therapeutic nutrition (double quantity) is given.

Nutrition and Health Education

Topics are given and workers are trained for this aspect.

Immunisation

Children and mothers are covered for U.I.P.

Health Check Up

This programme covers pregnant antenatal care, lactating postnatal care, IFA to lactating along with supplementary nutrition. Minimum 3 check ups are done. Children will have (a) Weight record (b) Mile stone observation (c) Immunisation (d) Every 3–6 months check up (e) Treatment for Diarrhoea, ARI (f) Deworming (g) Vit A prophylaxis and (h) Referral service.

Non Formal Education

This is for 3–6 age children to reduce dropouts from schooling.

FURTHER REFERENCES

1. Prabhakara, G.N. – Mimeographed notes on ICDS MO and CDPO and Dist Level Officers Training.
2. C.T.C. (AIIMS) – Monitoring and continuing education system, ICDS.
3. Integrated clinical skills course CSSM – GOI.
4. Research on ICDS, An overview – NIPCID, Delhi.
5. R.C.H. Training Modules.
6. Government of India annual reports 2002 & 2006.

12

Human Sexuality

Human sexuality is how people experience and express themselves as sexual beings. The study of human sexuality is comprised a broad range of behaviors, processes and societal topics. Biologically, sexuality can encompass sexual intercourse and sexual contact in all its forms, as well as medical concerns about the physiological or even psychological aspects of sexual behaviour. Sociologically, it can cover the cultural, political, and legal aspects; and philosophically, it can span the moral, ethical, theological, spiritual or religious aspects.

According to Foucault, sexuality began to be regarded as a concept part of human nature and sexuality began to be used as a mean to define normality and its boundaries, and to conceive everything outside those boundaries in the realm of psychopathology. According to the theories of Sigmund Freud sexuality was seen more as a "discontent of civilization".

In many historical eras, recovered art and artifacts help to portray human sexuality.

IMPORTANCE

Sex, a wide term, which do not mean aptly, play a dominant role in human life. It is an accepted creative and pleasurable force shaping human behaviour. It is not just equal to reproduction, but more than a biopsychosocial function.

It has positive aspects like:

- Pair bonding
- Fostering intimacy
- Providing pleasure
- Bolstering self esteem
- Reduction in tension etc.

It has negative aspects like:

- Asserting masculinity
- Asserting femininity
- Exploitation of sex
- Expression of hostility
- Psychological turmoil
- Emotional turmoil etc.

DEFINITION

According to WHO it is defined as "the whole range of behaviour associated with psychobiological phenomenon of sex".

It is dealt under family health where disciplines like psychology, gynaecology, urology, nursing, sociology interact in its problem management.

COMPONENTS

Biological

It is a biological component dealing right from birth till death through infancy, childhood, adolescence, adulthood and old age. It deals with sexual desire, male and female sex differences, sexual response, sexual behaviour and sexual functioning.

Psychological

Development of gender, sex identity, emotions, thoughts, feelings and personality traits are covered under psychological component.

Socio Cultural

It covers regulation of sex socialisation, regulation of sexual behaviour, sex role play, family practices and social pressures in sex life.

Understanding of human sexuality requires the study of these factors and their interaction and inter-relationships.

Socio cultural component of human sexuality: They influence sexual development through social learning. Subsequently it gives rise to sexual behaviour of an individual in a society. Culture approves certain norms of sexual behaviour to assure peace, to stabilise domestic relations and to facilitate procreation. Historical, ethical, economic and educational subcultures are packed up constraints in human sexuality. Culture moulds the expression of sexual drive. Some major factors influencing human sexuality are:

- Marriage and family
- Religion
- Social class
- Media and advertisement
- Contraception and abortion services
- Technological development
- Educational status
- Revolutions.

SEX EDUCATION

As a component of population education it was introduced in India through National Family Welfare Planning Programme during 1960. It includes mostly education on reproduction; however, it should also impart positive attitude to sex behaviour. Sex education can motivate people to change or to modify the existing negative attitude and misbehaviours.

Main goal of sex education is to develop an ability to merge biological impulses with socially acceptable norms of sex behaviour conducive to a satisfying family life as adult men and women.

It is going on as a learning process without our knowledge both in informal form (Home, peer group) and formal form (School, University). Feeling of love and affection that has to be from parents in role modelling and also by siblings is not a true sex in human sexuality. It is the learning of sex attitude and sex emotion which are responsible for family relation and family responsibility that needed to be imparted in sex education.

Parents need to attempt to satisfy the natural and anxious curiosities of their child from where sex education starts. During adolescence, physiology of body, sexually transmitted diseases are to be made understandable. Sex education and counselling for adult men and women is managed by family physicians.

Sex education is the introduction of sexual topics within an educational context. Almost all western countries have some form of sex education, but the nature varies widely. In some countries (such as Australia and much of Europe) "age-appropriate" sex education often begins in pre-school, whereas other countries (notably the USA) leave sex education to the teenage years and even the late teenage years. Sex education covers a range of topics, including the physical, mental and social aspects of sexual behavior.

Content of sex education in nursing care are:

i. Anatomy and physiology of reproduction.
ii. Physical and emotional changes during puberty.
iii. Behaviour towards opposite sex.
iv. Moral codes and cultural standards.
v. Responsibility of marriage.
vi. Planned parenthood.
vii. Small family norms.

Common health problems associated with human sexuality are:

i. Masturbation
ii. Emotional inadequacy
iii. Unwanted pregnancy
iv. S.T.D.
v. HIV/AIDS
vi. Infertility, sterility
vii. Divorce.

SEX THERAPY

The care of sex problem which need treatment are multidimensional. They are:

a. *Somatic Therapy*: Drug, hormone or surgical treatment for certain conditions (e.g. genital tract infection, impotency).
b. *Behavioural Therapy:* Required for changing attitude of patient.
c. *Psychoanalysis:* For cases of imagination and fantasies.
d. *Hypnosis:* It is to induce relaxation.
e. *Psychotherapy:* Emotional treatment.

COUNSELLING

Nursing profession has been giving guidance and advice on all matters of health problems associated with human sexuality. In family planning, sterilisations, abortions, S.T.D. it is part of general health service. Educational and counselling techniques are to be learnt to impart the art of communication and good listening. From this we can remove erroneous beliefs and taboos to promote positive attitude in human sexuality.

FURTHER REFERENCES

1. Sexual. medicine in Primary care by William and Maurice (Mosby).
2. Sexual Medicine—A handbook by R.N. Srivastava, G.D. Shukla, B.L. Verma (JP).

13

Preventive Obstetrics

REVIEW OF REPRODUCTIVE SYSTEM

Pelvis harbour female organ of generation. It is designed for its work of child bearing. For anatomical purpose it is upper part a shallow cavity formed by the iliac fosse which is called false pelvis and bony basin lower portion containing organs of generation called true pelvis.

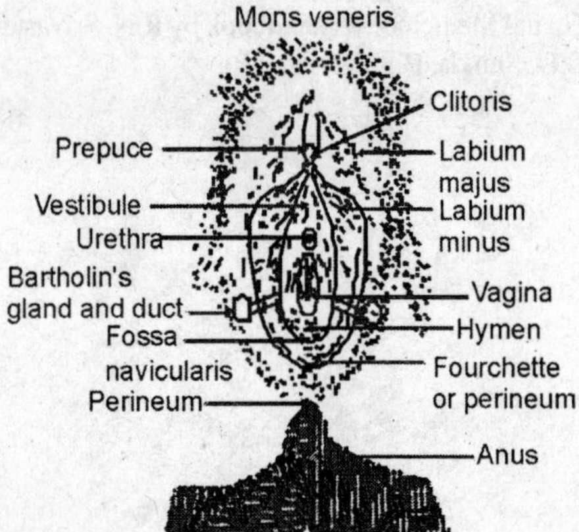

Fig. 13.1: External organs of generation

External organs of generation are mons pubis and vulva. Mons pubis is pad fat covering pubic bone and is covered with pubic hair. Vulva consists of labia majora, labia minora. Clitoris is situated at meeting point of labia minora. Urinary meatus is in the centre of a triangular surface 'vestibule'. Below this is the orifice entrance to vagina.

Internal organs of generation consist of vagina, uterus, fallopian tube and ovaries.

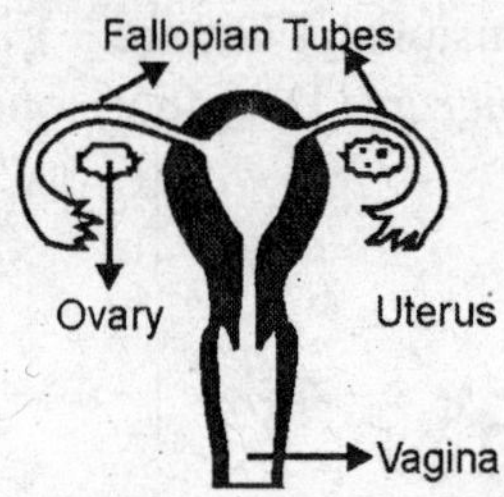

Fig. 13.2: Internal organs of generation

Vagina is a passage about 4" long sloping upwards and backwards from vulva to the cervix uteri. Its wall allows great expansion during labour. Uterus is pear shaped 3" × 2" x 1" with notable parts; body and cervix. It is tilted forward on the vagina and hence is antevertion in normal occurrence. Inner layer is endometrium, invests the fallopian tube and ovaries in the form of broad ligament. The fallopian tube leave the fundus of

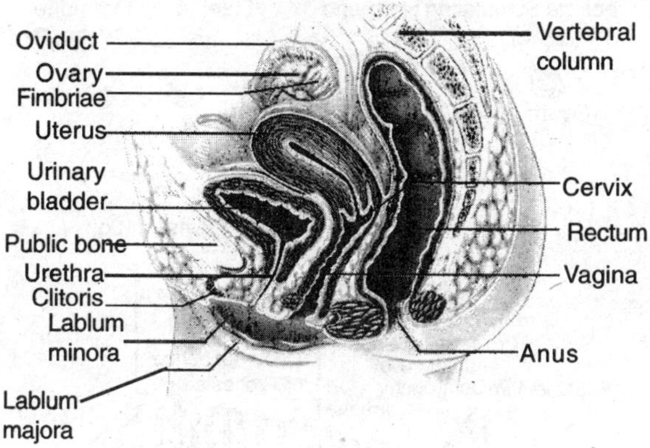

Fig. 13.3: Anatomical position of reproductive organs in sagittal section

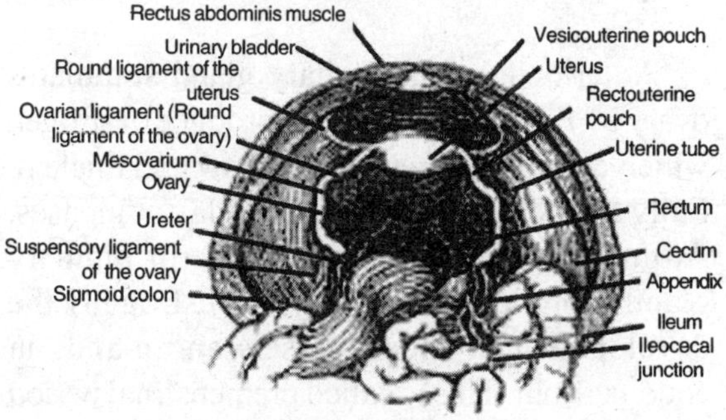

Fig .13.4: Internal reproductive organs seen from above

1. Bladder
2. Uterus
3. Rectum
4. Uterosacral ligament
5. Fallopian tube
6. Ovary
7. Ureter
8. Round ligament
9. Infundibulopelvic ligament

the uterus by tiny opening at either side. The cilia in the lining help the passage of ova along. Two ovaries on either side about the size and shape of almonds have 2 functions:

1. Produces internal secretions.
2. produces ova.

Anatomical relations of reproductive organs are shown in Figures 13.3 and 13.4.

Female Pelvis

The pelvic bone is made of 2 innominate bones, a sacrum and a coccyx.

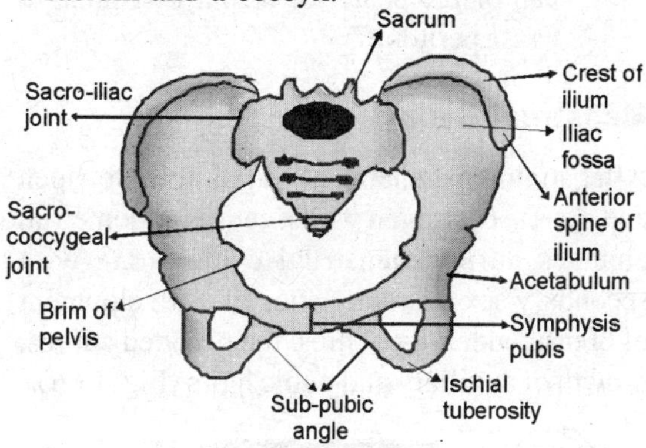

Fig. 13.5: Pelvic bone

Innominate bone is large, strong, irregular bone which has parts (a) Ilium and (b) Ischium and (c) Pubis. Upper expanded part of ilium is hip bone which presents a bony crest, iliac fossa, anterior prominence and posterior prominence. Ischium has large tuberosity which carry total load of body at rest. United front portion by a pad of cartilage form symphysis pubis. The sacrum which forms posterior wall of pelvis is a wedge shaped bone with five fused vertebrae. Extreme end of vertebral column is coccyx.

The relations of pelvic organs of reproduction enlarge as pregnancy advances and passes out to abdomen where they lie in relation to other abdominal organs.

Nursing care invites the following attention:

- Thorough clean of area before examination to avoid infection from rectum and bladder.
- Care in external /local infection to protect the spread of infection to peritoneal cavity through fallopian tube.
- Tear of vagina and cervix during labour can create fistulae.
- For correct, easy and painless introduction of vaginal speculum, upward and back-

ward slope of vagina should be remembered.

- Illegal abortion instruments in rural area can pierce posterior fornix of vagina to cause peritonitis.

Menstrual Cycle

After attaining menarche, ovarian follicle ripen and secrete oestrogen which causes endometrial changes during menstrual cycle along with secondary sex characteristics like development of breast, widening of hips, the rounded curves, growth of auxiliary and pubic hairs (Fig. 13.6).

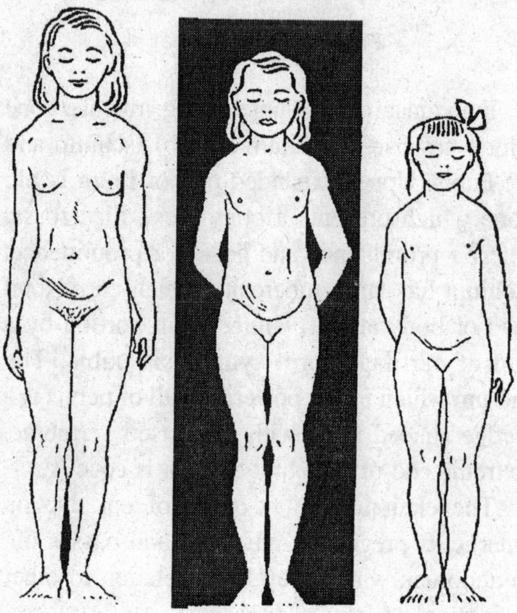

Fig. 13.6: Secondary sex characteristics in girls

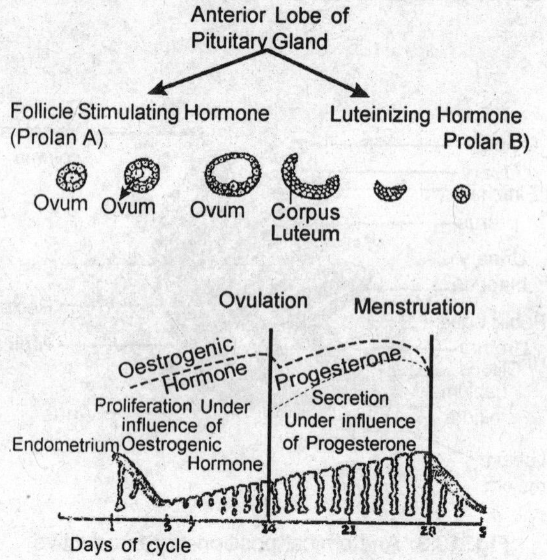

Fig. 13.8: Hormonal influence on menstruation

Anterior lobe of pituitary gland stimulates ovary by F S H to ripen and to produce oestrogen which cause endometrium to grow and thicken. Fully ripe follicle bursts on 14th day of menses. At that time, L H of anterior lobe of pituitary gland stimulates (along with oestrogen) the development of blood vessels and glands in endometrium. This is called premenstrual period which is ready to take up fertilised egg, if available. If there is no fertilisation, endometrium breaks down again causing menstrual flow which contains mucus and shreds of endometrium and unfertilised ovum. Average blood loss will be 100 to 300 ml lasting for 3-5 days.

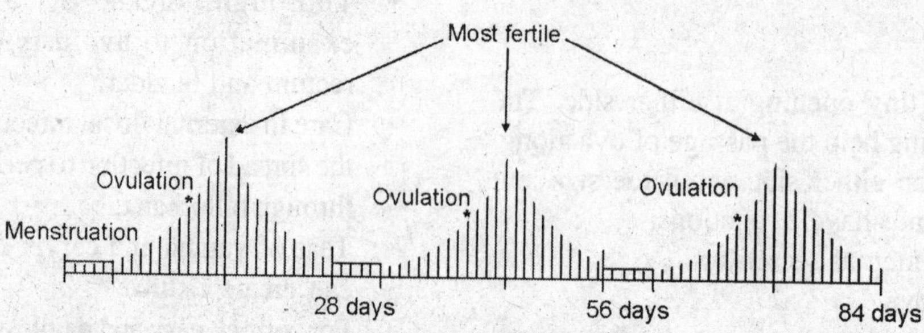

Fig. 13.7: Menstrual cycle

Fertilisation

By sexual intercourse, semen is deposited in vagina, sperm enters uterus and fallopian tube and fertilisation (union of ovum and sperm) occur in fallopian tube. When fertilisation takes place, sperm penetrates ovum usually in fallopian tube. Each of these cells contains 24 chromosomes. The result of union is the formation of a single cell containing 48 chromosomes (24 from sperm 24 from ovum). The fertilised cell enters uterus and gets implanted there; cell's differentiating stages like morula, tryphoblast and eventually embryo develops.

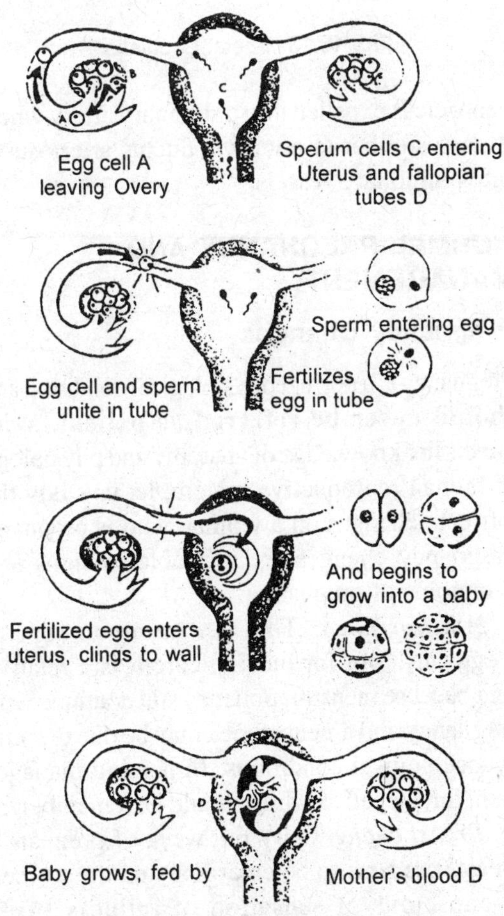

Fig. 13.9: Fertilization

Foetal Development

Fertilised cell undergoes cell division. At this stage it appears like mulberry and is called a morula. Further cell different-iation leads to outer layer tryphoblast concerning with absorbing nutrition and inner cells eventually become the embryo. Tryphoblast grows to primitive chorionic villi. Its surface is called syncitium. Two small vesicles appears, one with clear fluid (amniotic sac) and the other with opaque material (yolk sac). Between them the embryonic disc gets located with 3 distinguished layers:

1. Ectoderm – to form skin and appendages

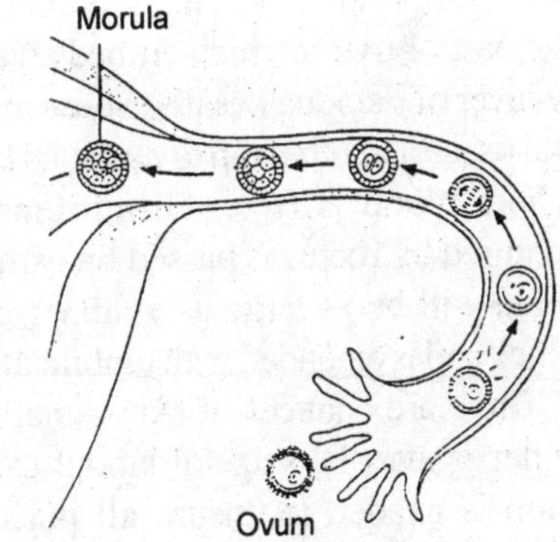

Fig.13.10: Morula

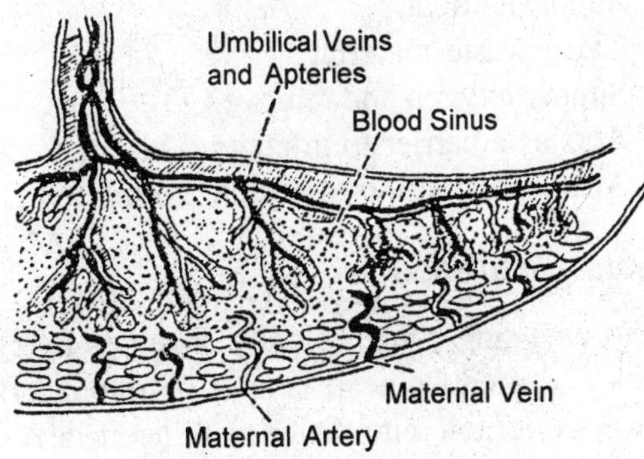

Fig. 13.11: Development of villi

2. Entoderm – to alimentary tract
3. Mesoderm – to connective tissue, muscle, vessels, nerves.

Placenta

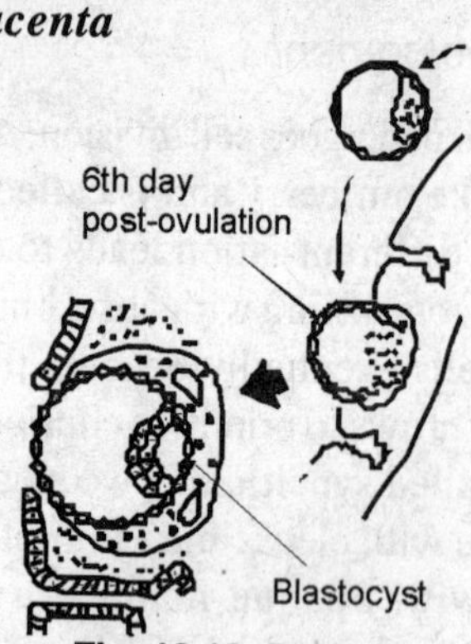

Fig. 13.12: Placenta

The placenta is firmly attached to uterine wall by 12th week of pregnancy. The true chorionic villi on the part of ovum which embeds burrow to spongy layer of decidua basalis. Some anchor to placental tissue and other dip to maternal blood spaces where blood is free. All nutrient and oxygen required by foetus is passed by osmosis. The placenta will be as large as a dinner plate, one inch thick and is extended with umbilical cord to foetus. There are chances of extra small placenta and hence after III stage of labour careful examination is needed to ensure all placental tissue has come away. Functions of placenta are:

- Supply nutrient
- Carry waste material
- Supply oxygen and remove CO_2
- Acts as a barrier to infection
- Acts as endocrine to secrete hormone.

Foetal Circulation

Heart as a single tube initially develops by 5th week and produce heart beat of 65/minute. By 11weeks definite circulation with heart beat of 140/min is established. In the mature foetal circulation (Fig. 13.12) about 40% of venous blood return entering the right atrium flows directly into the left atrium through foramen ovale. Blood pumped from right atrium into right

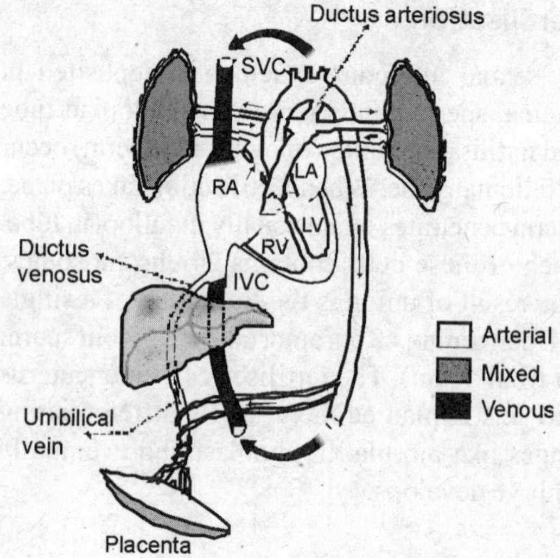

Fig. 13.13: Foetal Circulation

ventricle is expelled into pulmonary artery where it passes either to aorta via ductus arteriosis or into pulmonary vessels.

NORMAL PREGNANCY AND MANAGEMENT

Pregnancy Changes

Pregnancy is a normal physiological condition and **should never be referred as patient.** With our earlier knowledge of anatomy and physiology of human reproductive system, let us study the intricate changes on a woman who is pregnant. Pregnancy changes are referable to signs and symptoms of pregnancy.

Amenorrhoea: This is a common sign of pregnancy. But for nursing care it is a relative sign because menstruation may still continue with pregnancy and amenorrhoea may be due to some gynaecological conditions. In nursing management threatened abortion should be remembered.

Breast changes: By 6th week of pregnancy breasts are seen to be enlarging and the women is conscious of sensation of fullness. Area around nipple becomes pigmented. By 20th week, secondary areola occurs by whitish spots. It is a reliable sign in primigravida. But in nursing care pseudo-cyesis (false pregnancy) is to be noted.

Genitalia: Cervix becomes more secretary, vagina and vulva become purple. It is due to extra venous blood in 2nd month onwards.

Morning Sickness: Nausea and vomiting from 4th week which may be due to changing metabolism and extra cellular activity.

Frequency of Micturition: This is due to pressure on urinary bladder from 3rd month onwards. This also continues in late pregnancy when bladder is displaced upwards.

Abdomen: Per abdominal examination for the height of uterus which usually correspond to the period of amenorrhoea. It is obvious from 18th week onwards. About 12.5 kg will be the contribution to weight gain in pregnancy (Fig. 13.13).

Foetal Movement: After 18 weeks the foetal movement "quickening" is felt. From 6th month foetal heart sound is heard. The uterine "soufflé" a soft swishing sound as the blood enters the uterine arteries can be heard just above the pubes to the left of the midline.

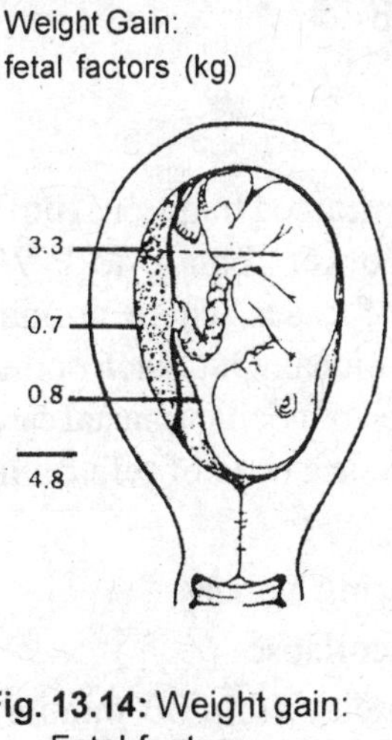

Fig. 13.14: Weight gain: Fetal foetus

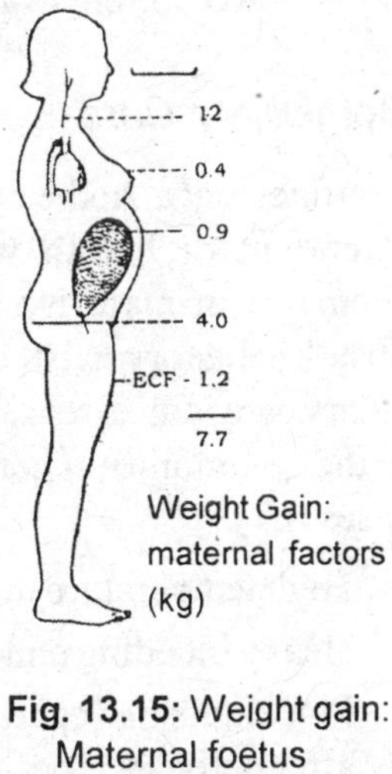

Fig. 13.15: Weight gain: Maternal foetus

Pregnancy Test: Urine examination for pregnancy test will be positive, usually on or after 40 days of conception.

Antenatal Care (ANC)

ANC is for achieving normal delivery with a healthy baby. This helps in high risk identification to foresee complications, remove anxiety of mother, teach element of mother care and personal hygiene. Minimum of 3 antenatal visits, 1 at 20 weeks, second at 32 weeks and third at 36 weeks are required. In first visit history taking, physical examination, examination of urine, blood and stool, blood grouping and Rh typing are done. On subsequent visits physical examination and laboratory test are done. The visits are used for IFA advice, TT immunisation and nutrition advice. Following conditions are considered high risk:

- Elderly primi
- Short stature primi
- Malpresentation
- APH
- Threatened abortion
- PET and toxaemia
- Anaemia
- Twins and hydromnios
- Previous bad obstetrical history
- Pregnancy with systemic disorders.

Above normal or away from normal findings are notable and have to be put in ANC record along with identification data.

Home visiting will win women's confidence which also help to observe social and environmental conditions.

Prenatal Advice

Nutrition: Average weight increase during pregnancy is around 12 kg. Her diet needs extra calorie and extra protein which is highlighted in nutrition chapter.

Food for pregnant women		*(Additional calories)*
Cereal	35 g.	118
Pulses	15 g.	52
Sugar	10 g.	10
Milk	100g.	83
	Total	293 calories

Personal Hygiene

It includes cleanliness, good bowl habit, and regular household work.

Drugs should be used only when essentially required but under doctor's supervision.

Pregnant woman should not be exposed to unnecessary X-ray.

Any warning sign like swelling feet, fits, headache, blurring vision, bleeding per vagina are to be reported for emergency obstetric care.

Specific Health Protection

Anaemia: I.F.A. containing 60 mg elemental iron and 500 microgram folic acid should be advised and minimum of 100 tablets during pregnancy is advocated.

Toxaemia: Early detection of risk in high blood pressure and urine albumin reduces the risk of morbidity and mortality.

Two doses of TT given, 1 dose at 16-20 weeks and the second at 20-24 weeks, protects from tetanus.

Specific diagnosis and treatment of RTI/STD prevents abortion and perinatal mortality.

German measles need attention because foetal anomalies like cataract, deafness and congenital heart disease are associated with Rubella in early pregnancy.

If the mother is Rh –ve and the child is +ve, it provokes an immune response in her so that she forms antibodies to Rh which can cross placenta and produce foetal haemolysis. Routine test and timely intervention prevents this Rh iso immune response.

HIV +ve mother can transmit disease to growing foetus. Precaution to check mother to child transmission is possible by specific protective measure.

Mental Preparation: Time and opportunity are given to mother for acceptance and cooperation for fruitful outcome of pregnancy.

Family Planning: In indicated cases small family norm through post partum centre is undertaken.

Child Component: In ANC check up presence of paediatrician help in paying attention to accompanied children, which boosts the morale of the RCH activities.

Intra Natal Care (INC)

Effective intranatal care is required to overcome complications of labour. Prevention of maternal and neonatal sepsis is overcome by:

a. Five Clean Practice:
   - Clean surface for delivery
   - Clean hands for cutting cord
   - New blade for cutting cord
   - Clean tie for cord
   - No application on cord stump.
b. Issue of Disposable Delivery Kit (DDK) which contain:
   - A piece of soap
   - A new razor blade
   - Two pieces of thread
   - Two cotton swabs.

Domiciliary Care

Confinement at home by trained traditional birth attendant or health worker female M.P.W. (Female) in majority of cases where normal obstetric history exist, is ideal. Out reach domiciliary care is an extension of good intranatal care to the community. There is a need of referral in cases of:

- High temperature during labour
- Heavy bleeding and collapse
- Placenta not separated within 30 minutes after delivery
- Cord prolapse
- Prolonged labour.

Labour

It is a series of increasingly strong and painful rhythmical contraction of the uterine cavity, assisted in the later stages by the abdominal muscles, which expel the foetus. Uterine contraction in labour is painful and not painful in pregnancy (before labour).

Nursing care need the understanding of terms used for an act in an emergency. Foetus lies in uterus in an attitude of universal flexion with the head at the lower pole and the back lying against the anterior abdominal wall. Head presentation is normal and all other presentations like occiput, face, brow, breech, cord are abnormal presentations.

LOA (left occipitoanteriror) where vertex position is the most common and the one is described in normal labour.

Stages of Labour

First Stage: It is from the onset of labour to full dilatation of cervix. Per vaginal examination is done to ascertain if the cervix has begun to dilate. There is little bleeding from torn capillaries, in the beginning then with mucus "The show" starts with fore water in front of head (liquor amnii). When tension rises, membrane ruptures, fluid escapes by which time foetal head starts getting brunt of the pressure. This may produce "Caput succedaneum" which, however is soon reabsorbed. The interval between the pains gives the mother rest and allows free flow of blood, through the uterine muscle to the placental site. The stage is 24 hours in primi and lesser (6-12 hour) in multi.

Second Stage: It is from full dilatation of cervix to the birth of baby. This takes 2 hours in primi and lesser in multi. Retraction of uterine muscle presses down from above and advances with each pain. Head descends through vagina, perineum is stretched, head passes through vulva and is delivered between contractions. The shoulders rotate and are born with the next contraction and rest of the body is delivered at the same time.

Third Stage: It is from the birth to the delivery of placenta. The baby breathes and often cries lustily immediately after it is born and the cord may be cut as soon as convenient. There is no need to wait until it has ceased to pulsate.

Table 13.1: APGAR scoring system

	Score		
Sign	*0*	*1*	*2*
Heart rate	Absent	<100/min	>100/min
Respiration rate	Absent	Weak cry	Strong cry
Muscle tone	Limp	Some flexion	Good flexion
Reflex irritability	No response	Some motion	Cry
Colour	White	Blue periphery	Pink all over

Interpretation of APGAR Score:

A normal score at 1 min is 7 – 10

Score of 4 – 6 at 1 min = moderately depressed baby

Score of 0 – 3 at 1 min = severe depression.

Hypothermia Prevention

Neonatal death can occur by hypothermia which is due to fall in body temperature since ambient temperature to which they are born is always by several degrees cooler than temperature in the womb. New born body temperature is 99.5° F and hypothermia occurs if room temperature is below 97.5°F.

Measures suggested are:

1. After birth, baby is quickly dried with clean cloth and wrapped with cotton clothing (turkey towel) (Two Towel method).
2. Skin to skin contact with mother at breast feeding is allowed.
3. Avoid bath to new born for one week.

Strong contraction which causes expulsion of foetus also results in separation of central area of placenta. The centre is bunched up and behind it is a pool of blood from maternal sinuses forming haematoma. Abdominal palpation revealing soft uterus concludes that contraction is over.

Nursing care should be vigilant on the following complications of labour:

- C.P.D. (Cephalo Pelvic Disproportion)
- Foetal abnormalities like breech, hydrocephalus
- Uterine inertia
- P.P.H. (Post Partum Haemorrhage)
- Retained placenta.

Rooming In:

For mental stability, self confidence and for early breast feeding baby is kept by the side of mother's bed. This is called "Rooming-in".

Post Natal Care

Care of the mother and the new born is attended as Post Natal Care services. This is combined area of perinatology which involves both obstetrical care and paediatrician care.

The puerperium is the time, approximately 42 days during which time the genital organs are returning to normal in their size and position after pregnancy and labour. This is called involution. The nursing responsibility includes:

- Checking healing of placental site.
- Checking involution of uterus.
- Establishment of lactation.
- Care of the new born.
- Teaching the mother, mother craft.

Routine observations are made and recorded daily at nursing duty. They include:

- Temperature, pulse, respiration
- Lochia
- Involution of uterus
- Excretions.

Establishment of Lactation (Exclusive Breast Feeding)

The advantage of breast feeding to mother and new born are emphasised to mother and at her earliest, she should start breast feeding. No other feed is allowed and there is no restriction to collostrum. Only breast feeding till 4 months and no other feed at that time constitute "Exclusive Breast Feeding".

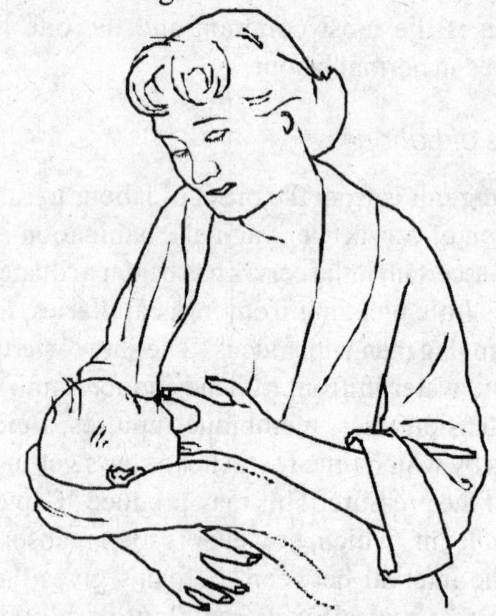

Fig. 13.16: Position at breast feeding

Nursing profession play a key role in ensuring 100 percent Exclusive Breast Feeding and make their institution a "Centre of Excellence".

Advice on postnatal exercise will build up muscular strength and early recovery from brunt of pregnancy and labour.

Nursing care include a vigilance on common puerperal complications. They are:

- Traumatic-perineal tears and fistulae.
- Puerperal sepsis
- Breast complications.

Good postnatal care takes care of the following:

- Prevention of complication of postnatal period.
- Care for recovering mother.
- Check exclusive breast feeding.
- Provide PPC service.
- Give health education.
- To control puerperal sepsis, thrombophlebitis and secondary haemorrhages.

Postnatal Care Measure

PNC Examination:

Post natal care involves examination twice a day during first 3 days, later once a day till cord drops off. Each examination should cover pulse, respiration, temperature recording, breast examination, uterus involution, examination of lochia, excretion position. At the end of 6 weeks, follow up for involution of uterus is done. Later monthly post natal examination for first 6 months, thereafter once in 3 months till 1 year, is done. In rural area, effort must be made to have minimum 3 post natal visits.

Anaemia is kept in mind and if found, correction with supplementation is advocated. Nutrition is looked after with additional allowance of calorie and protein:

Table 13.2: Additional calorie to lactating mother

	Additional	*Allowance (calories)*
Cereals	60 G.	203
Pulses	30 G.	105
Milk	100 G.	83
Fat	10 G.	90
Sugar	10 G.	40
Total calories		521

Post natal exercise is necessary to bring muscles back to normal as early as possible. Many known exercises are displayed in postnatal wards, which need to be appreciated by nursing students during ward work.

Psychological assurance to allay fear and insecurity help the mother to come to normal, which, otherwise would have precipitated by pregnancy and labour.

Social assurance by good family atmosphere is another requisite for women to have smooth and eventful post delivery period.

Basic education on health is given to mother for personal hygiene, environmental hygiene, infant feeding, pregnancy spacing, health check-up and birth registration.

FURTHER REFERENCES

1. Malcolm Symonds and Ian M. Symonds – Essential Obstetrics and Gynaecology (Churchill Livingstone).
2. Hilda M Gration and Dorothy L. Holland – Obstetric Nursing (Bailliere, Tindall and Cox).
3. Prabhakara G.N. – Short Text Book of PSM (JP).

14

Preventive Pediatrics

IMPORTANCE

This area takes care of children from conception to adolescence by averting diseases and disabilities among children. Prevention of disease and promotion of physical, mental and social well being of children are key success in preventive Paediatrics. A strategy of primary health care to paediatric age group through Growth monitoring, ORS, nutritional surveillance, promotion of exclusive breast feeding, UIP and regular health check is aimed at.

CHILD RIGHTS

Awakening of public all over the world has lead to many policies on child rights. United Nations Assembly passed a resolution in 1954 and later passed on to UNICEF to observe "Universal children's day on every year November 14th. Five years later, in 1959, UN adopted the declaration of the rights of the child which opened the gate for free education and special care.

During 1974 Government of India adopted a National Policy for children which declares:

"It shall be the policy of the state to provide adequate service to children, both before and after birth and through the period of growth, to ensure their full physical, Mental and Social development. The state shall progressively increase the scope of such services so that, within a reasonable time, all children in the country enjoy optimum conditions for their balanced growth".

Following this, many programmes like ICDS, Supplementary feeding. Nutrition education, National children award, welfare of the handicapped, CSSM, RCH etc., were introduced.

Child right policy is made and is in force through:

- Article 24 – prohibiting child labour
- Article 39 – prohibiting child abuse
- Article 45 – provides free education up to 14 years of age.

HUMAN CYCLE

Human development is intricate and has been studied in-depth. Most of the observations are recorded and available as scientific proof. One of the most revolutionized men "Homo Sapien" has out beaten nature by developing fertilized egg (Invitro fertilization) for the treatment of infertility and sterility.

During early development, human cycle passes through following stages:

	Fertilised egg (Embryo) 14-63 days
	Foetus 9th week to birth
	Early neonate birth to 7 days
Infant	Late neonate 7 days to 28
Neonate	days
	Post neonate 28 days to 1 year
	Preschool age 1 year to 5 years
	School age 5 to 14 years
Adolescent	14 – 18 years
Adult	18 – 45 years
Middle age	45 – 64 years
Old age	65 – 100 years

For the sake of understanding physical growth, mental growth and neuromuscular endowment the grouping is done as under:

0-1 month	– New born infant
1-12 month	– Infant
1-3 year	– Early childhood
3-5 years	– Late childhood
6-10 years	– School age
10-18 years	– Adolescent
18-45 years	– Adult
45-64	– Middle age
65 +	– Old age

Biological Principles

During 1 month of neonatal period natural adjustment to Biological growth is seen. Nutritional needs in terms of breast feeding and human activity for neonatal problems are attended.

Late neonatal period is associated with social and emotional development. In this period we notice common behavioural problems. Appraisal of infant through nutrition and physical protection is the felt need.

Early childhood period is influenced by nutritional availability. Care and training for the proper socialisation is called for.

School age group is vulnerable period for infection and social, emotional and intellectual development. Appraisal of child through school health is called for.

Adolescent and adult period is filled with social, emotional and intellectual development. Puberty changes allow changes in behaviour. Guidance during puberty and sex education has been found useful in human society. Recreation and vocational interest are added burden during this period. Special problems for the adolescent in society, if not tackled, leads to delinquent changes.

Adult life is period of getting acquaintance of maturity from all angle. There is little maladjustment which has medical answers. Preparation for marriage and Planned Parenthood for the job of good family pattern calls for attention.

Middle age and old age have their own events which are tackled in human geriatrics (Chapter 15).

Development of Personality

Hereditary plays a part in personality development. Environment plays a greater role in this aspect. It is difficult to get an ideal situation for all. Consequently we develop personality, strong in some aspect and weak in others. If it is socially acceptable it is judged as normal.

According to Erick Erickson, human development takes place in 8 stages. Through these stages physical, mental, social and spiritual developments go together. Certain situations illustrate how human development is intricate with social interaction.

- A girl overprotected, not given a choice to face difficulties, all wants are attended, no chance given to learn the art of house keeping and house management; she breaks down with "marriage".
- Basic need of a family like food, cloth, shelter, love and affection are zero; then children become deviants.
- A boy who lost his father, brought up by over anxious mother reacts like hostile dissatisfied.

Nursing role in human development has an obligation to work for the over all development of man.

Infancy

They are completely dependant for feeding, elimination, cleanliness, warmth and protection. Love and protection are needed for proper development.

Food satisfaction is fused with infection and malnutrition which severely affect mental growth and development.

Preschool (Toddler)

Rapid physical growth, muscular coordination and control over physical functions are seen. Family pattern and social regulation have an impact on their health. Foundation of future life, the basic blocks for a future personality are laid at this stage. Socialisation and spiritual health implicit good development.

School Age (5-14 years)

Rapid physical and mental growth are seen; proper nutrition protection from infection and injury are made available. Encouragement and help are need for emotional development. Life long attitudes and habits are formed at this stage. They are prone to fantasies; strong attachment is seen with same age groups irrespective of sex. Teachers also help in secondary socialisation. At this stage they are sexually latent.

Adolescent (15-18 years)

This is a crucial sage of development. There's transition from childhood to adulthood. Secondary sexual characteristics develop. Emotionally they are very sensitive to criticism and correction. At the same time they are insecure and unsure of themselves. To overcome inferiority they put up a show in dress, speech. Sexual feelings cause fantasies and attention seeking.

Early Adulthood (18-25 years)

They are at the zenith of strength and energy. Socially they are ready to assume competent role in life. Physical health and mental health make them to assure their role play in life.

Adulthood (25-45 years)

This is the height of productive life and achievements. Emotionally and spiritually they will be stable.

Late Adulthood (45-64 years)

Physical strength and attractiveness gets reduced. They are prone to sickness and infirmities if move for health is not obviated. Depressive episodes are common in this phase of human cycle.

Old Age (65 +)

Failing physical strength and sickness produce emotional insecurity. Geriatric problems make them upset at every stage and even they are worried about death.

An insight into the above eight stages of human development will help to get an insight to the nursing profession for an effective nursing care in day to day practice.

PREVENTIVE PAEDIATRICS

Certain specific biological and psychological needs must be met to ensure the survival and healthy development of a child. It needs recognition, diagnosis and timely management of health problems and rests on paediatric care and Nursing Paediatrics. Childhood period is a vital period for socialisation which transmits attitude, custom and behaviour. Children are susceptible to disease, disability and death.

Perinatology

This calls for professional care to the foetus at risk. Inborn errors of metabolism and birth defects are diagnosed through USG, amniocenteses, chorion biopsy and foetoscopy. The knowledge gained by perinatology is useful to prevent LBW, birth defects and birth asphyxia. Nursing care allows genetic counselling and Planned Parenthood in perinatology. Recent nursing care allows providing care for:

- Limitation of families
- Spacing of births
- Delaying women's first pregnancy
- Ensuring maternal nutrition
- Look to Intra uterine infections control.

Overall modern nursing care directs its effort in maternal nutrition, family planning and counselling of young couple.

Neonatology

Neonatal Nursing care concentrates on optimum newborn care through priority based scientific approach. Early neonatal period is crucial and hence great care is to be exercised for the prevention of preventable neonatal health problems.

Figure 14.1 gives an ideal plan, as a model, for a methodical approach to neonatal care. They include cardiopulmonary resuscitation, prevention of hypothermia, chemoprophylaxis and early detection of defects and disorders. Neonatology takes care of TORCHES in daily hospital procedures (Toxoplasmosis, rubella, herpes infection and syphilis).

Immediate natal care includes the following:

a. Airway:

Immediate attention to cardio-pulmonary function is given. Mucus and other secretions are cleared. Positioning of newborn with head low to drain secretions is tried. Intensive measures like suction, oxygen mask, intubation or assisted respiration should be ready.

Labour ward equipments for above items are attended by nursing staff.

b. APGAR Score:

This is a monitor done at 1 minute and 5 minutes after birth. A score of 7-10 normal, 4-7 mild depression and 0-3 severe depression allows for prompt action.

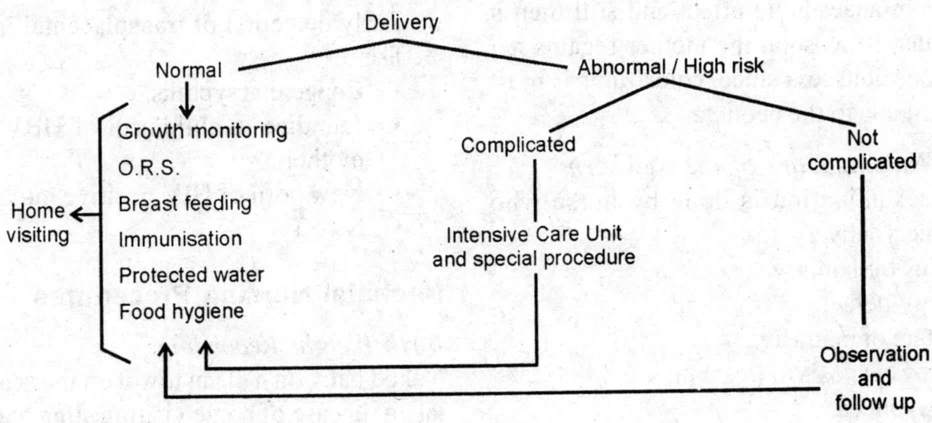

Fig. 14.1: Neonatal care model

c. **Care of the Cord:**
As soon as pulsation is stopped the cord is cut by sterilised instrument; there is no necessity to apply any antiseptic over the stump. It shrivels up and separates by necrosis in one week.

d. **Care of the Eyes:**
Eyes are cleaned. One drop of 1% freshly prepared silver nitrate solution prevents gonococcal conjunctivitis. Any discharge need to be attended by ophthalmologist. Because of immediate and good eye care Opthalmia neonatorum is greatly prevented.

e. **Skin Care:**
To prevent hypothermia, skin bath is avoided till one week. Neonate bath by nurse need special skill and is considered to be a professional gift.

f. **Protection of Body Temperature:**
Two towel method and rooming-in provide effective maintenance of newborn body temperature. Thermal control may be needed in severe hypothermia.

g. **Breast Feeding:**
Breast feeding is initiated at the earliest. In case of a caesarean there may be little delay till mother regains consciousness from anaesthetic effect and still then it must be as soon the mother regains her consciousness since, colostrums is most suitable to the neonate.

Special Nursing Care of the Newborn:

a. First examination is done by nurse who conducts delivery, for:
   - Any birth injury.
   - Any defect.
   - State of maturity.
   - Any cyanosis of lip, skin.
   - Dyspnoea.
   - Imperforated anus.
   - Persistent vomiting.
   - Twitching, neck rigidity, concussion
   - Body temperature variation

   Any deviation is to be brought to the notice of duty pediatrician for immediate attention.

b. Second examination is done within 24 hours of birth which should follow regular nursing protocol as under:
   - Body length (Crown-head-thoracic).
   - Body weight.
   - Body temperature.
   - Skin for cyanosis, pallor, jaundice, erythema, bullous lesions.
   - Thoracic cage retraction.
   - Respiratory rate over 60 per minute.
   - Absence of femoral pulse.
   - Central cyanosis.
   - Posture and muscle tone.
   - Signs of hydrocephalus.
   - Any signs of cataract, coloboma, conjunctivitis.
   - Any dysmorphism, accessory auricle, preauricular pits, hare lip, cleft palate.
   - Abdominal mass, distension, imperforate anus.
   - Joints, bones for deformity, dislocation.
   - Hypospadius, undescended testis hydrocele in male child.
   - Fused labia, enlarged clitoris in female child.

c. Early detection of transplacental infections like:
   - Congenital syphilis.
   - Jaundice in childbirth of HBV positive mother.
   - New born of HIV positive mother
   - N.N.T.

Neonatal Nursing Procedures

Birth Weight Recording:

Naked baby on a clean towel on the scale pan is taken. In case of home visiting sling bag using a Salter weighing scale is used. The measurement is done to nearest 100 grams.

Height Recording:
By infantometer with a fixed head piece on which the newborn is laid supine with legs fully extended, feet flexed at right angles to lower limbs. The measurements are done to nearest to 0.1 cm. At home visiting, one family member can help the nurse and a metallic tape is an appropriate technology.

Head Circumference Recording:
With the help of a measuring tape, measure is taken at the maximum circumference of the head in the occipito frontal diameter.

Theoretical and Research oriented parameters to be obtained by an attending nurse are:

Weight	–	Birth weight
Height	–	Total, sitting, knee length
Perimeters	–	Head circumference Chest circumference Abdominal circumference Arm circumference Calf circumference
Diameter	–	BiAcromial BiCristal BiEpicondylar BiStyloid BiCondylar
Skinfold Thickness	–	Subscapular Biceps Triceps Supra iliac

Neonatal screening procedures:
- APGAR scoring
- Blood phenylalanine for PKU
- T_4 or TSH assay for hypothyroidism
- Coombs Test for incompatibility
- Agar gel electrophoresis for G_6PD and thalassemia
- Snap test for congenital dislocation of hip

Identification of at risk infant:
- Birth weight below 2.5 kg
- Twins
- Birth order of 5 and 5+
- Artificial feeding
- Severe malnutrition (Grade III, IV)
- Failure to gain weight
- P.E.M.
- Diarrhoea
- Working mother.

LOW BIRTH WEIGHT

Table 14.1: Difference between pre term baby and small for date baby

	Preterm	*Small for Date*
Birth	Before 27 week of gestation	Pre term or full term
I.U. growth	Normal	Retarded
Prognosis	Easily brought back to normal	Difficult to bring back to normal
Weight	More than 10th percentile for gestational age	Less than 10th percentile for gestational age
Palmar and Plantar crease	Developed	Not developed
Areola of nipple	Developed	Not developed

LBW is calculated by:

$$\frac{\text{LB with} < 2.5\text{kg}}{\text{Total LB}} \times 100$$

While it is 4 to 8% in developed countries, in a developing country like India it is 26%. I.C.M.R. quotes that maturity, respiratory distress and feeding problem makes 2.5 kg nonacceptable as LBW among Indian children. But criteria is coming in the way that when applied the percentage comes down to nearing zero. For examples when 2.5 kg is criteria and prevalence is 26% the prevalence comes down to 5.5% with 2.0 kg criteria.

Causes	:	Malnutrition Infection Uncontrolled fertility
Association	:	Mental retardation I.M.R. Morbidity

Strong Association : Maternal nutrition
Length of pregnancy

Prevention:

- Dietary improvement of pregnant women.
- Control of maternal infections, diseases.
- Incubatory care to LBW.
- Proper feeding of LBW.
- Infection control of LBW.

Nursing observation and reporting of the following are called for, since they are leading causes of deaths among LBW babies.

a. Atelectasis
b. Malformation
c. Pulmonary haemorrhage
d. Birth trauma giving rise to intracranial bleeding and anoxia
e. Pneumonia.

INFANT FEEDING

The present paediatric concept is for exclusive breast feeding of infants. Breast milk is ideal and no other feed is required for the child. On an average Indian mother secrete 600 ml of milk, which yield 6.6 gram of protein which is more than sufficient for the baby. Chance of survival and reduction of infection are known with exclusive breast feeding.

Table 14.2: Advantages of breast feeding

Advantage	*Disadvantage*
Safe	NIL
Clean	
Hygienic	Except among
Cheap	Inverted nipple
Available at body temperature	Crack, fissure
Meets nutritional requirement	
Contain antimicrobial factors	
Easily digestible	
Promotes bonding	
No obesity	
No hypocalcaemia	
No hypomagnesaemia	
Natural spacing possible	

Artificial Milk:

It is indicated in mother's death, failure to breast feed due to defects of breast. It is done by dried whole milk powder and fresh milk from cow. For planning artificial feeding following principles are kept in mind:

- Calorie required is 100 per kg body weight.
- Protein required 2 g per kg body weight.
- Carbohydrate required 10 gram per kg body weight.
- After 4 months undiluted boiled cooled milk should be given.
- On an average child needs 6-8 feeding per day.
- During illness, calorie should be increased.

Table 14.3: Notable points in artificial feed

Dried milk powder	*Cows milk*
Safe	Natural source
Free from bacteria upto 2 months	Need humanization of milk
Fortified	
But expensive	

Table 14.4: Difference between breast milk and cow's milk

	Breast milk	*Cow's milk*
Protein	11 G/L	33 G/L
Non protein	0.32 G/L	0.32/L
Linoleic acid	3.5 G/L	1.0 G/L
Lactose	62 G/L	50 G/L
Calcium	0.3 G/L	1 G/L
Phosphorus	0.1 G/L	1 G/L
Iron	1.5 mg/L	0.5 mg/L
Vitamin C	60 mg/L	20 mg/L
Vitamin D	50 I U	25 I U
Calorie	640 calories	650 calories

WEANING

It is a gradual process of withdrawal of breast milk and substitution of weaning food. It is advocated after 4 months. They are cow's milk, fruit juice, soft cooked rice, dhal soup, vegetable soup. Weaning period is crucial and observation is advisable to prevent malnutrition and infection. At the age of one year supplementation with cereals, pulses, vegetables and fruits is necessary. It is always advisable to have home made weaning foods.

CARE OF THE PRESCHOOL CHILD

By virtue of their number, they need and are entitled to a large share of health service. Malnutrition is common and care for its detection through underfive care is accorded. Common morbid conditions are anaemia, Xerophtalmia, diarrhoea, whooping cough, measles, eruptive fevers, skin infections, eye infections, intestinal parasitism. Malnutrition and infection influence growth and development at this stage. Toddlers are not easily accessible and hence special inputs like day care centres, play centre and child park are needed.

HEALTH PROBLEMS IN CHILDHOOD PERIOD

1. Low birth weight (LBW)
2. P.E.M.
3. Micronutrient malnutrition
   - Vitamin A
   - Iodine
   - Iron
   - Calcium
   - Zinc.
4. Nutritional anaemia
5. Nutritional blindness
6. I.D.D.
7. Infections
8. Accidents
9. Poisoning
10. Behavioural problems

CONGENITAL MALFORMATIONS

Congenital malformations are subsequently determined before and during birth and commonly recognisable in early life. It refers to anatomical defects in childhood. In case of biochemical and functional disorders are seen, they are grouped under congenital anomaly.

Incidence of congenital malformations has been estimated to be 30 per 1000 live births, which causes 18% of I.M.R. in the world. As per WHO estimates global incidence of some selected malformations are as under:

Table 14.5: Global incidence of congenital malformations

Heart defect	6 per 1000 live births
Cleft lip	0.9 per 1000 live births
Cleft palate	0.5 per 1000 live births
Spina bifida	1.0 per 1000 live births
Other defects	17.0 per 1000 live births

Incidence of congenital malformation in India is estimated to be 20-28 per 1000 live births. It is the third leading cause of perinatal mortality in India.

Cause of Congenital Malformations:

- Down's syndrome
- Klinefelter's syndrome
- Turner's syndrome
- Phenylketonuria
- Tay Sachs disease
- Galactosemia
- Huntington's chorea
- Thalassaemia
- Sickle cell disease
- Haemophilia
- Rubella
- Cytomegalovirus infection
- Toxoplasmosis
- Drugs induced (Thalidomide).

  Possible risk factors are:
  - Late marriage of woman
  - Consanguineous marriage.

Diagnosis of Congenital Malformation:
During Prenatal period following laboratory tests are diagnostic of congenital malformations.

i. Maternal blood sample or amniotic fluid sample for specific protein called μ protein detection.
ii. U.S.G. (Ultra Sonography) helps to visualise malformations.
iii. Taping amniotic fluid during second trimester can help diagnosis of Down's syndrome and neural tube defect.
iv. Chorionic villi sampling after 9 to 10 weeks of pregnancy help in determination of chromosomal aberration.

Prevention:

a. Prevention of consanguineous marriage.
b. Prenatal diagnosis for chromosomal aberration in advanced maternal age.
c. Control in the use of teratogenic drugs.
d. Attention to environmental improve-ment than touching heredity for a successful normal reproduction.

HANDICAPPED CHILDREN

According to Last it is "the reduction in a person's capacity to fulfill a social role as a consequence of an impairment, inadequate training for the role, or other circumstances. Applied to children, the term usually refers to the presence of impairment or other circumstances that are likely to interfere with normal growth and development or with the capacity to learn".

Table 14.6: Handicap differentiated from impairment and disability

Handicapped	*Impaired*	*Disabled*
Cannot perform a social role	Abnormal structure and function	Unable to perform an activity

Current Problem: *(World)*

Mental retardation – 83 million (Estimate)
Hearing loss – 42 million (Estimate)
Polio lameness – 10 million (Estimate)

Current Problem (India):
It is estimated that 2.3 percent of the population (2001 population = 1.027,015 247) viz., 23.6 million (23,621,350) are physically handicapped. Among 0-6 age population (2001 census = 157,863,145) developmental delay is estimated to be 1.1% viz., 1.7 lakhs (1,736,494).

Types

Physically Handicapped: Blind, Deaf, Mute, Hair lip, cleft palate, Talipes, Lame, Cardiac defect, Accidents, burns and other injuries.
Mentally Handicapped: Moron, Imbecile, Mentally retarded.
Socially Handicapped: Orphan child, Destitute, Delinquent.
Prevention:

- Genetic counselling
- Identification and advice of at risk group in a population
- I.P.P.I.
- Rubella vaccination
- Proper nutrition of expectant mother
- Banning teratogenic drugs
- Avoiding unnecessary X-ray at early pregnancy.

Control:

- Detection and proper management of handicap in the community.
- Training and education of handicapped.

Institutions working for handicaps:

1. Occupational Therapy College, New Delhi.
2. Occupational Therapy School, Nagpur.
3. Occupational Therapy School, Mumbai.

4. Physical Therapy School, Mumbai.
5. All India Institute of Physical Medicine and Rehabilitation, Mumbai.
6. Institute of Physical Medicine and Rehabilitation, Vellore.
7. N.I.M.H. (National Institute for Mentally Handicapped), Secunderabad.
8. N.I.O.H. (National Institute for the Orthopaedically Handicapped), Kolkata.
9. Ali Yavar Jung National Institute for the Hearing Handicapped, Mumbai.
10. National Institute for the Visually Handicapped, Dehradun.
11. All India Institute of Speech and Hearing, Mysore.
12. Many other non Government voluntary organisations.

BEHAVIOURAL PROBLEMS IN CHILDREN

There are many types of behavioural problems in children. They are grouped as under:
Educational: Slow learner, School phobia, Repeat failure.
Habit: Bed wetting, Nail biting, Thumb sucking, Masturbation.
Personality: Jealous, Tantrum, shy, Hysteric.
Psychosomatic: Depression, Delusion, Hallucinations.
Antisocial: Stealing, Cruelty, Sexual offense, destructiveness.

One of the major behaviour problems in India is Juvenile Delinquency. It is described below:

Juvenile Delinquency

It is an offence committed by a boy below 16 years or by a girl below 18 years. It is high among boys between 15-16 years in India.

Causes:
Chromosomal anomalies
Broken homes
Urbanised life with poverty.

Prevention:
It is possible to prevent juvenile delinquency through:

a. Proper schooling to provide education.
b. Social welfare activities to facilitate deviation in behaviour; and
c. Family life improvement.

Others

Some of the concepts in child health are:

i. **Child Abuse:**
Physical violence on child, sexual abuse, mental and emotional maltreatment, neglect, Deprivation and Lack of opportunity are included under child abuse. Physical battering has lead to death, blindness and mental retardation.

ii. **Street Children:**
Children without family are living and working on the street, are at risk for malnutrition, Tuberculosis, drug abuse and criminal exploitation.

iii. **Battered Baby Syndrome:**
Children below 3 years received inexcusable violence resulting in mental and neurological complications.

iv. **Child Labour:**
Children below 15 years are obligated to work and earn.

GROWTH AND DEVELOPMENT

Child grows and develops which include physical growth and intellectual-emotional-social development. With optimal nutrition, optimum growth and development is possible.

Thus growth is defined as increase in Physical size of body and Development is defined as increase in skills and functions. Process of growth during 0-20 years is depicted in Figure 14.2.

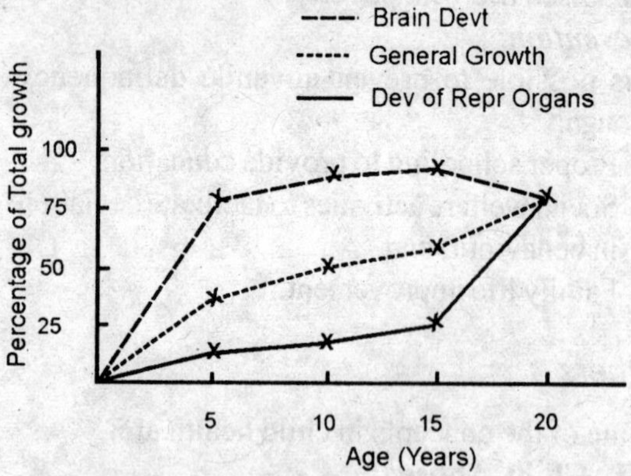

Fig. 14.2: Process of growth during 0-20 years

Reference Value:
For studies and comparison we use standard values as under:

1. Harvard standard
2. WHO standard
3. I.C.M.R. standards.

Measurement of Growth:
Weight Recording: Beam type weighting scale is used in clinics and hospitals. In the Field (Home visiting) a Salter spring machine is used.

Height Recording: Upto 2 years infantometer is used. Older children can stand and height is measured by the rod attached to the lever type machine or by anthropometer. In Home visiting measuring height against a wall is found quite satisfactory.

Mid Upper Arm Circumference: This measurement is done with a tape while the arm is relaxed at the side of the body.

Head and Chest Circumference: They are measured with the help of a tape.

Indian Standards:

Table 14.7: Mean weight and height of Indian children

	Mean weight		*Mean height*	
	Boys	*Girls*	*Boys*	*Girls*
	(Kg)		*(Cms)*	
Birth	3.1	3.0	49.2	48.8
6 months	7.5	6.9	66.3	64.5
1 year	9.5	8.7	73.4	72.1
2 years	11.7	10.6	84.5	82.1
3 years	13.6	12.6	92.7	90.0
4 years	14.9	14.3	98.1	98.0
5 years	17.0	16.0	106.7	104.4
6 years	19.5	17.2	114.6	109.4

Table 14.8: M.U.A.C. in Indian children

	Mean M.U.A.C.	
	Male	*Female*
	(Cms)	
1 year	14.9	14.4
2 years	15.1	14.5
3 years	15.3	14.8
4 years	15.5	15.0
5 years	15.7	15.4
6 years	16.2	15.7

Table 14.9: Weight increment in infants

Age	*Weight increment per week*
0–3 months	200 G
4–6 months	150 G
7–9 months	100 G
9–12 months	50-75 G

Table 14.10: Weight and height increment from 1 to 5 years

Weight increments per year	
1 – 2 years	2.5 kg
3 – 5 years	2.0 kg
Height increments per year	
1st year	25 cm
2nd year	12 cm
3rd year	9 cm
5th year	6 cm

Growth Pattern

Rapid growth occurs in infancy. All babies loose weight during first 4 days after birth. The same is regained in 8 days. It doubles in 5 months, trebles at 1 year.

Length of baby increases 1½ times by 1 year. Weight, height and M.U.A.C. are given in Tables 14.9 and 14.10.

Growth is a natural process and it is a sign of well nourishment. If there is loss of appetite, listlessness, decreased activity and peevishness it is reflection of illness and ill nourishment. Since weight is made up of height and fatness which is recorded in weight, the weight is the best indicator for the growth of a child. Each child varies in its weight according to local influencing factors. Hence a range is considered for fixing normal or abnormal. Following is the reference standard by N.C.H.S., USA (National Centre of Health Statistics). They are Harvard values considered as standard by WHO.

Age (years)	*Boys*		*Girls*	
	Median	*± 2 SD*	*Median*	*± 2 SD*
Birth	3.3	2.4 – 4.3	3.2	2.2 – 4.0
6 months	7.8	5.9 – 9.8	7.2	5.5 – 9.0
1 year	10.2	8.1 – 12.4	9.5	7.4 – 11.6
2 years	12.69	9.9 – 15.2	11.9	9.4 – 14.5
3 years	14.6	11.4 – 18.3	14.1	11.2 – 18.0
4 years	16.7	12.9 – 20.8	16.0	12.6 – 20.7
5 years	18.7	14.4 – 23.5	17.7	13.8 – 23.2
6 years	20.7	16.0 – 26.6	19.5	15.0 – 26.2

This uses concept of centile. Lower the percentile more the growth retardation and vice versa.

Growth Charts

We have growth charts for recording weight corresponding to a given age. Since under 6 years

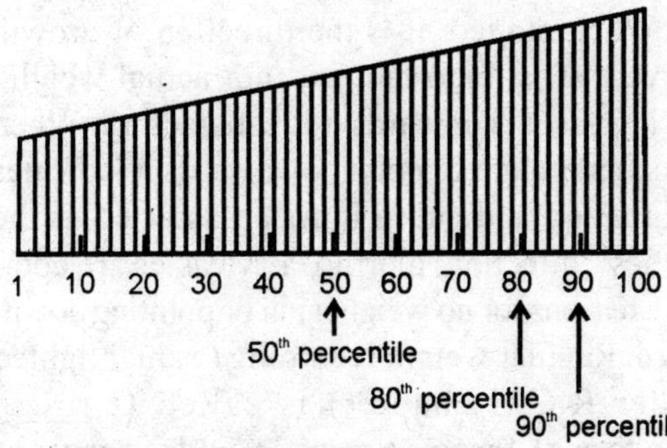

Fig. 14.3: Concept of centile marked in 100 values of height of 100 children *(Shortest to tallest arranged)*

are considered for growth monitoring R.C.H., in I.C.D.S. services, weight recording is done for 0-6 age children in the I.C.D.S. (Govt. of India) chart. The I.A.P. has recommended the following classification for child nutrition.

Normal: Up to 80% of median (reference curve).

I Degree

Malnutrition: Between 80-71% of median (reference curve).

II Degree

Malnutrition: Between 70-61% of median (reference curve).

III Degree

Malnutrition: Below 60% of median (reference curve).

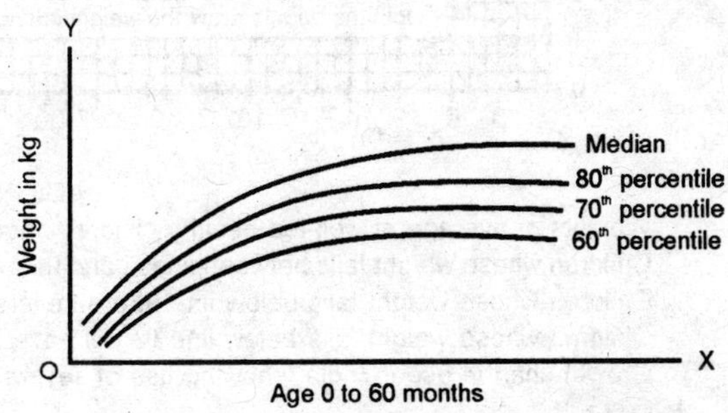

Fig. 14.4: I.A.P. grouping for malnutrition

When plotted, it is the direction of growth curve that is important and not actual weight. As long as it is upwards it is satisfactory. When remains straight or point downwards it indicates retardation and cause must be asserted at the earliest. Infection, diarrhoea, Measles are common reasons for no weight gain or pointing downward. Regular weight recording (as highlighted under R.C.H chapter) is called (Growth monitoring). Since we monitor, find out cause of growth faltering, discuss with mother for supplementation, it is better to use the word *Growth Monitoring and Promotion.*

Nursing care should make sure of the following in Growth monitoring and promotion.

i. Good reliable weighing scale
ii. Growth chart
iii. Knowledge on recording and interpretation of growth on the growth chart
iv. Two way discussion with mother of the child for action.

Growth charts are useful in diagnosis, education, take measure, evaluation, teaching and growth monitoring and promotion.

Commonly used I.C.D.S. Growth chart used by Anganwadi worker in Anganwadi is given in Figure 14.5:

I.C.M.R. Standards:

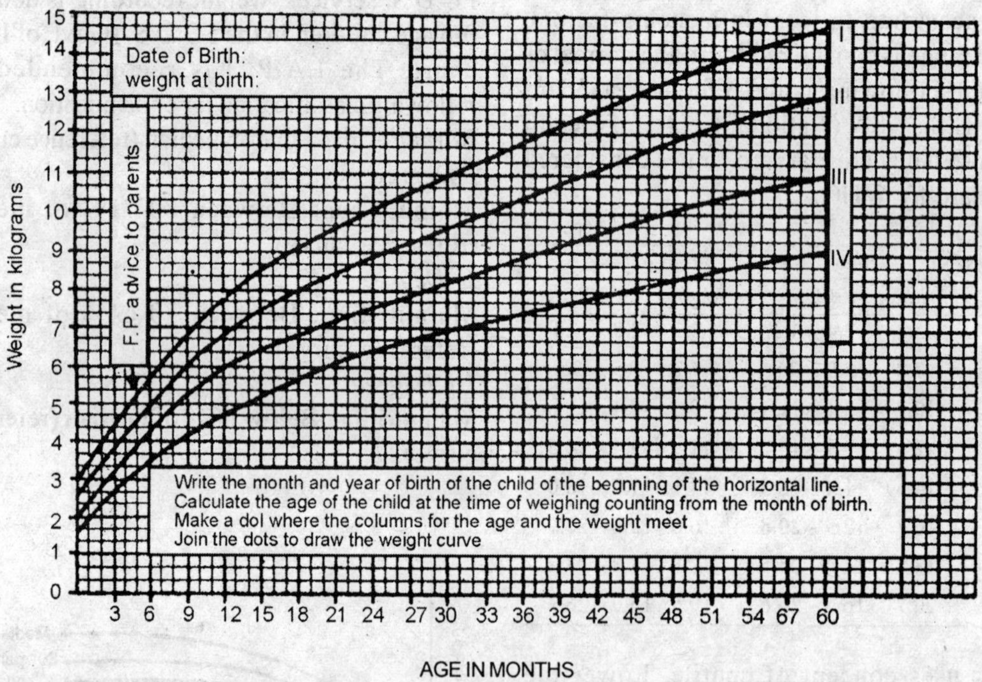

Weights of average of well-fed healthy children should be above the uppermost line I.
Children whose weight falls between lines I and III are under-nourished and require supplementary feeding at home.
Children whose weight falls below line III are severely malnourished. Consult the doctor and follow his advice.
Children whose weight falls below line IV will have to be hospitalized for treatment
Growth chart in use in India, showing use of several reference curves to indicate the nutritional status of the child

Fig. 14.5: I.C.D.S. growth chart used for growth monitoring

Table 14.11: I.C.M.R. standard for weight (boys and girls)

Age (year)	Male Child Mean weight Kg	Female Child Mean weight Kg
1	8.4	7.8
2	10.1	9.6
3	11.8	11.2
4	13.5	12.0
5	14.8	14.5
6	16.3	16.0

Table 14.12: I.C.M.R. standard for height (boys and girls)

Age (years)	Male Mean height (cm)	Female Mean height (cm)
1	73.9	72.5
2	81.6	80.1
3	88.8	87.2
4	96.0	94.5
5	102.1	101.4
6	108.5	107.4

Table 14.13: I.C.M.R. standard for head circumference (boys and girls)

Age (years)	Male Mean Head circumference (cm)	Female Mean Head circumference (cm)
1	44.4	43.6
2	45.9	45.2
3	47.3	46.2
4	48.0	47.1
5	48.5	47.8
6	49.0	48.3

Table 14.14: I.C.M.R. standard for chest circumference (boys and girls)

Age (years)	Male Chest circumference (cm)	Female Chest circumference (cm)
1	43.3	42.3
2	45.8	45.1
3	48.0	47.2
4	49.4	48.7
5	50.8	50.1
6	52.5	51.3

Table 14.15: M.U.A.C.circumference standard for boys

Age (years)	M.U.A.C. WHO Standard (Male)			Indian (Shanti Ghosh) (Male)
	100%	90%	80%	
1	16.3	14.4	12.8	14.9
2	16.8	14.7	13.0	15.1
3	17.0	15.3	13.6	15.3
4	17.0	15.3	13.6	15.5
5	17.0	15.3	13.6	15.7
6	17.3	15.6	13.8	16.2

Table 14.16: M.U.A.C. circumference standard for girls

Age (years)	M.U.A.C. WHO Standard (Female)			Indian (Shanti Ghosh) (Female)
	100%	90%	80%	
1	15.6	14.0	12.5	14.4
2	15.9	14.4	12.8	14.5
3	16.9	15.2	13.5	14.8
4	16.9	15.2	13.5	15.0
5	16.9	15.2	13.5	15.4
6	17.3	15.5	13.8	15.7

Factors influencing growth and development:

i. Genetic factors like inheritance
ii. Affordability and acceptability of nutrition
iii. Younger age
iv. Growth spurt at puberty
v. Physical surroundings
vi. Good parent child relation
vii. Infections
viii. Parasitism
ix. Standard of living
x. Birth spacing

Relation of Head and Chest Circumference in Preventive Paediatrics

At birth head circumference is larger than chest circumference. Cross over of these take place around 24th month among Indian children when compared to American children (Fig. 14.6).

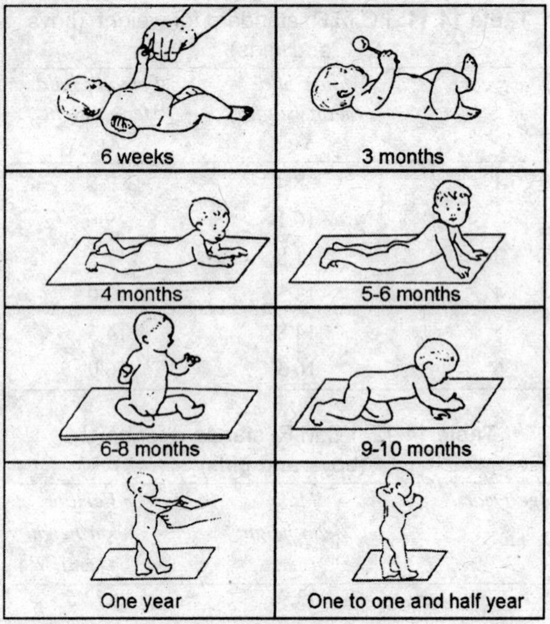

Fig. 14.7: Milestones

Milestones

Behavioural development in terms of (a) Motor (b) Personal (c) Adoptive and (d) Language developments are having specific landmarks of development in human life cycles. These are averages and hence are not absolute. Relative approach of fixing milestones for development is ideal, after studying individual cases, for fixing either normalcy or abnormalcy.

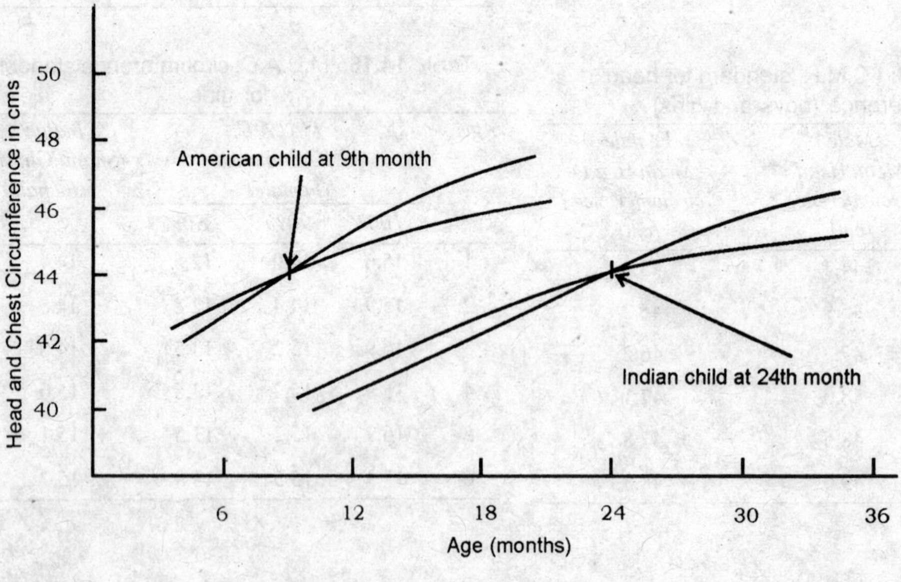

Fig. 14.6: Crossing over of head and chest circumference in American and Indian child

Motor Development

Table 14.17: Milestones in development of a child

6 weeks	–	Smiles, recognises
3 months	–	Holds object deliberately
4 months	–	Holds head without support
5-6 months	–	Lifts head, turns to see
6-8 months	–	Sits without support
9-10 months	–	Crawls
1 year	–	Stands with support
1-1½ years	–	Stands without support

Major Sociopersonal Developments:

6-8 weeks	–	Looks and smiles
4-5 months	–	Recognises mother
6-8 months	–	Enjoy hide and seek
9-10 months	–	Suspects stranger

Major Adoptive Developments:

4-5 months	–	Reaches for object
6-8 months	–	Transfer objects hand to hand
9-10 months	–	Releases objects
12-14 months	–	Builds the shape

Major Language Developments:

6-8 months	–	Experiments with noise
9-10 months	–	High sounding noise
10-11 months	–	First word "Ma, ma"
18-21 months	–	Joins words

CHILD GUIDANCE CLINIC

It was started in 1909 with an intention to deal juvenile delinquent child. Now other forms of child maladjustments are tackled through child guidance clinic.

Child guidance clinics are run in team spirit by child psychologists, psychiatrists, psychosocial workers, paediatrics speech therapists, neurologists and occupational therapists. Common methods employed in child guidance clinics are:

- Child counselling
- Play therapy
- Parental counselling.

UNDER FIVE CLINIC

Earlier years well baby clinics were running which took preventive care services. Now, of late, under five clinics have taken up the task of integrating treatment, prevention and surveillance activity in the community.

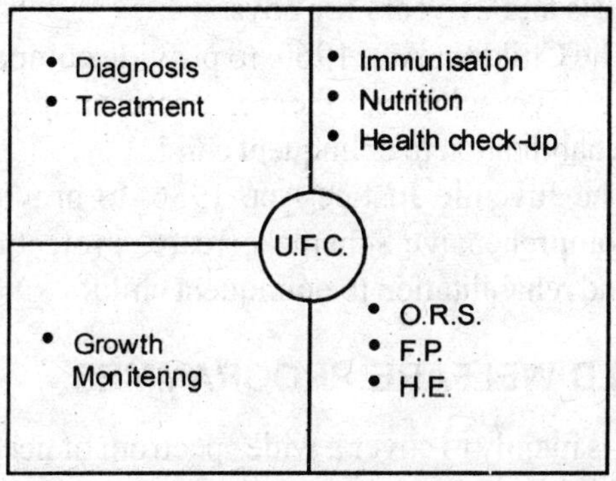

Fig. 14.8: Functions of under five clinics

CHILD PLACEMENT ACTIVITIES

Problem children and deviants are tackled through child placement procedures. Mainly they are as under:

i. *Adoption:* Childless couple can legally adopt which give a permanent placement for orphans.
ii. *Faster Homes:* Social work minded organisation run faster homes which are nearer to a family to provide love and affection.
iii. *Orphanage*: It is an institution where large number of broken home children, street children and begging children are placed.
iv. *Remand Home*: A child is kept under a trained person, psychiatrist and doctor to improve mental and physical well-being of a child. It also has elementary schooling.

v. *Borstal:* Deviant child, misbehaved in a certified school, usually above 16 years of age are sent to Borstal for training and reformation.

LEGISLATION FOR CHILD HEALTH

1. The Child Labour (Prohibition and Regulation) Act, 1986 to protect the child from Child Labour.
2. The Child Marriage Restraint Act, 1978, to raise legal age of marriage to 18 years for girls and 21 years for boys.
3. The Children Act, 1960, to provide comprehensive scheme of care, protection and rehabilitation to delinquent child.
4. The Juvenile Justice Act, 1986, to provide comprehensive scheme of care, protection and rehabilitation to delinquent child.

CHILD WELFARE PROGRAMMES

This is mainly to cover a wide spectrum of needs of children who are socially, economically, physically or mentally handicapped. These children will be usually under any one of the following categories:

a. Children of working mothers
b. Destitute children
c. Handicapped children.

Indian Council for Child Welfare (I.C.C.W.), Central Social Welfare Board, Kasturba Memorial Trusts and Indian Red Cross Society are organising the following child welfare programmes:

i. Nursery schools, balwadies, crèches, day care homes and day care services for working mothers.

ii. Holiday homes for 12 to 16 age group children for spending holidays for deviated healthy activities.

iii. Recreation facilities like park, children library, balbhavan, children film, children museum, hobby classes etc.

FURTHER REFERENCES

1. Prabhakara, G.N. Short Text Book of P & SM (JP).
2. Shanti Ghosh – Nutrition and Child Care (JP).
3. I.C.M.R. Standards – N.I.N. Hyderabad.
4. Mimeography notes of I.C.D.S. Consultancy work of author.

15

Geriatrics

IMPORTANCE

Aging process involves changes in physiological, pathological, social and psychological conditions of a person. Changing sociocultural trend is taking elderly off from joint family system to the old age homes (those who can afford). Slowly family life by bonding is weaning off creating chaos in health status, nutrition status, metabolic status and psychological status. Sometimes the elderly are left alone to feed themselves for their survival.

According to Sir James Sterling Ross "We cannot heal old age; we can protect it, promote it and extend it".

Now that expectation of life is increased, Geriatric age group is widening and we have nearing 3.8% of the population being above 65 years age. This comes to nearly 39 million people above the age of 65 years as per 2001 census. Current SRS estimates are 7.2% of total population are above 60 years of age.

HEALTH STATUS

Various studies have shown that illness among old age is multifactorial and multiorgan. Main illnesses seen are loss of vision (Cataract), non ambulatory (arthritis) Bronchitis, Vitamin deficiencies, Ear infections, Diabetes, Hypertension and accidents. ICMR study has shown that reported sickness is as under by proportion: (pooled observations)

- Gradual loss of vision 88
- Muscle joint disorders 40
- Neurological 18.69
- Cardiovascular 17.44
- Respiratory 16.13
- Skin infections 13.35
- G.I. tract 9.10
- Mental ill health 8.5
- Loss of hearing 8.2
- Genito urinary disorder 3.5

COMMON HEALTH PROBLEMS

Old Age Problems

The change in old age is called senescence which is a natural process. Common effects of old age are:

- Senile cataract
- Nerve deafness
- Osteoporotic changes
- Bronchitis with emphysema
- Changes in mental outlook

and many more old age changes.

Chronic Illness

Old people are prone to a few known chronic diseases. Of particular importance are:

- Atherosclerosis
- Heart attacks
- Hypertension
- Stroke
- Cancer
- Diabetes
- Accident and fractures
- Gout
- Rheumatoid arthritis
- Fibrocytis
- Neuritis
- Chronic bronchitis
- Asthma
- Prostate enlargement
- Fibroid of uterus.

Psychological Disturbances

Dependency, retired life and loneliness aggravate mental changes; cessation of reproductive activity lead to jealousy; social maladjustment leads to emotional disorders.

PUBLIC HEALTH ASPECT OF OLD AGE

At national and state level burden of pension, Medical service and social services increases, slackening the development of youth activities and health. Preparation for old age and retirement helps a lot for an active aging. As long as cultural bondage exist, utility of old age for socially useful productive work, care of children and guidance at family problems helps in reducing old age burden.

According to German and Fried old age preventive care can be grouped under 3 levels:

1. **Primary Level:**
   Good health habits like:
   - Good sleep
   - Good and required nutrition
   - Curtailing smoking, alcohol and fatty foods.
   - Avoidance of overeating (Obesity control)

   Avoiding risk factors like:
   - Care at routine to avoid accident, fracture.
   - Diet restrictions.
   - Periodic health check up.
2. **Secondary Level:**
   - Screening for hypertension
   - Early diagnosis and prompt treatment for infections.
3. **Tertiary Level:**
   - Rehabilitation for Physical defects
   - Rehabilitation for Cognitive defects
   - Rehabilitation for Functional defects
   - Use of care taker for support.

NURSING RESPONSIBILITIES OF OLD AGE CARE

- Advice, counselling, help for safe housing, good diet and happy surroundings.
- Help old person to overcome infection, mental strain and frustration.
- In case of bed ridden, there is a need for frequent visit for careful attention. She helps in bed sore prevention.
- Demonstrate feeding, bath and back care to the family in case of chronic patients (e.g. stroke).
- Help in development of favourable attitude towards elderly by youngsters.

NUTRITION OF ELDERLY

During aging process, certain inevitable degenerative changes occur that will result in functional decline. They are usually influenced by nutrition followed by genetics, psychosocial and economic conditions. Hence proper nutrition and health care are necessary for elderly to lead a normal life.

Ageing Process and Nutrition

Lack of physical activity, poor appetite, feeling of loneliness and sense of neglect herald old age changes. All old people have gastrointestinal changes. Some of them have diseases like diabetes, hypertension, heart disease, G.I. problem, kidney problems and arthritis.

ICMR has worked out the nutritional requirement of old people (1990). The requirement of energy is expected to be 10% less that of an adult.

Balance Diet for Geriatric Age

Foodstuff	*Requirement (Grams)*	
	Male	*Female*
Cereals	350	225
Pulses	50	40
Vegetables	200	150
Leafy vegetables	50	50
Roots, tubers	100	100
Fruits	200	200
Milk and milk products	300	300
Sugar	20	20
Fats and oils	25	25

Nutrient Required for the Old Age

Foodstuff	*Requirement (Grams)*	
	Male	*Female*
Calorie	2200	1700
Protein	65 G	50 G
Fat	50 G	40 G
Calcium	1 G	0.9G
Iron	38 mg	30 mg
Vitamin A (retinol)	1030 μg	930 μg
Thiamin	1.96 mg	1.45 mg
Riboflavin	1.78 mg	1.51 mg

Some dietary tips for the elderly:

The diet of the elderly may be modified according to physical activity of an individual and general health condition. The following tips are suggested for dietary management of the elderly. They are:

1. Take simple but nutritious diet
2. Improve the quality of diet by adding liberal quantity of green leafy vegetables, fruits and whole cereals
3. Take frequent but small meals
4. Take plenty of fluids and semisolids
5. Avoid dry foods
6. Reduce total fat
7. Reduce refined carbohydrate
8. Reduce salt intake
9. Avoid fasting.

Other Indirect Nutritional Advice

1. Maintain good social and psychological environment for normal health.
2. Do regular exercise like brisk walking
3. Avoid inactivity, loneliness and social isolation

SOCIAL WELFARE FOR ELDERLY

There are many social welfare schemes that are helpful to the positive health of elderly. They are:

- Old age homes when no dependents are there for security, food and shelter.
- Social assistance like pension, old age pension etc.
- Home services for attending to all physical requirements.
- Home care services for attending to all biological requirements.
- Meals on wheels services to supply fresh, hot food to home supply at appropriate time and at required frequent timings.
- Health check up camps for elderly for screening their health.
- Socioeconomic benefits to elderly like concession in rail, bus, and other benefits to senior citizens.

FURTHER REFERENCES

1. Cowdry – The care of the geriatric patient (CV Mosby).
2. NIN – Nutritional Tips to Elderly.
3. Health problems of specialized groups VHAI report 1997.

16

Personal Hygiene

IMPORTANCE

The word hygiene has come from Hygiea (The Goddess of Health) who was the daughter of a leader of Greek medicine Aesculapius. "Personal hygiene" is appropriately called as "personal health" mainly because it is not just cleanliness of body. It has other factors equally important to maintain the health of the individual. Positive health is something more than cleanliness and absence of disease. It is a positive state of well being of whole body which will enable the body to grow and develop normally to its full capacity and have the ability to enjoy all the opportunities that life may present.

DEFINITION

It deals with practices of an individual which help in maintaining and promoting his health physically, mentally, socially and spiritually.

Benefits of Personal Hygiene:

- Helps in maintaining good clean physique.
- Helps in muscular and bony strength.
- Helps in keeping health of oral cavity, tongue, teeth.
- Helps in maintaining skin integrity.
- Helps in the control of
  Genitourinary infections
  Skin infections
  Gastro intestinal disorders
  Musculoskeletal disorders.
- Helps in building up resistance.

COMPONENTS

Skin

It is a delicate organ. Apart from protection and insulation it helps in the process of excretion. Perspiration contains thrown out waste products which is evident after an act of heavy exercise. The sebaceous gland secretion acts as a natural coat to the skin. In high temperate climate and tropical countries where perspiration is high, skin cleaning becomes a paramount importance.

Skin needs regular bathing and appropriate clothing. If sebaceous glands are blocked with dirt, it leads to many complications like sebaceous cyst, impetigo, scabies, prickly heat and ringworm infection.

Bath with hard soaps is routine in human habits. Bathing cleans, increases circulation, give muscle tone, improve appetite, make free from infection and gives a sense of freshness and well being. If water temperature is between 35°C to 36°C it is warm bath, between 33°C to 35°C cold bath and 36°C to 43°C hot bath. Oil bath is common in traditional families which gives coolness and softness to the skin. Turmeric and sandal application has germicidal action.

Ritual bath like after menstruation, after childbirth, after hair cut, after a visit to graveyard are quite interesting to note and to be understood by the nursing community. Bathing in well, swimming pools are attached with exercises.

Sunbath is appropriated to allow sunlight (UV and cosmic rays) in early morning or late evening which is found to increase blood circulation. Care must be taken to avoid sunburn. Before and after seawater bath, sun bath is advocated which has a utility in personal health.

Clothing

It has many fold uses like protection from extreme climate, protection from insect bite; maintain body heat and personal value of decoration. Dress code from health point of view may not be suitable for civilisation point of view.

Material used in clothing has impact on skin. Cotton cloth is a good conductor of heat, absorbs moisture, easily washable and suitable for tropics. Khadi handwoven is economical and durable cotton. Wool is best for winter, it being bad conductor of heat. Silk is bad conductor of heat. Rayon and other synthetics are slightly warmer but are found to produce skin allergy.

Care of the Hand

Care of the hand is of paramount importance because it is an agent to contaminate food. Washing hands before eating is the first lesson of personal hygiene to avoid food borne infections. After visiting toilet and latrine, hands must be washed with soap and water.

In nursing care, washing hands is a must before any procedure. Nursing hand wash is to be followed as under:

"Wet the hands from elbow towards finger tips, soap well, wash the tips of fingers and thumbs turned in, then wash between fingers and arms with rotary motion. Then rinse from elbow downwards. This helps to remove dirt. It is repeated in case adherent dirt is there.".

Care of the Hair

Hair is an outgrowth of epidermis. It grows from hair follicle which will be situated in dermis. The composition of hair is dead thorny cell. The colour of the hair is due to pigment between the cells during its growth. Softness of hair is due to sebaceous gland secretions. The hair is reflection of personal health, which is seen as streaked yellowish brown among malnourished individuals.

Each person should have his/her own comb and brush for a better personal hygiene.

Care is needed at hair-cut, for; it may cause injury, infection or infestation.

In case of head louse infestation, application of 5% Benzylbenzoate overnight, headbath and proper grooming is advocated (also refer page 162 and page 372).

Body Sweating

Sweating affects the adolescent, who is inclined to be nervous, especially girls who get excited. It is not only embarrassing but also ruins clothes. Cheap and unreliable deodorants cause skin problem. A good anti perspirant when used though takes off perspiration; it causes irritation in the skin (if not used properly). Sweat allowed to decompose in woollen material is offensive. Repeated bath and hygienic practice are the only answer for bad excessive sweating.

Blackheads and Acne

This is common among adolescents. It particularly affects those with a greasy type of skin. The pores from sebaceous glands become blocked with sebum and a hard head forms on the top (Comedo). At the top infection may occur. Regular wash with soap, careful rinsing and drying, exposure to fresh air and sunlight, and evacuation of blocked pore by gentle pressure or by comedo remover will help to some extent in controlling acne and black heads. They may have to limit sweet and starchy foods since there is significant association of acne and diet.

Hygiene of Toilet

The kidneys excrete about 4 pints of water per day which helps in the excretion of urea, uric acid, creatinine and inorganic salts from the body. One to 1½ litre of water consumed per day help in good elimination process. Bladder control as an outcome of civilised life and social inhibitions should be avoided. It should be treated as a physiological function of the body (excretion).

Bowel Habit

Regular bowel habit avoids constipation. Too much or too little rigid regulations are harmful and emotionally put an individual in a dangerous position. Diet with high fibre help to overcome constipation. Since constipation is known to cause headache, tension, abdominal discomfort, gastro intestinal infections, it is advisable to develop a good and routine bowel habit.

Care must be taken at advice for flexible attitude in cases where a person is on liquid diet, on fasting etc. Where passing stool once in 3-4 days may be normal (for the given individual). In females, since there are chances to infect urethra or vaginal area from the bowel, it is advisable to educate them to clean from the vagina to rectum.

Menstrual Hygiene

This aspect is surrounded by taboos and superstitions. It should be looked as a physiological process in all female human beings. A young girl usually gets instructions from her mother. Recently, mass media is playing a very important role in educating the girls about menstrual hygiene. Traditionally, taking bath is considered as not advisable during menses. Actually washing and cleaning of groin and vulva is mandatory. Woman hygiene kit (natural or sanitary pad) should be changed regularly and should be disposed off hygienically. There is no need to feel unwell while girls are menstruating. Intravaginal tampons can be used if found comfortable. Vaginal douching is not necessary at the end of cycle. Nature takes care to see by itself by clearing all menstrual debris. It is the habit of cleanliness that accounts most in menstrual hygiene. For healthy couple (regarding intercourse) there is no sound medical reason for advising against intercourse during menstruation.

Care of Special Sensory Organ

Eyes

Eyes reflect health and is found dull when ill or fatigued. Eyes need correction and use of glass when there is impairment of vision. Care is needed at beautification of eyelash, eyelid and eyebrow. The colour, the chemical, the lotion, the substance used must be harmless. It is advisable to avoid common stick to apply Kajal since eye infection can spread very easily.

Light from above and left is advocated for reading and not to strain eyes. Whenever a touch or cleaning of eye is needed, hands and fingers must be washed thoroughly with a detergent soap. Washed hand and finger should not be dried with a dirty cloth.

Any headache, watering of eyes, fatigue on reading, eyes must be got tested.

Protective goggle at work and while riding a two wheeler avoids accidental injury to the eye by a foreign body or avoids pterygium which is an exposure effect.

Ears

There are no specific criteria that wax should be removed as a ritual. Since it is a normal secretion process and a protective phenomenon wax formation in the ear do not call for attention. In case of excess secretion it may need to be attended with wax solvent and ear syringing by a trained person. No external material including dirty finger be put inside ear lest it may cause otitis media. Cleaning the outer ear during bath is found sufficient. No hard substance is put to ear lest it may cause rupture of tympanum. In case of entry of an insect like ant, use of oil is preferred to make it flow and remove.

Care of the Nose

Breathing, air entry, dust entry and pathogen by air cause health hazards. Enlarged adenoids can lead to mouth breathing, which is found associated with frequent cold and frequent sore throat. Taking off the hair from nostril is not advisable because hair is necessary as a natural filtering agent.

While sneezing one should use handkerchief to avoid discharge at air which can cause air pollution.

At swimming blowing the nose gently is advocated.

Oral Hygiene

It implies good teeth, good gum and good healthy buccal cavity. Mastication produces and promotes saliva and gastric secretion which help in digestion. Emotional satisfaction of eating is associated with good oral hygiene.

Mouth

Mouth cleansing or rinsing is a good habit after each act of food consumption. Very hot, very spicy and extraneous substance like tobacco leaves irritates and produces ulcer and even malignancy. Poor oral hygiene can lead to periodontal diseases (Pyorrhoea) and loss of tooth. Halitosis (bad breath) is an indication of oral cavity fermented smell which can be totally avoided by good oral hygiene.

Mouth rinsing with drinking water is more than sufficient in 99 percent cases. In 1% of cases sodium bicarbonate gargling, desensitising oral rinse with either potassium nitrate or sodium fluoride, may be needed.

A very inexpensive dentifrice can be made by warm water with a pinch of salt (hypo saline) as a wash to mouth and gullet. Mouth can be a seat of many organisms. If care is not taken for oral hygiene septic tonsils, infected sinus can produce widespread mouth sickness and are preventable.

Teeth

Dental caries is common and worldwide problem. This can lead to cavity formation and tooth decay. Decay is by acids of mouth bacteria acting upon food particles in the mouth. Sweets, chocolates, biscuits are seen associated with occurrence of dental caries. Sweet as sticky substance and increased sugar consumption enhances dental caries. Soft proteinous material accumulating around neck of teeth constitutes dental plaque which is to be removed by daily habit of tooth brushing. It is seen that caries is dependent on fluoride content of water. Optimal level of fluoride in drinking water (0.5 – 0.8 mg per litre) prevents dental caries. Fluoride containing dentifrices can reduce dental caries by 20%.

Limiting refined carbohydrates, avoiding frequent chewing of snacks in between meal, disallowing smoking, alcohol and tobacco leaves bring about an improved dental hygiene in the coming days.

Patient's denture also need wash under running water, placed in a tooth mug of cold water and returned to the patient. In addition to regular cleaning, the patient should be given antiseptic mouthwash last thing at night and a bowl of antiseptic for dentures if they are not worn at night.

Nutrition

Knowledge of balanced diet, to suit the body needs in anabolism and catabolism is judged best under personal health. Roughage consisting of high fibre diet can reduce many gastrointestinal problems like constipation, mucous diarrhoea, intussessuption and intestinal polyposis. Junk foods are better avoided and a traditional food can help to increase a man's life expectancy.

Exercise

Depending on one's age, regular exercise is a must for a good personal health. At home active engagement in household duties, social useful productive work and ritual inevitable exercises do as much good as an exercise by a sportsman or gymnast. It is a tool to restore strength, correct deformity and to reduce body weight.

In hospital practice post operative exercise, post natal exercise and physiotherapeutic exercises are well known in keeping the body and mind fit for a positive personal hygiene.

Posture

Good posture in standing, walking, sitting and recumbent has an active role for positive health. Round shouldered position, dropped chest, protruding abdomen, are indication of ill health or deformity. Poor nutrition, chronic infection, bone defect, emotional maladjustment can cause poor as well as bad exposure. Personal hygiene in posture is meant to well adjusted emotional life and free from physical defects.

Sleeping Habit

The amount of sleep needed varies with age, occupation and habit. Physiologically 8 hours of sleep (1/3 of active life) is found sufficient for regaining bodily and mental fatigue. "Early to bed and early to rise" is a dictum found useful for an active life. There is no use in sleeping for 12-16 hours which are full of dreams and is superficial. Deep sleep of 4 hours without bodily strain by dreams is found healthy for active life.

Sleep is a natural process to overcome fatigue and to recuperate the energy, strength and vigour spent during days work. Developing good sleeping habit can reduce tiredness, body ache, headache, nausea and discomfort, provided it is undisturbed deep sleep for a limited time.

OTHER ASPECTS

Other aspect of personal hygiene for a better personal health:

- Wearing footwear while walking in an open field where open field defecation prevails can prevent hookworm infection.
- Observing *purdha*, avoiding even sunrays prone to cause certain respiratory infections like tuberculosis.
- Alcoholism, smoking and gambling do not allow cultivating good health habit in an individual. He also lacks in personal hygiene.
- Awareness at traditional barbering, tattooing, and circumcision can allow personal hygiene which can reduce the incidence of skin infection, AIDS, tetanus and scabies.
- Personal hygiene in the form of no spitting, no urination etc. in swimming pool can bring down certain infections. This needs an idea of swimming pool sanitation.
- Ritual purifications if not harmful, have an equal effect on a good personal hygiene.
- Poor personal hygiene can cause (autograde) thread worm infection which is overcome by

cleanliness after defecation and drug treatment.

- Care and observation of meat to be eaten can prevent tape worm infection, is a part of personal hygiene.
- Louse infestation and scabies are known fundamentals to personal hygiene.
- Worm infestations are avoidable if raw fruits and vegetables are washed and used at eating.

CONCLUSION

Personal hygiene, personal habits and personal health are interwoven in such a way that they are not separable from one another. Good habit and personal hygiene for health are known since age old days. But health by habit and health by hygiene needs culture imbibed motto in an individual for a positive health.

FURTHER REFERENCES

1. Priest MA – Modern Text of personal and Community Health for Nurses (Heinemann).
2. St. John Ambulance Association – Nursing Manual.
3. Freeman – Public Health Nursing Practice (W.B. Saunders).
4. Prabhakara G.N.—Research and Evaluation of Women Hygiene Kit Phase I in Dharwad District 2001 April (Govt. of Karnataka Research Grant) Study Report.
5. Prabhakara G.N.—Research and Evaluation of Women Hygiene Kit Phase II in Dharwad District 2002 Feb (Govt. of Karnataka Research Grant) Study Report.

17

General Epidemiology

Epidemiology has become basic science in understanding health and disease in the practice of modern medicine today. Substantial developments are seen in the fields of clinical epidemiology, serological epidemiology, epidemiology of communicable diseases, epidemiology of non communicable diseases and neuro-epidemiology. All other disciplines are engaging the scope of epidemiology in understanding their role through epidemiological studies.

The word Epi= among, demos = people and logos= study truly signify the role of epidemiology in maintaining positive health in the country.

IMPORTANCE

Epidemiology has its involvement in disease occurrence, causation, transmission and health-related event. Improved knowledge of Epidemiology has brought into focus the risk factors. Separate departments exist in:

a. Disease Epidemiology under National Institute of Communicable disease.
b. Cancer Epidemiology in oncology institutions.
c. Neuro Epidemiology in National Institutions of Mental Health.
d. Occupational Epidemiology in International and National Labour Organisation; and
e. Epidemiological units at National Institute of Speech and Hearing.

United States appointed W.H. Frost as first professor of epidemiology 76 years back and UK appointed Major Greenwood as first professor of Epidemiology 70 years back.

All descriptions available in present text books on health sciences are based on our knowledge of Epidemiology. Positive health of individuals and groups is main concern of modern Epidemiology. Knowledge of nutritional science, knowledge of bacteriology and Immunology has enhanced the progress of epidemiology.

Nursing profession at its nursing care process uses the knowledge of disease transmission, disinfection and causation, for efficient nursing. It is interconnected with the triad of Nurse-Ward-Patient in case of hospitals and Nurse-Health Centre – Community in case Public Health Nursing Activities.

DEFINITION

According to Mac Mohan it is defined as "the study of the distribution and determinants of disease frequency in man".

Twenty-eight years later John M. Last has given new definition to the word epidemiology as "the study of the distribution and determinants of health related states or events in specified populations and the application of this study to the control of health problems".

MAIN AIMS OF EPIDEMIOLOGY

International Epidemiological Association and Indian Epidemiological Association have endorsed 3 aims of Epidemiology as under:

i. To describe the distribution and magnitude of health and disease problems in human populations.
ii. To identify aetiological factors (risk factors) in the pathogenesis of disease.
iii. To provide the data essential to the planning, implementation and evaluation of services for the prevention, control and treatment of disease and to the setting up of priorities among these services.

APPROACHES TO EPIDEMIOLOGY

One approach is to ask questions like what? Where? When? Who? And Why ?.

Second approach is to make comparison and judge which is better?

DISEASE TRANSMISSION

Dynamics of disease transmission is represented in Figure 17.1:

Some of the terms that are to be known by their meaning are:

Reservoir: "Any person, animal, arthropod, plant, soil or substance in which disease agent live and multiply."

Case: "A person in the population or study group identified as having a particular disease, condition or disorder which is under investigation."

Carrier: "An infected person or animal that harbours a specific infectious agent in the absence

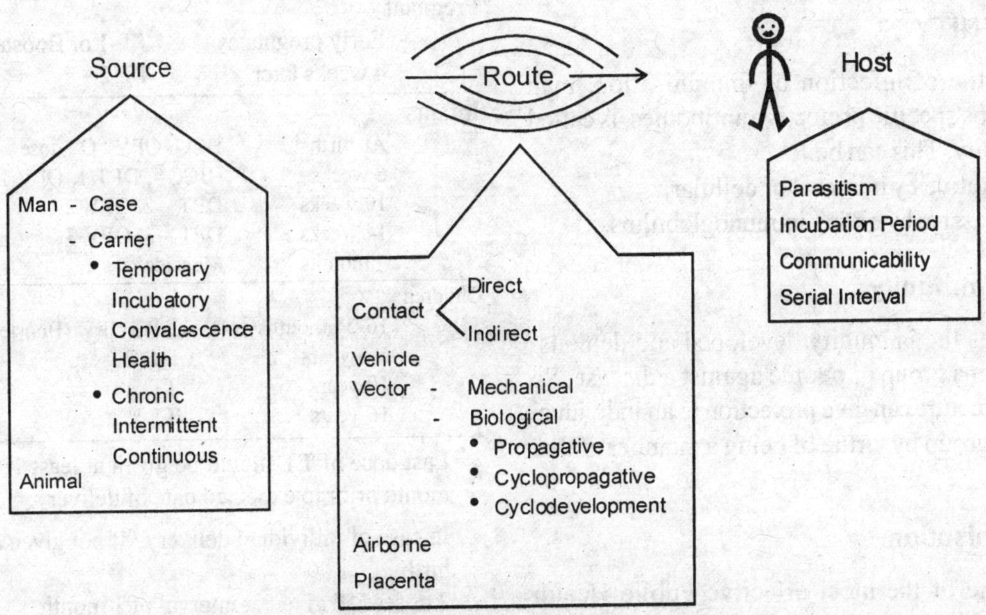

Fig. 17.1: Dynamics of disease transmission

of clinical manifestation and which serve as a potential source of infection to others.

Chronic Carrier: "Person who excretes disease agent for indefinite period". Chronic carrier state is known with Typhoid, Malaria, gonorrhoea and hepatitis.

Droplet Infection: When droplets of saliva and nasopharyngeal secretions are sprayed to the air, (it is forceful in cough, sneeze) droplet infection occurs. Respiratory infection and tuberculosis are typical droplet infections. If droplet is tiny 1-10 microns it is called droplet nuclei.

Incubation Period: "Time interval between invasion by disease agent to disease manifestation by signs symptoms". In non communicable disease it is called Latent period. If development occurs outside man (e.g., Malaria parasite in mosquito) it is called extrinsic incubation period.

Secondary Attack Rate (SAR): "The number of exposed persons developing the disease within the range of the incubation period following exposure to the primary case."

IMMUNITY

By virtue of infection or immunisation, man develops specific protective antibodies, is called immunity. This can be:

i. Active by humoral or cellular.
ii. Passive by giving immunoglobulins.

Herd Immunity

It means the immunity developed and demonstrated in a group of people against a disease. So herd structure can give protection to an individual in that group by virtue of being a member of that group.

Immunisation

It is one of the most effective Public Health Interventions to reduce childhood mortality and morbidity due to Vaccine Preventable Disease (VPD). It is very much cost effective. Nursing care lies in effective implementation and supervision of activities of the programme. Knowledge and skills in line with recent advances is required to strengthen nursing care in the field.

Following the successful global eradication of smallpox in 1979, vaccine use became an important tool for disease eradication. The programme named EPI (Expended Programme of Immunisation) was launched to control VPD's (Vaccine Preventable Disease). In the beginning DPT, OPV and BCG were covered. Later in 1985 it was renamed UIP (Universal Immunisation Programme). Measles vaccine was introduced in a phased manner. In 1990 India was covered with UIP to cover all pregnant and all new born with primary immunisation.

In 1992, UIP became part of CSSM (Child Survival and Safe Motherhood programme). In 1997 it became component of RCH (Reproductive and child health programme).

National Immunisation Schedule:

Pregnant		
	Early pregnancy	TT-1 or Booster
	4 weeks later	TT-2 ✲
Infants		
	At birth@	BCG+OPV "O" dose
	6 weeks	•BCG@, DPT 1, OPV 1
	10 weeks	DPT – 2, OPV 2
	14 weeks	DPT – 3, OPV 3
	9 months	Measles
Children		
	16-24 months	DPT OPV (Booster)
	5-6 years	DT m
	10 years	TT m
	16 years	TT m

✲ Last dose of TT should be given at least 1 month prior to expected date of delivery

@ In case of Individual delivery / if not given at birth

m 2 doses DT given at interval of 1 month

• If there is no past history of immunisation

Table 17.1: Syringe and needle specifications

Vaccine	*Syringe*	*Needle*
B.C.G.	1 ml syringe (BCG syringe)	26 gauge
Other vaccine	2 ml syringe	23 gauge
For reconstitution	5 ml syringe	20 gauge

Table 17.1 and Figure 17.2 give an idea of specifications and injection safety management. Figure 17.3 gives idea of injection site and angle of needle.

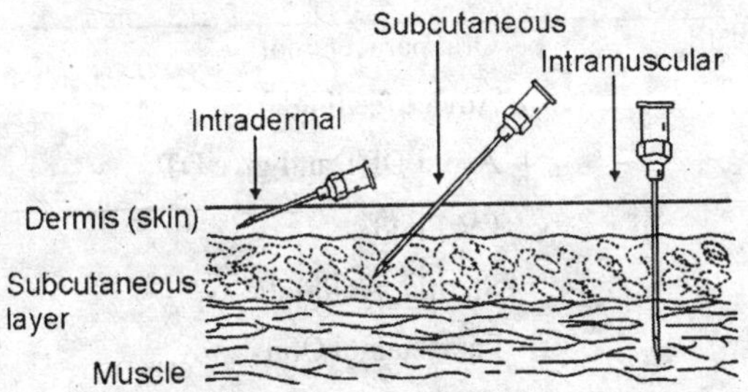

Note: The approximate angle of the needle to the injection site is:
Intradermal injection: 15° (BCG)
Subcutaneous: 45° (Measles)
Intramuscular: 90° (DPT, DT,TT, Hepatitis B)

Fig. 17.3: Injection site and angle

Adverse event which require caution:

Table 17.2: Adverse events requiring caution

B.C.G.	Osteitis, Dissemination of infection, lymphadenitis
D.P.T.	Prolonged convulsion, encephalitis, infantile spasm
Measles	Encephalitis, Fever, Transient rash, SSPE (Subacute sclerosing panencephalitis)
O.P.V.	Paralytic polio

If and when a previously healthy child gets severe adverse event following immunisation, the parents or community consider that the vaccine is the cause. Therefore, health personnel should immediately respond to public complaints. Immediate response by health personnel will allay public fear and maintain credibility, Further it prevents spread of rumour as well as adverse publicity by the media. It is the adverse, which causes major set back in the implementation of National Immunisation Programme.

Nursing care and nursing management of reactions due to immunisation are tabulated as under:

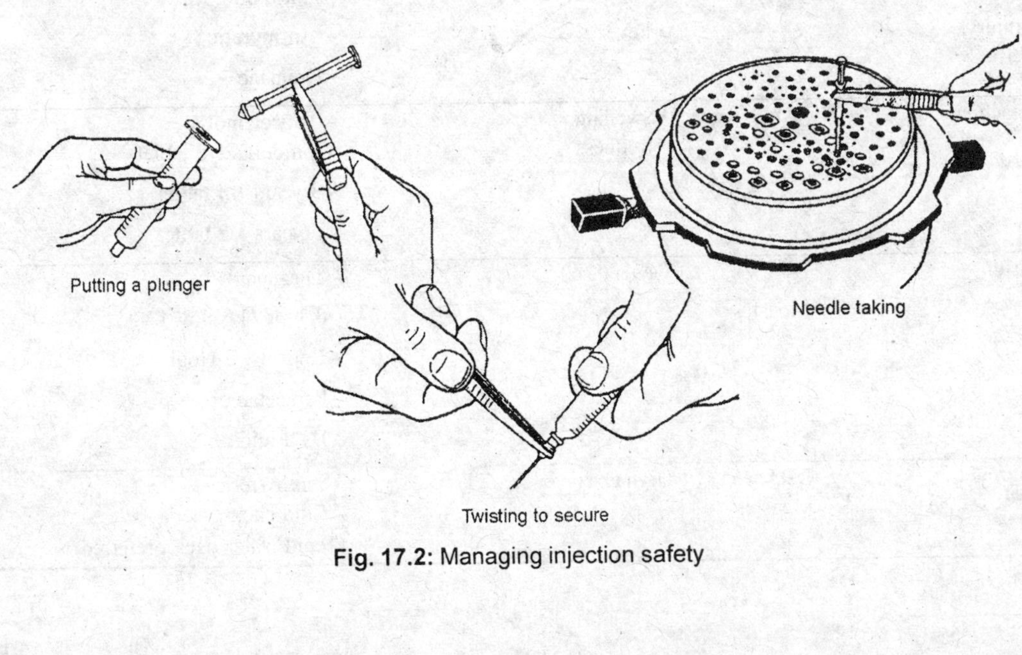

Fig. 17.2: Managing injection safety

Event	*Vaccine*	*Symptom*	*Nursing care and Nursing management*
Anaphylaxis	Any	• Acute decompensation of CVS • Hypovolemic shock • Altered sensorial • Larynx spasm/Oedema • Acute respiratory distress	– 1:10,000 adrenaline 0.01 ml per kg.(I.M.) – C.P.R. – I.V. Volume expanders – Oxygen – I.V. hydrocortisone
Hypotension	DPT	• Acute paleness • Loss of consciousness	– I.V. Fluid – Dexamethosone – Oxygen
Incessant cry	DPT	• Excessive inconsolable Cry	– Oral paracetamol – Advice feeding – Avoid DPT and give DT
Toxic shock Syndrome (Contamination!)	Measles (Staph aureus!)	• Mounting fever • Vomiting • Diarrhoea • Septic shock	– I.V. Fluid – Steroid, Antibiotic – Paracetamol Oral – Supportive Therapy
Lymphadenitis	BCG	• Firm axillary nodes • Soft nodes • Sinus, ulcer	– No treatment – Aspiration – INH 5 mg / kg once a day For 3 months
Abscess any Nerve injury	Any	• Abscess • Fever	– Antibiotic – Antipyretic – Drainage
Local reaction	Any	• Swelling • Redness	– Paracetamol < 3 months 1/8 tablet < 3 years 1/4 tablet < 5 years 1/2 tablet
Convulsion	DPT Measles	Generalised	– Diazepam 0.3 mg / kg slow I.V. – Repeat 1/2 Hour – Paracetamol – I.V. Fluids
Hyperpyrexia	DPT Measles	High fever	– Antipyretic – Cold pack (Tepid water pack preferred)

Other immunizing agents: They can be grouped as under:

Vaccine			
	Live attenuated	Bacterial	Typhoid, plague
		Viral	Yellow fever, rubella Mumps, Influenza
		Rickettsial	Epidemic Typhus
	Inactivated (killed)	Bacterial	Typhoid, cholera Pertussis (single), plague
		Viral	Rabies, Salk vaccine Hepatitis B, JE, KFD
Toxoid		Bacterial	Diphtheria, Tetanus

Immunoglobulin	
Human (normal)	Tetanus, Rabies, Measles, Hepatitis A, Mumps
Human (Specific)	Diptheria, Hepatitis B, Varicella
Non human (Bact)	Diptheria, Tetanus, Gas gangrene, Botulism
Non human (Viral)	Rabies

Combined Vaccines:

If more than one kind of agents is included in the vaccine it is called combined vaccine.

E.g.
- DPT
- DT
- DP
- DPT + Typhoid
- MMR
- DPTP (DPT + OPV)

It is different from poly-valent where 2 or more strains of same species are prepared.

Common immunoglobulins that are used are as under:

Rabies (RIG) (Rabies Immunoglobulin)	20 I u/kg body weight
Tetanus (TIG) (Tetanus Immunoglobulin)	4000-6000 units for treatment, 250 units for prophylaxis
Rh isoimmunisation (RhIG) (Rhesus factor immunoglobulin)	200 – 300 micrograms (1 vial)
Severe Measles (IG) (Human Immunoglobulin)	0.25 ml / kg body weight
Hepatitis B (HBIG) (Hepa B Immunoglobulin)	0.05 ml / kg body weight

Hazards due to immunisation are:

1. *Local reaction:* Pain, Swelling, Redness, Tenderness, Nodule, abscess.
2. *General reaction:* Fever, Headache, Malaise
3. Faulty technique to cause infection.
4. Neuritic manifestations.
5. Some latent infection becomes dominant.
6. Foetal damage in some cases.

The Cold Chain:

It is a system of storage and transport of vaccines at low temperature from the site of manufacture to the site of vaccination. Polio and Measles are stored in Freezer. Others (DPT, DT, BCG and Diluent) are stored in cold part of fridge. Ice line refrigerator (ILR) and Deep Freezers (DF) are used at higher level for long duration storage. Vaccine carriers and day carriers are used to carry small dose for short length of time.

CONTROL AND PREVENTION OF DISEASE

See Figure 17.4.

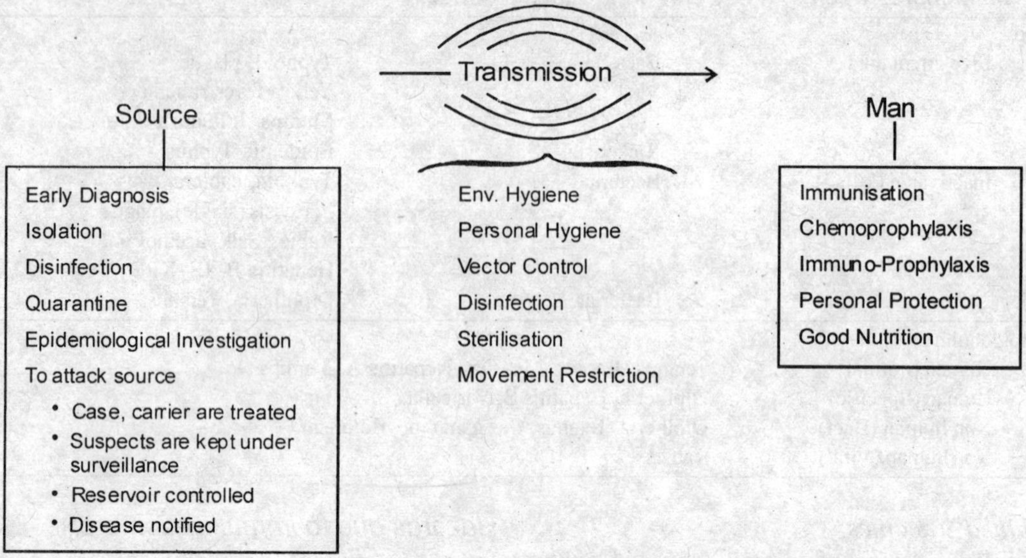

Fig. 17.4: Measures to be taken in the control and prevention of disease

EMPORIATRICS

This is described as a science of health of travelers. They are exposed to malaria, giardiasis, dengue, influenza, SARS, STD, HIV/AIDS, Amoebiasis, Typhoid, Hepatitis. Diagnosis and detecting the source help in interventions. Personal protection, health awareness, required immunisation help in preventing diseases of travelers.

Medical kit suggested for travelers contains disinfectant, dressings, sun cream, mosquito repellent, ORS and basic necessities.

W.H.O. provides guidelines through booklet "International Travel and Health, Vaccination requests and Health advice".

EPIDEMIC INVESTIGATION

When an epidemic occurs, which is beyond our imagination, procedure followed to examine, observe and analyse the disease occurrence is called "epidemic investigation". Following actions are taken in public health Activities:

- Diagnosis is confirmed.
- Innumerable cases occurring are confirmed.
- Geographic area is mapped.
- Contact search of cases done.
- Data is analyzed for time, place and people involved.
- A cause is suspected (Hypothesis).
- It is tested.
- After report preparation, measures to check spread is continued.

DISINFECTION

A method of killing pathogens is called disinfection:

Table 17.3: Difference between disinfection and antiseptic

Disinfection	*Antiseptic*
Kills outright	Prevent growth
Immediate action	Mild action
Short duration	Long duration
Can be antiseptic in low dilution	
Bactericidal	Bacteristatic

Detergents: Which lower surface tension and has cleansing property like soap, cetrimide.

Deodorant: That controls bad odours.

Disinfestant: That kills vermin (lice, bugs)

Common types of disinfection in nursing care are:

Concurrent disinfection: In the illness course; for sputum, vomitus, stool, urine, linen, hand, cloth, apron, and gown.

Terminal disinfection: At discharge or at death.

Prophylactic disinfection: Instruments at hospital, O.T. material, hand scrubbing, etc.

They are classified as under:

I. 1. Physical
   2. Chemical
   3. Natural

II. 1. Solid
   2. Liquid
   3. Gas

Hospital disinfection procedure:

Faeces, Urine	– 2 hours contact Phenol 10% Formalin 10% Bleaching powder 8% Cresol 5%
Sputum	– Burning Autoclave (20 min 20 Lb) Cresol 5%
Room	– Soap water wash Cresol 2.5% Phenol 5.0% Formalin 10% Formalin + $KMnO_4$ in water (200 G. / ½ Litre)
Linen	– Boiling Steam Cresol 2.5%
Dead body covered sheet	– Formalin 10% Phenol 5%
Instruments	– Boiling
Glove + Dressing	– Autoclave
Rubber, plastic catheter	– Boiling
Gum elastic catheter	– Formalin vapour
Cystoscope face mask	– Pasteurisation
Suture (Catgut)	– Lygol's iodine
Other suture	– Autoclave
Polythene tubing	– Gamma radiation
Urinals	– Hypochlorite solution
Bedpan	– Lysol
Blanket	– Hot formalin vapour

Operation theatre disinfections

i. Soap water clean, aeration, sunlight
ii. Wash with chlorinated lime (25 PPM)
iii. Wash with 1% Formaldehyde solution
iv. Wash with 2.5% cresol
v. 500ml formalin in 1 litre per 30 cub.mtr. as fumigation
vi. 200G. $KMnO_4$ in 500 ml formalin in 1 litre water for 30 cub.mtr.

EPIDEMIOLOGY– MEASUREMENT

Standardised measurement is necessary for epidemiological study, observation and analysis. When a case of stroke is admitted, the management of case does not require immediate epidemiological measurement for clinical management. But Epidemiological management needs more measurement for a community management of stroke.

Common measurement like:

i. *Rate:* Birth rate, IMR etc.
ii. *Ratio:* Sex ratio, Nurse population ration etc.
iii. *Proportion:* 22% scabies, 6% tuberculosis etc., are used in epidemiological measurements.
iv. *Mortality:* To form a uniform basis, international death certificate is proposed. Its usual format is as follows:

Cause of Death
Direct cause (a) ________________
Antecedent cause (b) ______(c)______
Significant condition________ _______

Mortality measurements are:
- Crude death rate
- Specific death rate (to sex, age, disease)
- C.F.R.
- Proportion mortality rate.
- Survival rate
- Standardised death rates

Morbidity measurements are:
- Incidence
  (new cases in defined population in a given time)
- Prevalence
  [All current cases (Old + New)].

EPIDEMIOLOGY– METHODS

i. *Descriptive:* They are first phase of any investigation. Procedures followed are depicted as under:
   a. Population to be studied is defined.
   b. Disease to be studied is defined.
   c. Time, place and personal factors are collected.
   d. Disease is measured.
   e. Compared with other similar studies.
   f. Cause of disease/condition is arrived.

   Descriptive studies have given us common epidemics of public health problems in the country. They are:

Common Source Epidemic ....Food poisoning (it is also called point source epidemic)

Common Source continuous epidemic ..... Outbreak of Pneumonia

Propagated epidemic .... Hepatitis A, Poliomyelitis

Cyclic Tread .... Measles, Rubella

Secular Trend .... Coronary Heart Disease Lung Cancer

ii. Analytic include case – control and Cohort They are highlighted under nursing research (Chapter 5).

In analytical study individuals are studies in the said population.

Case control is a retrospective studies through studying cases and controls, the exposure, analysis, interpretation of results.

$$\text{Relative risk} = \frac{\text{Incidence among exposed}}{\text{Incidence among non- exposed}}$$

$$\text{Attributable risk} = \frac{\text{Incidence rate among exposed — Incidence rate among non-exposed}}{\text{Incidence rate among exposed}} \times 100$$

$$\text{Odds ratio} = \frac{ad}{bc} = \text{A measure of strength of association between risk factor and outcome.}$$

Odds ratio is also called Cross Product Ratio.

Cohort study is an observational study for additional evidence. This can be prospective or Retrospective or combined. Cohort deals with subjects selection, data on exposure, study of comparison, follow up and analysis.

iii. *Experimental:* Randomised and Nonrandomised Trials and study designs and association.

They are highlighted under nursing research (Chapter 5).

EPIDEMIOLOGY – USES

There are wide varieties of uses which are applied in day to day patient care and public health activities. They are enumerated as under:

- Establish cause of health and disease.
- Help in community diagnosis.
- Gives clinical picture of disease.
- Provides the list of determinants and distribution of disease.
- Help General Practice.
- Help in the investigation of an epidemic
- It is a tool for mass survey.
- It establishes need and methods of control and prevention of disease.
- Chances of risk is measured.
- Syndromes are described by the knowledge of epidemiology.
- Temporal variation (seasonal) of a disease is established for health care management.
- Helps in establishment of a model of nursing care for any given disease.
- It gives an idea for promoting, protecting and rehabilitating for a given condition/disease/syndrome.

FURTHER REFERENCES

1. Last John M. – A Dictionary of Epidemiology (IEA).
2. Lilienfeld – Foundation of Epidemiology (Oxford).
3. RCH – Immunisation Trg. Modules I to VIII by GOI (2001).
4. Prabhakara G.N. – Short Text Book of Preventive and Social Medicine (JP).
5. Prabhakara G.N. – Policies and Programmes of Health in India 2004 (JP).

18

Communicable Diseases

IMPORTANCE

Council for international organisations of medical science under WHO has given a description for communicable disease as "an illness due to a specific infectious agent or its toxic products capable of being directly or indirectly transmitted from man to man, animal to man, animal to animal, or from the environment through air, dust, soil, water, food etc.; to man or animal".

Knowledge of communicable diseases helps nursing professionals in their professional care in nursing management of diseases. Nursing health administrators have to take note of information on communicable diseases both for nursing education and practical nursing care in hospital, health centre, home visiting, special health and nursing care services.

Because of the importance of period of communicability, secondary attack rate, selective isolation of infectious patient, personal protection of nursing profession and population movement within the country and outside the country, the descriptive study of these geographic pathologies are of utmost importance. As per standard regulations of administrative control of communicable diseases, uniformity of control measures takes into account the following:

i. *Preventive measures:* Applicable generally to individuals and groups when the particular disease may occur in sporadic endemic or epidemic form and whether or not the disease is an active threat at the moment.
ii. *Patient, contact and environment control:* These are designed to prevent infectious matter present in the persons and environment of infected individual from being conveyed to other persons, animals or arthropods in a way to spread the disease and to keep contacts under surveillance during the assumed period of incubation period of the disease, and, carriers under control until they are found to be free of the infectious agent of the disease. Specific treatment has to be included as a means of limiting the communicability.
iii. *Epidemic measures:* They are emergency measures which are designed to limit the spread of a communicable disease which has occurred in a community (beyond our expectation) or a nation.
iv. *International measures:* International sanitary regulations and conventions have recommended control of international travellers, immigrants, goods, animals,

animal products. These measures will protect population of one country against known risk of infection from another country.

v. *Reporting of communicable diseases*: Local Health Authorities after getting information will pass on to district, state and national level authorities. Finally, for certain prescribed diseases, report is made by National health authorities to WHO in Geneva. These come under 5 categories in accordance with desirability and practical benefits. They are:

Class 1: Case report universally required by International Sanitary Regulations.

Class 2: Case report regularly required whenever the disease occurs.

Class 3: Selectively reportable in recognised epidemic areas.

Class 4: Obligatory report of epidemics where no case report required.

Class 5: Official report not ordinarily justifiable.

MAJOR COMMUNICABLE DISEASES OF PUBLIC HEALTH IMPORTANCE

I. Diseases of international and national importance:
   1. SARS
   2. Anthrax
   3. Dengue
   4. AIDS
   5. Influenza

II. Vaccine preventable disease:
   6. Diphtheria
   7. Whooping cough
   8. Tetanus
   9. Poliomyelitis
   10. Tuberculosis
   11. Measles

III. Diseases under eradication process:
   9A. Poliomyelitis
   12. Leprosy
   13. Yaws
   14. Guinea worm
   15. Malaria

IV. Diseases not present but to be noted:
   16. Yellow fever
   17. Smallpox

V. Diseases under control measures:
   10A. Tuberculosis
   18. Filaria
   19. STD
   20. Kalaazar
   21. Cholera
   22. Diarrhoea
   23. Typhoid
   24. Meningococcal meningitis
   25. Food poisoning
   26. Plague
   27. ARI
   28. Chickenpox
   29. German measles
   30. Mumps
   31. Hepatitis
   32. Rabies
   33. Relapsing fever

VI. Protozoal infection:
   34. Amoebiasis
   35. Giardiasis

VII. Helminthic infection:
   36. Round worm
   37. Hook worm

VIII. Ectoparasitic infestation:
   38. Insect bite
   39. Jigger flea bite
   40. Leech bite
   41. Myiasis
   42. Scabies.

DISEASES OF INTERNATIONAL AND NATIONAL IMPORTANCE

SARS (Severe Acute Respiratory Syndrome)

SARS is a droplet infection by new corona virus

which is highly contagious and with high secondary attack rate and high case fatality rate. In early part of 2003, China, Hong Kong and Vietnam reported cases. Later the epidemic of SARS was reported from more than 20 countries. By Aug 2003, 8422 case and 916 deaths were reported around the world. This included the death of Dr. Carlo Urbani, a WHO expert who discovered and worked on SARS virus.

Ohio State University pointed out the relationship of SARS with cattle car-syndrome (shipping fever) where cough, pneumonia, drip mucous from eye and nose among cattle are seen.

It is known as "*shaheed haad Tanaffusi Alaiymia*" in *unani*. Herbal fumigation with *neem, tulsi, loban*, camphor and sandal is advocated.

In India suspected cases are reported from *Manipal, Kerala, Pune and Goa.* NICD has observed 10 out of 12 are negative and that "all flu is not SARS."

Hong Kong study's observation has reported cockroaches spread SARS infection.

WHO has recommended Infra-red "Fever sensitizing system" for the diagnosis of SARS under "SARS surveillance".

ICMR has stated that SARS is not a public health problem in India, since no single case fits to WHO criteria and as against this WHO declared India "SARS Free". India has only milder version of SARS since all cases are X-ray clear. National level screening committee is formed and Government of India has recommended "Watchdog Panel" in all the states. WHO case definition:

Suspect Case:

- High fever above 38° C.
- Cough or breathing difficulty.
- Close contact with a suspect or probable case of SARS.
- History of travel to an affected area.

Probable Case:

- A suspect case with X-ray finding
- Consistent Pneumonia (Clinical and Radiological findings).
- Respiratory Distress Syndrome (Evidence of infiltrates).
- A suspect case with pathological findings of RDS.

Global Picture:

Total of 8402 cases were reported with 772 deaths by June 2003 (which include atypical pneumonia).

Clinical Features:

High fever above 38°C.

Dry cough.

Shortness of breath or breathing difficulties

Changes in chest X-ray indicating pneumonia changes.

Associated symptoms like headache, muscular stiffness.

Loss of appetite, malaise, confusion, rash and diarrhoea.

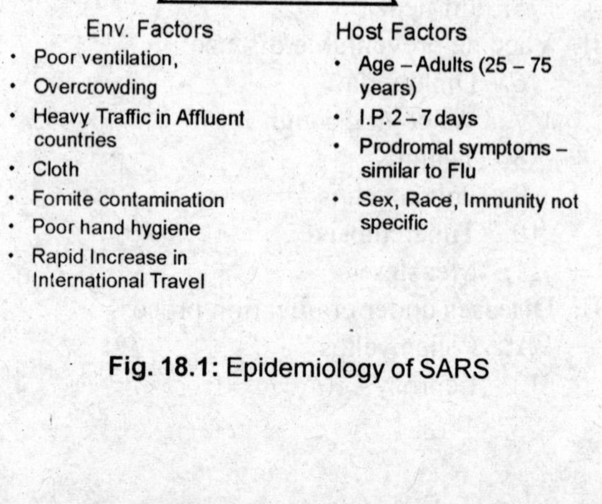

Fig. 18.1: Epidemiology of SARS

Transmission:

SARS can be transmitted in any season; overcrowding precipitates the spread. Epidemic outbreak of SARS is influenced by population density and population movement. It is transmitted from person to person by droplet infection. Contact with aerosolized (exhaled) droplets and bodily secretions from infected persons appear to be important. Hospital workers, Home contacts and nursing care personnel are high risk group. Hence for nursing care of SARS patient they are admitted in isolation hospitals. Robot to attend to SARS patient has been developed and is being tried.

Complications:

Severe pneumonia
Respiratory failure
C.F.R.: 3 percent.

Case Management by Nursing Care

Patient is kept in isolation. Respiratory and mucosal barrier nursing is recommended. Suspected cases are home isolated. Health care workers and nursing care workers wear efficient filter mask, goggle, apron, head cover and gloves.

Types suggested for mask are:

A71 Mask (Rs 80.00) to paramedical staff.

N95 Mask (Rs 230.00) to attending doctor and nurse.

NBC Mask (Rs 2000.00) to attending doctor and nurse in isolation hospital.

Treatment Protocol:

Stage 1: I.V. Cefotaxime / I.V. Levo-floxacin
Stage 2: Desaturation
Stage 3: Ribavirin+oral prednisolone
Or Hydrocortisone
Oxygen saturation in I.C.U.

Blood monitoring for leucopenia and thrombocytopenia.

Dose:

Oral Ribavirin 3.6 G / Day
Oral Prednisolone 1 mg / kg / day
I.V. Ribavirin 1.2 G per day
I.V. Hydrocortisone 100 mg q6h

Stage 4: Pulse steroid initiated
Serum therapy
Plasma exchange
Oxygen saturation in I.C.U.

Contact Management:

Contacts are categorized under (a) With definite contact history, (b) No definite contact history. WHO protocol is followed in contact management.

Hospital Guidelines for SARS control:

- Rapid diversion of suspected, in OPD and N95 mask to such patients.
- Staff involved in case management to wear N95 mask.
- Wash hands before each patient examination.
- In-patient isolated ward, should have independent air supply, exhaust system and bath room facility.
- Appropriate disposable equipment is used.
- Visitors are given PPE (Personal protective equipment).
- Restriction to non essential staff to SARS ward is followed.
- Alcohol based skin disinfectants are used.
- Special care is given in interventions like nebuliser, chest physiotherapy, bronchoscopy and gastroscopy.

International Action for containment:

i. Contain and control the outbreak.
ii. Identify the agent.
iii. Formulate treatment regimen.
iv. Ensure supply of drugs and health care workers, nursing care workers to epidemic area.
v. Arrange information supply to health officials and to the community.

SARS Control Initiative Programme

a. Strategy
   Administrative – I.E.C., policy and procedure enforcement
   Engineering – Good ventilation
   Protection – Mask and PPE
   Environmental – Disinfection
b. Prevention
   i. Early diagnosis: By clinical and laboratory tests.
   ii. Containment : Selective isolation, Home isolation, Segregation of suspects and limiting patient contact.
   iii. Personal protection: Mask, Goggle, Gown, Head cover, Shoe cover, Barrier nursing techniques and use of disposable equipment.
   iv. Handling of contaminated material
       Linen – Detergents, bleaching
       Waste – Hospital grade disinfectants (1:100 $CaOCl_2$)
   v. Hand hygiene: Soap wash, alcohol based hand rubs
   vi. Safe disposal of biohazard waste.

Anthrax

For centuries anthrax is know as diseases of livestock. It is caused by *Bacillus anthracis*. Historically we know that grazing lands remaining infective and elders advising to bury infected carcasses deeply to avoid soil contamination.

W.H.O. Case Definition:

Suspect: A case that is compatible with the clinical description and has an epidemiological link to confirmed or suspected animal cases or contaminated animal products.

Probable: A suspected case that has a positive reaction to allergic skin test (in non vaccinated).

Confirmed: A suspected case that is confirmed by laboratory procedure like:

a. Isolation of *B.anthracis* from specimen of blood, lesion, discharges.
b. Direct examination of bacteria in smear
c. Positive ELISA, western blot, toxin detection, chromatographic assay and F.A.T.

Incubation Period:

In animals 3–6 days
In man 1–7 days.

Mode of transmission:

a. Through cut or abrasion of skin.
b. Through contaminated meat.
c. Through inhalation of spores.

Clinical Manifestation:

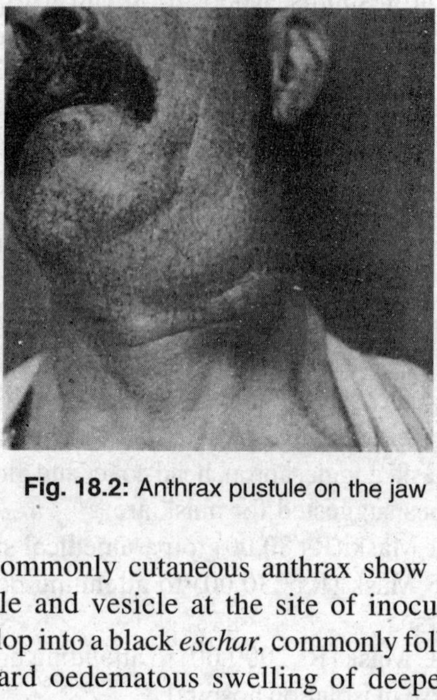

Fig. 18.2: Anthrax pustule on the jaw

Commonly cutaneous anthrax show initial papule and vesicle at the site of inoculation develop into a black *eschar,* commonly followed by hard oedematous swelling of deeper and adjacent tissues. Pain associated with the lesion is unusual and if present is related to oedema. If untreated infection extends progressively to regional lymph nodes and blood stream with overwhelming septicaemia and death.

Gastrointestinal anthrax, by uncooked meat, select the caecum as the seat of the infection which produce nausea, vomiting, anorexia, fever, followed by severe abdominal pain and bloody diarrhoea in 2-3 days. Toxaemia and death can occur rapidly thereafter.

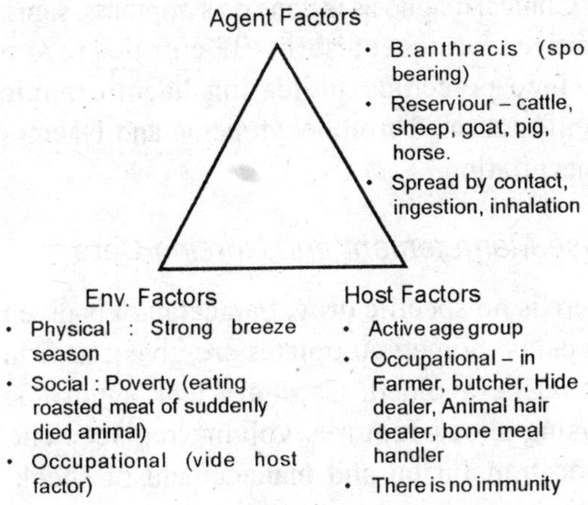

Fig. 18.3: Epidemiology of anthrax

Inhalation Anthrax is associated with Bioterrorism. If there is no rapid and aggressive treatment, patient dies in 90 percent of the cases. Fever, dyspnoea, cough, headache, septicaemia, widening of the mediastinum and pleural effusion in X-ray are common findings.

Case diagnosis – Culture from skin swabs
– Serological tests.

Case Management with Nursing Care

Skin lesion is readily curable with early diagnosis and prompt treatment. Treatment is started with ciprofloxacin 500mg daily until penicillin sensitivity result comes. Then change of treatment is 6 lakh unit penicillin-G Intravenously 6 hourly (or penicillin V 500 mg 6 hourly). Aggressive fluid resuscitation and addition of Aminoglycoside improve the condition. In pneumonia (of inhalation type) ventilatory assistance is needed.

Nursing staff and medical staff attending the case need prophylaxis with ciprofloxacin 500mg 12 hourly.

Preventive Measures

Animals suspected of anthrax are isolated and treated. Milk of infected animal should not be used. Animal died of Anthrax (carcasses) should be completely burned or buried deeply with quick lime. Animal inoculation with approved vaccine is done. Effluents and trade wastes of hair, wool, and hides are controlled. Health awareness on anthrax spread is created among occupational risk group.

Public Health Measure

Case reporting is obligatory to local health authorities. Isolation of cases till skin lesion is bacteriologically free is done. Concurrent and terminal disinfection are properly done. Pre processing disinfection of hair, wool, hides and bone meal is done.

International Measure

As per international measure, sterilisation of imported bone meal, imported hair and wool product disinfection before import are mandatory.

Dengue

First reported epidemics are recorded in Egypt and Indonesia nearly 230 years ago. Asia harbour cases as endemic countries. During II world war, increased travel of susceptible foreigners to endemic areas along with urbanization affected the emergence of newly emerged D.H.F. Increased transmission is seen with rainy season. Classical Dengue is rare among indigenous people who have herd immunity.

Now, clinical entitles are more and dengue fever is replaced by Dengue syndrome which constitutes.

- Undifferentiated dengue fever
- Actual Dengue fever
- D.H.F. without shock
- D.H.F. with shock.

Clinical Feature: 2 days of malaise and headache form prodromal symptoms. Acute stage is manifested by fever, backache arthralgia, headache, breakbone fever (generalised pain),

pain on eye movement, lacrimation, anorexia, nausea, vomiting, relative bradycardia, prostration, lymphadenopathy, depression and scleral injection. Fever is continuous or saddle back with break on 4th day, usually lasts for 10 days. On 3-5 days of illness scarlet morbilliform spreading centrifugally sparing palm and sole.

There are 4 sero types that cause Dengue that are transmitted by *Aedes aegypti* mosquito. Common breeding places of vector are discarded tin, broken bottle, fire bucket, flower pot, earthen pot, tree hole, tyre, overhead tank, water cooler, flower vase, defreeze container of fridge.

3 billion are living in geographical risk zone. About 50 million cases are occurring every year and about 12000 deaths are occurring in a year.

In South East Asian Region about 30 million cases per year in which 2 lakh haemorrhagic type of Dengue are occurring. The Case Fatality Rate in SEARO has been 3.5%.

There was an outbreak of dengue epidemic at Delhi in 1996. Later outbreaks are recorded in Rajasthan, Tamilnadu, Karnataka and Gujarat. After Delhi Epidemic, Government of India has given certain guidelines to control and prevent dengue. All 4 serotypes are seen in India. 18 States/UTs have reported Dengue. During 2005 about 11928 cases are reported and about 156 cases death from Dengue are reported.

Clinical diagnosis is done on symptoms, signs, positive tourniquet test (by BP cuff tied to arm produce petechiae indicating haemorrhagic manifestation, Thrombocytopenia and Haemoconcentration.

Case Management and Nursing Care

There is no specific drug. Paracetamol is given for pains. Sometime opiates are given; aspirin should be avoided. Capillary leak syndrome causing shock requires volume replacement, blood transfusion and management of shock; corticosteroids are not useful.

Incubation period is usually 5-6 days. Patients are infective for mosquito from the day before on-set to 5th day of disease. The Mosquito becomes infective 10 days after blood meal and remains for life.

Control Measures

Mosquito control measures including elimination of breeding places; protection from bite is possible by using mosquito repellents and screening of houses.

Reporting is obligatory to local health authorities. Isolation of patient for 5-6 days from onset of disease, followed by residual insecticide

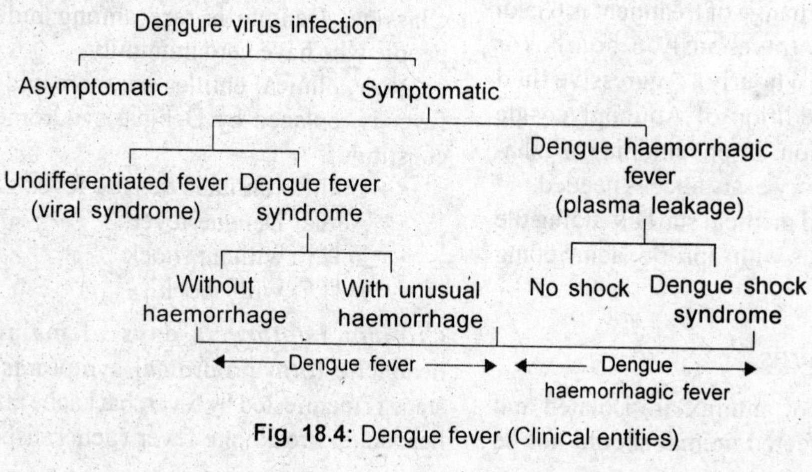

Fig. 18.4: Dengue fever (Clinical entities)

spray to patient's quarters is suggested measures to control spread of the infection.

Community survey, vectors density study and anti Aedes mosquito measures are suggested during epidemics.

Enforcement of provisions of International Agreements designed to prevent spread of the disease by persons and mosquito transfer by ships, airplane, and land transport from epidemic area to disease free area have been taken up.

AIDS (Acquired Immuno Deficiency Syndrome)

AIDS is caused by human Immuno deficiency Virus (HIV). It is a serious disorder of the body immune system in which the body normal defences against infection break down, leaving the body vulnerable to a host of life threatening infections and life threatening conditions including unusual malignancies.

World Picture:
95% of HIV/ AIDS patients are living in developing countries. Sub Saharan Africa appears to have stabilised with respect to new infections. Latin America and Caribbean countries harbour about 2 million cases. Eastern Europe and central Asia is relatively recent for HIV/AIDS.

Table 18.1: AIDS Epidemic – World

No. of people living with HIV/AIDS end of 2006	Total	39.5 million
	Adults	37.2 million
	Women	17.7 million
	Children <15 years	2.3 million
New infection HIV/AIDS In 2006	Total	4.3 million
	Adults	3.8 million
	Women	1.8 million
	Children <15 years	5.3 lakhs
AIDS Death in 2006	Total	2.5 million
	Adults	2.6 million
	Women	1.1 million
	Children < 15 years	3.8 lakhs

Indian Picture:
Since the detection of HIV in Tamil Nadu in 1986, there has been a steady increase in HIV/AIDS seeking treatment in hospitals. NACO has reported cases of 1,25,000 AIDS cases by Aug 2006. With estimated 5.2 million HIV infections, the Aids cases are likely to rise still higher.

Based on HIV prevalence states and union territories are grouped under 3 categories.

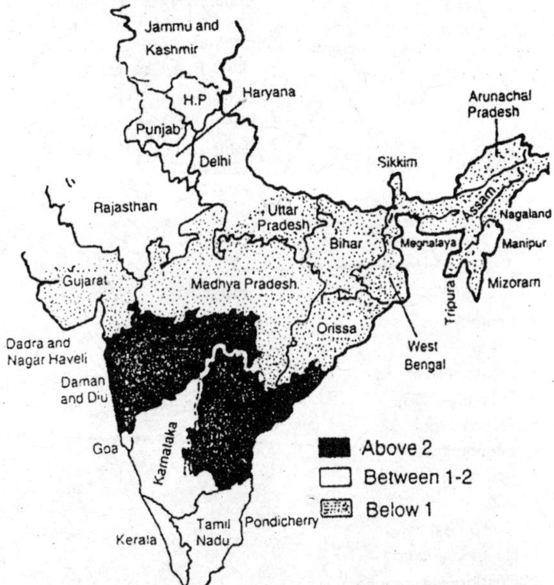

Fig 18.5: HIV prevalence in India among ANC cases

Table 18.2: 3 groups according to the prevalence

States	Group
Maharashtra, Tamilnadu, Karnataka, Andhra Pradesh, Manipur, Nagaland	High prevalence State – Group I
Gujarat, Goa, Pondicherry	Moderate prevalence State – Group II
Remaining States and Union Territories	Low prevalence State – Group III

Agent:

It is a virus (lentivirus) one of the subfamily of retroviruses. Its enzyme copies viral RNA to DNA which eventually integrates to host cell. Hence eradication of HIV/AIDS is not found possible. HIV-1 and HIV-2 are common types of infective agent.

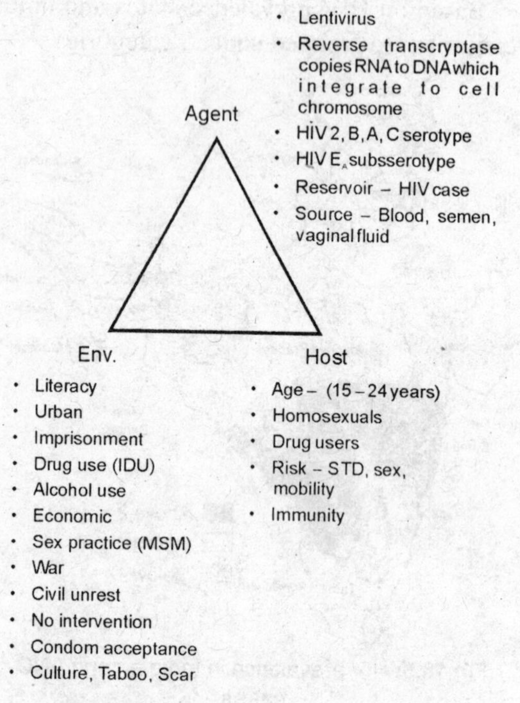

Fig. 18.6: Epidemiology of HIV/AIDS

Reservoir of infection is men suffering from disease. Source of infection are infected blood, semen and vaginal fluids. Infected breast milk may be source of infection from mother to child.

Saliva and Tears are not source of infection.

Following Figure (Fig. 18.8) and Table (Table of Source of infection) show a change in the trend of source of infection of HIV/AIDS (over a period of 4 years—2002 to 2006):

a. Sexual transmission has increased over a period of 4 years.
b. Remarkable reduction in Blood transmission.

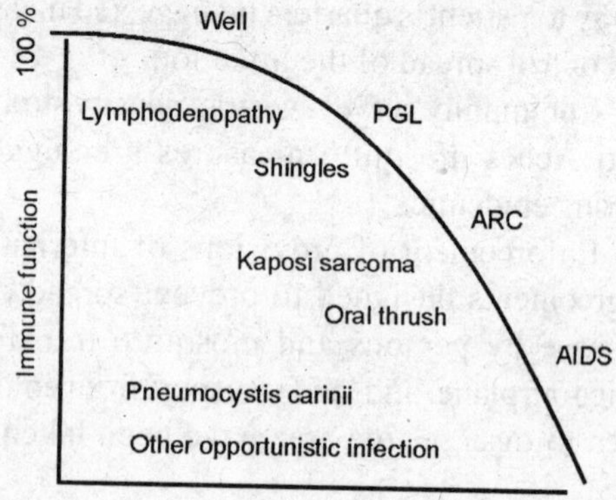

Fig.18.7: Immune function in the natural history of HIV/AIDS

c. Remarkable reduction in injecting drug users.
d. Perinatal transmission is raising.

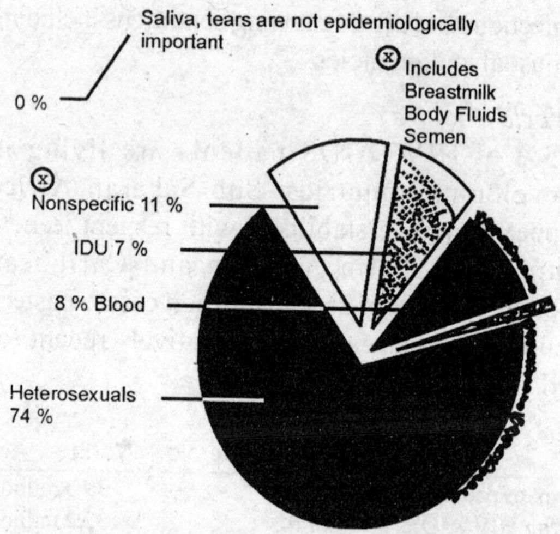

Fig. 18.8: Source of infection (2002)

Transfusion category	*No.*	*%*
Sexual	106669	85.34
Perinatal	4755	3.80
Blood, Blood Product	2563	2.05
IDU	2930	2.34
Not specified	8078	6.47
Total	124995	100.00

Source of infection as on (Aug 2006)

Host Factors:

Young people 20-30 years age in both sexes are found infected with HIV/AIDS. Certain group of people shows higher risk of infection. They are:

- Person suffering from RTI/STD
- Frequency of exposure of unprotected sex
- Mixing pattern of population
- Drug users
- Sex workers
- Profound lymphopenia.

Socioeconomic Factors:

Following socioeconomic factors influence the occurrence of HIV/AIDS:

i. Low literacy
ii. Urbanization
iii. Imprisonment
iv. High mobility
v. Migration and separation from family
vi. Drug use
vii. Alcohol use.

Mode of Transmission:

Both heterosexual and homosexual intercourses are major mode of transmission of HIV/AIDS; other modes of transmission are given in Table 18.3.

Table 18.3: Mode of transmission of HIV/AIDS

Sexual intercourse with infected person	85.7 %
Blood Transfusion by infected blood	2.2 %
Drug users by common syringe use	3.0 %
Perinatal	3.1 %
Non specific mode (Includes mother to child transmission)	6.0 %

Natural History of HIV/AIDS:

Stage 1: Infection with HIV results in rapid proliferation of the virus in blood and lymph nodes. The infected person may experience a sero-conversion illness, which usually resolves within weeks. The CD_4 cell count declines rapidly before virus is controlled by the immune system, whereupon the count returns to near normal.

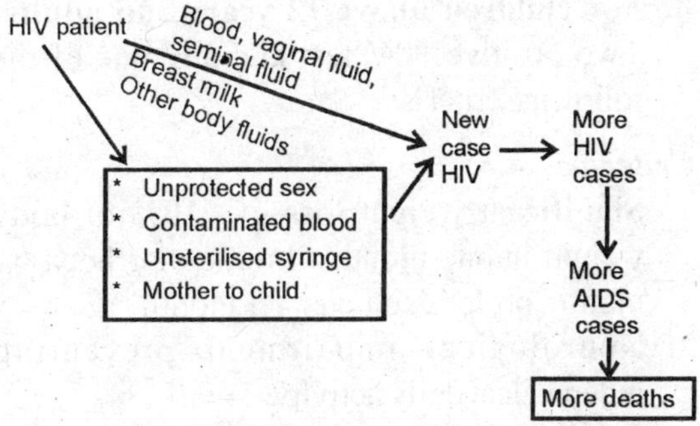

Fig. 18.9: HIV transmission cycle

Stage 2: During stage 2, the immune system has controlled the virus, which is largely restricted to lymphoid tissue. In this the damage inflicted by the virus is limited to the regenerative capacity of the immune system and people with HIV are usually without symptoms. CD_4 count will be above 500/ml in this stage.

Stage 3: In this stage viral replication is very high and CD_4 cell turnover is rapid. Subtle signs and symptoms indicating compromise of immune system begin to appear. CD_4 cell count will be 200-500/ml.

Stage 4: The virus which proliferate throughout the body, overcomes the immune system. Major opportunistic infections take an upper hand. CD_4 cell count will be <200/ml. This is the stage of advance immune deficiency.

Clinical Case Definition:

a. **For children below 12 years:** Two positive HIV test and presence of at least 2 major and 2 minor signs in the absence of known causes of immune suppression.

Major sign	*Minor sign*
1. Loss of weight without cause	1. Repeated pneumonia, otitis, pharyngitis
2. Chronic diarrhoea > 1 month	2. Lymphadenopathy (all)
3. Prolonged fever > 1 month	3. Oropharyngeal candidiasis
	4. Persistent cough >1 month
	5. Disseminated maculo-papular dermatitis

b. For children above 12 years and adults: Two positive HIV test and any one of the following criteria:

Criteria:

1. Significant weight loss of >10% of body weight in one month, chronic diarrhoea >1 month, prolonged fever > 1 month.
2. Neurological impairment preventing independent daily activity.
3. Candidiasis of oesophagus
4. Life threatening pneumonia
5. Kaposi sarcoma
6. Other conditions like cryptococcal meningitis, neuro toxoplasmosis, CMV retinitis, recurrent herpes zoster and disseminated molluscum.

Clinical Features:

Various systematic manifestations of HIV/AIDS patient include loss of weight of more than 10% of body weight, fever of more than 1 month duration, asthenia, diarrhoea and amenorrhoea in females.

As far as organ involvement is concerned, the manifestation is tabulated as under:

I. Cutaneous and Oral Manifestation:

a. Infections
   Herpes Zoster and simplex
   Fungal (Candidiasis)
   Cryptococcosis
   Histoplasmosis
   Molluscum contagiosum
   Folliculitis
   Polymyositis
   Hairy leukoplakia

b. Neoplastic
   Kaposi sarcoma
   Lymphoma
   Basal cell carcinoma

c. Others
   Pruritic popular dermatitis
   Seborrhoetic dermatitis
   Drug eruptions
   Vasculitis/Gingivitis

II. Gastro Intestinal Manifestations:

a. Persistent diarrhoea
   Cryptosporidiosis
   Isospora
   Shigella
   Salmonella
   E. histolytica
   Giardia, Microspora

b. Colitis
   Cytomegalovirus
   Kaposi Sarcoma

c. Dysphagia
   Oral and oesophageal candidiasis
   CMV Oesophagitis
   Oral hairy leukoplakia
   Gingivitis/Ulcer

d. Perianal discomfort
   Herpes viral proctitis
   Herpes viral ulceration

III. Respiratory Manifestations:

a. Persistent cough, dyspnoea, cyanosis, Tachypnoea, haemoptysis, pleural effusion by:
   M. Tuberculosis
   B. Pneumonia
   Streptococcus
   H. influenza
   Atypical mycobacteria
   Cytomegalo virus
   Pneumocystis carinii
   Legionella, candida
   Histoplasma
   Lymphoid interstitial pneumonitis
   Herpes simplex virus
   Kaposi Sarcoma

IV. Neurological Manifestations:

a. Headache, lethargy, dementia, ataxia, altered personality, convulsions, incontinence etc., due to:
   HIV encephalopathy
   Cryptococcal meningitis
   Lymphoma

Herpes virus
AIDS dementia complex

b. Meningism by:
Cryptococcal meningitis
Tubercular meningitis
Bacterial meningitis

c. Visual impairment by:
CMV retinitis
Toxoplasmosis
Kerato conjunctivitis
Microsporidia

d. Focal seizures, hemiplegia, peripheral neuropathy by:
Abscess due to Toxoplasma, Cryptococcus
HIV Vasculitis
Lymphoma

V. Haematological Manifestations
VI. Renal Manifestations
VII. Cardiac Manifestations
VIII. Endocrinal Manifestations
IX. Reproductive Manifestations.

Diagnosis:

i. Physical examination, weight, oral cavity, eyes, skin, lymphadenopathy and systemic examination
ii. Check for STD
iii. Tests
   - HIV 2 tests (western Blot is no longer required as a must in India)
   - CD_4 cell count
   - CD_4/CD_8 Ratio
   - TC, DC
   - Chest X-ray.

National Guidelines for HIV Testing:

1. Surveillance to monitor trend
2. Transfusion safety
3. Voluntary testing purpose
4. Research.

Legal and Ethical Consideration:

HIV testing has brought out both legal and ethical forefront. HIV/AIDS is more of a social problem rather than medical problem. People with HIV have a role to play if the social ills associated with HIV/AIDS are to be minimised. There have been allegations of human rights violation across the globe and HIV infected persons have been discriminated. There is also a need to reform laws which marginalize women and children who are the most vulnerable group in the HIV/AIDS epidemic.

Case Management and Nursing Care

Drug
1. Nucleoside analog: Zidovudine (AZT) (Retrovir) 500–600 mg orally daily in 3 divided doses.
2. Protease inhibitor Saquinavir (invirase) 600 mg orally 3 times daily.
3. Non nucleoside reverse transcriptase inhibitor Nevirapine (viramune) – 200 mg orally daily for 2 weeks, then 200 mg orally twice daily.

Counselling

It is face to face communication by which one can help the person to make decisions and act on them. It aims at preventing transmission of HIV and provides psychological support. Counselling is aimed at problem solving. It helps people to understand themselves better in terms of their own needs, strengths, limitations and the resources they can avail of. It brings about change through a supportive relationship aiming to make the client independent through interpersonal contact along with opportunity to ask questions and to meet frequently needed help greatly.

Nurse in her counselling, with the help of medical social worker, will listen, understands client's dignity, uses good communication skill and non-judgmental attitude. Pretest counselling is done before HIV test and post test counselling is done after HIV testing.

Blood Transfusion

Promotion of voluntary blood donation should get top priority.

AIDS Education: Health education on AIDS enables people to make life saving choices.

Health Care: Primary health care for HIV/ AIDS with an integration of R.C.H., F.W.P. and health education.

Nursing Management of Needle Stick Injury

Being risk group, nursing professionals have to deal with anticipated accidental exposures to HIV. Average risk is 1 in 300 (0.3%) and prevention is the main strategy to avoid occupational exposure to HIV.

Use of protective barrier

- Latex or vinyl gloves
- Heavy duty rubber glove at cleaning
- Gloves and apron at surgery
- Protective eye wear
- Safe handling of sharps.

If injury (after exposure)

- Wash injury with soap and water
- Splash to the nose, mouth, skin should be flushed with water
- Eyes are irrigated with clean water
- Don't put prinked finger into mouth
- Report to authorities
- Post exposure prophylaxis (PEP) may be recommended.

When source material are blood, bloody fluid or other potentially infectious material, determination of the Exposure code (EC) and determination of HIV status code (HIVSC) as EC_1, EC_2, EC_3, EC_4 and $HIVSC_1$, $HIVSC_2$ HIVSC unknown, will help in case management with recommended prophylaxis.

National AIDS Control Programme

This was launched in 1987. Main aim is to reduce the spread and strengthen India's capacity in terms of production and economics.

1992-95 AIDS control 100% was centrally sponsored scheme.

1996-2006 Phase II National AIDS Prevention Policy was launched as 100% centrally sponsored scheme in all States / UTs and 3 Mega cities.

In 2002 National AIDS prevention and control policy was brought out with the objectives of reducing impact of epidemic and to bring about a Zero transmission rate of AIDS by 2007.

The programme includes:

a. Blood safety programme
b. Policy on HIV testing
c. STD control programme
d. Condom promotion
e. HIV surveillance
f. HIV sentinel surveillance
g. IEC activities
h. Social mobilisation
i. Family health awareness campaign
j. Prevention of mother to child transmission.

International health is to be maintained from HIV epidemic and AIDS epidemic, which itself has become global problem and this needs research and future plan of action.

Tenth Five Year Plan Goals have been:

a. 80% coverage of high risk groups through targeted interventions.
b. 90% coverage of schools and colleges through education programme.
c. 80% awareness among the general population in rural areas.
d. Reducing transmission through blood to less than 1%.
e. Establishing at least one voluntary testing and counselling centre in every district.
f. Scaling up of prevention of mother to child transmission activities, up to the district level.
g. Achieving zero level increase of HIV/ AIDS prevalence by 2007.

HIV Surveillance:

ICMR blood screening was started in 1985 which gave first HIV case in 1986 in Chennai. Since then 62 sero-surveillance centres and 9 HIV Reference Centres are established in India. In 1993 Sentinel surveillance system was introduced. Here annual cross-section al survey of the risk group is done by unlinked anonymous serological testing procedure. Later Behavioural surveillance was initiated followed by Targeted interventions.

Anti-Retroviral treatment:

New initiative for priority categories like pregnant HIV women, children up to 15 years and full blown AIDS case ART is given in government hospital free of cost in high prevalence states.

Post exposure prophylaxis for health workers within 2 hours of exposure is given as per NACO guidelines.

AIDS Helpline:

For information and counseling a toll free helpline is set up by the government computerised voice response system is linked to help the community.

Influenza

Influenza is a specific acute illness caused by a group of myxoviruses-2. Common types are A and B. Type C is uncommon in epidemics of influenza. It has been pandemic, claiming high morbidity and mortality. Hence it is of International importance. Common strains are $A(H_1N_1)$, $A(H_3N_2)$ and B. Recently $A(H_5N_1)$ strain has been isolated.

Man is the reservoir and source of infection are discharges from mouth and nose of infected persons. It is transmitted through droplet infection and air borne.

Incubation period is 24-72 hours. The patient will be infectious from pre-clinical phase to 1 week after clinical onset.

Agent:

The virus is from orthomyxoviridae group. A, B, C are antigenically distinct and there is no cross immunity.

Influenza A is subjected to antigenic variation both major and minor. When there is sudden complete major change it is called a shift. When the antigenic change is gradual over a period of time it is called a drift. Man is the reservoir of infection; clinical or subclinical case is source of infection. Virus is present in the nasopharynx from 1 to 2 days before and 1 to 2 days after onset of symptoms.

Host:

Influenza affects all ages and both sexes. Human mobility helps in the spread of disease.

Environment:

It is common in winter and rainy seasons. Overcrowding enhances transmission. It is high in close population group like school, ship etc.

Clinical Feature:

Sudden onset of pyrexia associated with generalised aches and pains, anorexia, nausea and vomiting. Degree of ill health ranges from mild to rapidly fatal. Usually harsh unproductive cough is noticed among patients. Most patients do not develop complications and acute symptoms subside within 5 days but may be followed by post influenzal asthenia which can persist for several weeks. During epidemics the diagnosis is usually easy. Sporadic cases are to be diagnosed by viral isolation. Fluorescent antibody technique or sero-logical tests for specific antibodies are done for confirmatory purpose.

Complications:

Tracheitis, bronchitis, bronchiolitis and bronchopneumonia are manifested. Toxic cardiomyopathy may cause sudden death. Encephalitis and peripheral neuropathy are rare complications.

Case Management with Nursing Care

Bed rest is advocated until fever subsides. Paracetamol 0.5 to 1.0 gram 6 hourly can relieve headache and generalised pains. Amantadine and Rimantidine 100 mg BD for 3 days is found effective. Pholcodine 10 mg every 6 hours may be given to suppress cough. Specific treatment for pneumonia may be necessary.

Control Measures:

i. Good ventilation, avoiding overcrowding, encouraging patients to cover while sneezing or coughing.
ii. Vaccines
   - *Killed vaccine:* Chick embryo harvested formalin killed 0.5 ml subcutaneous single dose.
   - *Live attenuated:* Administered as nose drops
   - *Newer vaccines:*
     1. Split virus vaccine
     2. Neuraminidase specific vaccine
     3. Recombinant vaccine.
iii. Reporting to local health authorities are obligatory.

International Measures

- Prompt notification to WHO.
- Identification of virus type and reporting.
- Continued epidemiological studies and exchange of information.
- Continuing attempt to mobilise development and production facilities to permit rapid shipment and use of an appropriate vaccine when a new strain appears or when it threatens to become pandemic.

Influenza viruses that affect birds produce Avian Influenza. H5N1 like strain can adopt and can infect humans. This affected human in 1997 is in the record. Since 2003 the virus is producing pandemics.

VACCINE PREVENTABLE DISEASES

Diphtheria

It is an acute bacterial infection of Tonsil, Pharynx, larynx and Nasal mucous membrane caused by *C.diptheriae*. From Greek "Diphtherite" meaning skin or hide refers to the appearance of characteristic pharyngeal membrane. Local infection destroys tissue and distal infection by toxin affects vital organs. Death is always by airway obstruction, myocarditis or polyneuritis.

The known reservoir is man. It spreads from person to person. From case or carrier the disease spreads both by droplet infection and contact. Milk contamination can cause epidemics. Powerful exotoxin causes:

- False membrane
- Lymphadenopathy
- Toxaemia.

Case fatality rate is 10% which is reduced to 5% among treated cases.

World Problem: It is not a major public health problem because of effective preventive work. But reduced immunity in certain place is causing epidemics which would have been controlled by total coverage immunisation.

Indian Problem: There is total decline of cases in India. Still hospital data indicate on an overage 100 to 200 cases in a year are being treated. Suspected cases during 2005 were 10231.

Fig. 18.10 depicts the triad of epidemiology of diphtheria. In case of good disease control, we need a herd immunity of 70% in the child community. Common portal of entry is respiratory tract.

Incubation period – 2-6 days.

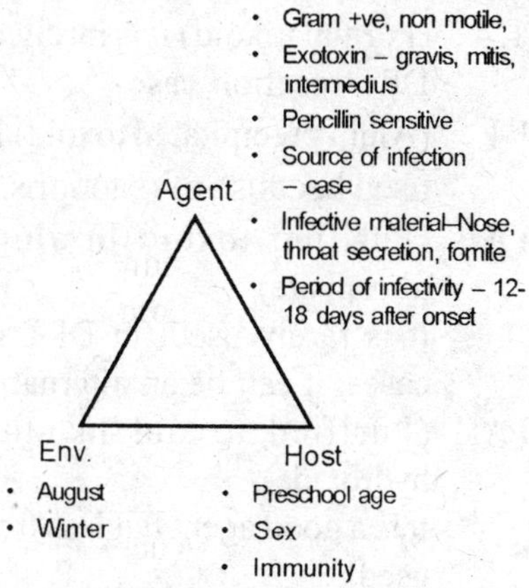

Fig. 18.10: Epidemiology of diphtheria

Clinical Feature:
It begins insidiously. Fever is seldom significant although tachycardia is marked. "Wash leather" elevated grayish green membrane on the tonsils is a diagnostic feature. The membrane has well defined edge, firm, adherent and surrounded by inflammatory zone. Bull neck and tender enlarged lymph node predominate.

In anterior nasal type blood stained nasal discharge is present.

In laryngeal type husky voice and high pitched cough is a signal of potential need for tracheostomy.

In untreated case circulatory failure occurs with in 10 days.

Complications:
- Laryngeal obstruction, paralysis
- Myocarditis
- Peripheral neuropathy.

Schick Test: It is done to find out susceptibility to infection and success of immunisation. 0.2 ml of Schick test toxin intradermally with control is tested.

Results:

-ve	*+ ve*	*Pseudo +ve*	*Combined*
Immune	10-50 mm Redflush in 24 hour maximum in 1 week Brown Desquamates "Susceptible"	Disappear in 4 days "Allergy"	Control is pseudo +ve Test is + ve "Susceptible"

Case Management with Nursing Care

Clinical diagnosis of diphtheria should be notified to local authorities. Swab is taken for confirmation and treatment is started at once. Regimen is:
- Antitoxin
- Antibiotic
- Isolation.

For mild case anti diphtheria serum (ADS) 4000-8000 units, moderately severe case 16,000-40,000 units and severely ill 100,000 units are given intra muscular route. Care is taken to see adrenaline is kept available for immediate type – reaction along (0.5 ml 1 in 1000 I.M.) with an antihistaminic.

Penicillin 1200 mg 6 hourly I.V or amoxicillin 500 mg 8 hourly should be administered for 2 weeks to eliminate bacteria. Erythromycin is a choice in penicillin sensitive cases. Patient is managed in strict isolation. Nursing management should adhere to strict nursing barrier. Patient is clear only when 3 swab 24 hour apart are culture negative.

Control of Diphtheria:
For case and carrier, early detection, isolation and treatment is suggested. For carriers Erythromycin is the most effective drug. Contacts are swab tested and depending on their immunity status primary or booster immunisation is

attempted. High level immunisation viz., above 90% among children by U.I.P. is attempted for community protection.

Vaccines:

Absorbed D.P.T. (Triple antigen) is available from Kasauli and Glaxo.

	Kasauli	*Glaxo*
Diphtheroid toxoid	30 Lf	25 Lf
Tetanus toxoid	10 Lf	5 Lf
B. Pertussis	32,000 million	20,000 million
Aluminum PO_4	3 mg	2.5 mg
Thiomersal	0.01%	0.01%

D.P.T. is stored at 4 – 8ºC. Immunisation is followed as per U.I.P. schedule (discussed under general epidemiology). Primary immunisation is started at 6 week after birth. Three doses with 1 month interval are optimal for effective immunisation. It is given deep I.M. Very mild reaction like fever may follow which is ignorable. No severe complications are seen in routine immunisation. But possibility of 1 in a million, convulsion, encephalitis, Reye's syndrome should be kept in mind.

There is no contraindication for DPT. Only acutely ill hospitalized child is excluded.

In case of children above 12 years, D.T. (paediatrics double antigen) is given 2 doses at 1 month interval and a booster at 12 month after second dose. For adults dT (adult double antigen) is used in the same manner.

Available vaccines are categorised as follows:

I Combined

- DPT (Diphtheria, pertussis, tetanus) for infants primary course
- DT Course (Diphtheria tetanus) (For children above 5 years)
- dT (Diphtheria, tetanus) For adult above 12 years

II Single

- F.T. (Formal toxoid) it is rarely used; in DPT reaction case
- APT (Alum precipitated toxoid) It is not used because of reactions.
- PTAP (Purified toxoid in aluminium phosphate) It is rarely used; in DPT reaction cases, it can be an alternative.
- PTAH (Purified toxoid in aluminum hydroxide) It is a good agent but less frequently used.
- TAF (Toxoid – antitoxin floccules) Alternate to DPT and DT; it can be used since no reaction is produced by TAF

III Antisera: Diphtheria Anti Toxin
It is passive agent 500 to 2000 units by I.M. as a prophylaxis. For therapy high dose is used 30,000 unit I.M. may be needed.

Whooping Cough

Whooping cough is caused by *Bordetella pertussis*, it is considered a disease of non-immunised children but can also occur in sporadic epidemics in middle life when immunity is weaned. After a short febrile tracheobronchitis (which itself is responsive to antibiotics). Severe episodic paroxysmal coughing bouts, associated with laryngospasm and often leading to inter costal muscle tears or fracture ribs may persist for many weeks.

In unimmunised children cough, whoop and vomiting are characteristic signs. Young infants do not whoop, although the cough is still spasmodic and is followed by vomiting. After a bout of coughing, apnoea may follow leading to unconsciousness. It can be complicated with pneumonia, malnutrition, conjuctival bleeding and rectal prolapse. Encephalopathy or respiratory complications are causes of mortality.

Thie triad of epidemiology is depicted in Fig. 18.11.

Incubation period 7-4 days.

The clinical course has a catarrhal stage lasting for 10 days, paroxysmal stage lasting for 20 days and a convalescent stage lasting for 2 weeks.

Control of Whooping Cough:

Cases are diagnosed, isolated and treated. Erythromycin 50 mg/kg body weight in 4 divided doses for 10 days is recommended. Alternatively ampicillin, cotriamaxzole or tetracycline as suggested by M.O.H. Epidemic Disease Hospital or an attending paediatrician should be considered.

Contacts of patient are given prophylactic course of Erythromycin or ampicillin treatment for 10 days.

The problem of cases and contacts do not occur if primary immunisation under U.I.P. is done with high coverage in the community.

Vaccines:

i. D.P.T. is used in active immunisation as per U.I.P. schedule.

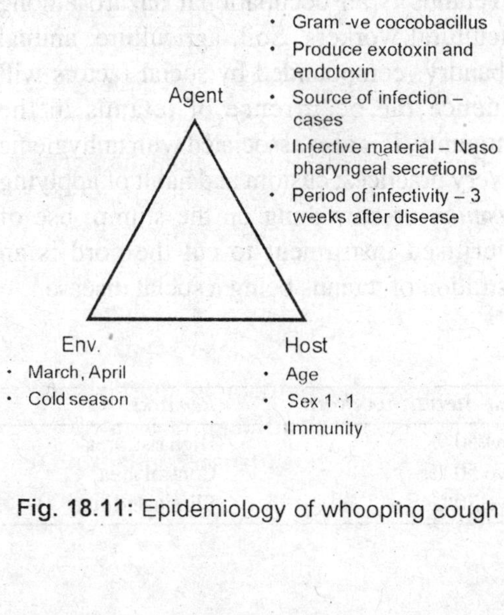

Fig. 18.11: Epidemiology of whooping cough

ii. Pertussis vaccine:
It is a killed whole cell preparation monovalent vaccine. 0.5 ml I.M. in 3 doses at 6 week interval starting in 2-3 months becomes a primary course. It has to be supplemented with 2 booster doses at 3rd year and 6th year. Side reactions of pertussis vaccine are persistent screaming, local reactions, fever and irritability. Contraindication is history of epilepsy or convulsions.

iii. There is no passive immunising agent. However, in practice (in E.D. Hospitals) practice of giving hyper immune globulin is observed which is still empirical.

With available weapon of U.I.P., problem of whooping cough is negligible in India.

Tetanus

Tetanus is caused by *clostridium tetani* bacteria which is a ubiquous organism in soil. Tetanus remains a leading disease in spite of available effective vaccine. Tetanus produces generalised or localized hypertonia of skeletal muscles, frequently accompanied by paroxysmal muscular spasm. Original Greek root teino (to stretch) gave a word tetanus meaning a muscular spasm.

Tetanus is of public health importance because of N.N.T. (Neonatal tetanus) causing Neonatal mortality in developing countries. Generalised tetanus from infected umbilical stump is characteristic of neonatal tetanus (Fig. 18.13).

The main causes of death are pneumonia, respiratory failure, circulatory failure, haemorrhage and septicaemia; even sudden death by severe spasm is recorded.

Epidemiological triad of agent host and environment in tetanus are depicted in Fig. 18.14.

World Problem: World neonatal mortality due to tetanus is reduced to 1.0 per 1000 live birth by available preventive care. Clinical cases

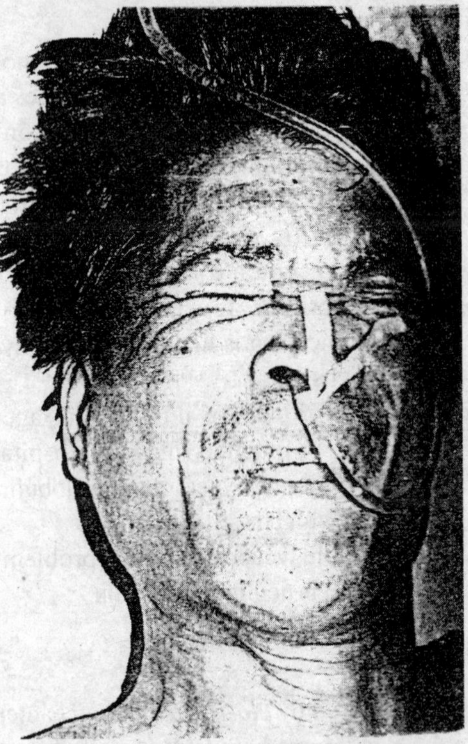

Fig. 18.12: Risus sardonicus with salivation

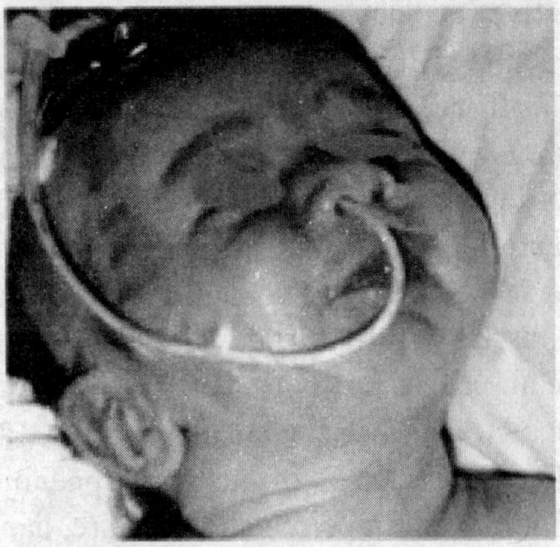

Fig. 18.13: Neonatal Tetanus

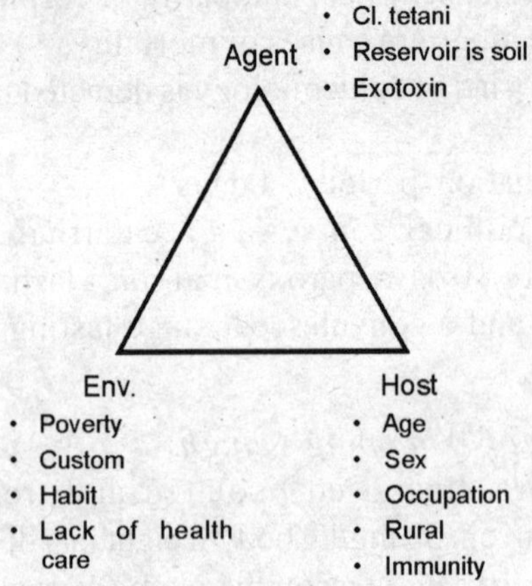

Fig. 18.14: Triad of epidemiology

which are hospitalized are adult cases and they carry 100% mortality in spite of specific treatment.

U.I.P. coverage by T.T. among A.N.C. cases has greatly reduced N.N.T. deaths. Further primary course and booster course have remarkable impact on adult tetanus.

In India, tetanus, being still a public health problem made the administration to gear up priority work. This gave rise to district grouping according to risk of N.N.T.

Tetanus is an occupational hazard among agricultural workers. Soil, agriculture, animal husbandry compounded by social factors will influence the occurrence of tetanus in the community. It is also associated with unhygienic delivery practices; custom and habit of applying *Bhasmum* or cow dung on the stump; use of unsterilised instrument to cut the cord is an illustration of tetanus being a social disease.

N.N.T. incidence	*Immunisation*	*Delivery by trained health workers*	*Remarks*
Above 1/100 LB	Below 70 %	Below 50 %	High risk area
Below 1/100 LB	Above 70 %	Above 50 %	Control area
Below 0.1/1000 LB	Above 90 %	Above 70 %	Eliminated area

Incubation period 6-10 days.

Types of clinical tetanus according to its source are:

1. Traumatic
2. Puerperal
3. Otogenic
4. Neonatal
5. Idiopathic.

Case Management and Nursing Care

Neutralise toxin by:

By I.V. injection 3000 I.U. human tetanus antitoxin.

Prevent further toxin by:

By Debridement of wound

Benzylpencillin 600 mg 1 V 6 hourly (Metronidazole as alternative).

Control the spasm by:

Nursing in a quiet room.

Avoid noise, light and other stimuli

I.V. diazepam for spasms.

General nursing by:

Hydration

Nutrition (tube feeding).

Treating secondary infections

Wound treatment strategy in hospital: Action is taken on the nature and type of injury or wound as under:

Vaccine:

1. D.P.T. as suggested under U.I.P
2. D.T. or dT as suggested under diphtheria management
3. TT 2 doses of 0.5 ml each I M at 1 month interval, Third dose is given at 1 year, Fourth dose after 5 years of primary dose. Immunologists and surgeons are of the opinion that frequent booster dose is useless and must be avoided.
4. Human tetanus hyper immunoglobulin is best prophylaxis. Dose is 250 I.U.
5. A.T.S. (Anti Tetanus Serum) prepared by horse blood, 1500 I.U. subcutaneously induces passive immunity
6. In non immune person, simultaneous active and passive immunisation are practiced
7. Active immunisation against tetanus is advised for international travellers.

Poliomyelitis

Poliomyelitis is a disease of early life in indigenous population in tropics, originally called infantile paralysis. Gentle passive movement of limbs will differentiate polio as it is the only condition in which pain is not aggravated and may even be relieved. Bulbar paralysis by polio is usually fatal.

The severity of polio is influenced by:

1. *Age:* Polio is severe in older than younger patients. Polio is severe in pre pubertal boys than girls.
2. *Injections:* If given during or just prior to onset cause provocative paralysis.

Death usually occurs by (a) Respiratory failure due to bulbar paralysis, (b) respiratory muscle paralysis, (c) cardio-respiratory failure and (d) pulmonary pathology like Atelectasis, oedema and pneumonia.

World Problem:

Poliomyelitis, though one of the preventable diseases yet cannot be under estimated. Countries are still reporting cases of polio. India

Table 18.4: Wound treatment strategy

	Less than 6 hours	*Other wounds*
TT taken before 5 years	No treatment	No Treatment
TT taken between 5-10 years	TT(1) dose	TT (1) dose
TT taken above 10 years	TT(1) dose	Active + passive Immunisation
TT history not known	TT course given	Immunoglobulin TT course given

is the only country reporting polio confirmed cases, which has caused concern in the world strategy of I.P.P.I. (Intensive pulse – polio immunisation).

Confirmed polio cases in 2001 and 2004

Region	*2001*	*2004*
Africa	69	845
America	10	0
Eastern Mediterranean	143	93
Europe	4	0
Only India (SEA)	268	109
Western Pacific	3	0
	497	1047

During 2006, number of endemic countries identified was 4 viz., India (66 cases) Pakistan (28 cases), Afghanistan (9 cases) and Nigeria (830 cases) totalling to 2033 cases in which wild polio identified were 1979.

Assessment of the situation shown that there were no cases in American region and European region. In Western Pacific one case was identified. In African regio0n about 995 cases and in SEARO region about 510 cases were reported.

Indian Problem:

Overall case reduction is noticed from 1995 by the initiated IPPI. But, India is getting confirmed polio cases till today causing anxiety in global eradication programme.

According to AFP surveillance report, AFP cases reported during 2006 have been 25286 and confirmed cases have been 490.

Epidemiological triad in polio is depicted in Figure 18.16.

A chimpanzee named Brunhilde, a place called Lancing and a boy named Leon gave us 3 serotype I, II and III in the history of polio.

N.H.D. of Polio

Clinical Feature

The incubation period is 7-14 days. With mild fever and headache many will recover. There

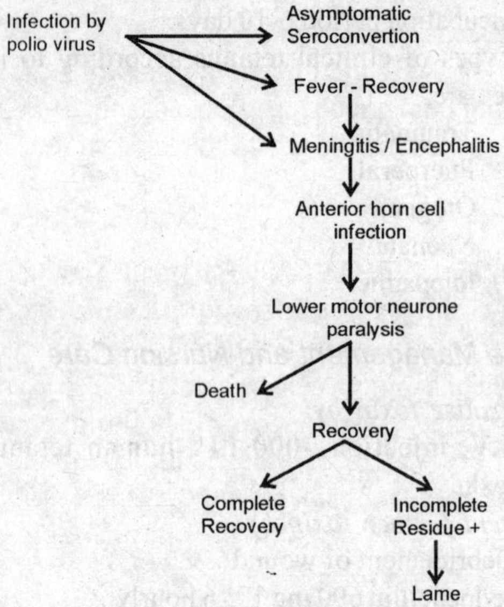

Fig. 18.15: N.H.D. of polio

may be recurrence of pyrexia, headache and meningism. Weakness may start later in one muscle group and can progress to widespread paralysis. Respiratory failure may supervene if intercostal muscles are paralysed or the medullary motor nuclei are involved. According to this response the case can be (a) Subclinical infection (b) Abortive polio (c) Non paralytic polio and (d) paralytic polio.

Mode of transmission is faecal oral route.

Prevention by Vaccine:

Two types of vaccine are available and in India oral (sabin) polio vaccine is used in eradication strategy.

Table 18.5: Difference between O.P.V. and I.P.V.

O.P.V. (Oral)	*I.P.V. (Injectable)*
Live attenuated	Killed formolised
Oral	I. M. or S.C.
Humoral and intestinal immunity is got	Only humoral
Prevents reinfection	Do not prevent reinfection
Useful in epidemic	Not useful
Cheap	Costly
Cold chain required	Not stringent

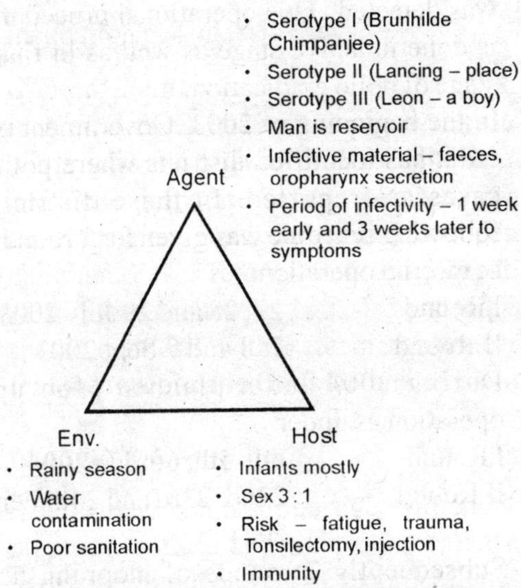

Fig. 18.16: Triad of epidemiology of polio

O.P.V.

O.P.V. contain live attenuated type I, II and III type virus grown in monkey kidney or human diploid cell cultures.

Table 18.6: Trivalent OPV constituents per dose

Type I	–	300,000 TCID – 50
Type II	–	100,000 TCID – 50
Type III	–	300,000 TCID – 50

Under U.I.P. programme O.P.V. is given as per schedule under primary course of immunisation. The dose is 3 drops per dose. WHO recommends a dropper for proper use. Tilt the child's back and gently squeeze the cheeks or pinch the nose to make the mouth of the infant to open. Let the polio drop fall from dropper onto the child's tongue. It has to be repeated if the child spits out the vaccine.

With the failure of OPV 3 dose regimen, paediatrician and immunologist advocate 5 dose regimen in clinic based programme as against 3 dose community based programme. In urban immunisation neonatal polio drops administered is called "Zero" dose polio. The vaccine must be stored at – 20°C in a deep freezer.

For passive immunity in acute infection, human normal immunoglobulin is used at 0.3 ml per kg body weight. But it must be used along with active immunisation.

Epidemiological Basis of Polio Eradication: In spite of hugh efforts, the vaccination coverage cannot reach 100 percent due to various reasons. Round the year routine immunisation has resulted in 80 % of child immunisation coverage. This 80% coverage is a community risk because we get more and more cases of polio by wild polio virus. This will be lurking in the intestine of un-immunised children. By epidemiological study, we could observe the following specific phenomena:

1. Man is the only host to get polio.
2. There is no chronic carrier state.
3. In the sewage, virus has 48 hours half life, and it spreads during this period of half life if at all it is spreading.
4. O.P.V. multiplies in intestine and interrupts the transmission of wild polio virus.
5. O.P.V. oral administration is easy for coverage.
6. O.P.V. is cheap and hence is cost benefit as well as cost effective.

Based on the above 6 noted phenomena, public health personal ventured for simultaneous administration of O.P.V. within a short period of time by mass immunisation. O.P.V. will interrupt the transmission of wild polio virus by displacing it from intestine where the wild polio virus is expected to multiply.

In the beginning, children up to 3 years of age were considered when eradication was planned in 1995. Later, it was felt that vaccination coverage of 100% of population at risk 0-5 years age will eradicate the polio from the world. Thus abrupt interruption of transmission of wild polio virus in the community became the epidemiological basis of polio eradication.

Many "lameness survey" done to map out prevalence and incidence of lameness due to poliomyelitis have shown that 80% of paralytic polio can be identified by house to house survey of lameness and muscle wasting among 5-10 year age children.

Epidemiological Investigation of Polio Case in the Community:
Even a single case of polio should prompt immediate active search for other cases. Now polio epidemic is defined as "Two or more local polio cases caused by same strain of virus within 1 month duration".

WHO guideline is followed in investigation as check list where selected essential data are collected at the time of epidemiological investigation of even single case of polio in the community. The check list is given in Appendix XVII.

Line listing of cases is done by visiting the children in the community. Line listing avoids duplication. If a polio case is reported, all contact children, 0-3 years in the said geographical area are listed in "line listing" which is a tool for planning, implementing mopping up operation, ring immunisation or pulse immunisation.

Under International Health regulations polio is subject to international surveillance. Even a single case must be reported to WHO and sent additional information like:

a. Type of virus
b. Number of cases
c. Number of deaths.

This should accompany a quarterly report by the country. Regarding polio virus isolation and serological techniques for polio surveillance, WHO has prepared guidelines.

Operational Terminologies:

i. **Mopping up:** involves door to door O.P.V. to below 5 year children in the village or a settlement where a case of polio was detected. This operational procedure is done in active stage as well as in final stage of polio eradication.
In the beginning of 2003, Government of India has identified districts where polio cases are reported. In these districts following schedule was given for 2 rounds of mop up operation:
I Round – 27, 28 and 29 July 2003
II Round – 7, 8 and 9 Sept 2003
During 2004 India planned Mop up operation as under
I Round – 4th, 5th, 6th Jan 2004
II Round – 22nd, 23rd and 24th Feb 2004
Subsequently 2 rounds of mopping up operation every year in National Immunisation Days were continued.
ii. **Ring Immunisation:** is a mopping up operation in cities where door to door O.P.V. to below 5 year children is done covering an area with a radius of 3 kms.
iii. **Pulse Immunisation:** O.P.V. is given to all 0-5 year children in a country on a single day regardless of previous immunisation. This is maintained as an annual event. Hence the name pulse.

Polio Eradication Programme

Along with global strategy, Government of India made its National Strategy for Polio Eradication in India. According to this even single case polio is treated as an epidemic. Preventive measures are initiated within 48 hours. Complete and timely reporting of cases is stressed in the programme. All cases of Acute Flaccid paralysis in children under 15 years are compulsory. Line listing of all reported cases is obligatory. Since 1992 all polio and non polio flaccid paralysis were included under active surveillance activity.

National polio eradication strategy included the following:

1. Pulse polio immunisation is done every year till it is eradicated.
2. Along with pulse polio, high level of routine immunisation coverage is sustained.
3. Monitoring of O.P.V. coverage is done at all levels.
4. Improve the surveillance capable of detecting all A.F.P. due to polio and non polio.
5. Rapid case investigation, and stool sample collection are ensured.
6. All cases are followed for 60 days to check residual paralysis.
7. To stop transmission, conduct outbreak control for cases confirmed.

I.P.P.I. (Intensive Pulse Polio Immunisation)

Polio eradication programme was called PPI (Pulse polio immunisation) from 1995 to 1999. Later with Intensification, it becomes IPPI from 2000 onwards. It is defined as sudden, simultaneous, mass administration of extra 2 doses of O.P.V. on a single day before the transmission season which is usually Jan-Feb of every year, to children below 5 years of age.

Despite PPI, due to non coverage of certain percentage of eligible children complete eradication has not been possible. Therefore, it was decided to Intensity this PPI in 4 rounds (Based on Brazil experience) through booth based on I day and house to house visit on II and III days. This intensified programme is called I.P.P.I.

Indian Expert Advisory Group on polio eradication (IEAG) recommended following measures during 2005 and 2006 period:

Use of mOPV1 and mOPV3 for targeted community.

Additional manpower for metropolitan cities

Social mobilisation for target

Mobile teams at transit points (bus stand, railway station etc.)

Accountability by political leaders

Zero dose or Birth dose at high risk areas.

AFP surveillance was strengthened by appointing about 248 SMOs (Surveillance Medical Officers) for a defined area.

The reason for changing PPI to IPPI are as under:

i. P.P.I. 2 rounds reduced polio cases not sufficient to reach eradication target, may be due to low routine coverage.
ii. Persistent wild virus circulation needs additional rounds.
iii. Eleven months between 2 usual PPI is large. Birth cohort and missed children in this period is large, which is a large susceptible group.
iv. More PPI round by IPPI will result in fewer chances for wild virus establishment.
v. IPPI is needed to flush out wild polio virus from the country (from the community and environment).

V.V.M. (Vaccine Vial Monitor) is made of heat sensitive material which change colour if the vaccine vial is exposed to high temperature than recommended.

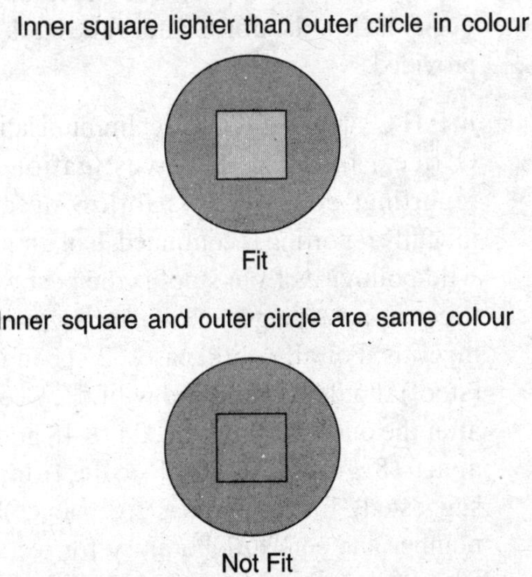

Fig. 18.17: Vaccine vial monitor (VVM)

V.V.M. is used in IPPI for good safety, clarity and purity of O.P.V.

Microplanning for social mobilisation, I.E.C. activities and coordination, has helped IPPI to be a success. Already existed PPI infrastructure and machinery have been mobilised as the resources for better IPPI.

A.F.P. Surveillance (Acute Flaccid Paralysis)

The eradication of polio is based on our knowledge about polio, effective vaccine and effective surveillance.

We have achieved highest vaccination coverage. We have successfully implemented nationwide mass immunisation. Now, we have to strengthen the surveillance of Acute Flaccid Paralysis so that all cases are detected, investigated and controlled.

It is carried out for all Acute Flaccid Paralysis along with polio.

i. Institutional surveillance (hospital). By visiting hospital, meeting with hospital staff, weekly hospital report is collected, its verification is done and feedback is provided.

ii. In P.H.C. area, DIO (District Immunisation Officer) initiates the investigation of reporting; does 60 days follow-up and monthly reporting is continued. Isolation of wild poliovirus from stool is the best way to confirm the diagnosis of paralytic poliomyelitis. For all A.F.P. cases, 2 specimen (stool) should be collected within 2 weeks after the onset of paralysis, 24 to 48 hours apart (8 grams of stool collection is suggested). Each sample is given an EPID number and sent to laboratory for test. It takes 28 days for isolation and identification of polio virus.

Following indicators are helping the A.F.P. surveillance, which is going on throughout the country.

a. Rates of A.F.P.
b. Monthly negative reporting.
c. Percentage of A.F.P. cases with 2 stool samples taken within 2 weeks after paralysis onset.

Tuberculosis

Tuberculosis is a chronic bacterial disease caused by Mycobacterium tuberculosis and an important cause of death in most parts of the word. When primarily it affects lung it is called pulmonary tuberculosis. Other than lung when it involves skin, lymph nodes, bone, joint, intestine, meninges and other tissues it is called non-pulmonary tuberculosis.

Tuberculosis principally involves cattle, sheep, goats, pigs. Man getting it from these vertebrate animals makes the disease as Zoonotic disease.

Tuberculosis is increasing alarmingly in the word. About 21.5 million new cases were notified by DOTT programme between 1995 and 2004. Annual risk of Tuberculosis is estimated to be 2%. Probable reason for this increase in the incidence of Tuberculosis in Developing countries could be due to: (a) HIV epidemic, (b) Population explosion, (c) Health care facility not accessible, (d) Poverty and civil unrest, and (e) Along with drug resistance, ineffective control.

In developed countries added reasons are immigration from high prevalence area, social deprivation and rising life expectancy.

Tuberculosis has a long and distinguished tradition, seen in mummies at Egypt, and for many centuries known to be a major cause of death, even when cause was known. In 1882 Robert Koch proved the specific cause. It is nearly 125 years are over, that we are struggling to control tuberculosis despite development in science, technology, and effective chemotherapy.

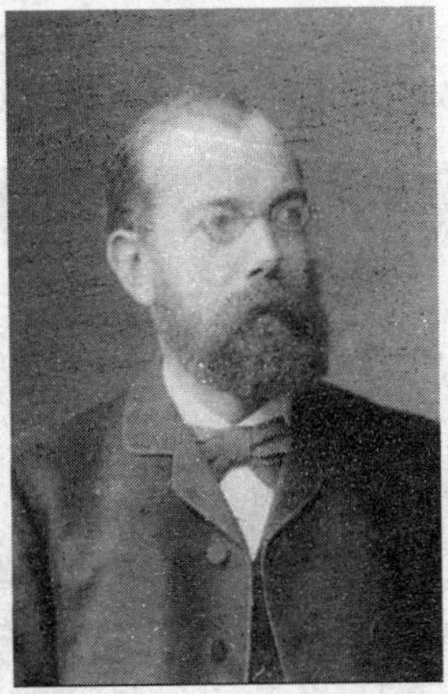

Photo: Robert Koch

Problem – World:

Every year 8 million new cases are occurring and 2.9 million deaths are occurring each year. The problem is acute in developing countries. 80% of cases are in economically productive age group of 15-49 years and is causing premature death. WHO has categorised countries for implementation of Directly Observed Treatment Short course (DOTS), (0 to 5 categories). All South East Asian countries have adopted DOTS. Poverty, economic recession and malnutrition make population more vulnerable to tuberculosis.

Problem – India:

Every year 2 million people are developing Tuberculosis and nearly 500,000 die from it – more than 1000 per day. Incidence has not changed over past 30 years. HIV associated TB and multidrug resistant TB are increasing the severity of TB epidemic. It is a major barrier of economic development costing 12000 crores rupees every year. More than 3 Lakhs children are leaving school because their parents have TB. More than 100,000 women with TB are rejected by their families. India has one third of global burden of tuberculosis. R.N.T.C.P. was initiated in 1993 with DOTS which is showing remarkable positive outcome in the country. In India, Drug resistant cases are about 3.0% which is very high. There is no difference in Rural or Urban areas. Prevalence of Tuberculosis (i.e. disease frequency) is 4/1000 population. Tuberculin judged finding is that prevalence of infection is about 30%.

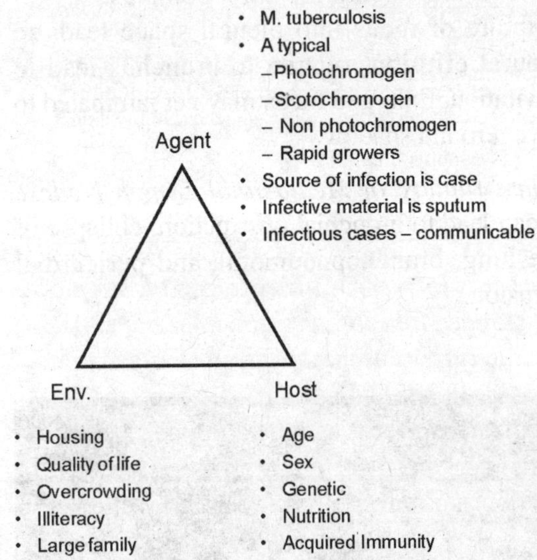

Fig. 18.18: Epidemiological trial in TB

Common Terms in Tuberculosis:

- i. **New Case:** Sputum +ve pulmonary TB who has never taken treatment.
- ii. **Failure Case:** Sputum +ve case, after 5 months treatment, still show +ve.
- iii. **Relapse:** Sputum +ve case declared cured show again sputum +ve.
- iv. **Defaulter:** One who left the treatment in between.
- v. **Cured:** Sputum + case after treatment show –ve on at least 2 occasion.

Agent, host and environment factors are depicted in Figure 18.18. Many social factors like poor housing, overcrowding, undernutrition etc., contribute to the causation of tuberculosis.

It is one of the social diseases which need both medical and social treatment.

Natural History of Tuberculosis:
Nearly 80% of population must have had their exposure one day or the other to tuberculosis. Many develop sero conversion and thus a few develop different adult variants of tuberculosis.

After Ghon Focus/ Primary Complex:
Rupture of focus into pleural space leads to pleural effusion, rupture to bronchus lead to cavitation. Enlarged focus may get laminated to give a round shadow.

When rupture of Mediastinal Lymph Nodes:
It can lead to bronchial obstruction, collapse of the lung, bronchopneumonia and pericardial effusion.

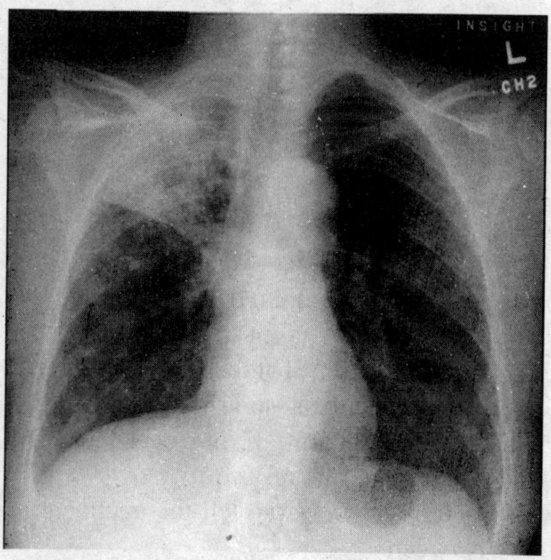

Photo: X-ray of pulmonary TB with cavity

As Sequelae of Bronchial Complications:
This lead to bronchial obstruction, bronchiectasis and fibrosis.

Latent period between primary infection and the development of pulmonary tuberculosis in adult life is longer in European countries and shorter in Asia and African countries.

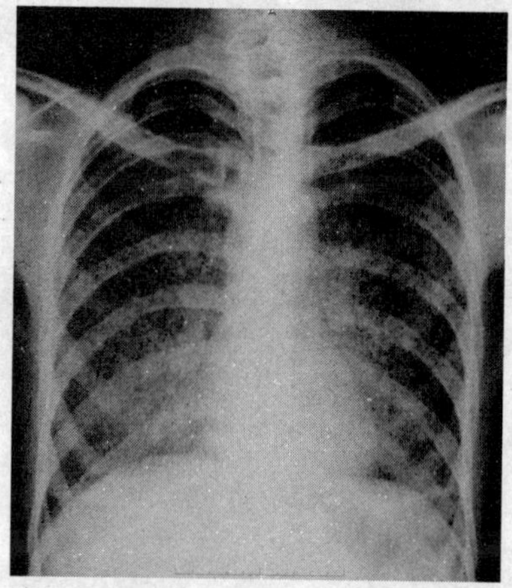

Photo: X-ray miliary TB

Tuberculin Test:
It is a skin test developed to find out the evidence of past or present infection with M.tuberculosis. Mantoux test is done by 0.5 ml P.P.D. (1 T.U.) intradermally on flexor surface of forearm. It is read after 72 hours. Result will be positive if 10 mm of induration is observed.

Incubation Period: 3 to 6 weeks will be the duration for infection to tuberculin +ve stage. For disease development the period is uncertain.

Mode of Transmission: Droplet infection and droplet nuclei.

Community Parameters:

a. Prevalence of infection – Tuberculin +ve = 30%
b. Incidence of infection – Newly infected (TB conversion index) = 2%
c. Prevalence of disease = AFB +ve = 0.4%
d. Prevalence of X-ray suspect = 2%
e. Prevalence of drug resistant = 10%
f. Mortality rate = 60 per 100,000.

Control of Tuberculosis

Tuberculosis control is said to be achieved when

the prevalence of natural infection in 0-14 year children is 1%. Control is by (a) Curative by case finding and prompt treatment (b) Preventive by B.C.G. vaccination.

Case finding Tools: Any case that show (a) Persistent cough of 1 month duration, (b) Continuous evening rise of temperature, (c) Chest pain and (d) Haemoptysis are subjected for sputum examination for A.F.B.

For chemotherapy we have major bactericidal and bacteriostatic drugs.

Bactericidal:

i. *Streptomycin:* It acts on rapidly multiplying A.F.B. Daily dose is 0.75 to 1.0 Gram in single injection. Vestibular damage and nystagmus are drug side effects.
ii. *I.N.H.*: It is the most powerful drug. It acts on bacilli. It is given as a single dose 4-5 mg/kg body weight (max. 300 mg). For intermittent therapy 700 mg twice a week is given.
Gastric irritation, neuropathy and liver damage are side reactions.
iii. *Pyrazinamide:* Acts on slow multiplying intra cellular A.F.B. Dose is 30 mg / kg body weight divided into 3 doses per day. Side reactions are liver damage and hyperuricaemia.
iv. *Rifampicin:* It permeates all tissue membranes and kills bacilli. Even extensive tuberculosis is curable with rifampicin. Dose is 10-12 mg/kg body weight taken 1 hour before or 2 hours after food. Daily convenient dose is 450-600 mg. For intermittent therapy 900 mg is given. Side reactions noticed are gastritis, thrombocytopenia and nephrotoxicity.

Bacteriostatic:

i. *Ethambutol:* It is used in combination to control drug resistance. Dose is 15 mg / Kg body weight given in 3 doses.
ii. *Thioacetazone:* In combination with I.N.H., it is used. Dose is 2 mg / kg body weight. Side effects are nausea, vomiting, blurring of vision and urticaria.
iii. Other bacteriostatic drugs are Ethionamide, PAS, Cycloserine, kanamycin and viomycin.

Earlier regimen was domiciliary or ambulatory treatment under (a) Daily regimen and (b) Biweekly regimen. But it is now totally replaced with short course therapy under R.N.T.C.P.

Technical organisation of tuberculosis programme is given in Figure 18.19.

D.T.C. is reference centre for diagnosis and treatment in the district. It is also responsible for training and supervision.

Figure 18.20 gives idea of flow chart for diagnosis and treatment of TB.

Figure 18.21 gives R.N.T.C.P. treatment regimen.

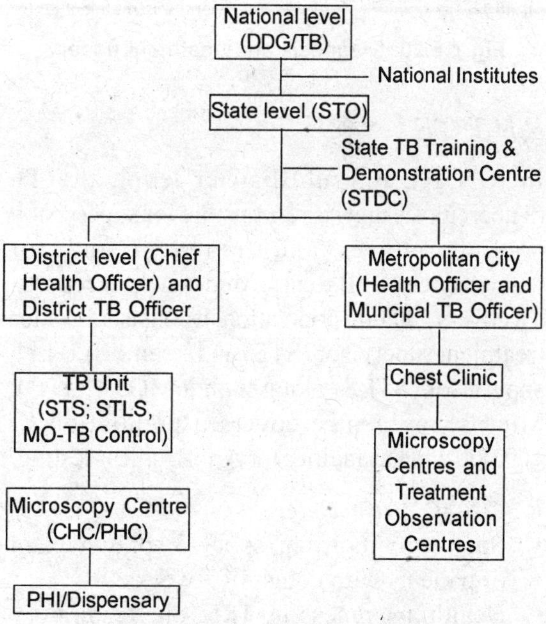

Fig. 18.19: Technical organisation of TB programme

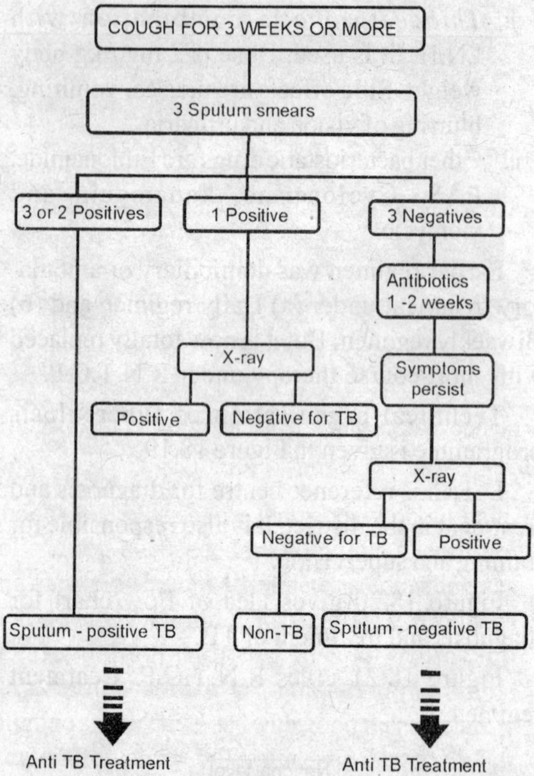

Fig. 18.20: Diagnosis and treatment under R.N.T.C.P.

R.N.T.C.P.

In R.N.T.C.P., sub district level, the Tu (Tuberculosis unit) is responsible for supervision of Laboratories and treatment and for maintenance of TB register and quarterly reports. Tu covers 500,000 population. It consists 1 senior treatment supervisor (STS) and 1 senior TB Lab supervisor (STLS) along with a MO (MOTC). Microscopy centre covers a population of 100,000 and has facility for A.F.B. smear testing.

R.N.T.C.P. Case Detection:

- Spot, early morning, spot – 3 sputum exam of patients with cough of 3 weeks
- Health awareness by H.E. on Respiratory symptoms
- Contact exam of AFB +ve children
- Evaluation of chest X-ray.

RNTCP Treatment Regimens:

Diagnosis is done as per flow chart shown as (a) Pulmonary +ve (b) Pulmonary –ve and (c) Extrapulmonary cases.

Treatment is instituted as per R.N.T.C.P. treatment regimen (Fig 18.21).

Category I: Initial phase extended by 1 mth of smear if +ve after 2 mths.

Category II: Retreatment cases. Initial phase extended by 1 mth if smear is positive after 3 mths.

Category III: If smear is +ve at 2 months categorised as failure case and treated afresh

RNTCP TREATMENT REGIMENS

TB Treatment	TB Patients	Intensive Phase	Continuation Phase
Category I	New smear-positive New smear-negative (Seriously ill) Extra-pulmonary**	2(HRZE)3*	4(HR)
Category II	Sputum smear-Positive – Relapse*** – Failure*** – Treatment After Defaults	2(SHRZE)$_3$ 1(HRZE)$_3$	5(HRE)$_3$
Category III	New smear-negative (Not seriously ill) Extra-pulmonary (Not seriously ill)	2(HRZ)$_3$	4(HR)$_3$

* The number before the letters refers to the number of months of treatment. The subscription after the letters refers to the number of doses per week. H: Isoniazid (600 mg), R: Rifampicin (450 mg), Z: Pyrazinamide (1500 mg), E: Ethambutol (1200 mg), S: Streptomycin (750 mg). Patients more than 50 years old receive streptomycin 500 mg. Patients in categories I and II who have a positive sputum smear at the end of the initial intensive phase receive an additional month of intensive phase of treatment.

** Examples of seriously ill extra-pulmonary TB cases are meningitis, disseminated TB, tuberculous pericarditis, peritonitis, bilateral or extensive pleurisy, spinal TB with neurological complications and intestinal and genito-urinary TB.

*** Very rarely, patients relapse with extra-pulmonary or smear-negative pulmonary tuberculosis; such patients are considered as "Other" and treated with the Category II regimen.

Fig. 18.21: R.N.T.C.P. Regimen

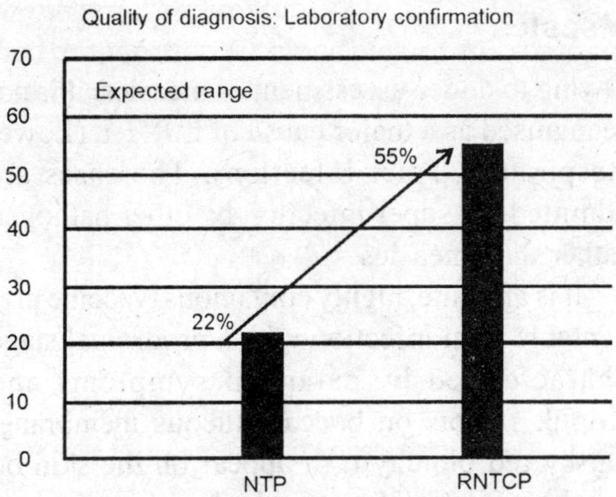

Fig. 18.22: Quality of diagnosis

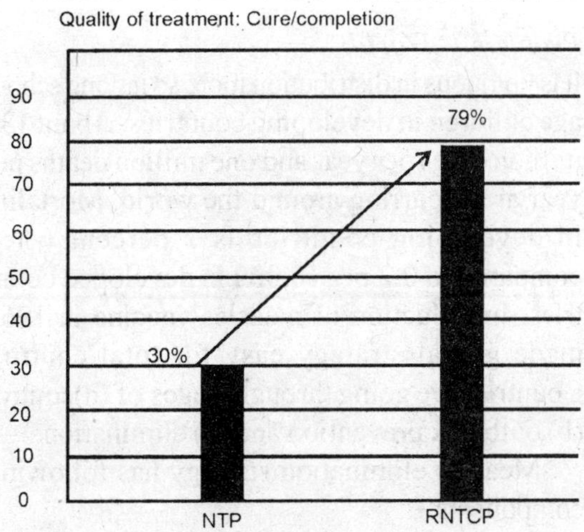

* Cure not assessed in NTP; 30 patients collect medicine for the prescribed duration

Fig. 18.23: Quality of treatment

Treatment result is announced as cured, completed, defaulted. failed, died, transferred etc.

It is expected that quality of diagnosis rises to 55% and that quality of treatment rises to 79% by instituting R.N.T.C.P. Figure (18.23).

DOTS Chemotherapy (Directly Observe Treatment, Short Course):

DOTS is a strategy to ensure that by providing most effective drug and confirming that the drug is taken.

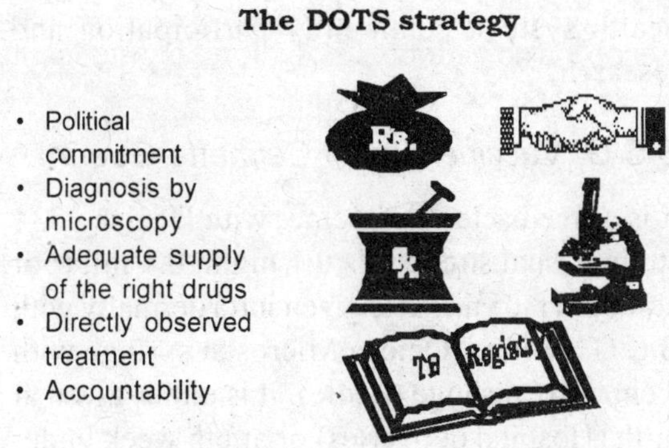

Fig. 18.24: The DOTS' s strategy

It is the only documented effective programme in the world. The DOTS strategy are (Fig. 18.24):

- Political commitment
- Diagnosis by microscopy
- Adequate supply of right drugs
- Directly observed treatment
- Accountability.

During intensive phase, Health worker watches as patient swallow the drug in his/her presence. During continuation phase patient is issued medicine for 1 week in multiblister combipack, of which the first dose is swallowed by patient in presence of a health worker. The pack is checked at return when patient comes to collect next pack. Drugs are packed in patient wise boxes with good shelf life. In DOTS, alternate day treatment is used.

Global Plan to Stop TB 2006-2015

This new Stop TB strategy was launched by World Health Organisation in 2006.

Diagnosis of 70% people with sputum positive and curing 85% of them was attempted till 2005. Reduction of global burden of TB was the main goal of Stop TTB Strategy by reducing death due to TB by 2015 to less than one million. Overall target of this plan to get 1case per million population per year by 2050.

Main components have been high quality DOTS, addressing drug resistance, strengthening health system, community participation and research.

B.C.G. Vaccine (Bacilli Calmette Guerin)

It is a live bacterial vaccine, with Danish 1331 strain. Usual strength is 0.1 mg in 0.1 ml. (For new born 0.05 ml). It is given intra dermally with B.C.G. syringe (Omega Microstat syringe with 1 cm sted 26 gauge needle). It is either given at birth (Hospital deliveries) or at 6th week under primary immunisation. BCG has protective value of 20 years and it prevents nonpulmonary serious complications of Tuberculosis. B.C.G. is not given for cases with eczema, hypogamma-globulinaemia.

Revised National T.B. Control Programme:
Details of National TB control programme is dealt in page 475. Government of India along with World Bank revised the National TB control programme in 1992. The main strategies under revised N.T.P. are:

- Achievement of not less than 85% cure rate among infectious cases of Tuberculosis through short term chemotherapy involving peripheral health functionary.
- Detecting 70% of estimated cases through quality sputum microscopy.
- Involvement of NGO's.
- Direct observed therapy short term (DOTS) as community based TB treatment and care strategy.

Tuberculosis and HIV

It is a lethal combination that accelerates tuberculosis progress from harmless infection to life threatening condition. Tuberculosis is an opportunistic infection that kills HIV +ve people. Tuberculosis with HIV can be treated effectively if early diagnosis is made.

International Measure: X-ray of individual prior to emigration to detect tuberculosis is a must as per Foreign Visa Regulations.

Measles

Owing to under-assessment of measles, it is not recognised as a major cause of L.R.T.I. (Lower Respiratory Tract Infection). The cases are admitted for super infection by other pathogen rather than measles.

It is an acute, highly contagious, vaccine preventable viral infection with a prodromal stage characterised by catarrhal symptoms and Koplik's spots on buccal mucous membrane. Dusky red blotchy rash appear on the skin on 4th day affecting face and body. Leucopenia is usual. Because of red spots on the body it is called Rubeola.

Problem – World:
It is ubiquous in distribution more so among school age children in developing countries. About 135 million cases per year and one million deaths per year are occurring around the world. Mortality in developing countries is 2 percent when compared to 0.2 per 10,000 in developed countries. Introduction of measles vaccine in 1963 made global strategy easy for total control. Countries are going through stages of (a)control (b) outbreak prevention and (c) elimination.

Measles elimination strategy has following components:

i. **Catch up vaccination:** One time nationwide vaccination of children 9-12 month of age under U.I.P.
ii. **Keep up vaccination:** Vaccinating above 95% of each successive birth cohort.
iii. **Follow up vaccination:** Nationwide vaccination of all children born after catch up vaccination once in 4 years.

Problem – India:
Measles is a major cause of morbidity and mortality. During 2005 an estimated number of cases have been 52454 and estimated deaths have been 55. CFR Case Fatality Rate is 1.8%. Many measles cases go unnoticed and not reported.

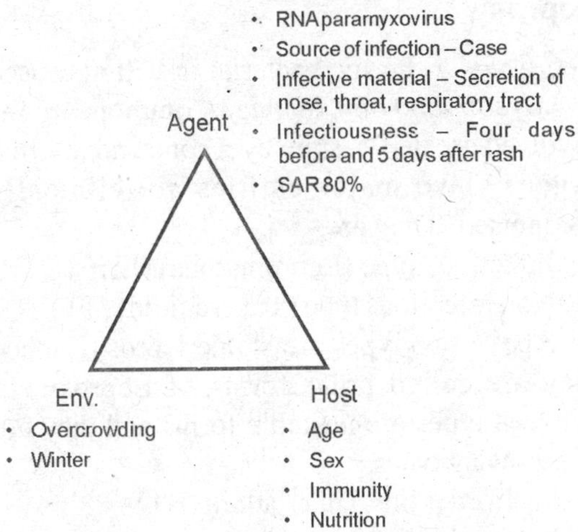

Fig. 18. 25: Triad of epidemiology in measles

Agent, host and environment factors are depicted in Figure18.25.

Mode of Transmission: Person to person by droplet infection and droplet nuclei. Incubation period is – 10 days.

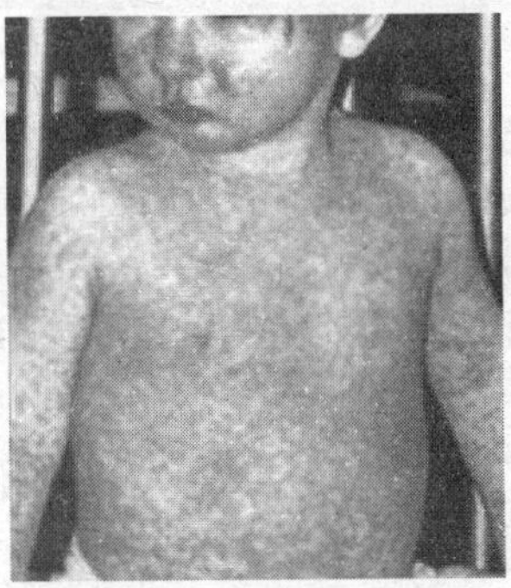

Photo: Measles rash

Clinical Features: Case will have usual prodromal phase of 3 days. Catarrhal stage is characterised by upper respiratory symptoms and presence of Koplik's spots on internal buccal mucosa, which is pathognomonic of measles. The child is irritable at this stage. Later, skin rash appear and lasts for 6 days, gradually fading with staining in the pale skinned children. Generalised lymphadenopathy and diarrhoea are very common. Bacterial pneumonia is seen in 4% of the cases. Very rarely S.S.P.E. (Subacute Sclerosing Pan Encephalitis) may occur. It is a serious infection along with malnutrition, among children.

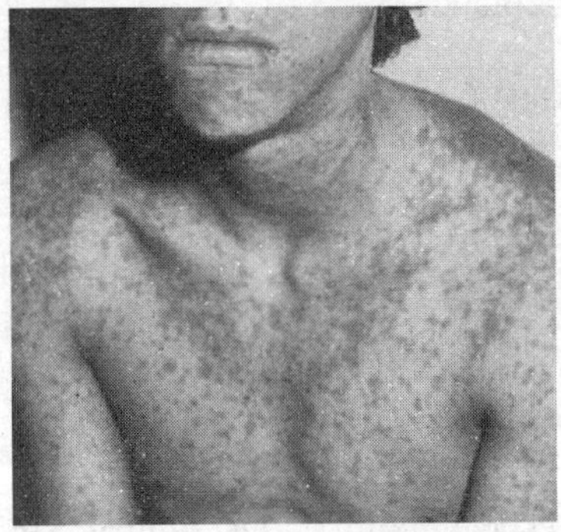

Photo: Koplik's spots in measles

Complications:

- Diarrhoea
- Pneumonia
- Respiratory complications
- Otitis media.

Management with Nursing Care

Only symptomatic treatment. Antibiotic should be given *only* if the child has clinical signs of pneumonia or other evidence of sepsis.

Control Measures:

- Isolation of cases for 7 days from rash.
- Immunisation of contacts within 2 days of exposure.
- Routine immunisation.
- Community measures against malnutrition.

Prevention

Measles is prevented by vaccine which is live attenuated vaccine. All are tissue cultured and are to be maintained at 2-8°C.

It is given at 9-12 months under U.I.P. 0.5 ml subcutaneous single dose is given. Except fever no other side reactions are observed in every day practice. It should, theoretically, give 95% immunity for life. Pregnancy is a contra-indication.

Measles vaccination combined with Mumps and rubella as M.M.R. is also made available on public demand.

DISEASES UNDER ERADICATION PROCESS

Poliomyelitis

Epidemiology, strategy for polio eradication in India through P.P.I. and I.P.P.I. are detailed in page 279.

In India NID's (National Immunisation Days) are largest campaign in the country. Since 1995, till 2003, 8 rounds of I.P.P.I. are covered by giving O.P.V. to all children below 5 years of age on a single day, regardless of their immunisation status. This is followed by subsequent supplementary door to door immunisation rounds. Approximately 200 million children are covered under I.P.P.I. 2002-2003 rounds under polio eradication campaign.

The eradication programme has not yet reached the point where the country can take up mop up work. Presently WHO experts have recommended to continue the I.P.P.I. rounds as under:

1. Nationwide I round in December every year.
2. Nationwide II round in January every year.
3. Sub nationwide round in October every year.

(1) and (2) are I day booth based, followed by II and III day house to house search for coverage.

In India, every year, 2 rounds of National Immunisation Days are conducted since 2004 till date.

The aim is to accomplish 100% O.P.V. coverage to eradicate wild polio in the world.

Leprosy

Leprosy is a chronic bacterial infection caused by *Mycobacterium leprae*. Common organs involved are nerve, skin, eye, bone and internal organs. Two major entities are clinically recognised. They are:

a. Infectious type (Lepromatous) (LL)
b. Non infectious type (Tuberculoid) (TT)

Above two types are stable leprosy. Hence they are called polar forms of Leprosy. In between types are unstable forms and they are of following types:

a. Border line Tuberculoid (BT)
b. Border line (BB)
c. Borderline Lepromatous (BL).

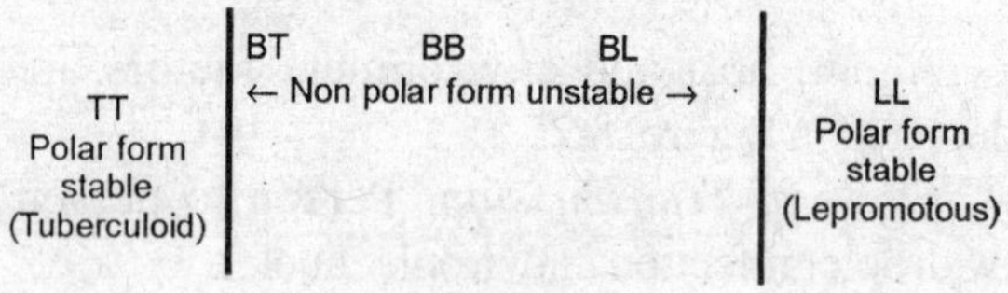

Fig. 18.26: Types of leprosy

For the purpose of treatment and prognosis, leprosy is classified according to Bacterial presence. They are:

a. Multibacillary: This contains LL, BL and BB.
b. Paucibacillary: This contains indeterminate (I), TT and BT.

Table 18.7: Difference between tuberculoid leprosy and lepromatous leprosy

	Tuberculoid leprosy	*Lepromatous leprosy*
Lepromin Test	+ve	-ve
Lion face	No	Yes
Bacteria in skin smear	No	Yes
Infectious	No	Yes
Sensation of lesion	Lost	Not Lost
Nerve thickening	Very early sign	Very late sign
Neural lesion sign	Always first sign	Never first

History of Leprosy – Major Milestones

Oldest disease of mankind got name from Greek word (Leper = Scaly), was known as *Kushta roga* in India.

1873 Hansen discovered M.leprae
1943 Sulphone drug was invented
1960 Shown multiplication in footpad of mice
1971 Experimentally produced in American Ant eater animal
1981 MDT – NLEP launched (Multi Drug treatment – National Leprosy Eradication programme)
1996 SAPEL were initiated (Special Action Projects for the elimination of Leprosy)
1998 MLEC (Modified leprosy eliminations campaign)
2000 World Bank supported project on NLEP
2003 Fifth MLEC
2005 Total elimination is targeted
2006 Global Strategy and National Action Plan.

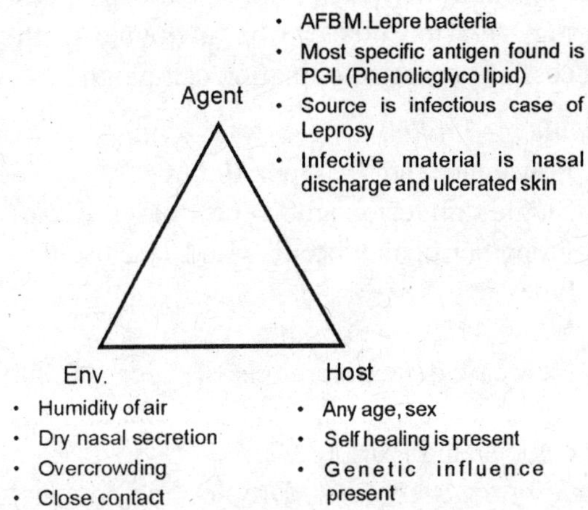

Fig 18.27: Epidemiological triad of leprosy

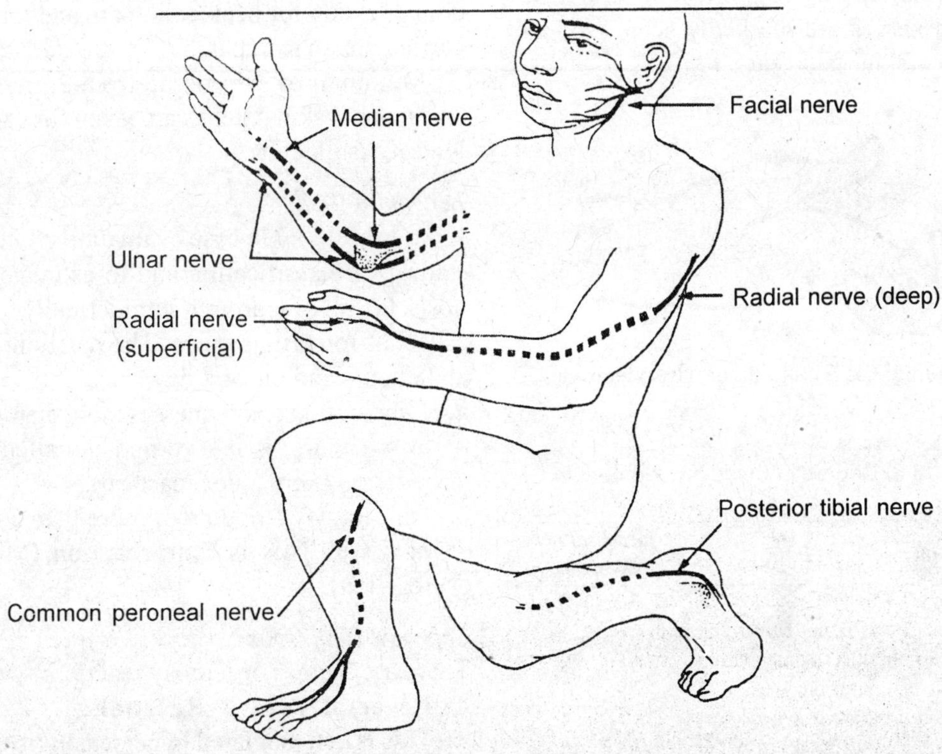

Fig. 18.28: Nerve thickening sites in leprosy

World Problem:

Leprosy is a public health problem in 15 countries which showed prevalence rate of more than 1 per 10,000, which includes India. Global increase during 1995 to 2000 can be attributed to the success of Leprosy elimination campaign.

Problem – India:

- Prevalence rate 0.84 per 10,000.
- Single skin lesion among new cases 4.1%.
- Proportion of multibacillary and paucibacillary type
  MB = 49.2% PB 50.8%.
- New case detection rate is 14.3 per 100,000
  Agent host and environment factors are depicted in Figure 18.27.

Mode of transmission – Droplet and contact.

Incubation period – 3-5 years.

Clinical Features:

Hypopigmented anaesthetic patches and thickened nerves are markedly seen. Nodules are seen on skin, face, ears.

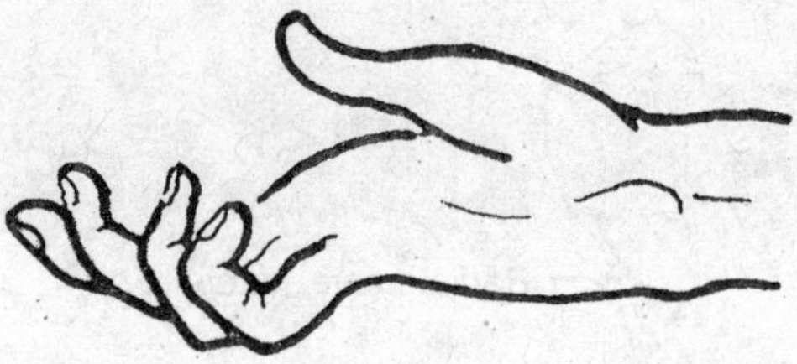

Fig. 18.29: Claw hand deformity in leprosy

Table 18.8: Degree of nerve involvement in leprosy

Criteria	*Grade of nerve involvement*
No pathology	0
Thick, Tender, Painful, no loss of function	1
Partial sensory loss, Loss of function	2
Full anaesthetic, no muscle weakness	3
Partial sensory loss, partial weakness	4
Full sensory loss, Full weakness	5
Muscle paralysis for 1 year	6

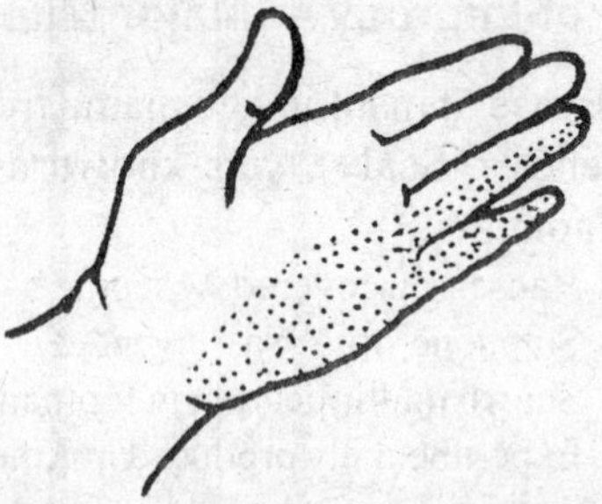

Fig. 18.30: Site of sensory loss in ulnar nerve damage

In late phase of Leprosy, loss of fingers, nasal depression, foot drop, claw toes, plantar ulcers are seen.

Specific precaution is taken in leprosy case detection. They include proper history of present illness and past history. Whole body is inspected in good natural light for lesion, presence of thickening of common cutaneous nerves are done. Testing for heat, cold, pain and touch are carried out on skin patch.

Minimum of skin tissue from 2 ears, nasal smear and 4 skin patches are taken for bacteriological examination.

Lepromin Test:

It is a useful tool in case evaluation on immune status, for classification and to estimate prognosis. 0.1 ml of lepromin intradermally to inner aspect of forearm is given. The reaction is read at 48 hours and on 21st day.

a. If induration and redness is more than 10 mm at 48 hours, it is +ve and is called early reaction (Fernandez reaction).
b. On 21st day a nodule of more than 5 mm is positive. This is Late reaction (Mitsuda reaction).

Leprosy Reactions:

There are 2 types of leprosy reaction:

A. **Reversal Type–1 Reaction:**

This is cell mediated hypersensitivity and is called Arthus Phenomenon. Clinically it shows painful tender nerves, loss of function, swollen skin lesions, new skin lesions and rarely fever. Loss of nerve function is sudden, with foot drop by overnight. Recovery is good with M.D.T. regimen.

B. **Erythema Nodosum Leprosum Type–2 Reaction:**
This is due to immune complex deposition. Clinically it shows tender nodules and papules. They may ulcerate. Painful tender nerve, loss of function, iritis, orchitis, myositis, lymphadenitis, fever and oedema are other reactions.

Treatment of Leprosy Reaction:

Arthus Phenomenon:

a. Aspirin 600 mg 6th hourly
b. Prednisolone 40-80 mg tapered in 9 months.

Erythema Nodosum Leprosum:

a. Aspirin 600 mg 6th hourly.
b. Prednisolone 20-40 mg tapered in 6 months.
c. Local treatment for eye involvement.

National Leprosy Eradication Programme:
In India NLCP was started in 1955. Later in 1983 Government of India declared to eradicate leprosy by 2000. This included population survey, school survey, contact examination and voluntary referral. This also includes MDT, Health education, ulcer and deformity care and rehabilitation.

MLEC was launched with public awareness and house to house search for cases. Staring in 1997, five campaigns were covered. During Fourth campaign, States were divided into 3 categories as under:

Category 1: endemic states like Bihar, UP, Chhattisgarh, MP, WB, Uttaranchal and Orissa.

Category 2 : Moderate to low endemic states like AP, Arunachal Pradesh, Goa, Gujarat, Karnataka, Maharashtra, TN, Chandigarh, Daman and Diu, Dadra, Nagar Haveli, Pondicherry, Andaman Nikobar, Delhi and Lakshadweep.

Category 3: Low endemic states like Haryana, Punjab, HP, Nagaland, Sikkim, Tripura, Meghalaya, Mizorram, J and K, Assam, Manipur, Rajasthan and Kerala.

During 5th Campaign (2003-04) following strategy was followed:
Urban — VRC and LEC in slum areas
Rural — VRC and SAPEL in selected pockets

Above campaigns were carried out through 1440 SAPEL/LEC

Now the goal is to reduce prevalence rate to below 1 per 10,000 during Tenth Five Year Plan.

National Leprosy Elimination Campaign:

N.L.E.C. has the following objectives:

a. To carry out intensive awareness campaign about leprosy involving the community in the campaign.
b. To give 1 day training to MOH, HS, MPW (M) and (F), VHG, AWW etc., to appraise them about the case detection procedure is adopted.
c. To give 3 days training to PHC staff who have joined the service recently.
d. To give I.E.C. training to Media officers, B.E.E., H.E. and H.S.
e. To detect hidden leprosy cases by active house to house search for 6 days or at fixed voluntary reporting centres on 2 previously fixed dates.
f. To confirm and treat all the detected cases with M.D.T.

Strategies of N.L.E.P.:

1. Early diagnosis and prompt treatment.
2. Disability prevention.
3. M.D.T is made accessible to all.
4. Treatment of all registered cases.
5. Improving quality of care.
6. Ensuring regular and complete treatment with M.D.T.
7. Enlisting community support.

Accelerated approach for Leprosy elimination was brought out by L.E.C. and S.A.P.E.L.

L.E.C.: Leprosy Elimination Campaign is an initiative to detect leprosy that remained undetected and to cure them. Elements involved in L.E.C. are:

i. Capacity building measures for local health workers to improve M.D.T.
ii. Increasing community participation and
iii. Diagnosis and curing leprosy patients.

S.A.P.E.L.: Special action projects for elimination of leprosy is an initiative aimed at providing M.D.T. services to patients living in "special difficult to access areas" or situation or to those belonging to "neglected population groups".

WHO "MDT" Regimen

A. Clinical Grouping:

Lesion	*PB Single skin lesion (Patch)*	*PB Paucibacillary*	*MB Multibacillary*
1. Skin lesion	1	2-5	6 and above
2. Nerve involvement	No	Only one	More than one
3. Skin smear	-ve	-ve	+ve

B. Treatment:

	Drug	*Dose*	*Frequency*	*Criteria for cure*
M.B.	Rifampicin Dapsone Clofazimine	600 mg 100 mg 300 mg 50 mg	Once monthly Daily Once monthly Daily	Completion of 12 monthly pulses Within 18 months
P.B.	Rifampicin Dapsone	600 mg 100 mg	Once monthly Daily	Completion of 6 monthly Pulses Within 9 months
Single Skin Lesion	Rifampicin Ofloxacin Minocycline	600 mg 400 mg 100 mg	Single dose	Single dose treatment

Proposed Strategy Beyond 2000:

a. Leprosy service to integrate with general health service.
b. All new cases will be brought under M.D.T. with probably better regimen than the current one.
c. The old cases: Disabled will continue to receive health care service especially for their disabilities.

Surveillance:

A. Single patch and 1-5 patches are followed once a year upto 2 years.
B. 6 and above 6 patches are followed once a year upto 5 years.

Under N.L.E.P., leprosy control units and SET centres play vital role. Major points are tabulated as under:

Table 18.9: Difference between LCU, SET

L.C.U. (Leprosy control treatment unit)		*S.E.T. (Survey education unit)*
800	Number	6000
1%	Prevalence	0.5 to 1.0%
a control unit	Status	a sub centre
1 M O	Staff	1 non medical supervisor
12 paramedical workers		5 PM worker
150,000 population	Coverage	10,000 population

National Action Plan 2006-07 under NLEP: Director General of Health Services, Government of India have released Action plan for the period April 2005 to March 2007 to continue the efforts, to continue the achievement, to continue efforts with quality leprosy service with the strategies of decentralization, strengthen service delivery, IEC activities and training.

Tenth Five Year Plan goals for leprosy elimination:
The strategy recommends to bring prevalence rate to below 1 per 10000 population through horizontal integration of programme to general health care system, manpower development for effective public health care, training component incorporation, adoption of reconstructive surgery, with rehabilitation and with NGO involvement.

Global Strategy for Leprosy Control activities during 2006-2010:
To change attitude of health care providers and beneficiaries global strategy for further reducing the leprosy burden and to sustain leprosy control activities, following elements are recommended and incorporated:

- To sustain control activities in endemic areas.
- Case detection rate has to be main indicator for monitoring.
- Quality service in diagnosis and treatment is maintained.
- Strengthening both routine and referral service component.
- To discontinue campaign approaches.
- To follow community based procedure in leprosy service.
- To utilize support from other agencies.

Yaws

A non venereal trepanematosis by yaws is caused by a *spirochete treponema.* Pertenue is the common endemic trepanematosis in tropical and sub tropical countries. Yaws was predominant in pre-antibiotic era. Long acting penicillin which is cheap, safe and curative is best cost effective known in the medical field. Yaws is very well differentiated by the following characteristics from syphilis and other trepanematoses. They are:

i. It is not sexually transmitted
ii. Mainly attack children
iii. Poverty and overcrowding are significantly related
iv. Do not transmit through placenta
v. Do not involve C.V.S.
vi. Do not involve C.N.S.

Yaws is found in warm, humid, tropical, rural areas. During rainy season, it increases in occurrence with more of skin lesions than before. Incubation period – 3-5 weeks.

Agent, host and environmental factors are highlighted in Figure 18.31.

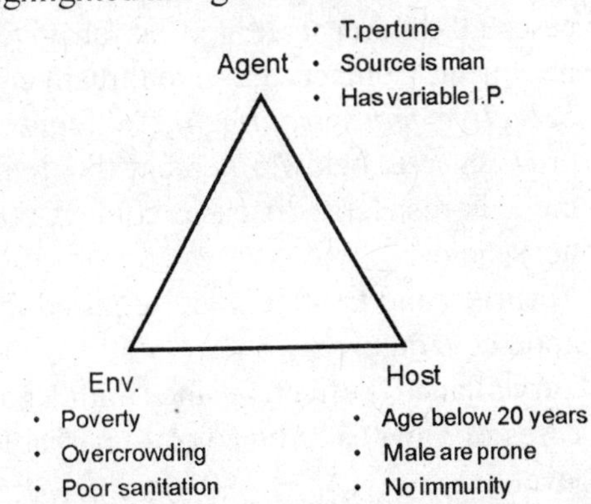

Fig. 18.31: Triad of epidemiology of yaws

Clinical Features:

Early Yaws: The primary lesion is called "Mother Yaw" appear on buttock or leg. In about 4 weeks crops of papilloma around the mouth follows. If it appears on sole, walking becomes painful. Untreated lesions will subside automatically.

Latent Yaws: For over 5-10 years there may not be any clinical signs of yaws. They may be serological positive by laboratory test. Hence the name latent yaws.

Late Yaws: Nodule or ulcer on skin, hyperkeratotic lesion of palm or sole and gumma of bone develop. Lesion of a face and palate give bad disfigurement called gangosa.

Treatment:

Single intra muscular injection of 1.2 million units of long acting Benzathine Penicillin G is given.

Control Measures:

i. Survey is done for case detection.
ii. Long acting penicillin is given to cases. 1.2 million units for adults and 0.6 million units for children are advocated. Under eradication strategy 3 treatment policies are recommended:

a. *Total mass treatment:* Wherever prevalence is more than 10 percent, entire population is given treatment.
b. *Juvenile mass treatment:* Whenever prevalence is between 5-10 percent, all cases, all children under 15 years are given treatment. Contacts are given treatment.
c. *Selective mass treatment:* Whenever prevalence is below 5 percent the treatment is restricted to case, contact and households.
d. Resurvey and treatment are required for good coverage.
e. Surveillance is effective since number of cases of yaws is reduced to remarkable level.
f. Improvement of personal hygiene, water supply, facility for skin bath with soap and water, better housing etc., reduces the risk of exposure to yaws.

In India, yaws is endemic disease but no more a public health problem. Low transmission of yaws is occurring which has to be detected by serological survey.

Old cases and resurgence of yaws are 2 types seen in the community.

Yaws Eradication: India considered its epidemiological situation and resources to take up eradication of yaws in the country.

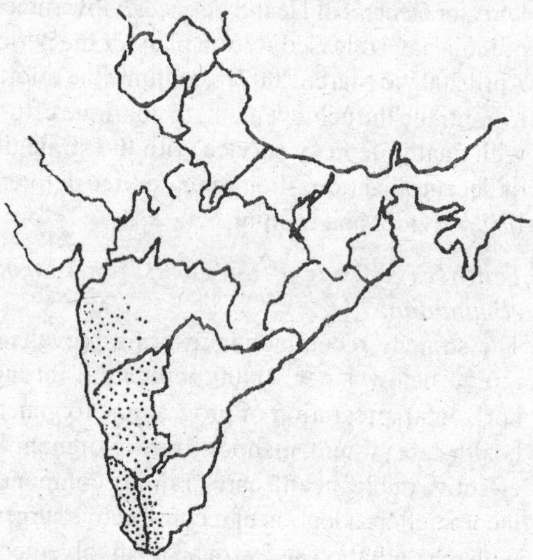

Fig. 18.32: Guinea worm endemic areas in India

Experience on the eradication measures for Yaws, public health authorities have noticed two major practical problems which are:

- Arriving at accurate diagnosis by field worker is a problem.
- There is no long lasting immunity.

Guinea Worm Infection

In global epidemiology guinea worm infection predominance in guinea and medina gave the names guinea worm and medina worm respectively.

It is caused by one of the longest nematode *Dracunculus medinensis*. It is transmitted through drinking water from unsafe sources like step well, pond etc., which contains Cyclops (water flea). Infection incapacitates man causing economic and productive loss to the family. When patient enters unsafe water guinea worm emerges and discharge embryos to water which are taken up by Cyclops. When healthy man drinks this water he gets the disease after a period of one year.

It is distributed in west coastal area of India and Sudan, Mali and Ghana of Africa; seasonally it occurs during rainfall days. Traditionally it is pulled, tied to a stick and rotated to extract from the leg (Fig. 18.33).

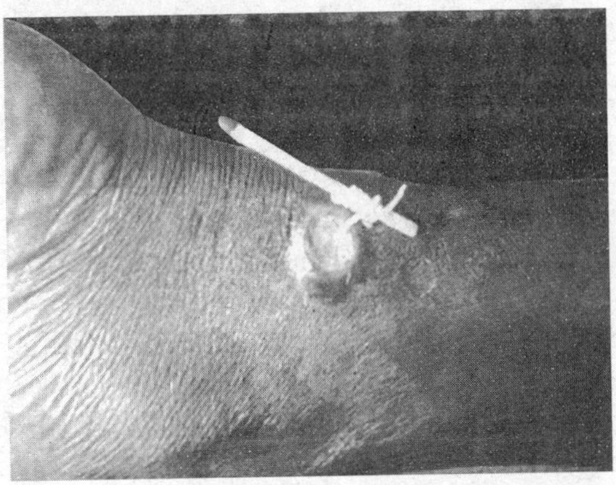

Fig. 18.33: Traditional removal of guinea worm

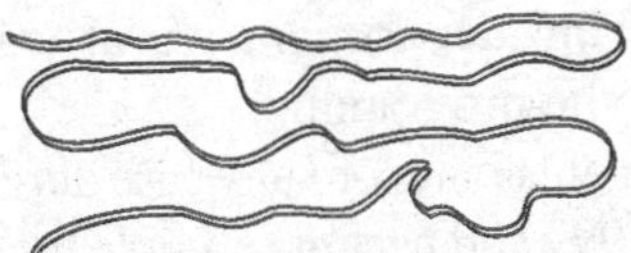

Fig. 18.34: Adult guinea worm

Adult worm measures up to 1 meter as thin slender long worm (Fig. 18.34)

Problem – World:
Remarkable reduction to the tune of 89.2% is observed with number of cases occurring in the world. Total cases during 2005 are 10674 which occurred from 9 African countries. Sudan, Mali and Ghana have reported more number of cases.

India – Problem:
It is limited to western and north western area of the country. Assam, Bengal, Bihar and Orissa are free from the disease. Cases have come down drastically to zero from thousands of cases.

1984 – 39792 cases
1996 – 9 cases
1998 – zero till 2005

The last case reported was July 1996 in Aau village in Peelwa P.H.C. area of Jodhpur district in Rajasthan. With 3 years zero incidence, India was declared free of Guinea Worm Disease in 2000.

The life cycle is depicted in Figure 18.35 and the life cycle is between man and Cyclops in the presence of water which has cycle to repeat and to reinfect the man.

Agent, host and environmental factors are depicted in Figure 18.36.

Mode of Transmission: Drinking contaminated water containing infected Cyclops. Incubation period – 1 year.

Control and Eradication:

i. Health education to public not to use contaminated step well or pond, to use boiled water or filtering through muslin cloth for use. Particularly an infected person should not enter water source.
ii. Cyclops control measures (Chapter 9)
iii. Provision of piped water, hand pumps
iv. Treatment of cases with mebendazole or metronidazole. Niridazole 12.5 mg per kg

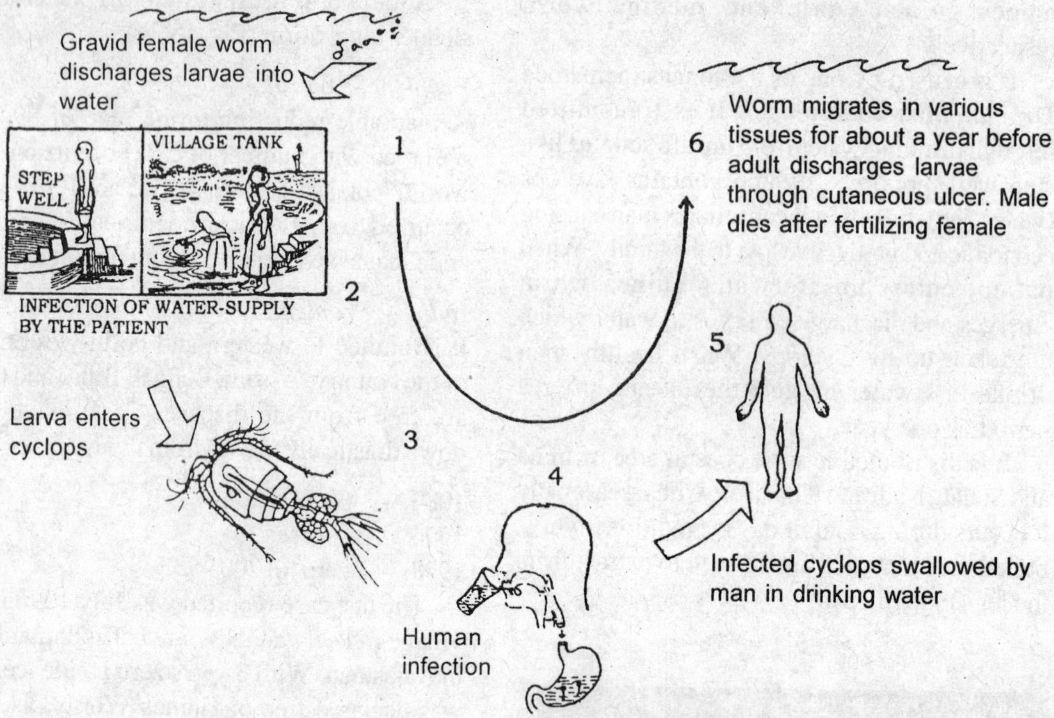

Fig. 18.35: Life cycle of guinea worm

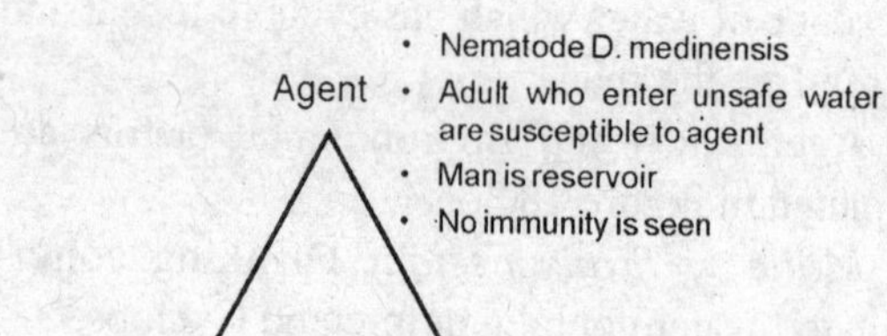

Fig. 18.36: Epidemiology of guinea worm

body weight reduces local inflammation and helps in worm extraction.

v. Active search for cases

Eradication Programme:

Public health experts identified guinea worm as potentially eradicable disease (next to smallpox). Epidemiological basis were (a) Its simple life cycle (b) Cyclops is present only in unsafe water (c) Tools for control is available (d) No deaths are reported.

In 1983-84 Government of India launched guinea worm eradication programme in the country. State Health Directorates, Ministry of Rural Development, state public health engineering department (rural water supply) assisted the programme.

India did not record any case during July 1996 to July 1999 and became eligible for certification by the ICCDE (International Commission for Certification of Dracunculiasis Eradication). WHO team visited India in Nov. 99 to validate the zero guinea worm disease status. Guinea worm eradication is a milestone in disease control programme.

Government of India declared India free of Guinea Worm disease based on the report of International Commission for the certification of Drucunculosis eradication in India. It also has recommended continuing following activities:

- Health education.
- Investigation of any rumor with Guinea Worm disease.
- To continue this under notifiable diseases.
- To continue surveillance in previously infected areas.
- Provision of safe water through bore wells.

Malaria

Malaria means "bad air" from Italian is a well known disease of mankind since antiquity. It is most important parasitic disease of a man, a protozoan infection of RBC transmitted by the bite of female anopheles mosquito. Ronald Ross discovered the life cycle of malaria parasite, when he was in India.

There are 4 species of plasmodium that produce malaria. They are:

1. P. vivax
2. P. malariae
3. P. ovale
4. P. falciparum.

Global Malaria Problem:

All most all countries have malaria cases. About 3 million are dying every year of whom 1 million are children under five years. About 40% of world population is exposed to varying degrees of malaria in some 100 countries. Modern rapid means of travel make people to get exposed which may only seriously affect them after they have returned home. DALY's lost by malaria is least in Europe and highest in African countries. The endemicity of malaria is expressed in terms of spleen rate and parasite rate in children aged 2-9 years.

Table 18.11: Endemicity of malaria

Spleen rate Or Parasite rate	*Endemicity*
0-10%	Hypoendemic
10-50%	Mesoendemic
50-75%	Hyperendemic
75% above	Holoendemic

Morphology of Malaria parasite is depicted in Figure 18.37 and Table 18.10.

Vector Bionomics

Urban area – Anopheles stephensai, which breed in used well overhead tank, transmits malaria.

Rural area – A.culicifacies, which breeds in stagnant or slow running water, transmit malaria.

Hilly area – A.fluviatilis which breeds in slow running water, transmits malaria.

Table 18.10: R.B.C. changes in M.P. smear

	RBC changes in malaria					
	Size	*Shape*	*Ring stage*	*Schuffner dot*	*Merozoites*	*Band form*
P. vivax	Increase	Round	–	Present.	30-40	–
P. malariae	No change	Round	–	Absent	10-15	Present
P. ovale	Irregular	Oval Irregular	–	Present	8-10	–
P. falciparam	No Change	Round	Present	Absent	8-10	–

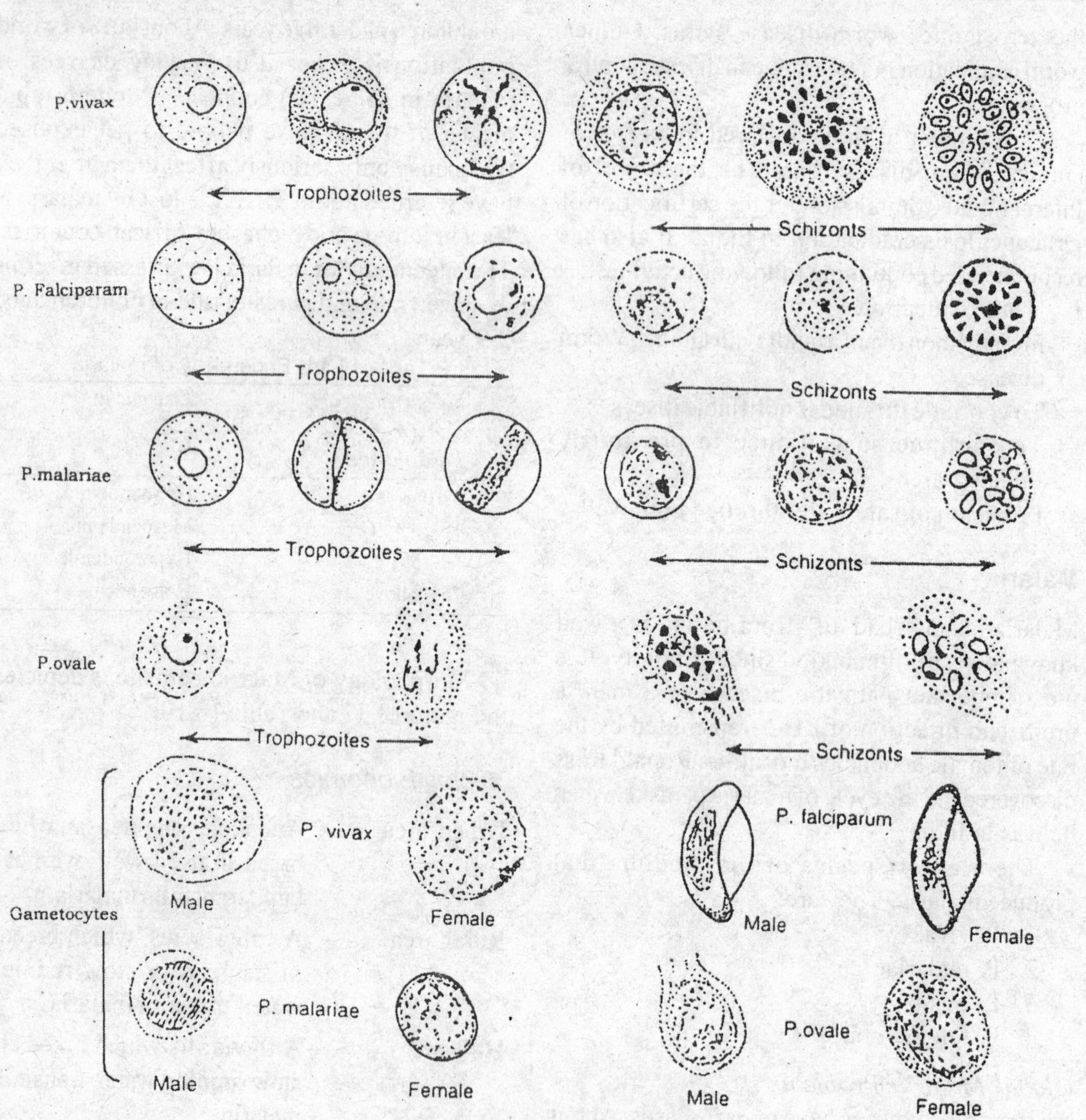

Fig. 18.37: Malaria smears differentials

Sea coastal area	–	A.sundaicus which breeds in salt water, transmits malaria.
Tea plantation area	–	A.minimus which breeds in slow running water, transmits malaria
Water logging area	–	A.philippinensis which breeds in high level subsoil water, transmits malaria.

Malaria Problem in India:

Upto 1976 there was a good improvement in malaria situation. But after 1977 resurgence of

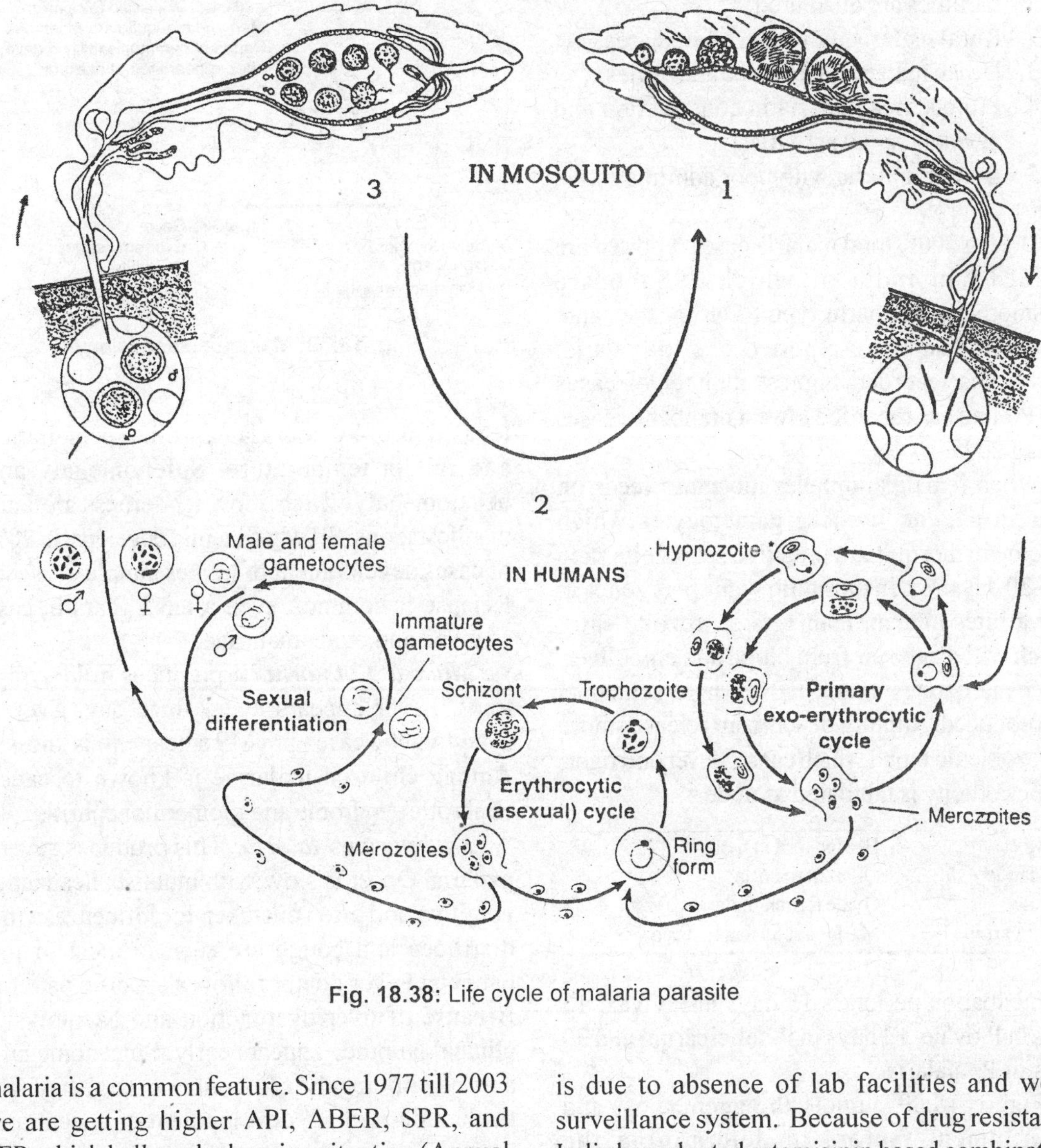

Fig. 18.38: Life cycle of malaria parasite

malaria is a common feature. Since 1977 till 2003 we are getting higher API, ABER, SPR, and SFR which hall mark alarming situation (Annual Parasite Incidence, Annual Blood Examination Rate, Slide Positive Rate and Slide Falciparum Rate). Severe malaria due to P.falciparum is also increasing.

Under reporting, drug resistance and insecticide spray are major field problems encountered in malaria control in the country. Under reporting is due to absence of lab facilities and weak surveillance system. Because of drug resistance India has adopted artemisinin based combination therapy (ACT). Insecticide treated nets are introduced to supplement indoor residual spray.

In the course of anti malaria measures, following epidemiological types of malaria are observed:

1. Tribal malaria more with forest related activities where women and children

succumb to deaths. Lack of drugs and facilities are attributed.

2. Rural malaria more in irrigated areas
3. Urban malaria in metropolitan cities.
4. Project area malaria in construction and developmental activities.
5. Border malaria with poor administrative control.

During 2005, total malaria cases reported are 1808217 in India of which 798546 are Plasmodium falciparm type. During the same year 940 deaths are reported due to malaria. Orissa has recorded highest number of cases and Punjab has recorded lowest number of cases during 2005.

When female anopheles mosquito feeds on malaria patient, it sucks gametocytes which develop in mosquito to infective sporozoite state in 7-20 days. When mosquito with sporozoites in saliva bites human, man gets sporozoite entry which will disappear from blood and enter liver. Later merozoites attack RBC where schizonts are produced. Rupture of schizont releases more merozoities to blood which causes fever and rigor; the periodicity is tabulated as under:

P. vivax	–	Benign tertian malaria
P. malariae	–	Quartan malaria
P. ovale	–	Ovale tertian malaria
P. falciparum	–	Malignant tertian malaria

Incubation period is 15 days in P.vivax, 15 days in P.ovale, 12 days in P. faliciparum and 30 days in P. malariae.

Figure 18.39 depicts the agent, host and environment factors in determining the prevalence of malaria in a community.

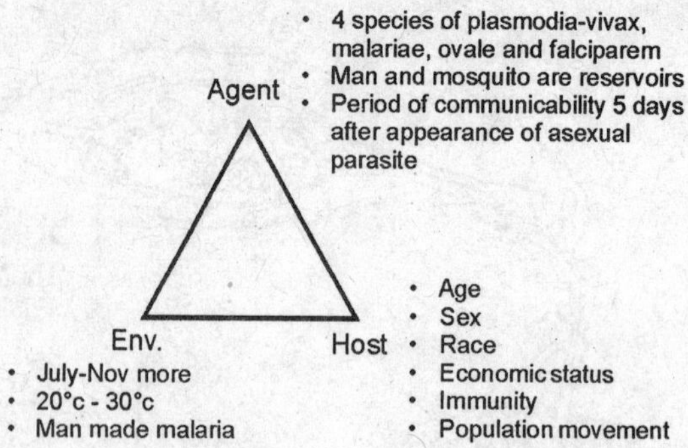

Fig. 18.39: Malaria epidemiology

Clinical Features:

Vivax and Ovale Malaria: Illness starts several days of continued fever before classical fever on alternate days. Fever starts with rigor. Patient feels very cold but body temperature rises to 40°C. Hot phase is followed after 30 minutes of temperature. 4-6 hours later profuse perspiration and fall in temperature. Splenomegaly and hepatomegaly which show tenderness are later manifestations. Slowly anaemia develops. In 20% of cases development of herpes simplex is seen. Relapse is common even after 2 years in case of vivax and ovale malariae.

Malariae Malaria: It produces mild symptoms. Fever appears every third day. Even a symptomatic case with MP smear +ve is known. Among children malariae is known to cause nephrotic syndrome and glomerulonephritis.

Falciparum Malaria: This produces severe malaria. Onset is slow with malaise, headache, vomiting and often mistaken for influenza, Mild diarrhoea and cough are seen in most of the patients. Fever do not follow a specific pattern. Because of liver dysfunction and haemolysis, clinical jaundice appears early. Spleenomegaly and hepatomegaly are common and they are tender. Very rapid, development of anaemia is seen with falciparum malaria. A patient with severe falciparum malaria present with confusion, drowsiness, extreme weakness, prostration. The following clinical entity is noticed with severe malaria which needs special nursing care in day to day practice.

- Cerebral malaria, defined as unarousable coma not attributable to any other cause in patient with falciparum malaria

- Generalised convulsions
- Severe normocytic anaemia
- Hypoglycaemia
- Metabolic acidosis with respiratory distress
- Fluid and electrolyte disturbances
- Acute renal failure
- Acute pulmonary oedema and adult respiratory distress syndrome (ARDS)
- Circulatory collapse, shock, septicaemia (algid malaria)
- Abnormal bleeding
- Jaundice
- Haemoglobinuria
- High fever
- Hyper parasitaemia.

Malaria Measurement in the Community

i. **Spleen rate:** Percentage of children 2-10 years who show spleenomegaly.

ii. **Parasite rate:** Percentage of children 2-10 years who shown M.P. smear +ve.

iii. **Infant parasite rate:** Percentage of infants (0-1) who show M.P. smear +ve.

iv. **Proportional case rate:** It is number of malaria cases out of 100 attending hospital patients.

Parasitological indicators of malaria in a community.

i. A.P.I.=
(Annual Parasite Incidence)

$$\frac{\text{Confirmed cases during 1 year}}{\text{Population under surveillance}} \times 1000$$

ii. A.B.E.R. =
(Annual Blood Examination Rate)

$$\frac{\text{No. of slide examined}}{\text{Population}} \times 100$$

iii. A.F.I. (Annual Falciparum incidence)

iv. S.P.R. (Slide Positive Rate)

v. S.F.R. (Slide Falciparum rate).

Case Management and Nursing Care

P.vivax, P.ovale, P.malariae infections should be treated with chloroquine 600 mg base followed by 300 mg base in 6 hours, Later 150 mg base 12 hourly for 2 more days. Relapse is overcome by antimalarial drugs in suppressive doses. Primaquin 15 mg daily for 14 days will destroy hypnozoits phase in liver. Haemolysis and cyanosis are common but not dangerous.

P. falciparum is best treated with quinine 10mg/kg body weight 8 hourly by mouth till clinical improvement and till M.P. smear is –ve. This is followed by single dose of sulfadoxine 1.5 G combined with pyrimethamine 75 mg. In pregnancy 7 days Quinine is given. Alternatively Atovaquone 250 mg + Proguanil 100 mg 4 tablets once daily for 3 days is given.

Nursing Care

Good nursing care of the patient with severe malaria is of vital importance.

i. Ensure meticulous nursing care. This can be life saving for unconscious patient. Maintain clear air way. Nurse the patient in the lateral or semiprone position to avoid aspiration of fluid. Insert a nasogastric tube and suck out the stomach contents to minimize the risk of aspiration pneumonia. Since aspiration pneumonia is fatal, it is dealt with by attending nursing staff by giving:

   a. Parenteral antimicrobials
   b. Change position of patient
   c. Give physiotherapy and
   d. Give oxygen. Turn the patient every 2 hours. Do not allow him to lie in a wet bed. Pay attention to pressure points.

ii. Keep a careful record of fluid intake and output. If this is not possible, weigh the patient daily in order to calculate the approximate fluid balance.

iii. Note any appearance of black urine (Haemoglobinuria).

iv. Check the speed of infusion of fluids frequently. Too fast or too slow infusion can be dangerous.

v. Monitor temperature, pulse, respiration and blood pressure every 4 hours.

vi. Monitor level of consciousness.

a. Glasgow coma scale for adults:

Eyes open	Spontaneously	4
	To speech	3
	To pain	2
	Never	1
Best verbal response	Oriented	5
	confused	4
	In appropriate word	3
	In comprehensible sound	2
	None	1
Best motor response	Obeys commands	5
	Localises pain	4
	Flexion to pain	3
	Extension to pain	2
	None	1
	Total	3 to 14

If score is 10 it is unrousable coma.

It has to be done repeatedly to assess improvement or deterioration.

b. Paediatric coma scale for child: (Blantyre coma scale)

Best motor response	Localises pain stimuli (Rub knuckle on child sternum)	2
	Withdraw limb from pain (Firm pressure on thumb-nail bed with pencil)	1
	No response	0
Verbal response	Appropriate cry	2
	Moaning	1
	None	0
Eye movement	Directed (Follow mother face)	1
	Not directed	0
	Total	0-5

Score of 3 is unarousable coma.

It has to be repeated to assess either improvement or deterioration.

vii. Report level of consciousness, convulsions or change in behaviour to duty doctor. All such changes need additional treatment.

viii. Rectal temperature if above 39^{0}C, rectal paracetamol is given, tepid sponging is done. Fanning continued.

As duty nurse, never allow duty doctor to give chloroquine to treat severe falciparum malaria, in view of chloroquine resistance in severe malaria.

Special Nursing Care in Severe Malaria of a Child

Nursing care should include all well established principles of the care of unconscious child. Every 2 hours frequent turning of the child; careful attention to airways, eyes, mucosae, skin and fluid requirements. The child should be nursed in the lateral or semi-prone position.

Special paediatric nursing care should include:

- Insert nasogastric tube to minimise risk of aspiration pneumonia
- Correct hypoglycaemia
- Restore circulating volume
- Treat anaemia.

Special Immediate Nursing Care of Complications of Malaria

All cases are attended with suggested chemotherapy for severe malaria.

Apart from that, immediate nursing management of complications includes the following:

1. Hyperpyrexia
   - Paracetamol 15 mg /kg
   - Tepid sponging
   - Fanning

2. Spontaneous bleeding, coagulopathy
   - Transfuse fresh whole blood
   - Transfuse clotting factor
   - I.V. Vit-K 10 mg.
3. Shock due to algid malaria
   - Suspect gram –ve septicaemia
   - Take blood sample for culture
   - Give parenteral antimicrobial
   - Correct hemodynamic disturbances
4. Acute pulmonary oedema
   - Avoid excess rehydration
   - Prop up the patient
   - Give oxygen
   - Give frusemide 15 mg I.V.
   - Withdraw 3ml/kg by venesection into donor bag.
5. Metabolic acidosis
   - Treat hypoglycaemia
   - Treat hypovolaemia
   - Treat septicaemia
   - Give isotonic saline 20ml/kg rapidly
   - Give whole blood 10ml/kg over 30 min
   - Do not allow Hb% fall below 5 G%.
6. Hypoglycaemia
   - R.B.S. take blood and check
   - 50% dextrose 50 ml followed by 5 or 10% dextrose infusion.
7. Acute renal failure
   - Exclude dehydration
   - Maintain fluid balance
   - If indicated dialysis.
8. Severe anaemia
   - Whole blood transfusion
   - Packed cell transfusion.
9. Hyper parasitaemia
   - Parenteral antimalaria therapy
   - Exchange transfusion
10. Malaria haemoglobinuria
    - Continue antimalaria treatment
    - Fresh blood transfusion.
11. Convulsion
    - Maintain airway
    - I.V. Diazepam (0.15mg/kg)
    - Intrarectal (0.5mg/kg)
    - I.M. Paraldehyde (0.1mg/kg).
12. Coma
    - Maintain airway
    - Exclude hypoglycaemia, exclude bacterial meningoencephalitis
    - Avoid corticosteroids
    - Avoid heparin
    - Avoid adrenaline.

National Level Malaria Control Programmes

- 1953 N.M.C.P. initiated
- 1958 N.M.E.P. initiated
- 1961 Focal outbreaks started
- 1976 Resurgence of malaria because of:
  a. Administrative failure
  b. Technical failure
  c. Operational failure
- 1977 Modified plan of operation launched
- 1995 Malaria action programme initiated
  a. To create awareness on malaria
  b. To encourage community participation
  c. Diagnosis and treatment through antimalaria month
- 1997 Enhanced Malaria Control Programme
- 1998 Roll back malaria initiative with World Bank assistance for:
  a. Better delivery
  b. Better insecticide
  c. Better training
  d. Use of other effective drugs
- 1999 Renamed as National Anti Malaria Programme
- 2001 Focus on epidemiological types of malaria:
  – Urban malaria
  – Rural malaria
  – Tribal malaria
  – Border malaria
  – Project area malaria

- 2005 Intensified Malaria Control Project.

Malaria Effective Control

a. **Case Management:**
Case detection: all fever cases are subjected to M.P. smear examination (under surveillance).
Active surveillance: Fortnightly visit by health worker, who detects fever, collects blood smear for M.P.
Passive surveillance: All health care institutions detect fever cases, collect blood smear for M.P.

Treatment:

i. Presumptive treatment with chloroquine in low risk areas:

Age	*Chloroquine*	*Remarks*
Below 1 year	75mg (½ Tab)	– Blood smear
1-4 years	150mg (1 Tab)	taken to all
4-8 years	300mg (2 Tab)	
8-14 years	450mg (3 Tab)	– P. T. given
Above 14	600mg (4 Tab)	after food

ii. Presumptive treatment with chloriquine and primaquine in high risk areas:

Age	*Chloroquine (mg)*			*Primaquine(mg)*	*Remarks*
	I day	*II day*	*III day*	*I day*	
Below 1 years	75	75	37.5	–	– Blood smear Taken to all
1-4 years	150	150	75	7.5	
4-8 years	300	300	150	15	– PT given after Food
8-14 years	450	450	225	30	– No primaquine for pregnant and infant
Above 14 years	600	600	300	45	

iii. Radical treatment for vivax, malariae, ovale:

Age	*Chloroquine (mg)*	*Primaquine(mg)*	*Remarks*
Below 1 year	75	–	
1-4 years	150	2.5	– No primaquine for pregnant and infant
4-8 years	300	5	
8-14 years	450	10	
above 14 years	600	15	

iv. Radical treatment for faliciparum and malaria:

Age		*Chloroquine (mg)* *I day*		*Primaquine (mg)* *II day*	*Remarks* *III day I day*
Below 1 year	75	75	37.5	–	– No primaquine for pregnant and infant
1-4 years	150	150	75	7.5	
4-8 years	300	300	150	15	
8-14 years	450	450	225	30	
Above 14 years	600	600	300	45	

v. Chloroquine resistant cases (Adult dose) :

1. Presumptive

Amodiaquine	600 mg
OR	
Sulphaline	1000 mg
Pyrimethamine	50 mg

2. Radical

Sulphaline	1000 mg	Single dose
Pyrimethamine	50 mg	
Primaquine	45 mg	

Malaria Chemoprophylaxis:
Person should take any one of the following till he moves in endemic areas:

i. Chloroquine – 500 mg weekly
ii. Chloroquine – 300 mg weekly + proguanil – 200 mg daily
iii. Chloroquine–300 mg weekly + Pyramithamine – 500 mg daily.

b. Public Health Measures:

Area with A.P.I. Above 2

- Spraying 2 rounds D.D.T./3 rounds H.C.H.
- Entomological assessment.
- Surveillance
- Case management.

Area with A.P.I Below 2

- Focal spraying
- Surveillance
- Case management
- Follow up
- Epidemiological investigation

c. Integrated Vector Control:

Following are the major measures through integrated vector control:

- Residual spray
- Antilarval measures
- Personal protection
- Control of breeding places by intermittent irrigation and source reduction.

d. Malaria Vaccine:

Trophozoites, Merozoites and sporozoites are used in the preparation of vaccines. Research with SPf 66 and PfS 25 vaccines on experimental animals are ongoing. But they are not available for community prevention.

Set Goals for Tenth Five Year Plan
Set goals are Annual Blood Examination Rate over 10%, Annual Parasitic Index 1.3 or less and 25% reduction in morbidity and mortality due to malaria by 2007 and 50% by 2010 as per National Health Policy.

DISEASES NOT PRESENT BUT NEED TO BE NOTED

Yellow Fever (India Does Not Have)

Yellow fever is not present in India. Its knowledge is very much required on two grounds.

a. It is an International Quarantinable disease
b. India has suitable climate, suitable vector and susceptible population and if it gets, it is disasterous.

Yellow fever is found in the tropical forest of Africa and South America (Fig. 18.40).

West Africa was probably the original home of yellow fever, which might have been transported to the Americas by ships carrying infected mosquitoes in the post Colombian period. Although potential vector is there in India, Asia, Australia, Europe, it has never been established there. Epidemiologists predict that catastrophic epidemic will occur if it enters above mentioned countries.

Agent, host and environment factors are depicted in Figure 18.41.

Mode of Transmission:
There are two main cycles of transmission:

a. The jungle (sylvan) cycle
b. Urban cycle (Fig. 18.42 and Fig. 18.43).

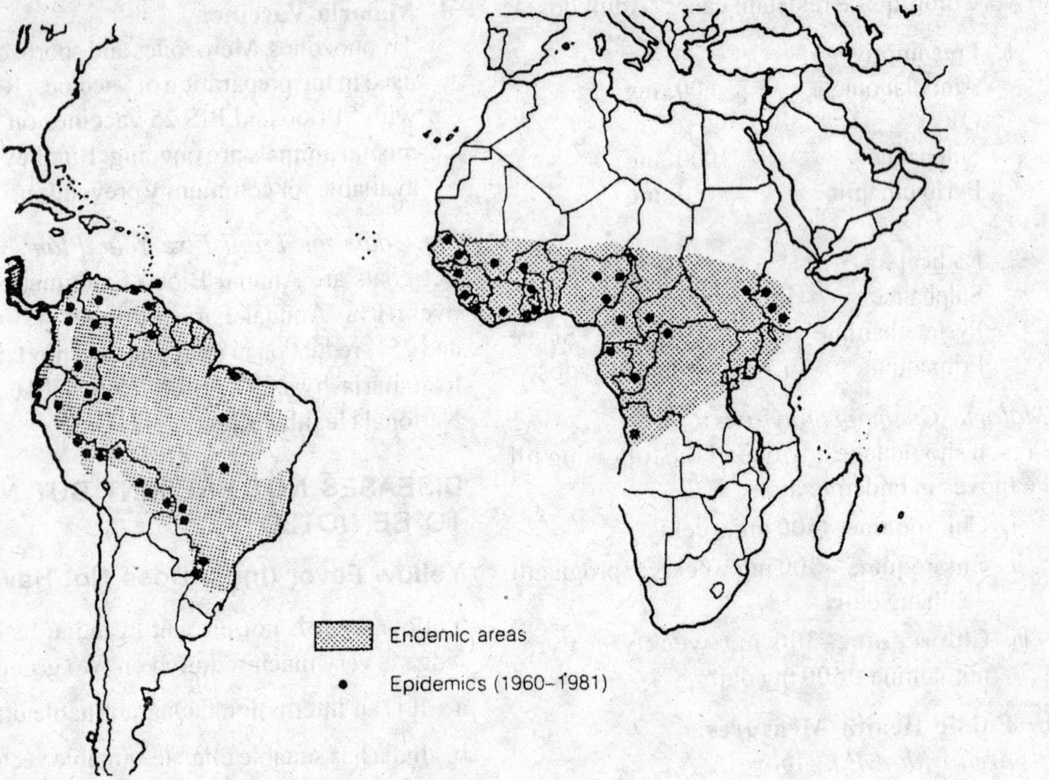

Fig. 18.40: Geographical distribution of yellow fever

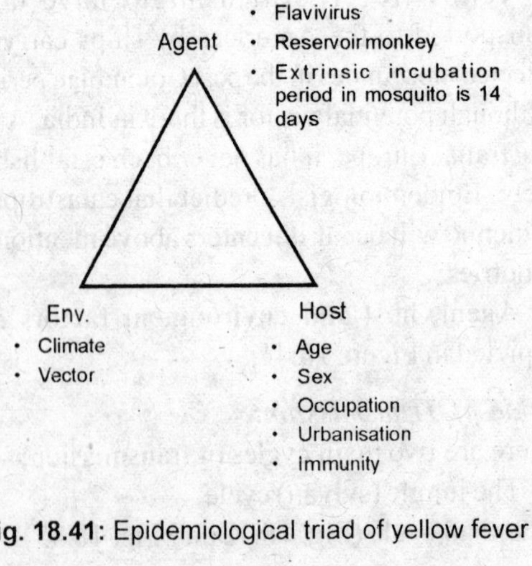

Fig. 18.41: Epidemiological triad of yellow fever

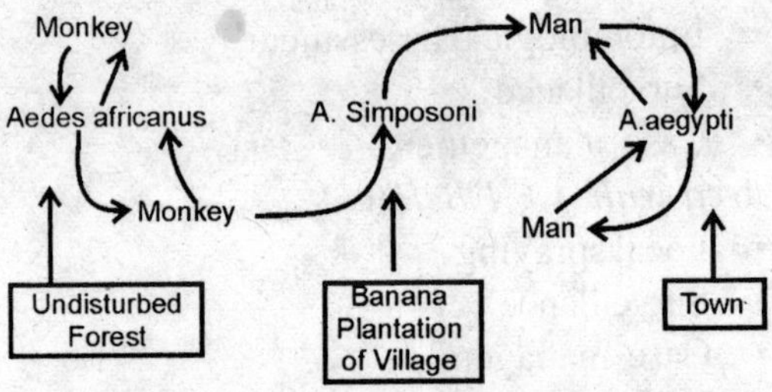

Fig. 18.42: Yellow fever ecosystem in Africa

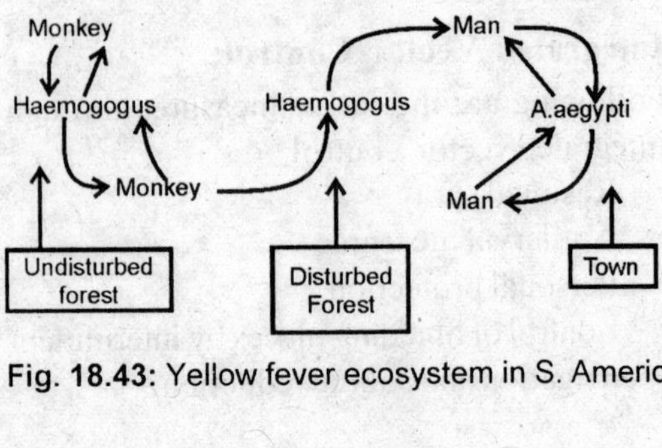

Fig. 18.43: Yellow fever ecosystem in S. America

Incubation period is 3-6 days.

Clinical Features:
It is mild fever lasting for one week. It starts with rigors and high fever. Backache, headache and bone pains are severe, Nausea, vomiting develops later. Bradycardia and leucopenia are common. Fever returns with acute hepatic and renal failure. There is jaundice and a haemorrhagic diathesis with Petechiae haemorrhages into the mucosa and G.I. bleeding plus oliguria.

Nursing Management

Whole treatment is supportive, with meticulous attention to fluid and electrolyte balance. B.P. and urine output need to be recorded. There may be requirement of Blood transfusion, plasma expanders and peritoneal dialysis. Patient is infectious and must be isolated during illness.

Control of Yellow Fever:
Jungle yellow fever is very difficult to control. People who go to deep forest are given yellow fever vaccine.

Urban Yellow Fever Control:

a. Immunisation of people at risk and of people who live in endemic area.
b. Intensive Aedes mosquito control.
c. Yellow fever surveillance.
d. Aedes aegypti index is maintained below 1.0 (The percentage of houses and their premises in a limited well defined area showing actual breeding of Aedes aegypti larvae is called aedes aegypti index).

India and Yellow Fever:

i. Quarantine (airport, sea port regulations).
ii. Ecological barrier is not answered.
iii. India is yellow fever receptive.
iv. Care is taken when given with other vaccine to travellers.
v. Pune and Kausali are referral centres on yellow fever

Yellow Fever Vaccine: It is a live attenuated vaccine called 17 D vaccine. Dose is 0.5 ml. subcutaneous route on deltoid give protection from 10th day up to 10 years.

International measure include (a) Case notification by telegraph to WHO, (b) Ship, aircraft, land transport regulation, (c) Animal quarantine and (d) Vaccination certificate to people travelling to America and Africa.

Travellers from infected area and even in transit need yellow fever vaccination. The validity is from 10th day of vaccination to 10 years. Re vaccination validity starts on the day of vaccination.

Two yellow fever reference centres one in Pune and the other is in Kasouli are developed under yellow fever containment activities.

Smallpox (World Does Not Have)

We do not have smallpox today. World has declared smallpox free in 1977 when a case from Somalia was last reported.

Similarly India was declared smallpox free in 1977 when a case from Bihar was last case reported.

With the eradication of smallpox we have prevented annual occurrence of 15 million smallpox cases, 2 million deaths by smallpox and 500,000 blindness due to smallpox. The strategy used is worth highlighting which is based on the following epidemiological basis.

They are:

- No animal reservoir
- No carrier stage
- Life long immunity after smallpox
- Diagnosis easy
- Subclinical case do not transmit
- Vaccine is 100% effective
- There was international cooperation.

Current Status

i. As per amendment by WHO assembly
   - All reference to smallpox deleted
   - Smallpox vaccination is discarded.

ii. WHO has identified 2 potential sources
   - Laboratory viral stock
   - Animal pox virus
     a. Human monkeypox
     b. Tanapox.

Smallpox rashes are compared with chickenpox for academic differentiation (See Table 18.21).

DISEASES UNDER CONTROL MEASURES

Tuberculosis

A chronic bacterial disease caused by M.tuberculosis is an important cause of death in the world. One third of world population is infected and it is the cause of 2.5 million deaths annually. Both pulmonary and non pulmonary tuberculosis have become public health problem. Its epidemiology and control measures are discussed in page 284.

Sexually Transmitted Diseases (STD)

They are contagious bacterial, viral, protozoal, fungal and ectoparasite infections of man whose principle mode of transmission is by intimate sexual contact. Earlier five classical venereal diseases viz., syphilis, gonorrhoea, chancroid, lympho-granuloma venerium and granuloma inguinale are added with many more sexually transmitted diseases which formed a giant group called STD's. They are enumerated in Table 18.12.

Global prevalence of STD is varying from 1 to 14 percent in the vulnerable population. Gonorrhoea and primary syphilis are on the increase. STD's are showing antimicrobial resistance which is a concern to the case management.

Table 18.12: Sexually transmitted diseases

First generation STD:	
1.	Syphilis
2.	Gonorrhoea
3.	Chancroid
4.	LGV (Lympho granuloma venerium)
5	GI (Granuloma inguinale)
Second generation STD:	
1.	Trichomonos vaginalis
2.	Scabies genitalia
3.	Thrush
4.	Herpes simplex
5.	Warts of genitalia
Third generation STD:	
1.	HIV/AIDS

Syphilis

The incidence of syphilis has declined steadily. Serological test has shown that syphilis is still being recognised in Antenatal screening procedure. About 12 million cases are Annual estimate of incidence of syphilis. In India, among ANC cases it is about 2.4 percent.

Syphilis is caused by *Treponema pallidum* (a spirochaete) and is sexually acquired with the entry of treponema through abrasions in skin and mucous membranes. Clinically it is manifested in primary, secondary and territory forms.

Primary Syphilis: The incubation period is 9-90 days. Chancre at the site of genital area develops which gets eroded to form an indurated ulcer. Lymph nodes will be enlarged, mobile, discrete and rubbery. Without treatment, this will become an atrophic scar. In 10% of cases extra genital lesions on finger, lip, tongue, tonsil, nipple, anus and rectum are seen.

Secondary Syphilis: After 2 months of development of chancre multisystem disease is noted. Fever, malaise, headache are common. About 75% manifest rash. These popular rashes coalescing to plaque are called condyloma lata.

In 50% of cases lymphadenopathy are seen. Other features of cranial nerve palsy, meningitis, hepatitis, periostitis are common. Later the disease enters a phase of latency and is called latent syphilis.

Tertiary Syphilis: This stage develops after 3-10 years of infection. Skin, mucous membrane, bone, muscle and viscera are involved. Gumma is characteristic of syphilis. Gumma of various organs are known. Aortic incompetence, aortic aneurysm, Tabes dorsalis (Meningovascular diseases), General Paralysis of the Insure are common patterns.

Congenital syphilis can lead to stillbirth, syphilitic baby, early congenital syphilis and late congenital syphilis.

Non-specific laboratory tests are VDRL and RPR (Venereal Disease Research Laboratory and Rapid Plasma Regain Test). Specific antibody tests are (a) EIA (Trepanomal antigen based enzyme immunoassay for IgG and IgM, (b) TPHA (T.pallidum Haemaglutination Assay), (c) FTA-ABS (Fluorescent Treponemal Antibody Absorbed Test).

Procaine Benzyl penicillin G 6 lakh units I.M. daily for 17 days or Benzathin penicillin G 2.4 million unit I.M. weekly for 3 doses are recommended. Doxycycline 100 mg 12 hourly for 14 days and Erythromycin 500 mg 6 hourly for 14 days are alternatives.

During nursing care Anaphylaxis, Jarish Herxheimer reaction (malaise, headache, myalgia, optic neuritis etc.) and procaine reactions are to be attended as per hospital procedures.

Gonorrhoea

Nearly 65 million annual incidence is reported globally. It is more common than syphilis. It is caused by *Neisseria gonorrhoea* and clinically Urethritis, Cervicitis, Epididymis salpingitis, PID and neonatal conjuctivitis are manifested. It is the common STD causing genital discharge. I.P. is 2-10 days. Gram negative intra-cellular diplococci under microscopy are diagnostic. Untreated cases go for complications like Prostatitis, Epididymoorchitis, Bartholin abscess, PID and Opthalmia neonatorum.

Ciprofloxacin 500 mg stat, floxacin 400 mg orally stat, or Ampicillin 3 G with Probenecid 1.0 Gram orally stat, are recommended specific treatments.

Chancroid

Chancroid, a soft sore is a disease causing genital ulceration caused by *Haemophilus ducreyi* (Gram –ve bacteria). It is highly prevalent among prostitutes. Single or multiple painful ulcers with ragged undermined edges are seen. Inguinal nodes are enlarged. I.P. is 3-10 days. Microscopy and culture of scraping of ulcer gives diagnosis.

Treatment choices are:

1. Azithromycin 1 gram orally once.
2. Ceftriaxone 250 mg I.M. once.
3. Ciprofloxacin 500 mg 12th hourly orally for 3 days.
4. Erythromycin 500 mg 6th hourly orally for 7 days.

L.G.V.

It is caused by *Chlamydia Trachomatis* types L_1, L_2, L_3. This is confined to the tropics. It is five fold more in men than women. In India it is reported in south India. I.P. is 3 to 30 days. Genital lesion is small, transient, painless ulcer. Vesicle and papule often are unnoticed. Inguinal nodes are enlarged and tender. Serological tests are diagnostic. Case is managed with Doxycycline Hydrate 12 hourly orally for 21 days or Erythromycin 500 mg 6 hourly orally for 21 days.

Granuloma Inguinale (G.I.)

Granuloma Inguinale was first recognised in India by Donovan who observed bodies in oral lesion of G.I. Hence they are called Donovan bodies. The disease is strongly associated with low socio economic state and prostitution. It is common in south India. It is caused by *Klebsiella Granulomatis* (Donovan bodies) and has an I.P. of 3-40 days. Hypertrophic granulomatous painless ulcers on genitals are common findings.

Inguinal lymph node enlargement, abscess and ulceration follow at a later stage. Identification of Donovan bodies is specific and diagnostic tool. Case is managed with Azithromycin 1 G. weekly orally or 500 mg daily orally is suggested. Alternatively Doxycycline Hydrate 100 mg 12 hourly is recommended.

T.V. Infection

Trichomonas vaginalis is a pathogenic protozoan in lower female genito urinary tract. It is world wide in distribution, both in rural and urban situation. High prevalence is in high level sexual activities. It is a common cause of Nongonococcal urethritis. Microscopical examination for T.V. and specific treatment with Metronidazole 400 mg orally 12 hourly for 5 days are measures for effective control of T.V.

Scabies of Genitalia

This is attributed to sexually transmitted disease. Poor personal hygiene and prostitution are contributing factors. Its diagnosis and case management are discussed in the Chapter 9 and chapter 18.

Thrush

Vulvovaginal condition or Balanitis condition is fungal (candidiasis) infection contracted through sexual activity. Cardinal clinical features are pruritus vulvae and vaginal discharge (curd like plaques adherent to vaginal wall. Case is managed with:

i. Clotrimazole 500 mg pessary once at night
ii. Clotrimazole cream 12 hourly
iii. Econazole pessary 150 mg for 3 nights
iv. Fluconazole 150 mg orally stat.

Herpes Simplex

Herpes (genital) by HSV-1 or HSV-2 are known, Asymptomatic primary course followed by asymptomatic general viral infections are recorded. Irritable vesicles rupture and ulcerate on genitalia. Fever, malaise, headache are common clinical features of herpes. Tissue culture and typing are diagnostic of Herpes Simplex infection.

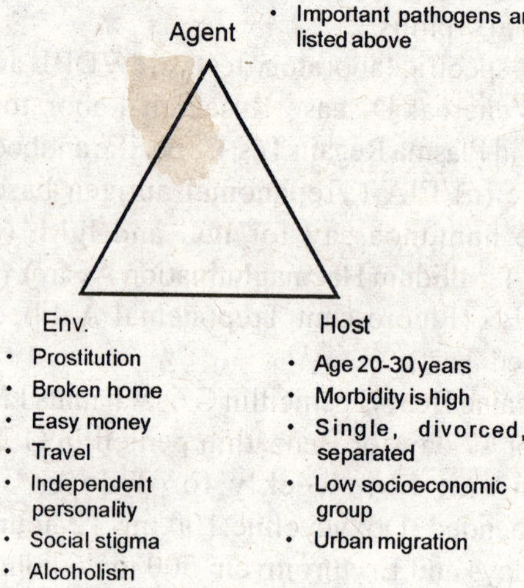

Fig. 18.44: Epidemiological triad in STD's

The treatment will be:

i. Aciclovir 200 mg 5 times a day
ii. Famciclovir 250 mg 8 hourly
iii. Valaciclovir 500 mg 12 hourly.

Normally the course is for 5 days, may be continued if necessary. For severity or intolerance I.V. therapy is suggested.

Community problem of STD are:

- Still birth
- Birth defects

- Premature birth
- Neonatal mortality
- Neonatal blindness
- Infertility
- Ectopic pregnancy.

S.T.D. Control in the Community

For the control of STD, prevailing situation in terms of local endemicity, survey reports analysis, national resources for the implementation, set objectives and strategies are necessary.

Case detection is done by screening, contact tracing and cluster testing. After confirmation, case is held for complete course of treatment. All contacts must be tested and positive are treated (epidemiological treatment). Health education of the community for personal prophylaxis is undertaken.

STD clinics are established which is found useful to maintain confidentiality, free treatment, counselling and integrated essential care services.

Lab facilities like VDRL, serological examination, smear examination and microscopic facilities are requirement in case finding activities.

STD activities are integrated with primary health care through VHG, MPW at sub centre and PHC, help in overcoming social stigma attached in hiding the disease.

Surveillance of STD

"Surveillance is the continuous scrutinising of factors involved in the distribution and trends of STD through systematic collection, consolidation and evaluation of mortality and other relevant data. This is linked to a system of feedback and action."

STD surveillance is collection of information on STD for community action. Surveillance systems are of 2 types:

1. **Routine Reporting:** S.T.D. case detection and reporting by health personnel include routine report and sentinel report. Surveillance is passive when a case attends clinic is recorded in STD register, entered in tally sheets and reported to authorities. But when health worker visits and finds a case of his reporting it becomes active surveillance.

Table 18.13: Advantage and disadvantage of routine case report

Advantage	*Disadvantage*
– Simple	– Not easy to handle enormous data
– Can be universalized	– Often no denominators
– Can be integrated	– Incomplete data
	– Patients attended by general practitioners are excluded.

2. **Sentinel Reporting:**
   It is the selection of a few reporting units to participate in the process of surveillance. These chosen units conduct serially repeated cross sectional studies (prevalence studies) on selected groups within the population. Following specific criteria are considered for selection of sentinel centre:
   a. Large number of S.T.D. cases is seen.
   b. Accurate diagnosis is possible by specialists and by support service.
   c. They use standard case definition.
   d. Willing to participate in surveillance.

Table 18.14: Advantage, disadvantage of sentinel reporting

Advantage	*Disadvantage*
1. Accurate	1. No definite population by Sentinel centre
2. Complete	2. Cannot be extrapolated to general population
3. Regular	
4. Timeliness of data	
5. Few units	
6. Simultaneously we get age, sex and use of condom	

Special studies by (a) Epidemiologists (b) Investigators and (c) Trained health staff will help to: (i) Measure magnitude of a disease (ii) to determine special characteristics with reference to cause and management (iii) Evaluate reliability of routine on sentinel surveillance itself. They are of 2 types:

1. Cross-sectional studies on a given population over a short period of time to determine the prevalence of a particular disease or condition in that population within the same period of time. It is not possible to calculate incidence rates from a single cross sectional study.
2. Community based survey by village based informants at the community, which could be by:
   - Syndrome approach.
   - Aetiological approach.

Syndrome Approach:
Syndrome approach is a method of management and control of STD's where diagnosis and treatment is based on a group of symptoms and signs. Treatment is targeted towards all diseases that could cause that syndrome. It allows diagnosis without extensive laboratory tests and treatment within a single visit. This approach is relevant in the context of Indian condition where laboratory facilities' for diagnosis is limited. Syndrome approach for "5 field-approach" is given in appendix for the following areas (Appendix VII):

- Genital ulcers.
- Vaginal discharge (no speculum examination)
- Vaginal discharge (with speculum examination).
- Urethral discharge.
- Lower abdominal pain in the female (PID).

Aetiological Approach:
Aetiological approach is a system of management of STD's where specialist service is available and laboratory facilities are available.

Under National STD control programme following steps are undertaken in STD surveillance:

Step 1 – Plan for surveillance.
Step 2 – Collection, compilation of data.
Step 3 – Analysis of the data.
Step 4 – Action taken.
Step 5 – Feedback is provided.

Legislation under the Immoral Traffic (Prevention Act) 1986 covers all persons whether male or female who are exploited sexually for commercial purpose, for punishment.

Social welfare schemes for rehabilitation of prostitutes, provision of recreation facilities in the community and marriage counselling are undertaken.

National STD Control Programme:
It is linked with HIV/AIDS and is existing since 1946. Diagnosis and treatment, condom promotion, STD surveillance, IEC activities and family health awareness campaign are detailed under National Health Programmes (Chapter 29).

Kalaazar

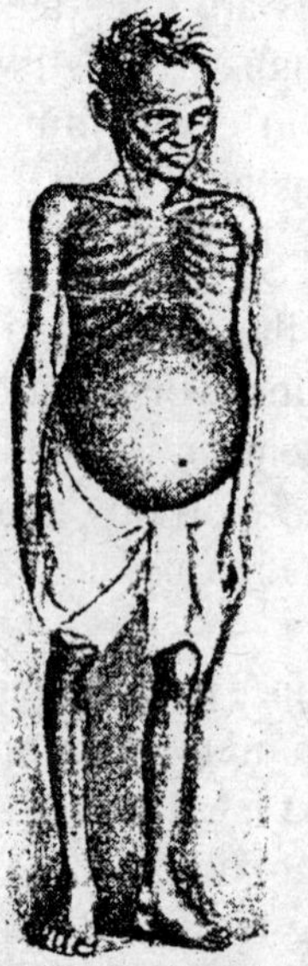

Photo: Patient of kalaazar

Since a group of diseases manifest under this category, Kalaazar is renamed as Leishmaniasis which is caused by Leishmania Donovan bodies. The entities are:

- Visceral Leishmaniasis (VL)
- Cutaneous Leishmaniasis (CL)
- Mucocutaneous Leishmaniasis (MCL)
- Anthroponotic Cutaneous Leishmaniasis (ACL)
- Zoonotic Cutaneous Leishmaniasis (ZCL)
- Post Kalaazar Dermal Leishmaniasis (PKDL).

Leishmania infection in man is of 3 types:
L.donovani cause Kalaazar
L.tropica cause oriental sore
L.brasiliensis cause espundia.

In India vector of transmission of leishmania are by following sand flies:

- Phlebotomus argentipes
- P. papatassi.

The disease is influenced by sandfly breeding, type of housing and occupation. Visceral type (kalaazar) is present in Assam, West Bengal, Bihar, UP, Sikkim, Tamil Nadu and Orissa.

Even now annual occurrence of Kalaazar case are 10 to 15 thousands annually and deaths are around 10 to 200 per year in India as per annual reports from DGHS chronicle. During the period Jan 2005 to July 2006 cases reported have been 50041 and deaths reported have been 219.

Incubation period range from 12 days to 2 years.

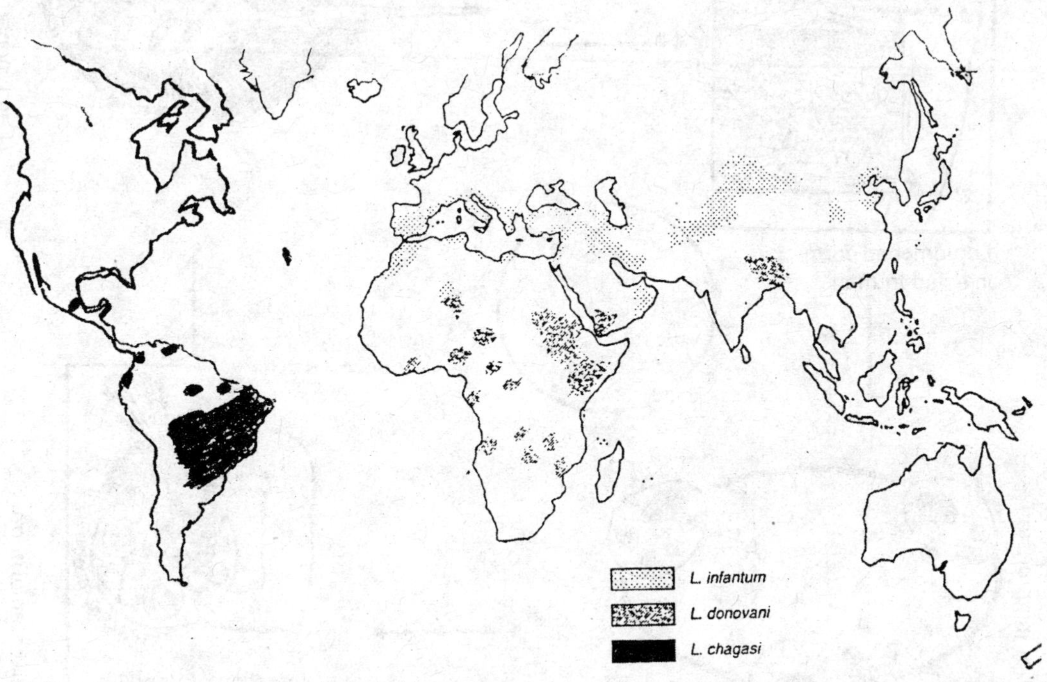

Fig. 18.45: World picture

Clinical Features:

Visceral (Kalaazar)	*Cutaneous (Oriental sore)*	*Mucocutaneous (Espundia)*
1. Fever	1. Mild fever	1. Mild fever
2. Splenomegaly	2. Painful ulcer on exposed parts	2. Ulcer in margin of mouth
3. Hepatomegaly		3. Ulcer in margin of nose
4. Anaemia		4. Face mutilation
5. Weight loss		
6. Skin darkening		

Life Cycle:

From kalaazar patient, sandfly sucks blood, containing L.donovani. This develops to Leptomonad form in sandfly. During blood meal these leptomonad are injected to a new host infecting a new host.

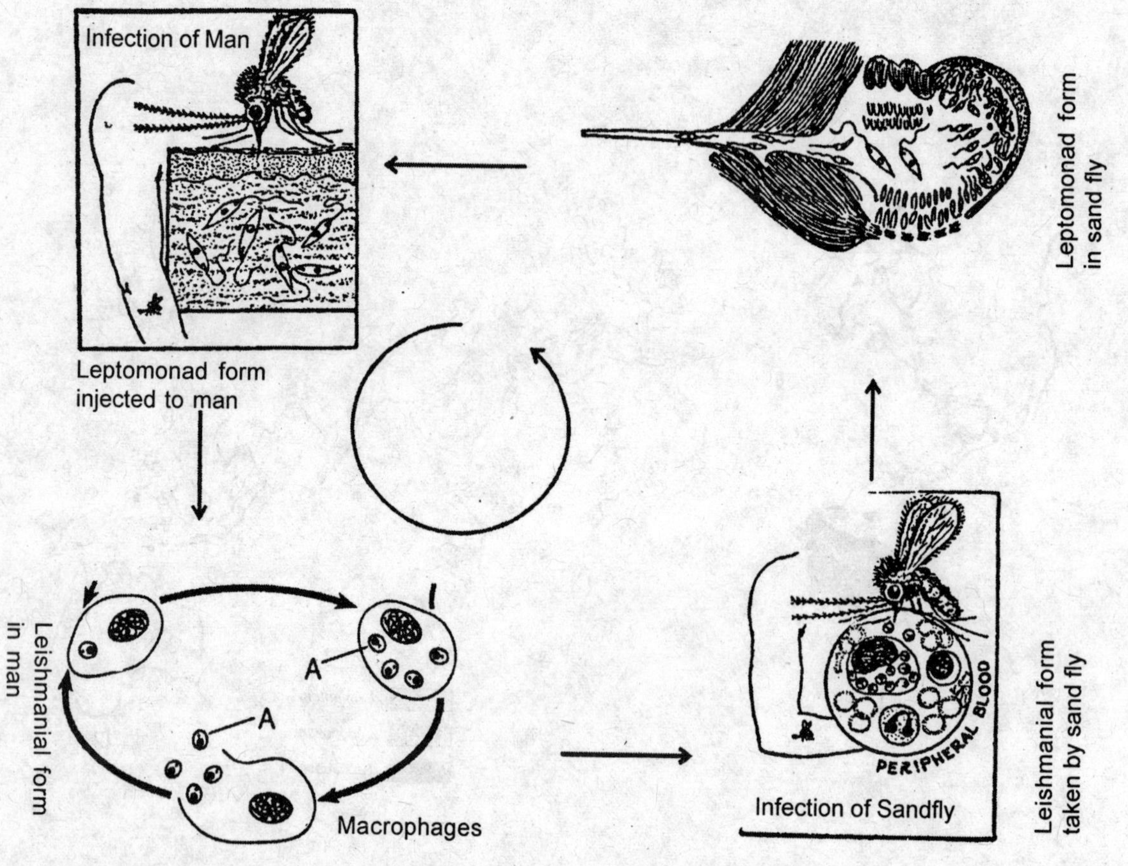

Fig. 18.46: Life cycle of L. donovani

Laboratory Diagnosis:
Blood examination for blood picture, microscopic examination and serological examination are done to establish diagnosis of kalaazar.

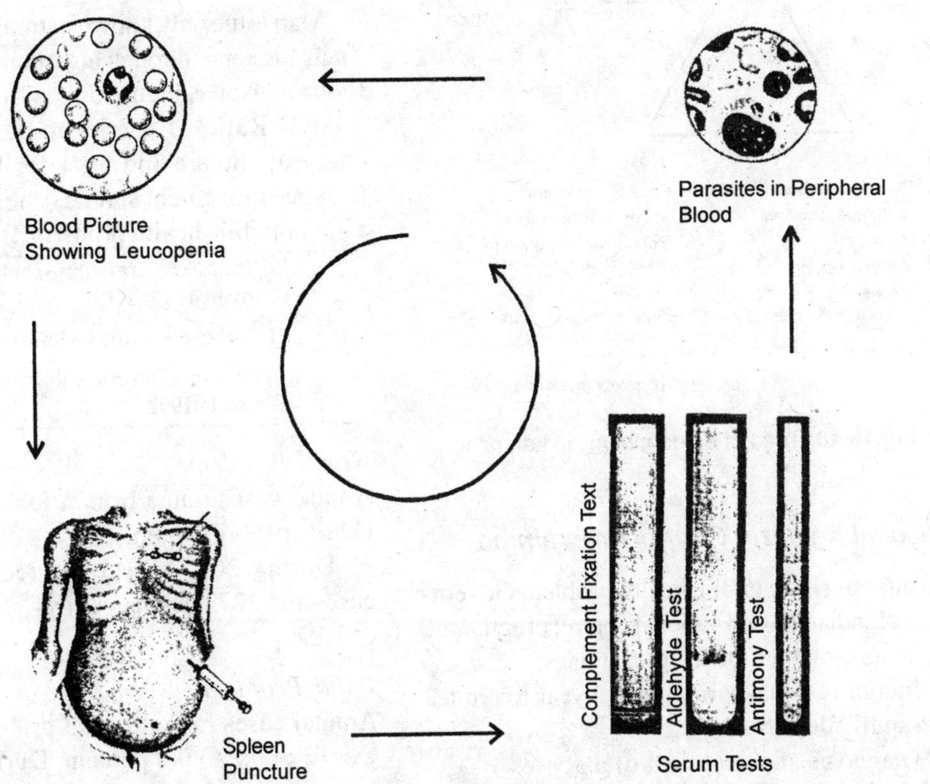

Fig. 18.47: Laboratory tests for kalaazar

Control of Kalaazar:

i. *Case management:* Drug resistance has become a problem in India. Where resources permit, Liposomal Amphoterecin B 2-3 mg/kg equivalent to 21-24 mg/kg of body weight total dose is given over 10 days. Pentavalent antimonials are drug of choice when cost, availability, efficacy and familiarity are considered. Meglumine antimoniate 85 mg sb/ml is also available; the dose is 20 mg sb/kg I.M. daily for 20 days. If there is no tolerance, the dose can be reduced progressively by 2 mg sb/kg. Side effects noticed are cardiac toxicity, myalgia and pancreatitis. Indian trail on oral Miltefosine for 1 month course has shown 100 percent cure rate.
ii. Animal reservoir (dog) is attended with appropriate measures.
iii. Sandfly control by use of insecticide and eliminating breeding places.
iv. Health education for the use of repellent and curtains to protect from the bite of sandfly are advocated.

Epidemiology:
It is depicted in Figure 18.48.

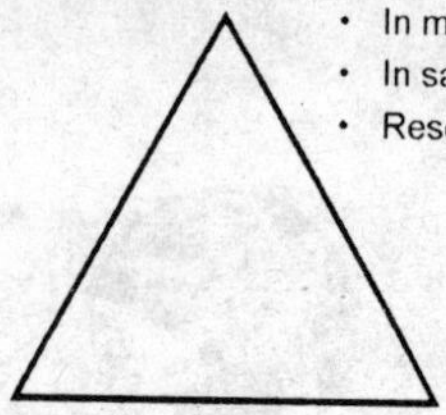

Fig.18.48: Triad of epidemiology in kalaazar

National Kalaazar Control Programme

Because of rising public health problem Government of India initiated national control programme for kalaazar with following strategies:

- Indoor residual spray twice a year to reduce sandfly density.
- Diagnosis and treatment of all cases.
- Health education on kalaazar.

It was initiated in West Bengal and Bihar followed by other states where cases were reported. During 1990 budget provision was made from National malaria eradication programme.

India has come up with a Memorandum of Understanding with Bangladesh and Nepal with the intention of bringing annual incidence below 1 per 10000 by 2010.

Since 2003, one hundred percent centre support by Government of India to achieve elimination of kalaazar by 2010.

Cholera

Cholera, one of the International Quarantine diseases is known to start from its natural home in Ganges plain and delta to the entire world. In world history 1817 pandemic is associated with Indian epidemic which devastated cities and rural India.

Man is the only known natural host of cholera. Transmission is through ingestion of contaminated food and water. Incubation is from few hours to 5 days. Ratio of carrier to case is 50: 1 for classical cholera and 5 : 1 for El Tor cholera. Refugee movement spreads cholera and creates a major public health problem.

- Classical cholera (Vibrio cholera) known even early to 1817.
- El Tor cholera (Eltor vibrio) was found in 1961.
- 0139 strain cholera (cholera of new era) was found in 1992.

World Problem:

Annual cases range from 4 to 6 thousand with C.F.R. of 3-4 percent.

During 2005 world has recorded 131000 cases and 2272 deaths with a Case Fatality Rate of 1.72.

India Problem:

Annual cases range from 3 to 4 thousand with C.F.R. of 0.2 to 0.4 percent. During 2005 India has recorded 3156 cases and 6 deaths with a Case Fatality Rate of 0.19. Agent, host, environment are depicted in Figure 18.49.

Special characteristics of cholera:-

i. Environmental sanitation is greatly associated with cholera.
ii. Seven pandemics are described in global epidemiology

I	–	1817–1823
II	–	1826–1837
III	–	1842–1862
IV	–	1865–1875
V	–	1881–1896
VI	–	1899–1923
VII	–	1964–2003

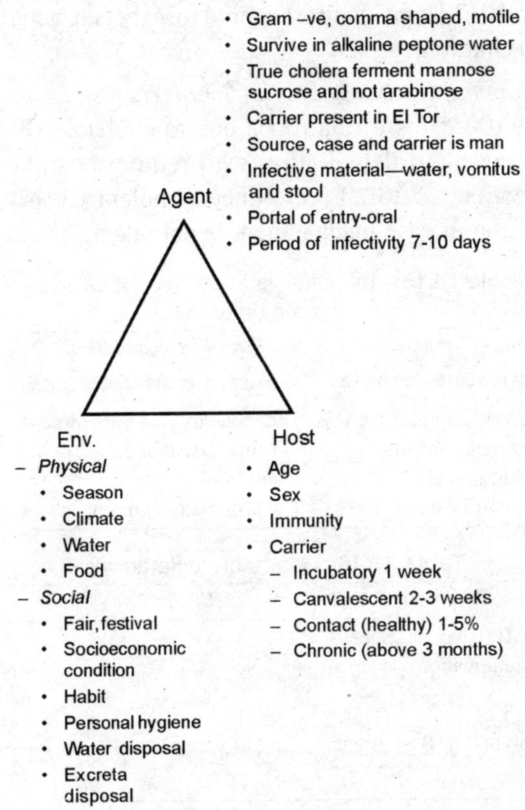

Fig. 18.49: Epidemiology of cholera

iii. It spreads fast and kills many.

iv. Water transmission and person transmission are powerful forces of infection.

v. Absolute differences between classical type and EL Tor type are recorded.

vi. All 3 strains classical, El Tor and 0139 are causing epidemics, deaths and acute public health problem.

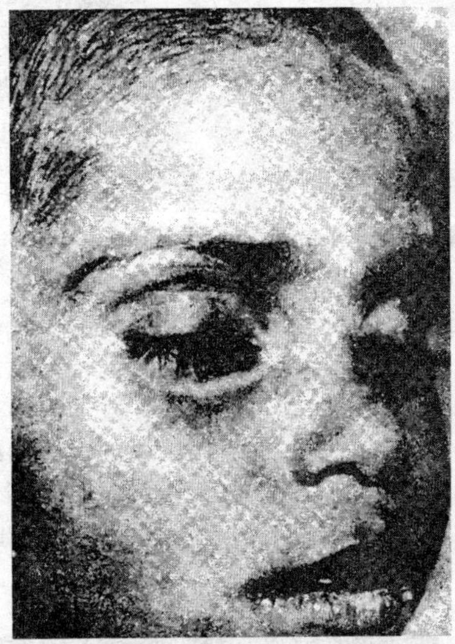

Photo: Sunken eyeball, dry lip and drowsy in cholera

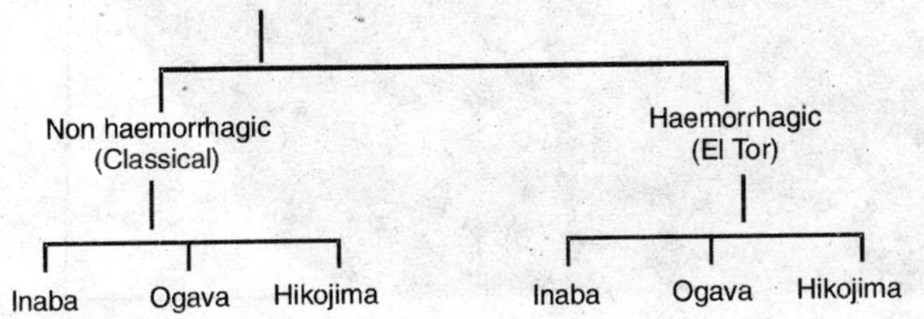

Fig. 18.50: Serological types in cholera

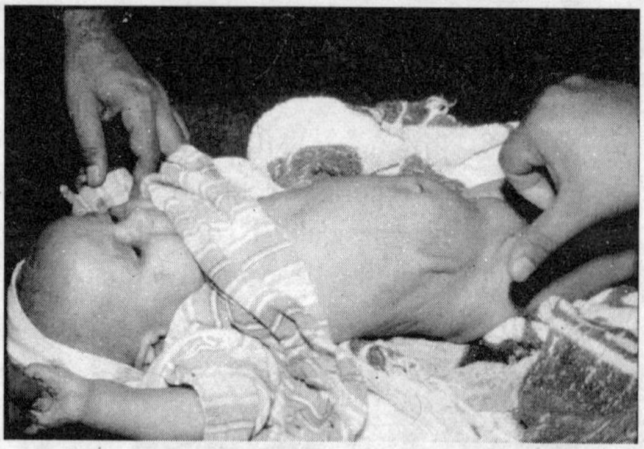

Photo: Skin pinch goes back slowly in dehydration

Clinical Features:
Sudden onset of severe diarrhoea without pain, colic and is succeeded by vomiting. Clear fluid and flecks of mucous characterise diarrhoea as "Rice water" stools. Classical type produces severe dehydration by loss of fluid and electrolytes and lead to muscular cramps. Oliguria shock develops with good mental clarity. Acute circulatory failure causes death. El Tor and 0139 type manifest in mild form but are acute in children.

Community Diagnosis of Cholera:
In 100 cases of diarrhoea due to cholera, 70% show rapid dehydration who require hospitalization. 15 to 20% die due to cholera if early action in case management is not taken.

Table 18.15: Differentials in cholera types in the community

Vibrio Classical	*Vibrio El Tor and 0139*
Severe cases are more	Mild cases are more
Secondary cases are less	Secondary cases are more
Not resistant to environment	More resistant to environment
No carrier stage	Carrier stage present

Table 18.16: Laboratory differentials

	Classical	*El Tor*
RBC (Chicken, Sheep) Agglutination	No	Yes
Phage IV resistance	No	Yes
Polymyxin B resistance	No	Yes
V P reaction	+ve	-ve

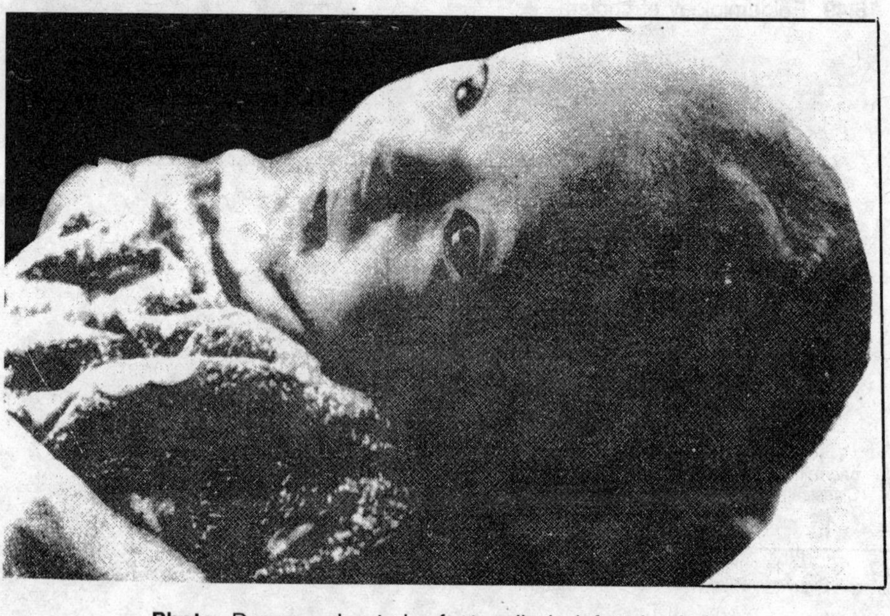

Photo: Depressed anterior fontanelle in infant in cholera

Stool sample collection in isolation wards:

- Fresh sample must be collected
- Should be collected before giving antibiotic
  - i. *Rectal swab:* 20 cm. Long wooden stick with one end wrapped with absorbent cotton, Sterilised by autoclaving, is dipped into holding medium before introducing into rectum. This is placed in a sterile plastic bag, sealed and sent to laboratory with details.
  - ii. *Rubber catheter:* No.26-28 soft rubber catheter is Sterilised by boiling. It is lubricated with liquid paraffin. This is introduced to rectum for a 4cm length. The stool is collected to VR medium and sent to laboratory with details.

Case Management

For sever cases I.V. Ringer Lactate is best fluid. When vomiting stops, oral fluid is started. This may be 5 litres per day in humid climate.

Three-day treatment with Tetracycline 250 mg 6th hourly is recommended. To make Bacterial load to minimum, a single dose of 300 mg Doxycycline or 1 gram of Ciprofloxacin is highly recommended. Children (paediatric ward) nursing care should include to check hypoglycaemia and careful attention to fluid balance.

Cholera Control:

As per WHO guidelines following steps are recommended for cholera control:

a. Confirmation of cholera
b. Notification to local, National and to WHO
c. Early diagnosis and prompt treatment
d. Rehydration by
   - Oral rehydration
   - I.V. rehydration
   - Maintenance therapy
e. Chemotherapy
f. Epidemiological investigation
g. Environmental sanitation
h. Vaccination
i. Health education
   - Confirmation of case of diarrhoea, due to cholera is first task before taking public health measures. Laboratory service is essential.
   - It is internationally quarantinable and notifiable. Notification to local authorities is done who in turn do the further needful.
   - Early diagnosis reduces mortality and early treatment reduces both mortality and morbidity. Isolation hospital, Epidemic disease hospital and treatment centres take care of these as special measures.
   - Rehydration:
     i. Assessment of dehydration:

Table 18.17: Assessment of dehydration

Sign	*Dehydration* *Mild*	*Severe*
Appearance	- Alert - Restless - Thirsty	- Unconscious - Cannot drink - Cold skin (shock)
Skin	- Normal elasticity	- Poor elasticity
Pulse	- Present	- Very weak
Eye, Fontanelle	- Normal	- Sunken
Urine flow	- Normal	- Little
Fluid lacking	- 50ml/kg	- 100ml/kg

During nursing care, check the following at your assessment of dehydration:

- Blood in the stool
- Fever
- Spleen palpable
- Unconsciousness
- Convulsion
- Difficult, fast, deep breathing
- PEM in children

ii. Rehydration

Dehydration	What Fluid	How Much	How Fast
Mild			
a. Who can drink	glucose – salt solution (Breast feeding to continue for infant)	Till they refuse	Within 6 hours
b. Nasogastric tube	Glucose saline or Glucose salt solution	120 ml/kg	6 hours
Severe	Ringer lactate (Hartmann)	100 ml/kg	Within 6 hours
IV fluid	Or		
	Darrow's solution With 2.5% Glucose	150 ml/kg	6 hours
	Or		
	Normal saline	100 ml/kg	6 hours

Oral Fluids

O.R.S. (Oral Rehydration Solution):

Sodium chloride (Table Salt)	3.5 G
Sodium Bicarbonate (Baking soda)	2.5 G
Potassium chloride	1.5 G
Glucose (dextrose)	20.0 G

Home made solution: (for emergency)

Table salt - Thumb and 2 finger pinch

Water Or Orange juice Or Tea — ½ litre

iii. Sustenance takes care of (a) Serious problems that cause or complicate dehydration (b) Maintaining rehydration and (c) Helps in nutritional rehabilitation. During this period nursing care should check:

- Pneumonia
- Otitis media
- Tonsillitis
- Skin infection
- Deep sighing breathing
- Malaria
- Unconsciousness
- Convulsions
- High fever.

Sustenance of rehydration is tabulated as below:

During diarrhoea following medicines are avoided:

- Neomycine (harm intestine)
- Streptomycin (harm intestine)
- Purgative (Worsen dehydration)
- Opium (harm children)
- Epinephrine (do not treat shock in diarrhoea)
- Coramine (do not treat shock in diarrhoea)
- Steroids (harmful).

Situation	Fluid given	How	How much
a. Can drink	Glucose salt solution	Oral	2-3 litres 100-200 ml / kg per day
b. Severe plus one stool every 2 hours	Glucose salt solution	Oral	15ml / kg per hour
c. Severe Diarrhoea persist	I.V. Ringer lactate	I.V.	10 ml / kg per hour + oral fluid

- Kaolin (no value)
- Pectin (no value)
- Lomotil (no value)

iv. Prevention
- Educating mother
- Solving problem of water supply
- Solving problem of sanitation.

Making Oral Fluid in Nursing Care:
One litre glucose salt solution should contain:

Sodium chloride	3.5 G
Sodium bicarbonate	2.5 G
Potassium chloride	1.5 G
Glucose	20.0 G

They are measured, pre packed in aluminum foil and sealed by drug companies. They are distributed through health service network. The above packet is dissolved in 1 litre of drinking water which is suitable size for use in Home visiting.

For clinics, hospitals, bags or bottles containing 10 times this amount for dissolving in 10 litres of water is more practical.

Standard measure is used at dispensing. Once prepared, the O.R.S. should be used within 24 hours. Every 24 hours, fresh solution is prepared. It should not be boiled.

Nutritional Care during Diarrhea

Breast milk is best food for infants and should be continued in diarrhoea also.

Earlier it was believed that undernutrition is due to inadequate food consumption alone. But the role of diarrhoea and other infections in causing undernutrition is now well recognised.

During diarrhoea, following nutritional advice is of paramount importance:

- Soft, easily digestible food which will be almost totally absorbed even if diarrhoea is present.
- Small frequent meals instead of a single large dish:
  - Energy dense food like, oil, ghee or sugar which in small quantity provide more energy and reduce the bulk in food.
- Chemotherapy

Drug	Dose	
Tetracycline for children 500 mg for adults	12.5 mg/kg a day for 3 days	4 times
Doxycycline adults	300 mg	
Trimethroprim	5mg/kg	Children twice daily 3 days
Sulfamethoxazole	25 mg/kg	

- Epidemiological investigation considers source detection, sanitary survey and contact tracing.
- Under environmental sanitation water control, excreta disposal, food sanitation and proper disinfection of patients' secretion and excretion are advocated.
- *Vaccination:* Cholera vaccine is killed vaccine preserved in phenol. Two doses 0.5 ml subcutaneously each at 6 weeks interval give protection for 3-6 months.
- Health education on reporting, food hygiene, vaccination, breast feeding in diarrhoea phase and nutritional care during diarrhoea are advocated.

Cholera Control Programme

The strategy is discussed under Chapter 11, 29 and page 324. It is now under Diarrhoeal Disease Control programme. (C.D.D. programme = Control of Diarrhoeal Diseases Programme).

Diarrhoea

Diarrhoea is a predominant symptom which signifies passage of loose, liquid or watery stools usually more than 3 times a day.

According to WHO, acute diarrhoea is an attack of sudden onset diarrhoea, lasting to 3-7 days or even up to 10-14 days, which is also called "G.E.". Common organisms causing acute watery diarrhoea are:

- Rotavirus
- Astrovirus
- Adenovirus
- Campylobacter jejuni
- Salmonellosis
- Listeria
- E.coli
  - Enterotoxigenic (ETEC)
  - Enteroinvasive (EIEC)
  - Enteropathogenic (EPEC)
  - Enteroagregative (EAEC)
  - Enterohaemorrhage (EHEC)
- Cl.difficile (Antibiotic associated)
- Yersinia
- Cholera.

In case of acute bloody diarrhoea, following pathogens are commonly found in the diagnosis.

- Shigella (Bacillary dysentery)
- Giardiasis
- Amoebiasis
- Cryptosporidia
- Cyclosporia.

Nowadays new entry "Travellers diarrhoea" has emerged which is self-limiting with oral fluid and salt replacement.

There are a few conditions which cause chronic diarrhoea. They are:

- Giardiasis
- Strongyloidiasis
- Hypolactasia
- E.Coli
- Tropical malabsorption
- HIV enteropathy
- Intestinal flukes.

Epidemiological importance of community history directs to the aetiology of diarrhoea.

i. Fever and bloody diarrhoea suggest invasive dysenteric process.
ii. Incubation of below 18 hours suggests food poisoning.
iii. Incubation above 4-5 days suggests protozoal or helminthic.

Problem – World:

WHO estimates about 2 million deaths are occurring annually due to diarrhoea.

Problem – India:

Diarrhoea is a major public health problem causing morbidity and mortality. S.E.A.R.O. has observed that every child below 5 years suffer from diarrhoea twice in one year. Diarrhoea per child per year under five age is 1.7 as per recent survey findings. Proportions of pathogen identified are as under:

No pathogen found	20.0%
Rota virus	15.0%
E.coli	10.0%
C. Jejuni	10.0%
Shigella	5.0%
Vibrio	5.0%
Crypto sporidium	5.0%
Salmonella	1.0%
E.P.E.C.	1.0%
Others	28.0%

Epidemiology:

Agent, host and environmental factors are depicted in Fig 18.51.

Mode of Transmission – Faecal Oral Route:

Inflammatory diarrhoea is charcterised by Abdominal pain, tenesmus and fever. Stool will be small volume, frequent, blood stained, pus cells and mucus are present. Usual site of inflammation is distal small intestine and colon. Mechanism of inflammation is by invasion of enterocytes leading to mucosal cell death and inflammatory response.

Non inflammatory diarrhoea is characterised by nausea, vomiting, abdominal pain and fever (all are mild symptoms). Stool will be voluminous and watery in nature. Site of non inflammatory changes is proximal small intestine. Pathogenesis of symptoms are osmotic or secretary changes.

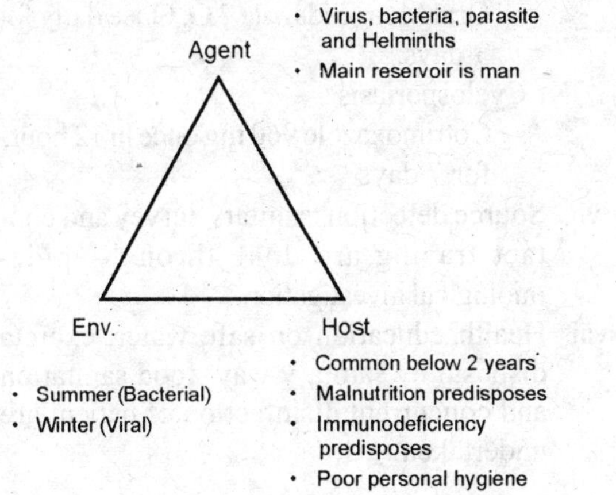

Fig. 18.51: Epidemiological triad in diarrhoea

Nursing diagnosis based on clinical symptoms can be represented as under:

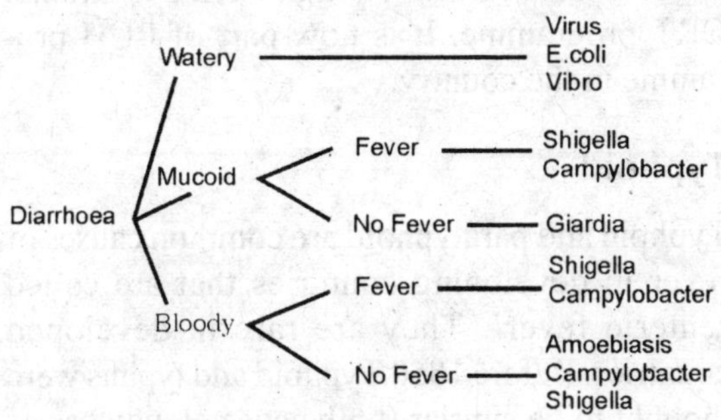

Fig. 18.52: Nursing algorithm in diarrhoea

Control and Prevention of Diarrhoea:

i. *Confirmation of cause of diarrhoea:* With available laboratory facility, cause is ascertained for case management and for public health measures.

ii. *Notification:* Depending on local health authorities, the given cause of diarrhoea has to be notified.

iii. *Early diagnosis and prompt treatment:* Assessment of dehydration, special check during assessment, rehydration, oral fluids, sustenance of O.R.S. and medicines that need to be avoided are detailed under Chapter 18 under rehydration.
Specific treatment depending on the causative agent is recommended.

iv. *Prevention:*
- Educating mother to promote breast feeding
- Food hygiene
- Improved water supply
- Provision of sanitary latrine.

v. Making of ORS is detailed in chapter 18 under making oral fluid, in nursing care.
In diarrhoea only 10 percent of cases show signs of dehydration, which require ORS. Only 1 percent of diarrhoea cases require hospitalization for I.V. followed by O.R.S. (Figure 18.53).

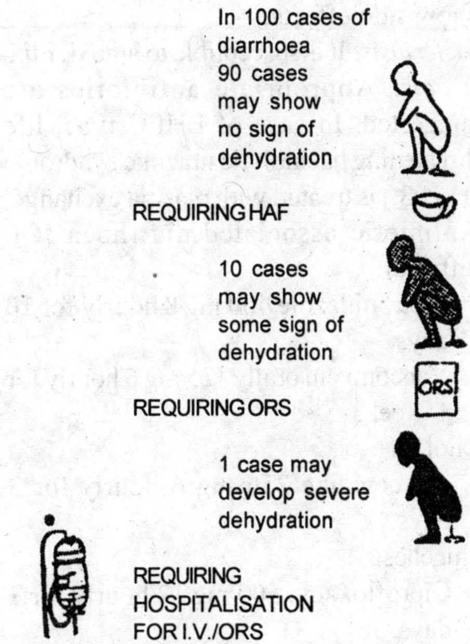

Fig. 18.53: Requirement of HAF, ORS and I.V. fluid (Home available fluid, oral Rehydration solution and Intravenous fluid)

Table 18.18: Minerals and Calories in ORS

	Na	*K*	*Cl*	*Calorie*
WHO	90	20	80	160
Orange juice	0.2	49	-	440
Breast milk	22	36	28	670

Nutritional care during diarrhoea is detailed under Chapter 18.

vi. *Chemotherapy*

A. Rota virus–Adenovirus: Self limiting, need rehydration only.
Other virus: Only in case of severity it is managed by symptomatic treatment.

B. *Campylobacter jejuni:* Self limiting after 1 week. 20% of cases require antibiotics such as ciprofloxacin or a macrolide.

C. *Salmonellosis:* There is no clinical benefit with antibiotics. Instead antibiotic may prolong confirmation of diagnosis and show side effects.

D. *Listeriosis:* It is susceptible to amoxicillin.

E. *E.coli:* Appropriate antibiotics are suggested. In case of EHEC type, life threatening haemolytic uraemic syndrome (H.U.S.) is treated with plasma exchange.

F. Antibiotic associated diarrhoea (Cl. difficile)
- Metronidazole 400 mg 8 hourly for 10 days.
- Vancomycin orally 125 mg 6 hourly for 1 week.

G. Cholera
- Tetracycline 250 mg 6 hourly for 3 days.

H. Shigellosis
- Ciprofloxacin 500 mg 12 hourly for 3 days.

I. Amoebiasis
- Oral metronidazole 800 mg 8 hourly for 5 days.

J. Giardiasis
- Oral Metronidazole 2 G. Once daily for 3 days.

K. Cyclosporiasis
- Cotrimoxazole 960 mg once in 12 hours for 7 days.

vii. Source detection, sanitary survey and contact tracing are done through epidemiological investigation.

viii. Health education on safe water, excreta disposal by sanitary way, food sanitation and concurrent disinfection of patient are undertaken.

Diarrhoeal Disease Control Programme (C.D.D.)

To reduce mortality and morbidity C.D.D. (Control of Diarrhoeal disease) was initiated in 1978. In 1985, it was strengthened by National ORT programme. It is now part of RCH proramme in the country.

Typhoid

Typhoid and paratyphoid are common causes of fever in developing countries that are called 'enteric fever'. They are rare in developed countries. Before 1850 Typhoid and typhus were thought to be similar (both cause cloudiness of mind) and were differentiated only after 1850. It is endemic in Indian subcontinent. Faecal carriers and urinary carriers are known. The carrier state is higher among women and in elderly.

Problem – World: Africa, Asia and Latin America show huge number of cases as well as deaths. Every year 17 million cases are occurring and death are about 6 lakh a year.

Problem – India: It is endemic and every year about 6.5 lakh cases and 400 deaths are occurring in India.
Incubation period – 10-14 days.

Mode of Transmission: Faecal oral route or urine oral route. Directly by ingestion of

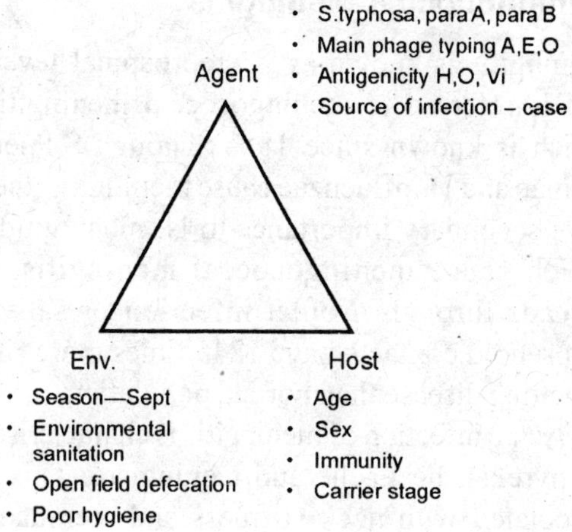

Fig. 18.54: Epidemiology of typhoid

contaminated water, food or flies and indirectly by contaminated hands.

Agents, host and environmental factors are depicted in Figure 18.54.

Clinical Features:

During first week of infection, fever, headache, myalgia, relative bradycardia, constipation, (Diarrhoea and vomiting in young patients) are common.

During second week of infection, Rose spots on trunk, splenomegaly, cough, abdominal distention and diarrhoea are common.

During third week, in untreated cases delirium, complications, coma and death are noticed.

In case of paratyphoid, symptoms are milder, onset is abrupt with acute enteritis, rashes will be abundant and complications are rare.

Complications:

- Perforation and haemorrhage of intestine.
- Septicaemic foci cause bone infection, joint infection, meningitis and cholecystitis.
- Toxic pneumonia.
- Myocarditis.
- Nephritis.

Investigations:

W.B.C. count for Leucopenia
Blood culture in first week
Stool culture in second week
Widal test in second week.

Case Management and Nursing Care

i. Ciprofloxacin 500 mg 12 hourly.
ii. Cotrimoxazole 2 tablet 12 hourly.
iii. Amoxicillin 750 mg 6 hourly.
iv. Chloramphenicol 500 mg 6 hourly.

In resistance case, third generation antibiotics like Cephalosporins, Ceftriaxone and Cefotaxime are used with caution.

The treatment is continued for 14 days. Pyrexia persists for 5 days with treatment. Chronic carriers are treated with ciprofloxacin for 4 weeks. In some cases of carrier's stage, cholecystectomy may be needed.

Control of Typhoid:

i. Case management by early diagnosis. Selective isolation of patient till three Bacteriologically negative stools is checked. Specific treatment course with sensitive drugs are given. Stool and urine of patient is disinfected with 5% cresol for 2 hours. Attending nurse should wash her hands before attending to next patient or for personal work. Follow up of patients reduces the development of carrier stage.
ii. Carriers are given one course of drugs as suggested under case management. In chronic carriers like legendary typhoid Mary (who was responsible for thousands of cases in her life time) need cholecystectomy with ampicillin treatment. Surveillance and health education on personal hygiene adds to specific line of management.
iii. Sanitation:
    - Water purification
    - Food hygiene
    - Environmental hygiene

iv. *Immunisation:* Monovalent, Bivalent and trivalent vaccines are available. Monovalent is preferred to traditional TAB vaccine. Dose is 0.5 ml. subcutaneous at an interval of 6 weeks (2 doses are given). Booster dose is required once in 3 months. Except for local reaction, there is no side effect with typhoid vaccine. It is stored at 2-4°C.

Oral vaccine is available (Typhoral). It contains Ty21 strain. It is available in enteric coated capsule form. One capsule on 1st, 3rd and 5th day one hour before meal in tepid water; gives protection from 15th day to 3 years.

Prevention:

Improved sanitation and improved living condition reduces the incidence. Travellers visiting endemic area are immunised to overcome the infection.

Meningococcal Meningitis

Meningitis is known as "Cerebrospinal fever" and is referred to meningococcal meningitis, which is known since 1887. Though S.Pneumoniae and H.influenzae cause meningitis, they have secondary importance to N. meningitidis which cause meningococcal meningitis. It spreads through droplet infection or saliva. Household contacts have 1245 times more risk in getting disease than normal population.

Acute infection of meningitis is characterised by pyrexia, headache and meningism. This is associated with neck stiffness and meningeal irritation, which is demonstrated by:

i. *Kernig's sign:* With the hip joint flexed, extension at the knee causes spasm in the hamstring muscles.

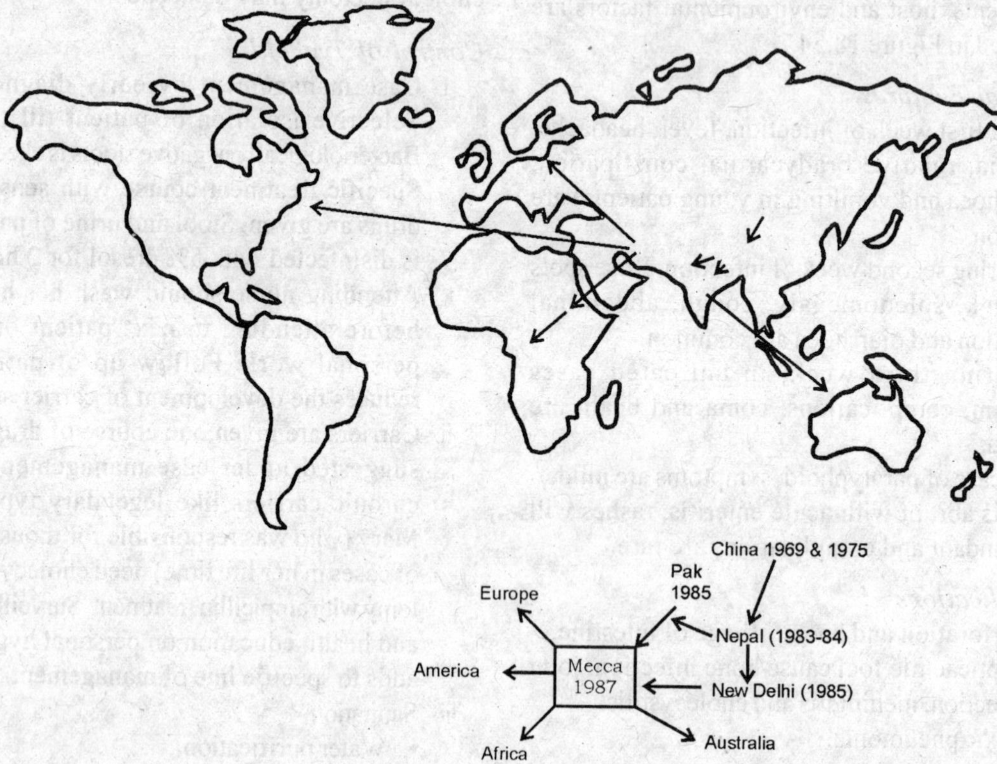

Fig. 18.55: Epidemic of meningococcal meningitis (Mecca epidemic of 1987 – Route)

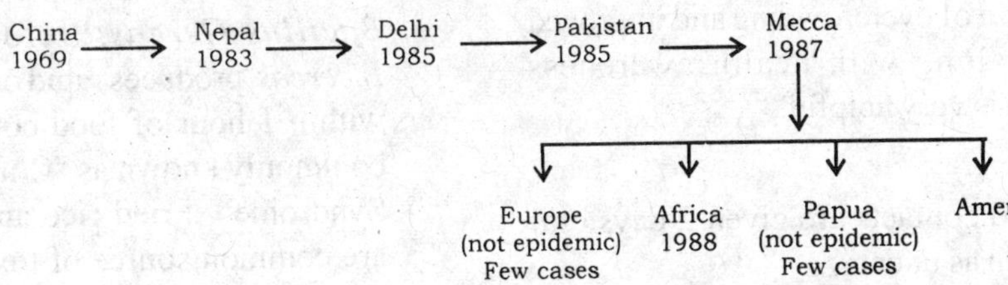

Fig. 18.56: Route of spread of "Clone III 1" meningitis

ii. *Brudzinski's sign:* Passive flexion of the neck causes flexion of the thighs and knees.

Untreated meningitis has 80-90% CFR where as with treatment it reduces to less than 10% CFR.

World – Problem:

1 to 2 million cases are occurring every year with 2 to 3 lakh annual deaths.

India – Problem:

Sporadic meningitis cases are being reported. Annual case is about 7 to 8 thousand and annual death is about 4 to 5 hundred.

Incubation period – 3 – 4 days.

Mode of transmission is by droplet infection.

Agent, host and environmental factors are depicted in Figure 18.57.

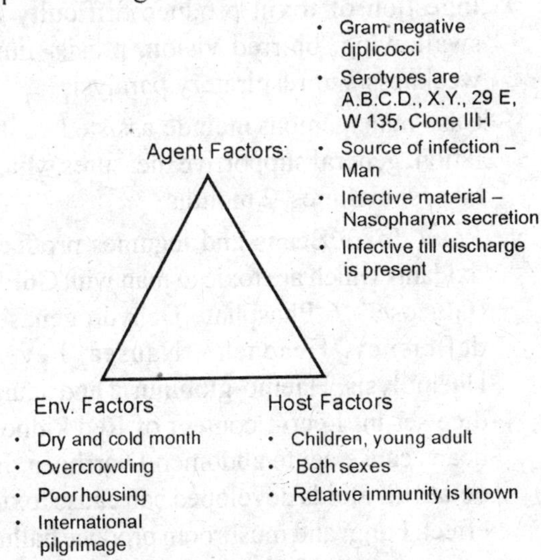

Fig. 18.57: Epidemiology of meningitis

Clinical Feature:

Headache, drowsiness, fever, neck stiffness, signs of cerebral oedema due to endotoxin /cytokine release, purpuric skin rash and circulatory failure.

Investigation – Lumbar puncture (L.P.).

Case Management and Nursing Care:

Benzylpenicillin 2.4 G. I.V. 6 hourly even before hospital admission is advocated. Hospitalisation, regular nursing care and C.S.F. analysis for any treatment regimen change, are advocated. Steroid therapy is useful in paediatric patients.

Control Measures:

i. **Case Management:**
Life saving penicillin is given as suggested under case management. Isolation has limited use.

ii. **Carrier Management:**
Rifampicin or more powerful antibiotics are advocated to eradicate organisms in carriers.

iii. **Contact Management:**
They need chemoprophylaxis. Rifampicin 600mg BD for 2 days for adults is given.

iv. **Mass Management:**
In international religious congregations (e.g. Mecca), medically supervised chemoprophylaxis is undertaken.

v. **Vaccination:**
Monovalent or polyvalent vaccines are administered to risk group or visiting group which gives 3 years immunity. It is not recommended to below 2 years children.

vi. **Prevention** of overcrowding and improved housing along with health awareness campaign is very helpful.

Prevention:

i. Household contacts are given 2 days oral Rifampicin as under:

3-12 months 5mg / kg	12 hourly
1 year – 12 year 10mg / kg	
Adults 600 mg	

ii. Other close contacts
Similar to household contacts

iii. Single dose 500mg Ciprofloxacin is alternative in adults

iv. Index case is made noninfectious

v. Meningococcal vaccine A and C is given to the risk group.

Food Poisoning

Food poisoning is an acute gastroenteritis by bacterial toxin, chemical toxin, plant toxin or by animal toxins. It is characterised by a common source, many will have same symptoms at one time.

Food poisoning is still a public health problem in the world. It is much more so in developing countries like India.

i. *Staphylococcal Food Poisoning:*
Poor personal hygiene allows the *staph. aureus* into dairy products, cheese and cooked meat. This also can be by boils, Furuncle and carbuncle. It produces enterotoxin A and B.
I.P. 1 – 6 hours
Nausea and profuse vomiting develop within 1 to 6 hours after ingestion. Diarrhoea is not marked. It is intra-dietetic toxin that produces toxic effect.
Antiemetic and fluid replacement are advocated. Suspected food is sent for laboratory examination. If food vending is involved, public health authorities are informed.

ii. *Bacillus Cereas:* Preformed toxin of *B.cereas* produces rapid on set of vomiting within 1 hour of food consumption. It is commonly known as "Chinese Restaurant Syndrome". Fried rice and vanilla sauce are common source of toxin. Enterotoxin is liberated during storage. Significant enterocolitis occurs if viable bacteria are swallowed and toxin is liberated in the gut. Rapid and judicious fluid replacement and appropriate notification are mandatory.

iii. *Clostridium Perfringens:* This is common by contaminated meat, or incompletely cooked meat and when stored in anaerobic condition. Reheating causes sporulation of clostridia and enterotoxin liberation. Diarrhoea and cramps are common. I.P. is 6-12 hours. It is common in school, party and get-together eating. Usually it is self limiting.

iv. *Cl. Botulism:* It is due to neurotoxin of *Cl.botulinum* which is manifested in paralysis and neurological dysfunction. It is common in canned meat and preserved vegetables. Contaminated honey also can cause toxin production and symptoms.
Ingestion of toxin produce difficulty in swallowing, blurred vision, ptosis, limb weakness and respiratory paralysis.
Case management include assisted ventilation, general supportive measures which take, sometimes, 2 months.

v. *Plant Toxin:* Beans and legumes produce oxidants which are toxic to man with G6PD (Glucose – 6 Phosphate Dehydrogenase) deficiency. Headache, Nausea, Fever, Haemolysis, Haemo-globinuria and Jaundice set in. Lectin content of Red kidney beans cause acute abdomen Diarrhoea. In potato alkaloids developed can cause toxic effect. Fungi and mushroom produce hallucinogens. Death head mushroom causes hepatorenal failure.

vi. *Chemical Toxin:* Saxitocin produced from shellfish and oysters can cause acute G.E. With G.I. symptoms, it can cause respiratory paralysis within 30 minutes. Ciguatoxin from some fishes or histidine in some fishes cause acute gastro enteritis. Heavy metals like Thallium and Cadmium cause G.E.

vii. *Norwalk like Agents:* These virus are faeco-oral transmitted, cause nausea, vomiting, diarrhoea after 48 hours of incubation period. It is common in nurseries.

viii. *Salmonella Poisoning:*S. Typhimurium from contaminated meat, milk and milk products produce symptoms with an I.P. of 12 to 24 hours. Fever, nausea, vomiting and watery diarrhoea are common. Reservoir is poultry and farm animals.

Investigation of an Epidemic of G.E.:

i. List of people involved is done.
ii. They are subjected for laboratory tests.
iii. Survey of eating places; kitchen and food handlers are done.
iv. Data is analysed for time, place and person distribution.
v. In all epidemics of Acute G.E, cholera is ruled out at investigation. Differences between cholera and food poisoning are as under:

Table 18.19: Differences between food poisoning and cholera

	Cholera	*Food Poisoning*
History of common meal	No	Yes
Incubation period	5 days	1 day
Onset	Diarrhoea	Vomiting
Nausea	Absent	Present
Stool	Rice watery	Offensive mucus and blood
Dehydration	Marked	Not marked
Muscle cramp	Severe	Less
Fever	No	Yes
Urine	Suppressed	Not suppressed
Differential WBC count	Leucocytosis	Normal

Control and Prevention of Food Poisoning:

i. Food sanitation includes meat hygiene, milk hygiene, food hygiene, sanitary method of preservation and food handling techniques. Health education on personal hygiene is essential.
ii. *Refrigeration:* Keeping food in cold storage (below 4°C) prevent bacterial growth and toxin liberation.
iii. *Food surveillance:* Periodic and suspected food analysis help in preventing food poisoning.

Plague

Well known to ancient people as "black death", plague is a Zoonotic disease transmitted by infected Rat flea. Over hundreds of years, the clinical entities are Bubonic plague, pneumonic plague, septicaemic plague, meningitis, Pharyngitis, Tonsillitis and Asymptomatic plague. World has recorded 3 great pandemics.

First – 6th century, all countries, death swept across the globe.
Second – 14th century, whole of Europe killing nearly one third of population.
Third – In 1860 in China, Hong Kong, South East Asia, India, Africa and America, Killing millions of people.

Global epidemiologists have observed the death toll in India from 1860 to 1920 period as 10 to 12 million.

*India–Problem:*Last plague reported was in 1966. For 28 years up to 1994 no confirmed plague could be seen India. In 1994, epidemic of plague started in Maharashtra (Beed), Gujarat (Surat), Delhi, Mumbai, Kolkata and Karnataka. As per Media, during 1994 epidemic about 5000 suspected cases were reported, about 170 proved positive and a death of 53 cases. During 2002, WHO has recorded epidemic of plague, Pneumonic type in Himachal Pradesh with 16 cases and 4 deaths.

Incubation period:

Pneumonic plague 1 to 3 days.

Bubonic and septicaemic plague 2 to 7 days

Mode of Transmission

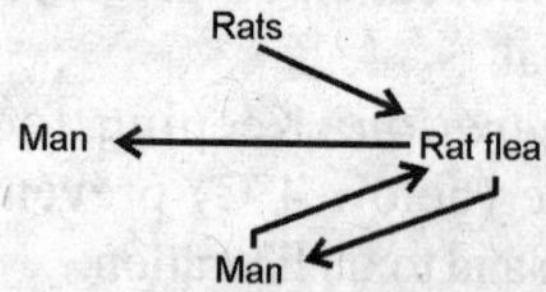

Fig. 18.58: Mode of transmission

Clinical Picture:

Bubonic	*Septicaemic*	*Pneumonic*
Rigor	Meningitis	Sudden onset
High fever	pneumonia	cough
Dry skin	Blood stained sputum	dyspnoea
Severe headache		Copious sputum (blood)
Lymphnode enlargement in groin		Cyanosis
Rapid pulse		X-ray lobar opacity
Hypotension		Death
Mental confusion		
Splenomegaly		

Agent, host, environmental factors are depicted in Fig 18.60.

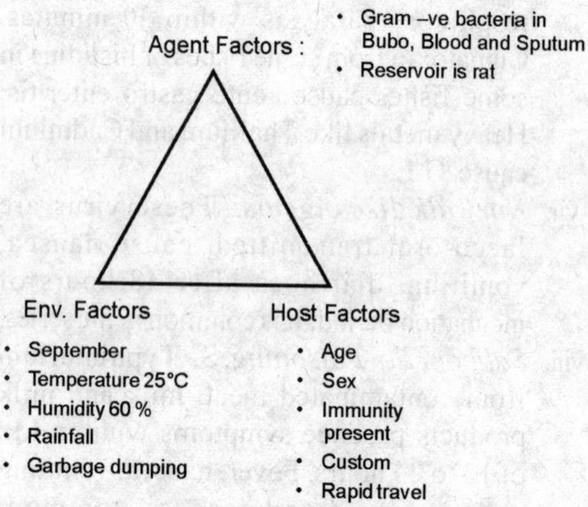

Fig. 18.60: Epidemiology of plague

Vector of Plague Transmission:

Rat flea xenopsylla cheopis, when infected with plague bacilli, bites the man and introduces *pasturella pestis* and cause plague. Millions of

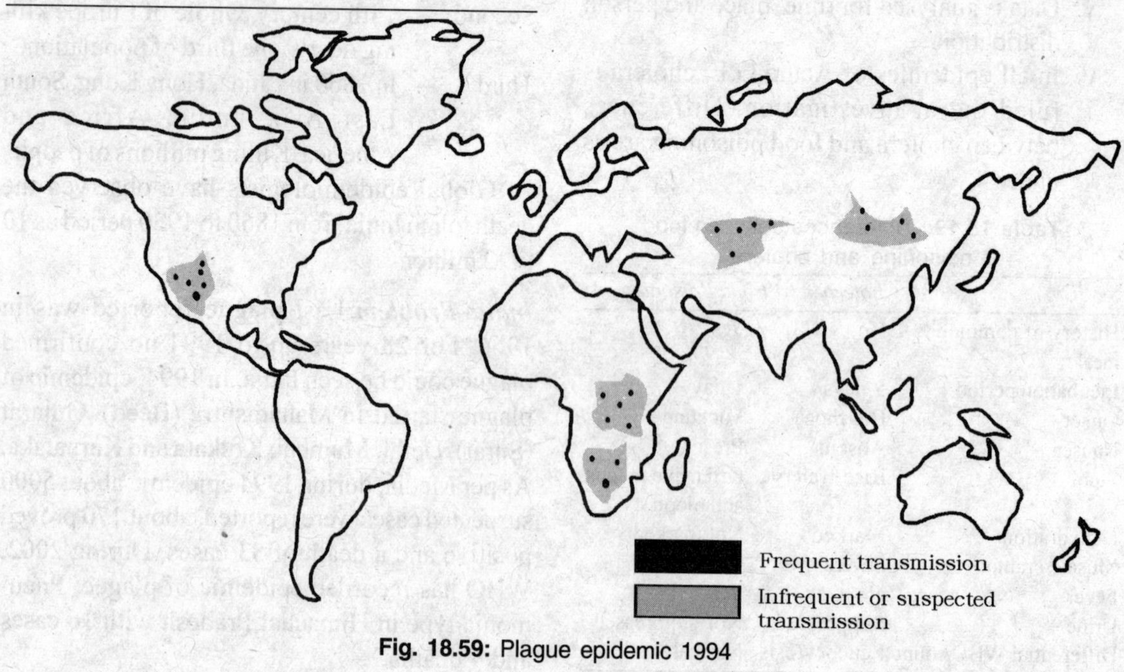

Fig. 18.59: Plague epidemic 1994

plague organism block the gut of flea which is called "Blocked flea" and is dangerous because it spreads plague in an enormous way.

Rat flea indices:

i. Cheopis index

$$= \frac{\text{No of x cheopis counted to Rats}}{\text{No. of Rats examined}}$$

ii. Total flea index

$$= \frac{\text{No of Rat Flea counted to Rats}}{\text{No. of Rats examined}}$$

iii. Cheopis percentage

$$= \frac{\text{No of x cheopis counted}}{\text{Total no. of Rat Flea counted}} \times 100$$

iv. Burrow index of cheopis

$$= \frac{\text{No of x cheopis counted}}{\text{Total Burrows examined}}$$

Case Management and Nursing Care

i. Streptomycin 1 G 12 hourly
ii. Gentamycin 1mg/kg 8 hourly
iii. Tetracycline 500 mg 6th hourly
iv. Chloromphenicol 12.5 mg/kg 6 hourly
v. Management of acute circulatory failure
vi. Management of disseminated intravascular coagulation
vii. Management of hypoxia.

Animal Plague

Death of rats causes concern in the community. In rats wild plague and domestic plagues are seen. They are natural foci for disease transmission. Epidemics in rats are called epizootic. When report of unexpected deaths of rats is received following action is mandatory.

- Collection and forwarding rats to nearest laboratory.
- Autopsy of rats is done.
- Plague bacilli in them are demonstrated.
- Appropriate public health measures are taken.

Control of Plague:

Early diagnosis and specific treatment are substituted. It is to be notified to the authorities, since it is a notifiable disease. Disinfection of sputum and articles of patients are carried out. Dead bodies (of plague) are carefully handled.

Specific Rat flea control and Rat control measures are undertaken.

Prevention:

With the help of Insecticide and Rodenticide, rats and fleas are controlled. One should be careful in handling and skinning animals. A formalin killed vaccine is available for prevention of plague among contacts. Contacts should be protected by Tetracycline 2 G. per day or Co-trimoxazole 1 tablet daily for 7 days. Health education, surveillance and chemoprophylaxis are recommended as supplements to prevention.

Vaccine:

Plague vaccine is formalin killed vaccine given subcutaneously at 14 days interval. First dose is 0.5 ml and second dose is 1.0 ml. Single injection of 1.0 ml is given during epidemic.

Acute Respiratory Infection (ARI)

It is a common cause of morbidity among elderly and common cause for mortality among young children. Depending on the site of infection, upper and lower respiratory tract infections are classified. Organs involved are depicted in Figure 18.61.

Clinically the entities are grouped under (a) Very severe (b) Severe (c) Pneumonia and (d) No pneumonia for the case management. Common sequelae are (a) Ear problems and (b) Sore throat.

Problem – World:

It is estimated that A.R.I. annual occurrence is about 238 million cases and about 39 million deaths are occurring every year.

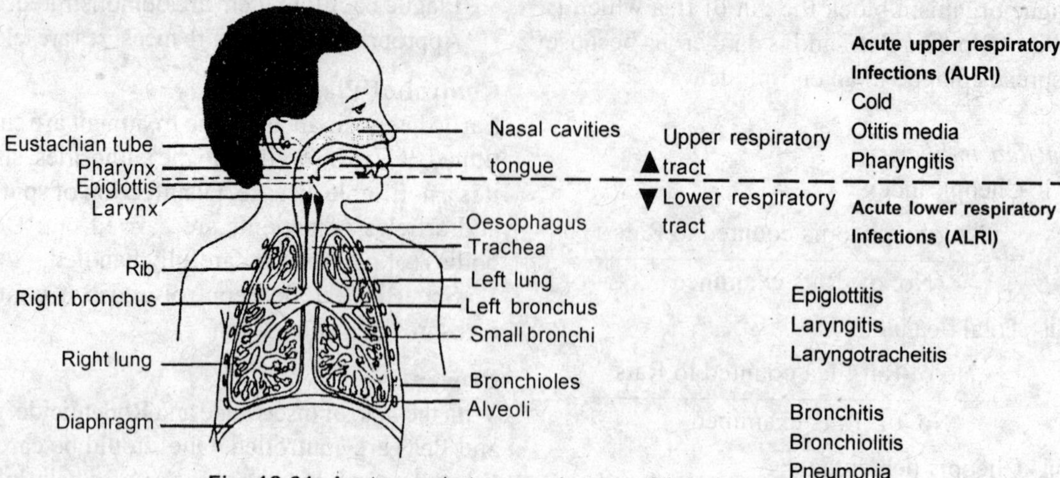

Fig. 18.61: Acute respiratory syndromes: Clinical syndromes

Problem – India:

A.R.I. is one of the major causes of I.M.R. in India. Hospital data show that about 13 to 14 percent of paediatric out patient load is by acute respiratory infections. 13% of in patient deaths in paediatric ward are by ARI. Two problems are encountered with respect to the case management. They are:

i. Inappropriate antibiotic use.
ii. Mother or parents do not know the correct home care.

Classification:

I. Aetiological classification
   1. Viral
   2. Bacterial
   3. Other causes
II. Anatomical classification
   1. U.R.I.
   2. L.R.I.
III. Management oriented classification
   1. Severe (unable to feed, chest retraction, respiratory rate above 70 and strider).
   2. Moderate (respiratory rate 50 to 70).
   3. Mild (cough, respiratory rate below 50 and no chest retraction).

Agent, host and environmental factors are depicted in Figure 18.62.

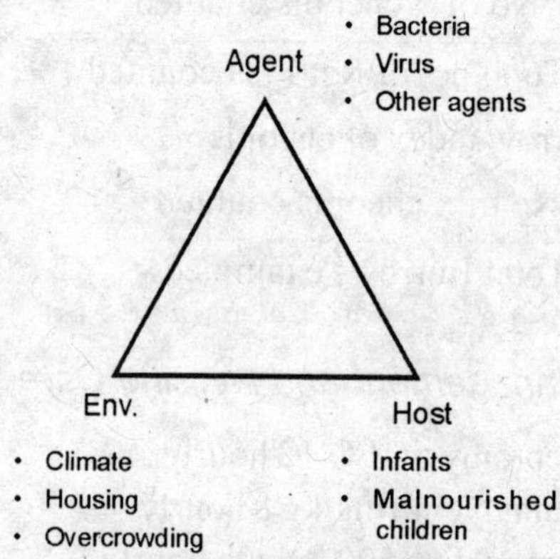

Fig. 18.62: Epidemiology of A.R.I.

Common causative agents of A.R.I. are as under Table 18.20.

Table 18.20: Common pathogens causing A.R.I.

Virus	*Bacteria*	*Others*
Adenovirus type 2 and 5	Bordetella	Chlamydia Type B
Influenza B	Klebsiella	Mycoplasma
Measles	Streptococci	
Respiratory syncytial		
Corona		

Mode of Transmission:

It is airborne and by person to person contact.

Management of the child with cough or difficult breathing

ASSESS

ASK

- How old is the child?
- Is the child coughing? For how long?
- Age 2 months upto 5 years: Is the child able to drink?
  Age less than 2 months: Has the young infant stopped feeding well?
- Has the child had fever ? For how long?
- Has the child had convulsions?

LOOK, LISTEN

(Child must be calm)

- Count the breaths in one minute.
- Look for chestin drawing.
- Look and listen for stridor.
- Look and listen for wheeze.
  Is it recurrent?
- See if the child is abnormally sleepy or difficult to wake.
- Feel for fever; or low body temperature (or measure temperature).
- Look for severe malnutiriton.

CLASSIFY THE ILLNESS

	THE YOUNG INFANT AGE LESS THAN 2 MONTHS
Signs	• Stopped feeding well • Convulsions • Abnormally sleepy or difficult to wake • Stridor in calm child • Wheezing or • Fever or low body temperature
Classify as	VERY SEVERE DISEASE
Treatment	• Refer urgently to hospital • Keep young infant warm • Give first dose of an antibiotic

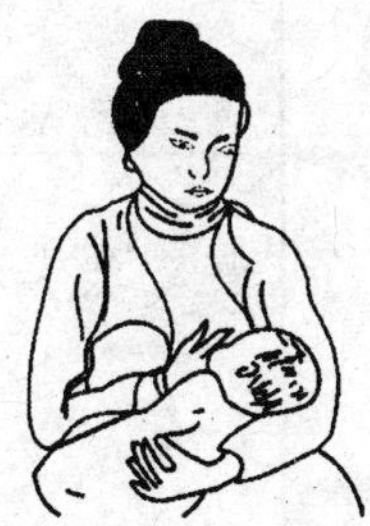

Signs	• Severe chest indrawing Or • Fast breathing (60 per minute or more)	• No severe chest indrawing and • No fast breathing (Less than 60 per minute)
Classify as	SEVERE PNEUMONIA	NO PNEUMONIA : COUGH OR COLD
Treatment	• Refer urgently to hospital • Keep young infant warm • Give first dose of an antibiotic (If referral is not feasible: treat with an antibiotic and follow closely)	• Advise mother to give the following home care • Keep young infant warm • Breastfeeding frequently • Clear nose if it interferes with feeding – Return quickly if: – Breathing becomes difficult – Breathing becomes fast – Feeding becomes a problem – The young infant becomes sicker

THE CHILD AGE 2 MONTHS UP TO 5 YEARS

Does child have danger signs?		
	SIGNS	• Not able to drink • Convulsions • Abnormally sleepy or difficult to wake • Stridor in calm child or • Severe malnutrition
	CLASSIFY BY	VERY SEVERE DISEASE
	TREATMENT	• Refer URGENTLY to hospital • Give first dose of an antibiotic • Treat fever, if present • Treat wheezing, if present • If cerebral malaria is possible, give an antimalarial

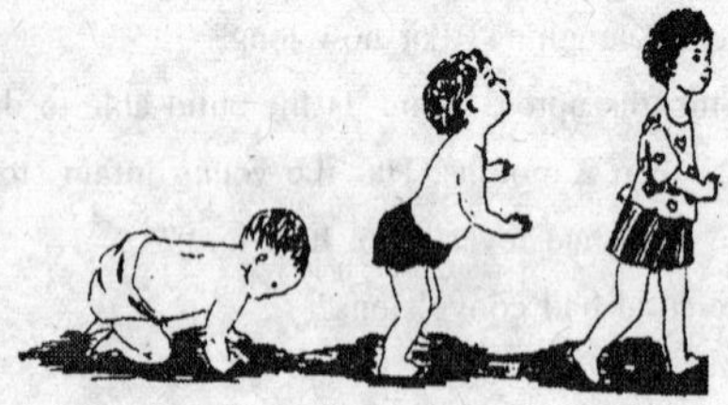

Does child have pneumonia?			
SIGNS	* Chest indrawing Or (If also recurrent go directly to • **Treat Wheezing**	• **No** chest indrawing and • Fast breathing (50 per minute or more if child 2 months upto 12 months; 40 per minute or more if child 12 months upto 5 years	• **No** chest indrawing and • No fast breathing (Less than 50 per minute if child 2 months upto 12 months; Less than 40 per minute if child 12 months upto 5 years)
CLASSIFY AS	SEVERE PNEUMONIA	PNEUMONIA	NO PNEUMONIA COUGH OR COLD
TREATMENT	• Refer URGENTLY to hospital • Give first dose of an antibiotic • Treat fever if present • Treat wheezing, if present (If referral is not feasible, treat with an antibiotic and follow closely)	• Advise mother to give home care • Give an antibiotic • Treat fever if present • Treat wheezing, if present • Advise mother to return with child in 2 days for reassessment, or earlier if the child is getting worse	• If coughing more than 30 days refer for assessment • Assess and treat ear problem if present (see chart) • Assess and treat other problems • Advise mother to give home care • Treat fever, if present • Treat wheezing, if present

	Reassess in 2 days a child who is taking an antibiotic for pneumonia		
SIGNS	WORSE * Not able to drink * Has chest indrawing * Has other danger signs	THE SAME	IMPROVING * Breathing slower * Less fever * Eating better
TREATMENT	* Refer URGENTLY to hospital	Change antibiotic or refer	Finish 5 days of antibiotic

TREATMENT INSTRUCTIONS

- ***Give an Antibiotic***
    - Give first dose of antibiotic in clinic
    - Instruct mother on how to give the antibiotic for five days at home (or to return to clinic for daily procaine penicillin injection).

AGE or WEIGHT	COTRIMOXAZOLE (Trimethoprim + sulphamethoxazole) • Two times daily for 5 days			AMOXYCILLIN • Three times daily for 5 days		AMPICILLIN • Four times daily for 5 days		PROCAINE PENICILLIN • Once daily for 5 days
	Adult Tablet Single strength (80 mg trimethoprim + 400 mg sulphametho-xazole)	Pediatric (20 mg trimethoprim + 100 mg sulphametho-xazole)	Syrup (40 mg trimethoprim + 200 mg sulphametho-xazole per 5 ml)	Tablet	Syrup	Tablet	Syrup	Intramuscular Injection
Less than 2 months (<5 kg)♦	1/4*	1	2.5 ml*	1/4	2.5 ml	1/2	2.5 ml	200,000 units
2 months up to 12 months (6-9 kg)	1/2	2	5 ml	1/2	5 ml	1	5 ml	400,000 units
12 months up to 5 years (10-19 kg)	1	3	7.5 ml	1	10 ml	1	5 ml	800,000 units

- Give oral antibiotic for 5 days at home only if referral is not feasible.
- If the child is less than 1 month old, give 1/2 pediatric tablet or 1.25 ml syrup twice daily. Avoid cotrimoxazole in infants less than one month of age who are premature or jaundiced.

• Advise Mother to Give Home Care

(For the child age 2 months upto 5 years)*

- **Feed the child**
    - Feed the child during illness
    - Increase feeding after illness
    - **Clear the nose if it interferes with feeding**
- **Increase fluids**
    - Offer the child extra to drink
    - Increase breastfeeding
- **Soothe the throat and relieve the cough with a safe remedy**
- **Most important: In the child classified as having no pneumonia: Cough or Cold, watch for the following signs and return quickly if they occur:**
    - Breathing become difficult
    - Breathing becomes fast
    - Child is not able to drink
    - Child becomes sicker

    } This child may have pneumonia
- See section on young infant for home care instructions for that age group

- **Treat Fever**

• Fever is high (39° C)	In a falciparum malarious area: • Fever is not high (38-39° C)
• Give paracetamol	• Advise mother to give more fluids

• Any fever, or • History of fever
• Give an antimalarial (or treat according to your malaria programme recommedation)

• Fever for more than five days
• Refer for assessment

PARACETAMOL doses → Every six hours		
AGE OR WEIGHT	100 mg tablet	500 mg tablet
2 months upto 3 years (6-14 kg)		1 1/4
3 years upto 5 years (15-19 kg)		1 1/2 1/2

FEVER ALONE IS NOT A REASON TO GIVE AN ANTIBIOTIC EXCEPT IN A YOUNG INFANT (AGE LESS THAN 2 MONTHS)

- ***Treat Wheezing***

Children with First Episode of Wheezing

If in respiratory distress	→	Give a rapid-acting bronchodilator and refer
If not in respiratory distress	→	Give oral salbutamol

Children with Recurrent Wheezing (Asthma)

Give a rapid-acting bronchodilator

- Assess the child's condition 30 minutes later:

IF :	THEN :
RESPIRATORY DISTRESS OR ANY DANGER SIGN	Treat for SEVERE PNEUMONIA or VERY SEVERE DISEASE (Refer)
NO RESPIRATORY DISTRESS AND :	
FAST BREATHING →	Treat for PNEUMONIA Give oral salbutamol
NO FAST BREATHING →	Treat for NO PNEUMONIA: COUGH OR COLD Give oral salbutamol

RAPID-ACTING BRONCHODILATOR	
Nebulized Salbutamol (5 mg/ml)	0.5 ml Salbutamol plus 2.0 ml sterile water
Subcutaneous Epinephrine (adrenaline) (1:1000 = 0.1 %)	0.01 ml per kg body weight

ORAL SALBUTAMOL • Three times daily for five days		
AGE or WEIGHT	2 mg tablet	4 mg tablet
2 months upto 12 months (< 10 kg)	1/2	1/4
12 months upto 5 years (10-19 kg)	1	1/2

MANAGEMENT OF THE CHILD WITH AN EAR PROBLEM OR SORE THROAT

EAR PROBLEM

ASSESS

ASK	LOOK, FEEL :
• Does the child have ear pain ? • Does the child have pus draining from the ear ? For how long ?	• Look for pus draining from the ear or red, immobile eardrum (by otoscopy). • Feel for tender swelling behind ear.

CLASSIFY THE ILLNESS

SIGNS :	• Tender swelling behind the ear	• Pus draining from the ear LESS than two weeks, or • Ear pain or • Red immobile ear drum (by otoscopy)	• Pus draining from the ear two weeks or MORE
CLASSIFY AS :	**MASTOIDITIS**	**ACUTE EAR INFECTION**	**CHRONIC EAR INFECTION**
TREATMENT :	• Refer URGENTLY to hospital • Give first dose of antibiotic • Treat fever, if present • Give paracetamol for pain	• Give an antibiotic for five days, as for pneumonia • Dry the ear by wicking • Reassess in five days • Treat fever, if present • Give paracetamol for pain	• Dry the ear by wicking • Treat fever, if present • Give paracetamol for pain

SORE THROAT

ASSESS

ASK	LOOK, FEEL :
• Is the child able to drink ?	• Feel the front of the neck for nodes • Look for exudate on the throat

CLASSIFY THE ILLNESS

SIGNS :	• Not able to drink the ear	• Tender, enlarged lymph node on neck and • White exudate on throat
CLASSIFY AS :	**THROAT ABSCESS**	**STREPTOCOCCAL SORE THROAT**
TREATMENT :	• Refer to hospital • Give benzathine penicillin • Treat fever, if present • Give paracetamol for pain	• Give benzathine penicillin • Give safe, soothing remedy for sore throat • Treat fever, if present • Give paracetamol for pain

TREATMENT INSTRUCTIONS

- ***Give an Oral Antibiotic for an Ear Infection***
  - Give first dose of antibiotic in clinic.
  - Instruct mother on how to give the antibiotic for five days at home.

AGE or WEIGHT	COTRIMOXAZOLE (Trimethoprim + sulphamethoxazole) • Two times daily for 5 days			AMOXYCILLIN • Three times daily for 5 days		AMPICILLIN • Four times daily for 5 days	
	Adult Tablet Single strength (80 mg trimethoprim) + 400 mg sulphametho-xazole)	Pediatric (20 mg trimethoprim) + 100 mg sulphametho-xazole)	Syrup 40 mg trimethoprim) + 200 mg sulphametho-xazole per 5 ml	Tablet	Syrup	Tablet	Syrup
Less than 2 months (<5 kg)♦	1/4*	1	2.5 ml*	1/4	2.5 ml	1/2	2.5 ml
2 months up to 12 months (6-9 kg)	1/2	2	5 ml	1/2	5 ml	1	5 ml
12 months up to 5 years (10-19 kg)	1	3	7.5 ml	1	10 ml	1	5 ml

- Give oral antibiotic for 5 days at home only if referral is not feasible.
- If the child is less than 1 month old, give 1/2 pediatric tablet or 1.25 ml syrup twice daily. Avoid cotrimoxazole in infants less than one month of age who are premature or jaundiced.

- ***Dry the Ear by Wicking***
  - To dry the ear:
    - Roll clean, absorbent cloth into a wick
    - Place the wick in the child's ear
    - Remove the wick when wet
    - Replace the wick with a clean one until the ear is dry

Treat Fever

• Fever is high (39° C)	• Fever is not high (38-39° C)	In a falciparum malarious area: • Any fever, or • History of fever	• Fever for more than five days
• Give paracetamol	• Advise mother to give more fluids	• Give an antimalarial (or treat according to your malaria programme recommedation)	• Refer for assessment

PARACETAMOL doses
→ Every six hours

AGE OR WEIGHT	100 mg tablet	500 mg tablet
2 months upto 3 years (6-14 kg)	1	1/4
3 years up to 5 years (15-19 kg)	1 1/2	1/2

FEVER ALONE IS NOT A REASON TO GIVE AN ANTIBIOTIC EXCEPT IN A YOUNG INFANT (AGE LESS THAN 2 MONTHS)

- ***Give Benzathine Penicillin***

for suspected streptococcal sore throat:

BENZATHINE PENICILLIN IM

A single injection

< 5 years	600,000 units
≥ 5 years	1,200,000 units

Or amoxycillin, ampicillin or penicillin V for ten days

- ***Sooth the throat with safe, simple remedies***
- ***Give paracetamol for pain and fever***

A.R.I. Control Programme:

It was initiated in 1990. When C.S.S.M. programme was launched in 1992, the ARI control programme becomes the part and parcel of CSSM. Since 1997 it is part of RCH programme at National level.

Training of health workers to recognise and treat at first contact, distribution of cotrimoxazole supplied to RCH drug kit are main activities under ARI control programme.

Home Care Instructions for Mother

i. Infant below 2 months
   - Keep infant warm
   - Breast feed frequently
   - Clear nose if it interferes with feeding
   - Take the child to doctor if
     a. Breathing becomes difficult
     b. Breathing becomes faster
     c. Feeding is not possible
     d. Infant seems to be really sick.

ii. Infant from 2 months to 5 years

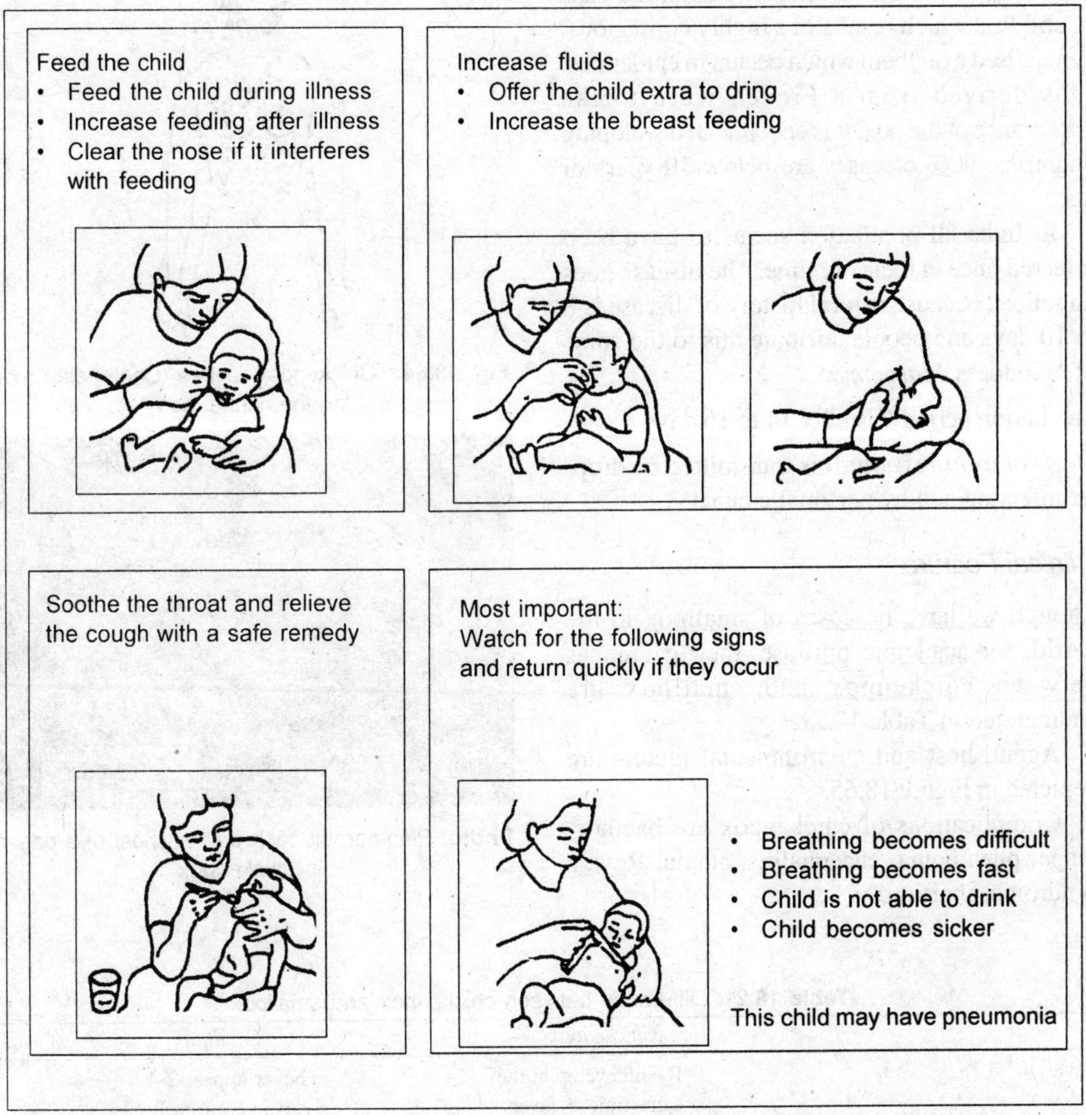

Fig 18.63: Home care instructions for children aged 2 months upto 5 years with acute respiratory infections

Fig 18.63 gives specific idea for home care of children from 2 months to 5 years. Mother or patients must take precaution to:

a. Feed the child.
b. Fluid intake is maintained by extra drink and breast feeding.
c. Safe remedy for cough and throat irritation is given; and
d. Watch for warning signs and to take the child to doctor, if they occur.

Chickenpox

Chickenpox is a viral infection, a primary disease of children which results in a highly contagious, generalised exanthem which occurs in epidemics. It is derived from a French word to the appearance of the pox. It is endemic in developing countries. 90% of cases are below 10 years of age.

In India all population seems to have been infected once in their life time. The disease goes unnoticed because natural history of disease is 8 to 10 days and people attribute this to the curse of "Goddess *Maramma*".

Incubation period: Usually 14 to 16 days.

Mode of transmission: It is transmitted by droplet infection and by personal contact.

Clinical Feature

Though we have no cases of smallpox in the world, for academic purpose, the differences between chickenpox and smallpox are enumerated in Table 18.21.

Agent, host and environmental factors are depicted in Figure 18.65.

Complications of chickenpox are haemorrhage, pneumonia, encephalitis, ataxia, Reye's syndrome, abortion.

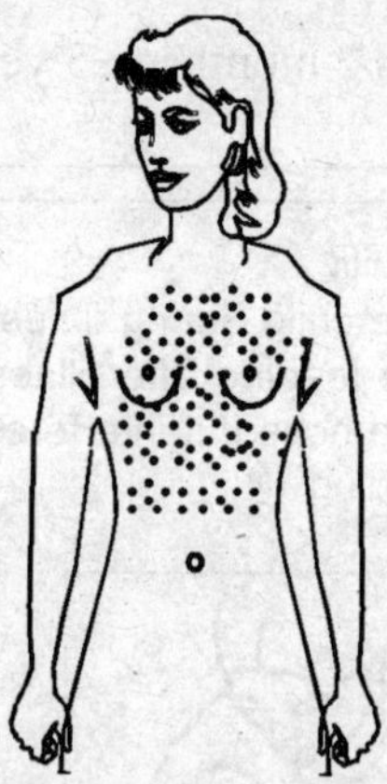

Fig. 18.64: Chickenpox rashes (Centripetal) more on the central body

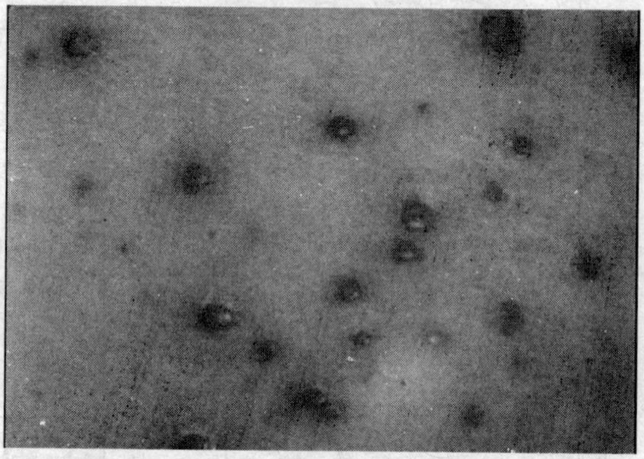

Photo: Pleomorphic rash on the chest of a patient in chickenpox

Table 18.21: Difference between chickenpox and smallpox

		Chickenpox	*Smallpox*
Fever		Rash develop at the same time as fever	Fever appear 2-4 days before rash
Rash	Appearance	Pleomorphic (Pocks are several stages) at a given point of time	Monomoryhic (Pocks are same stage) at a given point of time
	Development	Rapid	Slow
	Distribution	Centripetal (More in centre)	Centrifugal (More in periphery)
	Palm and sole	Absent	Present
	Mortality	Nil	High

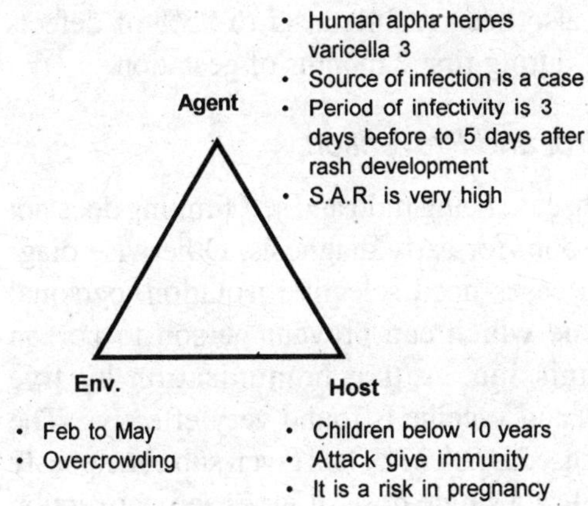

Fig. 18.65: Epidemiology of chickenpox

Clinically it is very easy to diagnose on features mentioned above. Aspiration of vesicular fluid for P.C.R. or tissue culture will contain will confirm the diagnosis. Recurrence of chickenpox is a common feature in developing countries like India.

Case management: It is a self limiting disease which needs selective isolation of case for preventing the spread to others. Human varicella Zoster Immunoglobulin may be used to attenuate the infection in highly susceptible contacts of chickenpox. In all other aspect the case management is purely symptomatic.

Control : Notification, selective isolation of case and personal hygiene.

Prevention:

i. V.Z.I.G. (Varicella Zoster Immunoglobulin) 2-5 ml I.V. before 72 hours of exposure.
ii. Chickenpox vaccine (a live attenuated) has given 90 percent seroconvertion.

German Measles

Large number of studies on German measles were conducted in Germany by German scientists and hence the name German measles. The name German measles has nothing to do with measles. By the manifestation of pink macular rash on the body, the name "Rubella" is derived (Latin word "Rubellus" means "reddish").

It is world wide in distribution. Epidemics occur in early spring. Epidemics once in 10 years and major epidemic once in 30 years are reported in global epidemiology. In 1941 Sir Norman Gregg recognised the association between Rubella and congenital abnormalities. The risk is pointed out as under:

Rubella in pregnancy	*Malformation of foetus*
1-2 months	85%
3rd month	35%
4th month	10%
After 5 months	Rare

Occasional deafness is observed in infection at the 5th months of pregnancy. Agents, host and environmental factors are depicted in Figure18.66.

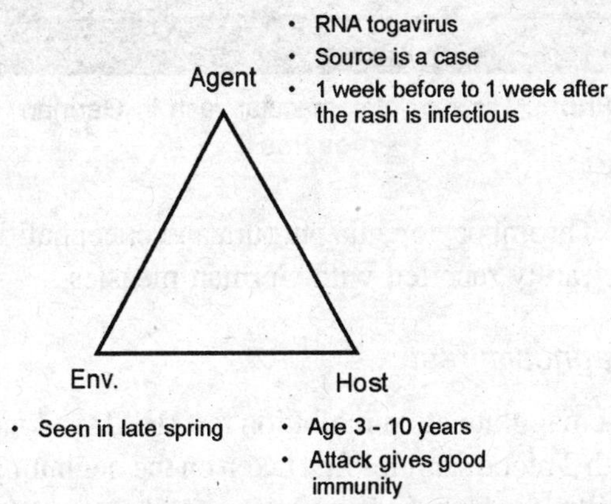

Fig. 18.66: Epidemiology of rubella

Incubation period – 2 to 3 weeks

Mode of Transmission: By droplet infection and by person to person contact.

Clinical Feature

Lymph nodes like post auricular, post cervical and suboccipital gets enlarged which lasts for several weeks. In 30 percent of cases splenomegaly is seen. A maculo papular non confluent rash starts simultaneously on the face and trunk. Petechial lesions (called "Forchheimer's spots") are seen on soft palate. Symptoms of coryza often confuses in the beginning of illness. Rubella is associated with mild conjunctivitis. Fever and rash start together and fever subsides on second day.

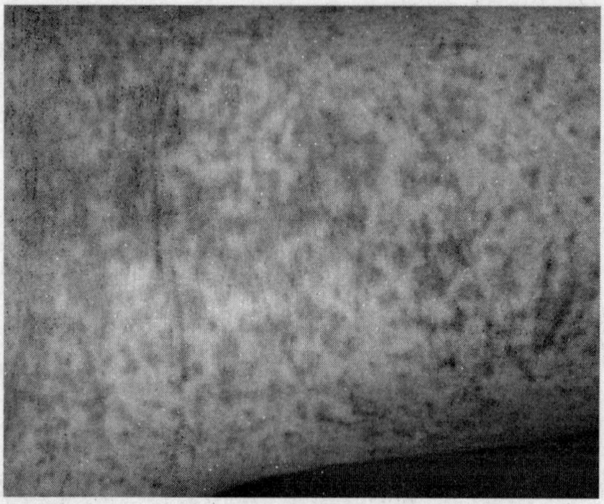

Photo: Discrete pink macular rash in German measles

Thrombocytopenia purpura and encephalitis are rarely reported with German measles.

Diagnosis Test

Haemagglutination inhibition test (HAI) is done with 2 blood samples first taken on the beginning of illness (first 5 days) and second sample 15 days later. A 4 fold rise in HI antibody titre in paired sera is diagnostic of Rubella.

Congenital Rubella Syndrome

Rubella infection in pregnant woman inhibits cell division of embryo and hence congenital defects like deafness, cardiac anomalies and congenital cataract are seen; microcephalus and retinopathy have also been reported. 85 to 95% of defects occur during first 2 months of gestation.

Control and Prevention

The disease being mild and self limiting does not give room for early diagnosis. Otherwise diagnosed cases need selective isolation, personal hygiene which can prevent person to person transmission. Active immunisation by live attenuated vaccine is found very effective. The strain used is RA 27/3. It is given sub cutaneously 0.5 ml as a single dose. It gives seroconversion in about 95 % vaccines.

In developed countries like USA, UK and Canada strategy used is as under:

First – Women of child bearing age (15 to 39) are immunised.

Second – All children 1-14 years age are immunised.

Third – All children at 1 year age are immunised.

In India it has not been possible to bring in to effect the above strategy. It is given on voluntary request since UIP load under national programme for 6 preventable diseases is high and since detection of risk population has been cumbersome.

In mega cities, MMR (Measles, Mumps and Rubella) is available and is found equally effective weapon against German measles.

Mumps

In history of medicine, we come a cross the description of mumps as "Swelling behind ear accompanied by swelling of testes", by Hippocrates in 5th century B.C. It is common in winter months among children of 5 to 14 year age who are school age group. If it is not complicated with meningitis, encephalitis or orchitis, no mortality will be reported. Peak risk is seen in prepuberty period among boys.

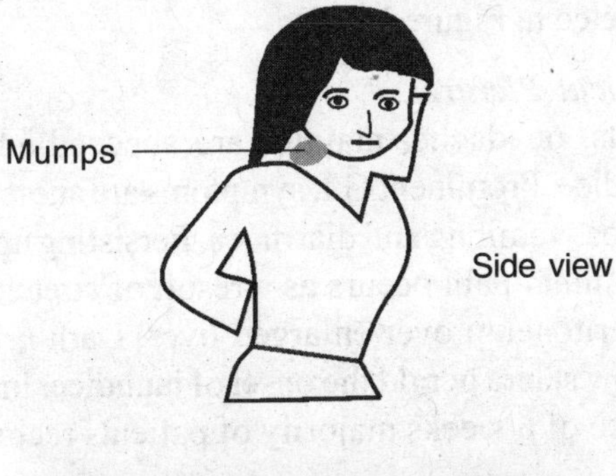

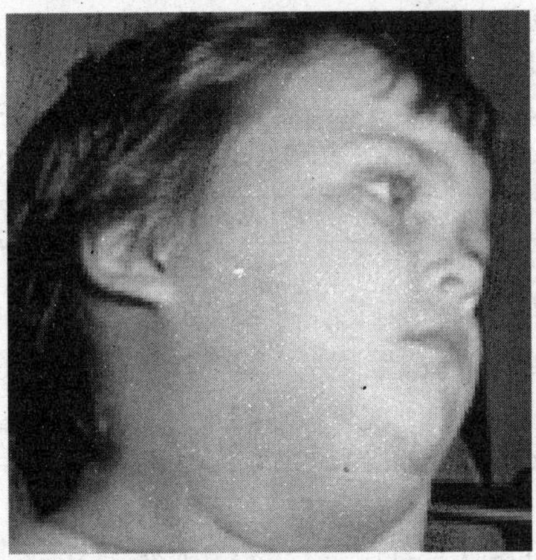

Photo: Unilateral mumps

Mumps primarily infects 5 to 9 years old children. In developing countries like India where there is no programmed vaccination, older teenagers are also affected. Infection is by droplet or direct salivary spread and initial infection is though URI.
Incubation Period: 16-18 days.
Period of infectivity: 1 week.

Clinical Picture:

Fever and malaise are the beginning symptoms and they are prodromal symptoms. This is followed by either unilateral or bilateral parotid swelling. In 10 % of cases other salivary glands may also be infected. Oophoritis and orchitis are complications in post puberty period manifested with abdominal pain or testicular pain. Sterility and meningitis are observed complications of mumps. Transient hearing loss, labyrinthitis and measurable deafness have been recorded. During pregnancy abortion is observed.

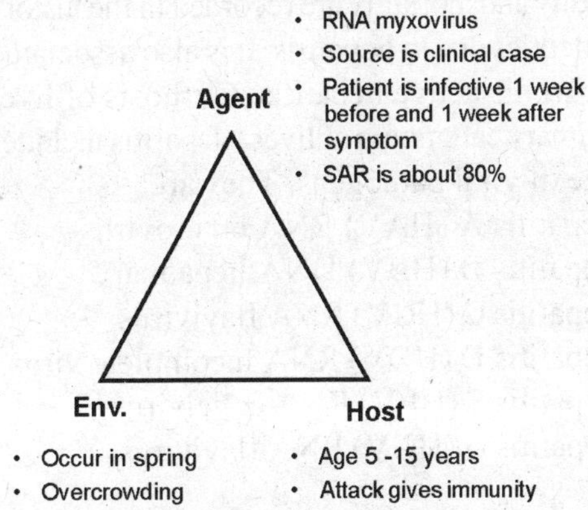

Fig. 18.67: Epidemiology of mumps

Triad of epidemiology is depicted in Fig. 18.67.

Case Management:

Most of the cases are treated with symptomatic treatment. In case of discomfort by orchitis or oophoritis (only when diagnosed) require 40 mg prednisolone orally for 4 days.

Control Measures:

There is no specific control measure advisable for mumps control. Selective isolation, proper disinfection of articles used by the patient and surveillance of contacts are useful tools for control of mumps.

Prevention:

i. Mumps immunoglobulin (MIG) is available, but not found satisfactory in protective action.
ii. Live attenuated mumps vaccine I.M. 0.5ml as single dose gives good detectable antibodies in 90% of cases.
iii. MMR (Measles – Mumps – Rubella) a combined vaccine is also found equally effective in the prevention of mumps.

Hepatitis

Over the part 35 years there has been an explosion in knowledge of viral hepatitis which is a major public health problem in India. Both morbidity and mortality are recorded in the history of epidemics due to hepatitis. It is also associated with chronic active hepatitis, Cirrhosis of liver and primary carcinoma of liver. Hepatitis includes a range of viral pathogens. They are:

1. Hepatitis A (HAV) RNA enterovirus
2. Hepatitis B (HBV) DNA hepadna
3. Hepatitis C (HCV) RNA flavivirus
4. Hepatitis D (HDV) RNA incomplete virus
5. Hepatitis E (HEV) RNA calicivirus
6. Hepatitis G (HGV) RNA flavivirus.

Hepatitis A (Infectious Hepatitis, Epidemic Jaundice)

It is endemic in developing countries producing epidemics. Annual global incidence is about 50 per 100,000. Poor personal hygiene and poor environmental hygiene are facilitators of the illness. Nearly 30% of hepatitis are caused by HAV infection. India has experienced many epidemics in many cities, colonies and in camps.

Incubation Period: 15 to 45 days.

Mode of transmission: Faecal oral route.

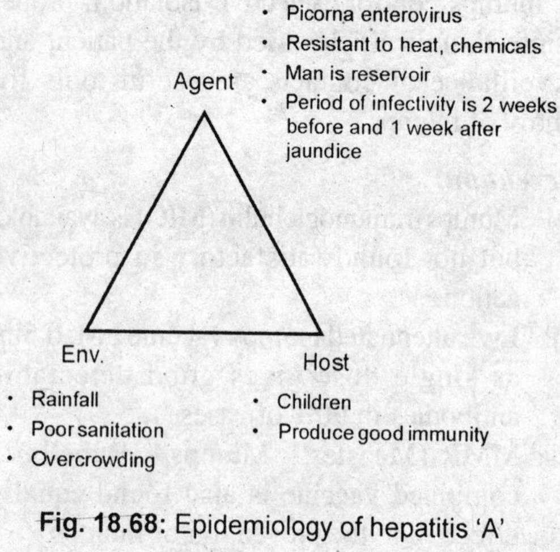

Fig. 18.68: Epidemiology of hepatitis 'A'

Agent, host and environmental factors are depicted in Figure 18.68.

Clinical Picture:

Chills, headache, malaise are succeed-ed by jaundice. Prominent G.I. symptoms are anorexia, nausea, vomiting and diarrhoea. Persisting upper abdominal pain occurs as a result of stretching of peritoneum over enlarged liver. Dark urine, yellow sclera herald the onset of jaundice. In the course of 6 weeks majority of patients recover.

Diagnosis:

i. Liver function tests (LFT).
ii. Anti HAV of IgM type (Immunoassay) is diagnostic of acute infection.

Investigation	*Reference Range*
Total protein	6.0 – 7.5 G%
Albumin	3.5 – 5.3 G %
Globulin	2.0 – 2.5 G %
A:G ratio	2:1
Serum Bilirubin	0.1 to 1.0 mg %
Direct Bilirubin	0.0 to 0.35 mg %
Indirect Bilirubin	0.1 to 0.65 mg %
SGOT	0 to 40 I.U./Lt
SGPT	0 to 38 I.U./Lt
Serum Alkaline Phosphate	100 to 290 I.U./Lt
GGT	5 to 38 u/Lt (male) 5 to 29 u/Lt (female)

Common laboratory tests for hepatitis infections

Case Management and Nursing Care

Acute cases (severe) need hospitalization for required nursing care to allow early detection of acute hepatic failure. Reassurance is needed for post hepatitis syndrome. Balanced diet should provide 2000 to 3000 calories per day which should have light diet supplemented by fruit drinks and glucose. The diet should be as per wish of patient for taste. This should take care of high protein intake. I.V. fluid and glucose may be needed in some of the patients.

Drugs like sedatives and hypnotics should be avoided. Oral contraceptives are avoided during illness. Except for life saving surgery no surgery is allowed in hepatitis patients. Mortality of acute viral hepatitis is about 0.5%.

Control and Prevention:

i. Case finding, notification, disinfection of stool with 0.5% sodium hypochlorite are recommended.
ii. Personal hygiene, environmental hygiene reduces the incidence of HAV infection.
iii. Passive immunity by human immunoglobulin (0.2 ml/kg) is advocated for contacts.
iv. Hepatitis A vaccine 2 doses are given at 6 months interval.

Hepatitis B (Serum Hepatitis)

Hepatitis B is transmitted by parenteral route and is an acute viral infection of liver parenchyma. In 5% of cases they become carriers. Liver cancer is associated with HBV infection.

It is distributed worldwide. It is estimated that there are 350 million chronic carriers and a global load of 2 billion people with disease.

In India "type 2" pattern of HBV infection is seen which accounts for 5-6% of general population.

Incubation Period – 45 to 180 days.

Mode of Transmission: Essentially it is blood borne infection, though other routes are demonstrated.

Clinical Picture:

Apart from clinical picture of HAV infection, HBV infection has arthralgia during prodromal stage, serum sickness syndrome with skin rashes, urticaria and poly arthritis.

Diagnosis:

In acute infection, surface antigen (HBS Ag) is a reliable marker of HBV infection. Chronic carriers show presence of HBS Ag and anti HBC (IgG) in the blood.

Following medical and nursing personnel are at risk group, who merit Hepatitis B vaccination.

- Dentist
- Surgeon
- Obstetrician
- Casualty department
- ICCU
- ICU
- IPCU
- Liver unit
- Endoscopy unit
- Oncology unit
- Laboratory staff handling blood.

Agent, host and environmental factors are depicted in Figure 18.69.

Case Management and Nursing Care

Nursing care should focus attention on monitoring acute liver failure. There is no specific treatment. Interferon 5 Mu daily for patients with high serum transaminase is advocated..

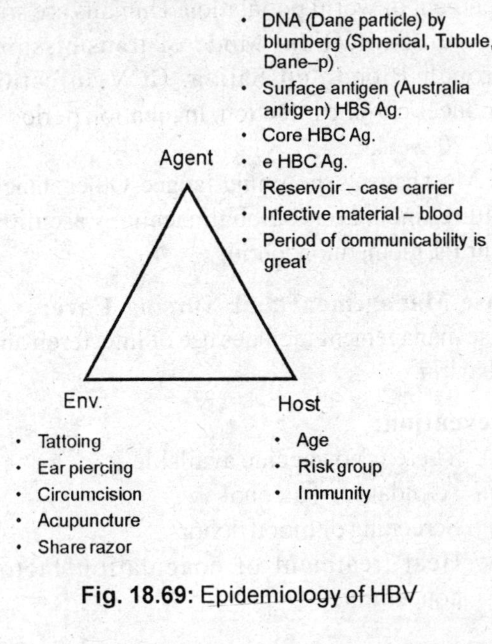

Fig. 18.69: Epidemiology of HBV

Interferon is found useful and helpful in HBV infection to maintain high level concentration of serum transaminase. Lamivudine, an anti HBV nucleoside drug 100 mg per day for 1 year can cause suppression of serum HBV-DNA among 90% of patients. Diet, drug, surgery etc. need special nursing care similar to HAV infection. There is no specific control measure.

Prevention of HBV Infection:

i. Hepatitis B vaccine:
   It is formalin inactivated sub unit viral vaccine for I.M. at 1.0 ml dose in 3 doses (0 month, 1 month and 3rd month).
ii. Recombinant DNA yeast derived vaccine 20 micrograms initially and later at 1 month and 6 month interval gives good protection.
iii. HBIG (Hepatitis B Immunoglobulin) 0.05 ml/kg per dose, 2 doses are given at 1 month interval for passive immunity.
iv. Blood donor screening for HBV.
v. Adequate sterilisation of instruments

Hepatitis C (HCV)

WHO estimate show the HCV infection as 2 to 3 percent of world population. Humans are sole source of infection. Mode of transmissions through Blood and Saliva. HCV infection produces chronic infection. Incubation period is 4 to 20 weeks.

Most patients show mild fatigue. Other clinical features include cryoglobulinaemia, Vasculitis, arthritis, glomerulonephritis.

Case Management and Nursing Care:
Case management includes use of Interferon and Ribavirin.

Prevention:

i. There is no vaccine available
ii. Avoidance of alcohol
iii. Screening of blood donors
iv. Heat treatment of coagulation factor concentrate.

Hepatitis D (HDV) (Delta Hepatitis)

This does not have an independent existence. This requires HBV infection for its replication. Source of infection and mode of infection are the same as HBV infection. The combined infection will be very severe. Close contact and vertical transmission of mothers who carry HBV is common. Drug abuse is a civilized source of infection.

Diagnosis depends on demonstration of anti HDV.

Mode of Transmission:
Through blood, sexual and vertical transmission. Chronic infection stage is present
Incubation period: 6-9 weeks

Prevention is by effectively preventing hepatitis B viral infection.

Hepatitis E (HEV)

It spreads through faecal oral route. It is associated with water pollution to spread as waterborne epidemic. Clinically it mimics HAV infection. Recovery is usually 100 percent.

Demonstration of anti HEV is diagnostic of HEV infection.

There is no vaccine available for prevention.

Control measures are similar to hepatitis A infection.

Hepatitis G (HGV)

It is caused by flavivirus through blood. Blood transfusion is blamed for its spread. Research over past 8 years has not revealed any practical findings in public health aspect of illness in the community.

Other Viruses

Viruses under group which cause hepatitis are:
Major ones

- Cytomegalovirus
- Epstein Barr

Minor ones

- Herpes simplex

Rare ones

- Chickenpox
- Measles
- Rubella
- HIV infection.

Rabies

Rabies virus belongs to Lyssavirus group under Rabdovirus.

Lyssa means "Rage" or "Frenzy" in Greek. Literature reference to rabies is recorded before 2000 BC. It is also available in many historical documents.

Rabies attack all warm blooded animals; particularly Fox, Jackal, Wolves, Dog and bat population. Incidence of rabies in a country is related with its National Rabies control programme. Global epidemiologists have recorded high incidence of 3.3 per 100,000 population both in India and Mexico.

Rabies infect CNS and salivary glands of mammals. It is transmitted through saliva by bite or lick on aberrations. Humans are normally infected from dogs.

Incubation period is 4 to 8 weeks, but it ranges from 9 days to many months. Severe bite on head or neck is associated with shorter I.P.

Clinical Picture:

At the site of bite paraesthesia and fever lasting for 1 to 8 days during which period the patient show anxiousness. Attempt to drink water provokes violent contractions of inspiratory muscles and diaphragm, making the person "fear of water". Hence the name "Hydrophobia" which is synonym with rabies. Delusion, hallucination, spitting, biting and mania are manifested with rabies patient. Terminal patients show hyperpyrexia. Mortality is 100 percent which will be within 8 to 10 days from the start of symptoms.

Epidemiological characteristics are depicted in Fig 18.70.

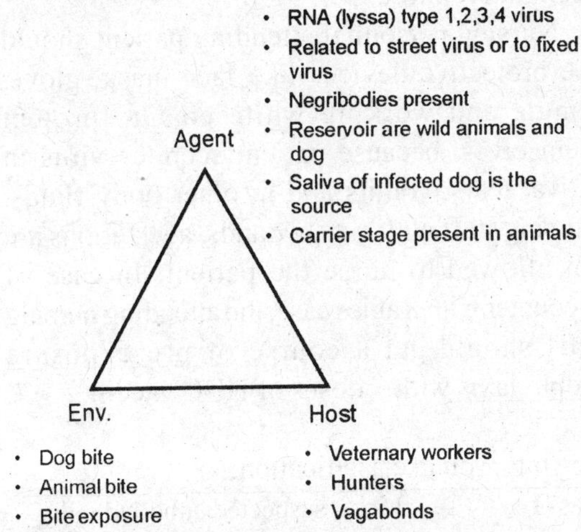

Fig. 18.70: Epidemiology of rabies

Diagnosis:

Usually diagnosis is made on clinical history and clinical examination. But early diagnosis is made with rapid immuno-fluorescent technique which can detect antigen in corneal impression smear or in skin biopsy.

Case Management and Nursing Care

As soon as a case of a dog bite by an infected dog is received, steps are taken to assure patient and his family to overcome unnecessary anxiety state. At the earliest post exposure prophylaxis with ARV is the need of the hour. In all cases post exposure prophylaxis must be started before 5 days from the day of bite to save the life of patient.

When once symptoms are started, only palliative treatment is ascertained. The patient is sedated with diazepam 10 mg 6 hourly. This is supplemented by chlorpromazine 100 mg. Nutrition and fluids are given intravenous route or through gastrostomy. The patient is kept in dark room and silent zone to avoid external stimulus. The patient may need intensive care with facilities to control cardiac failure and respiratory failure.

Nursing personnel attending patient should use protective devices like face mask, glove, goggle and working white coat to protect themselves, because patient secretes virus in saliva, tears, vomits and in other body fluids. Nursing staff with cuts, wounds, aberrations are not allowed to nurse the patient. In case of encounter with Rabies case, the attending nursing staff should get a course of pre exposure prophylaxis with 3 doses of HDC vaccine.

Dog bite wound classification:

Class I	–	Licks, suspected unboiled milk consumption, scratches
Class II	–	Fresh cut, oozing blood, minor wound
Class III	–	Wound on neck, face, palm, lacerated wound

Dose of BPL inactivated vaccine schedule (Pasteur Institute Coonoor):

Wound	*Adult*	*Child*	*Duration*
I	2 ml	1 ml	7 days
II	3 ml	3 ml	10 days
III	5 ml	3 ml	10 days

Available vaccines are:

i. BPL inactivated nervous tissue vaccine.
ii. Suckling mouse brain vaccine.
iii. Duck embryo vaccine.
iv. Human Diploid cell vaccine.
v. Second generation animal cell vaccine.

Vaccination of Persons Bitten by Infected Dog (Post Exposure Prophylaxis):

a. Initially local treatment of wound by cleaning with water and soap – Alcohol or povidone iodine is preferred – Wound suturing should be avoided – Local application of ARS is advocated – Mean while antibiotics are started – If possible bitten dog is observed for 10 days.
b. BPL inactivated nervous vaccine is administered in India since it is cheap, available and cost benefit. The regimen is suggested in table.

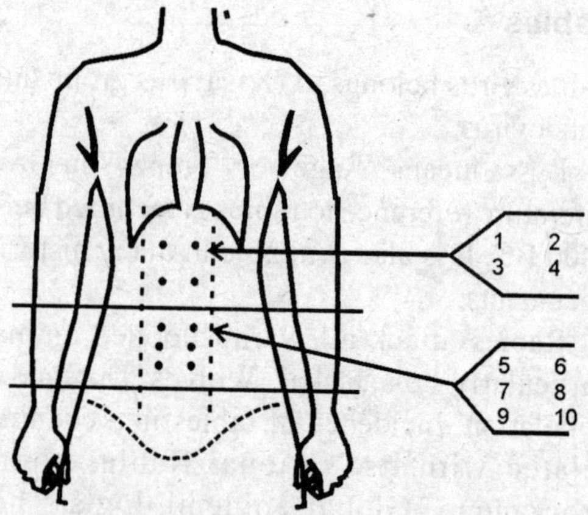

Fig. 18.71: Site for BPL inactivated ARV

BPL vaccine is given deep subcutaneously by lifting a fold of skin between thumb and other fingers, by injecting to base of the fold by 37 mm long needle. Different sites are used for different injection as shown in Figure 18.71.

Booster dose is imperative when combined "serum and vaccine treatment" is employed. It is as under:

Class I wound	-	No booster dose
Class II wound	-	One 21 days after 10th injection
Class III wound	-	2 doses booster I Booster 7 days after 10th injection II Booster 15 days after10th injection

c. ARS (Anti Rabies Serum)
Horse ARS 40 i.u./kg on day zero
Human ARIG (Human Rabies Immunoglobulin)
20 i.u./kg (½ I.M. ½ local site)

Side Reaction of ARV (BPL Vaccine)

- Commonly itching, irritation, pain, redness, swelling, headache, palpitation and diarrhoea.
- Often, urticaria, syncope, angio-neurotic oedema and anaphylactic shock.
- Rarely neuroparalysis.

d. Cell culture vaccine and duck embryo vaccine WHO Intra Muscular regimen is as under:

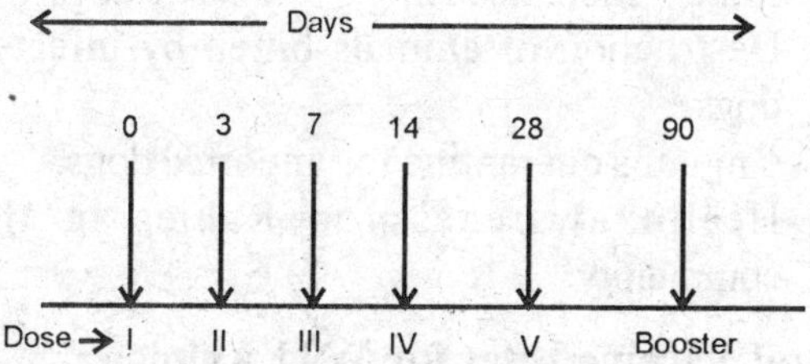

6 doses on 0, 3, 7, 14, 28 days and a booster on 90th day are recommended by I.M. to Deltoid muscle.

Other alternate methods are advocated for cell culture vaccine, for better immunogenic property. They are:

- Reduced multisite I.M. regimen

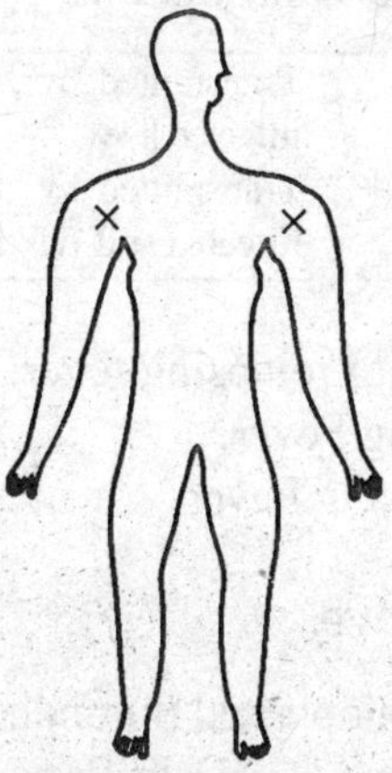

0 day - 1 dose left arm
1 dose right arm
7th day- Deltoid
21st day- Deltoid
(It is 2-1-1 regimen)

Fig. 18.72: Reduced multisite I.M. regimen

* 2 site intradermal schedule

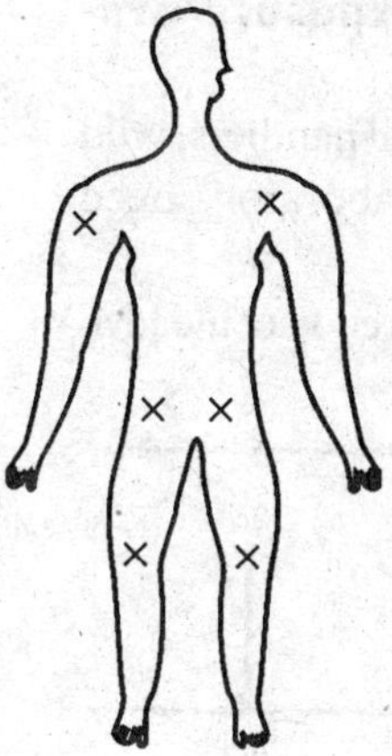

0 day – 1 dose left arm
1 dose right arm
3rd day – 1 dose left lower quadrant abdomen
1 dose right lower quadrant abdomen
7th day – 1 dose left lateral thigh
1 dose right lateral thigh
28th day – 1 dose left arm
90th day –1 dose right arm
(It is 2-2-2-0-1-1 regimen)

Fig. 18.73: Two site intradermal schedule

* 8 site intradermal schedule

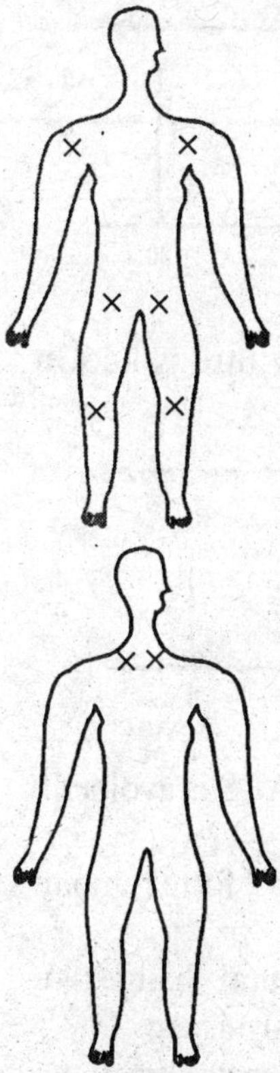

0 day – 0.1 ml in all 8 site i.d.
2 Deltoid
2 lateral thigh
2 supra scapular
2 lower quadrant abdomen
7th day – 0.1 ml in 4 site i.d.
2 deltoid
2 lateral thigh
28th day– 0.1 ml i.d.
Rt: lateral thigh
90th day – 0.1 ml i.d.
Lt: Lateral thigh
(It is called 8-0-4-0-1-1- regimen)

Fig. 18.74: 8 site intradermal schedule

Vaccination of persons who are exposed to the risk of dog bite (Pre-exposure prophylaxis):

People like veterinary staff, animal handlers, wild life staff, and staff at Rabies laboratory need pre-exposure prophylaxis.

They are given 1 ml cell cultured vaccine I.M. on 0, 7 and 28 days as under:

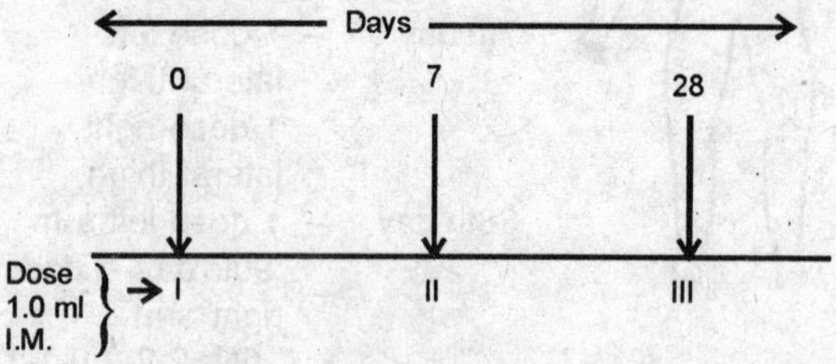

Vaccination of Previously Vaccinated People:

* Bite is severe, antibody titre not known then 3 doses are given

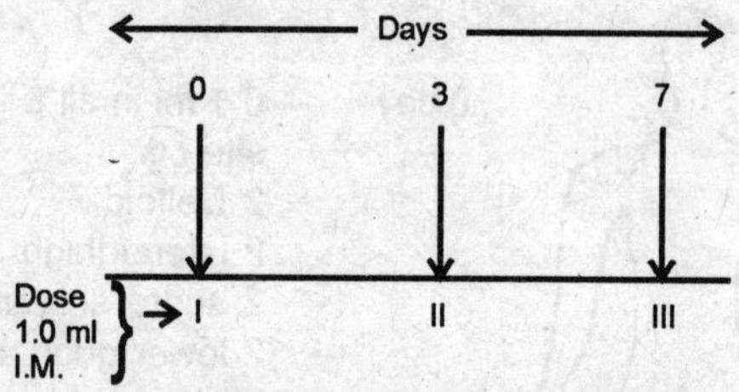

* Bite is not severe; antibody titre is known then 2 doses given as under.

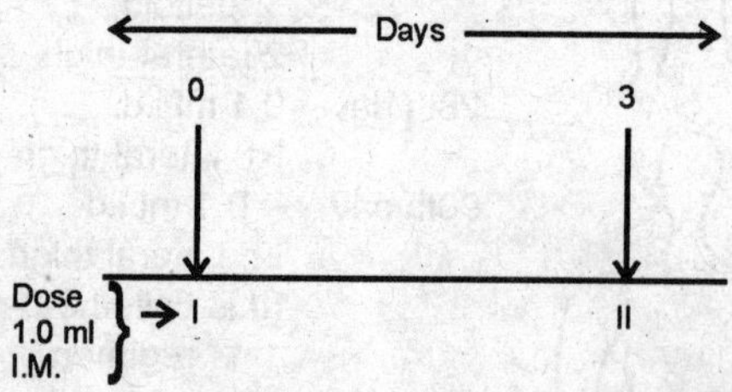

* Passive immunisation with ARS is avoided.

Rabies in Dogs:

Clinically rabies is manifested in 2 forms among dogs:

i. Furious type with behavioural change like running amuck, voice paralysis etc.
ii. Dumb type with quite and spending all the time in sleep state.

Suspected died dog's head can be sent to laboratory, packing in ice in air tight container. If brain is sent, it should be immersed in 50% glycerol saline.

Dog Vaccine:

- BPL vaccine
  Single dose 5 ml for dogs, 3 ml for cats. Booster dose at 6th month is advocated. Later once in a year they are revaccinated.
- Chick embryo vaccine
  3 ml by single injection given once in 3 years.

Public Health Measures for Dog Menace:

- Elimination of stray dogs.
- Registration, licensing of domestic dogs.
- Destruction of animals bitten by infected dogs.
- 6 months quarantine for imported dogs.
- Health awareness on Rabies in the community.

Oral Vaccine Bites for Wild Animals:

This is used in Canada, Germany and Switzerland to overcome Fox menace and found very effective in the control of animal rabies.

Relapsing Fever

Since fever relapses it is called "Relapsing fever" or "recurrent fever" caused by spirochaete *Borrelia recurrentis and Borrelia duttoni.*

Relapsing Fever	by B. recurrentis	Transmitted by infected lice
Relapsing Fever	by B. duttoni	Transmitted by infected soft tick

Hence we have two type of relapsing fever:

1. Louse borne Relapsing Fever.
2. Soft tick borne Relapsing Fever.

Louse borne Relapsing Fever

High endemicity is seen in Ethiopia and Burundi. Low endemicity is seen (Fig. 18.75) in Peru, Bolivia, North West Africa, East Africa, India,

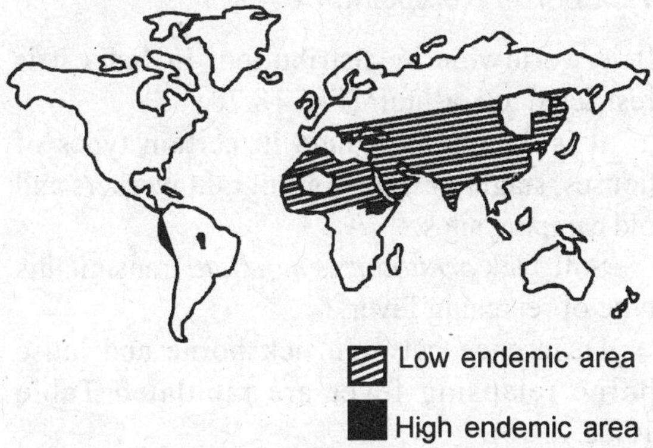

Fig. 18.75: Distribution of louse borne relapsing fever

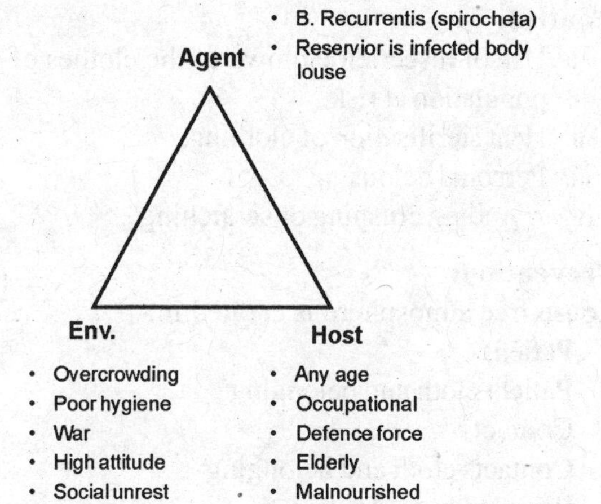

Fig. 18.76: Epidemiology of relapsing fever (louse borne)

Asia and China. Relapsing fever is associated with social unrest, war and suitable environmental conditions.

Relapsing fever coexists with Louse borne typhus. Migration, refugee and overcrowding favour epidemics. It is encountered in high altitude places of tropics, where head louse play a major role in transmission of disease.

Mode of Transmission:

Human body louse (Pediculus Corporis Humanus) causes itching. From infected body louse, the causative agent B. recurrentis are liberated. This is common when body louse is crushed during scratching, which also inoculates the pathogen into the skin.

Clinical Picture:

Sudden fever 39.5–40.5° C accompanied by rapid pulse, headache, body ache, injected conjunctivae, petechial rash, epistaxis and herpes labialis. Hepato-splenomegaly follows which is tender and clinical jaundice is manifested. There may be intestinal bleeding. Fever ends by crisis with profuse sweating, hypotension and circulatory failure. After 1 week, relapse of fever occurs ones or twice; without treatment mortality is 45 percent.

Diagnosis: By demonstration of organism by dark ground illumination of a wet film.

Epidemiological determinants are depicted in Fig. 18.76.

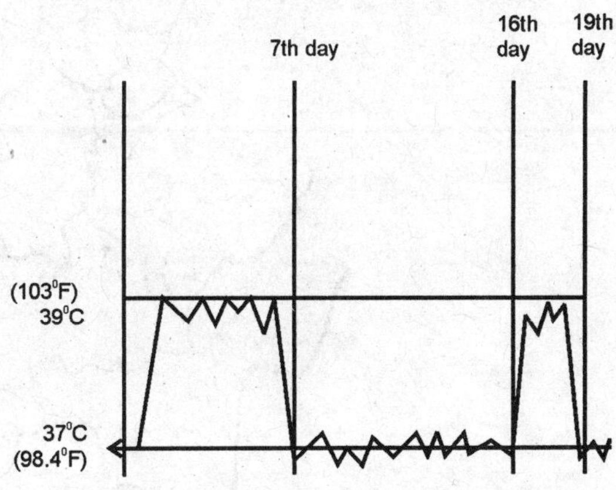

Fig. 18.77: Temperature chart in relapsing fever. Unusually there will be **one** relapse. Maximum relapse could be **four**

Case Management and Nursing Care

i. Procaine Benzylpenicillin 300 mg I.M. followed by next day 500 mg Tetracycline. Doxycycline 200 mg orally is alternative to tetracycline
ii. Since it produces Jarish Herxheimer reaction, the case is best managed in a high dependency unit with expert nursing care.

Control:

i. Use of insecticide blown to the clothes of population at risk.
ii. Heat sterilisation of clothing.
iii. Personal delousing.
iv. Avoiding crushing or scratching.

Prevention:

Louse free atmosphere is created in:

- Patient
- Patient cloth and belonging
- Contacts
- Contacts cloth and belonging
- Personal hygiene.

Tick borne Relapsing Fever

It is worldwide in distribution. In India it is restricted to Kashmir (Fig. 18.78).

It is commonly found in certain types of houses, staging camps for migrant workers and old camping sites.

Soft Tick *ornitodorus moubata* transmit this type of relapsing fever.

Difference between tick borne and louse borne relapsing fever are tabulated Table 18.22.

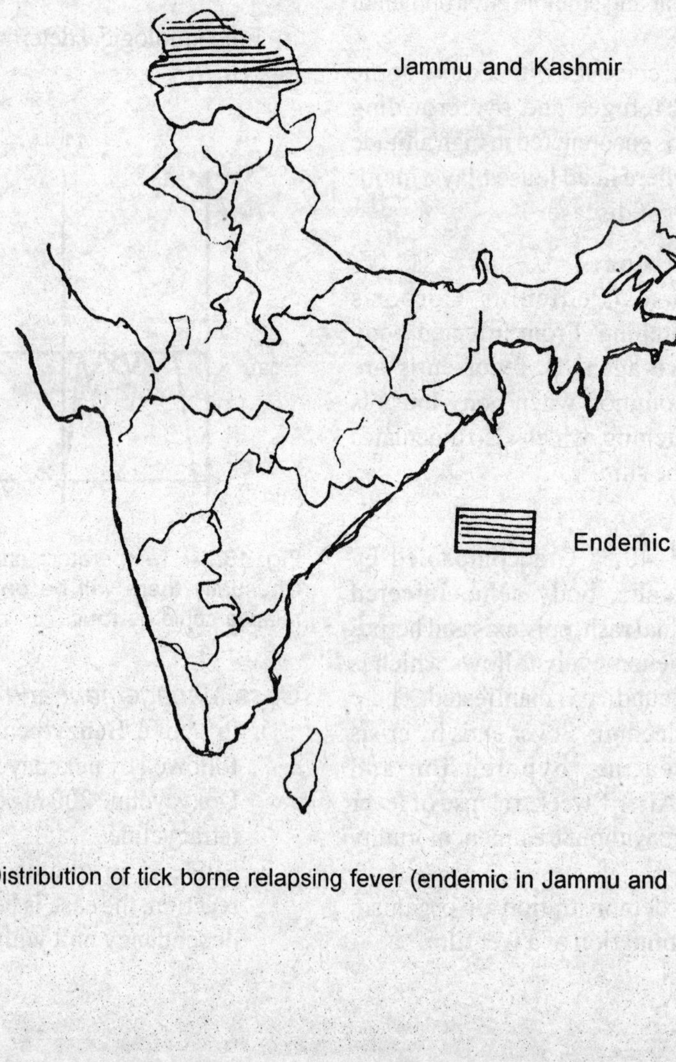

Fig. 18.78: Distribution of tick borne relapsing fever (endemic in Jammu and Kashmir)

Table 18.22: Difference between louse and tick borne relapsing fevers

	Louse borne	*Tick borne*
Parasite in blood smear	Plenty	Few
Paraxysms	Upto 10 days	Upto 5 days
Relapse	One or none	Two or more
Vomiting	Common	Only at meningitis
Other clinical symptom	Diarrhoea, jaundice, coma, haemorrhage	Loss of weight debility lethargy
Neurological complication	Nil	Cranial nerve palsy
Ocular complication	Nil	Papilloedema common
Illness	Severe	Not severe
Mortality	40%	6-8%

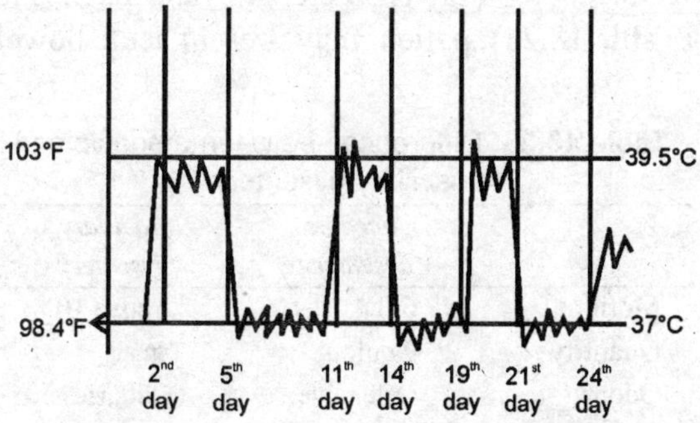

Fig. 18.79: Temperature chart of tick borne relapsing fever. See more than 3 relapse

Clinical Picture:

Headache, fever up to 40°C relapse more than 2 times; spleenomegaly, diarrhoea, bronchitis and haematuria are seen. Seventh cranial nerve is commonly involved. Opthalmoplegia and deafness are also seen as clinical features.

Diagnosis is done by blood smear examination.

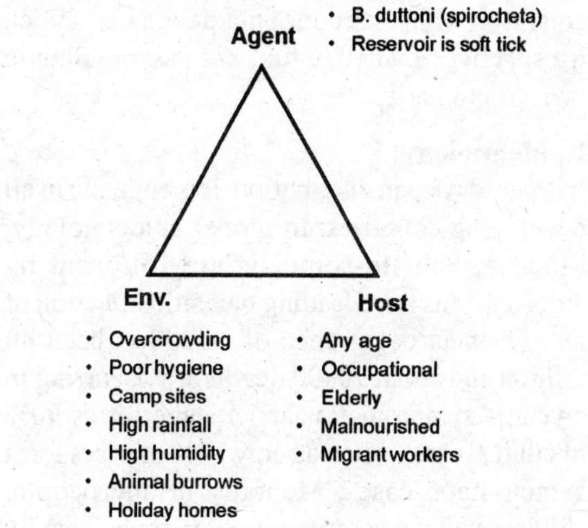

Fig. 18.80: Epidemiology of tick borne. Relapsing fever

Treatment: Is similar to that of louse borne relapsing fever

Control Measures:

i. Effecting concrete floors in the house.
ii. Improved walls in the house.
iii. Use of BHC 20 mg/900 cm^2 as dusting to the floor.
iv. Not sleeping on the floor.

Prevention:

Tick free atmosphere is created in:

- Patient
- Patient belongings
- Contacts
- Contact belongings
- Personal hygiene.

PROTOZOAL INFECTION

Amoebiasis

Intestinal amoebiasis is very common and ubiquitous in distribution, Extra intestinal amoebiasis is seen in tropics and subtropics as minor entity. WHO has defined this as a clinical condition which harbour entamoeba histolytica irrespective of whether the case is symptomatic or asymptomatic.

Epidemiology:

It is world wide in distribution. It is endemic in all developing countries. In global epidemiology, Malaria, Schisto-somiasis are followed by amoebiasis as third leading parasitic infection of man. Annual occurrence of cases has been 40 million and about 70000 deaths are occurring in a year. Asymptomatic carrier stage forms 90% of clinical cases whereas only 10% of cases form symptomatic cases. Mentally insane people, children under day care centres are found heavily infected with intestinal amoebiasis. Following category, if found infected with intestinal amoebiasis; seems to manifest severe infection.

- Those who are on corticosteroids
- Malnourished individuals
- Pregnant women
- Very young children

It is surprising to note that AIDS patient do not show increased risk of infection.

Known faeco-oral infection probably is an expression of food and drink becoming contaminated through exposure to human excreta.

Wherever human excreta is composted and used, prevalence of amoebic infection seems to be high.

India – Problem:

Filed studies have shown that prevalence of amoebiasis is about 15 percent.

Figure 18.81 gives epidemiological triad in precipitating amoebiasis.

Life Cycle:

E. histolytica passes its cycle in man in 2 phases of development (Fig. 18.82):

a. Trophozoite stage and
b. Cystic stage.

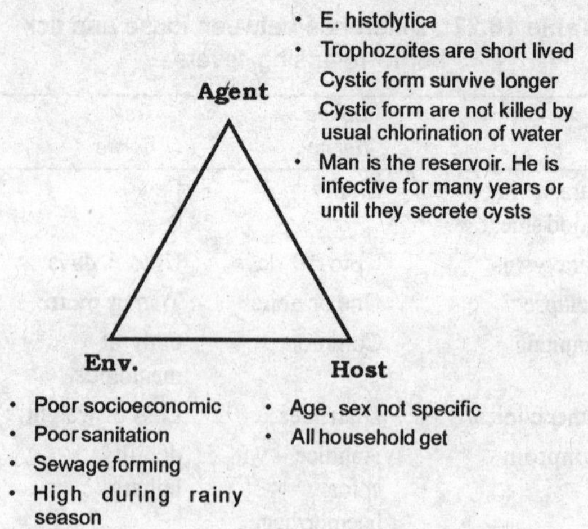

Fig.18.81: Epidemiological triad in amoebiasis

Mode of Transmission: Faecal oral route:

Clinical Feature:

Incubation period is 15 days to few years. Grumbling abdominal pain, 6-8 motions a day, alternating diarrhoea and constipation are features. Stools are characteristics and diagnostic (Table 18.23); patient may present acute bowel

Table 18.23: Differences between amoebic and bacillary dysentery

	Amoebic dysentery	*Bacillary dysentery*
Motion	6-8	Above 10
Quantity	Copious	Small
Odour	Offensive	Odourless
Colour	Dark red	Bright red
Nature	Stool+blood +mucous	Blood+mucus
pH	Acid	Alkaline
Adherent property	-ve	+ve
R.B.C.	Clump	rouleaux
Pus cell	-ve	+ve
Microphage	-ve	+ve
Eosinophils	+ve	-ve
Infective agent	Parasite	Bacteria

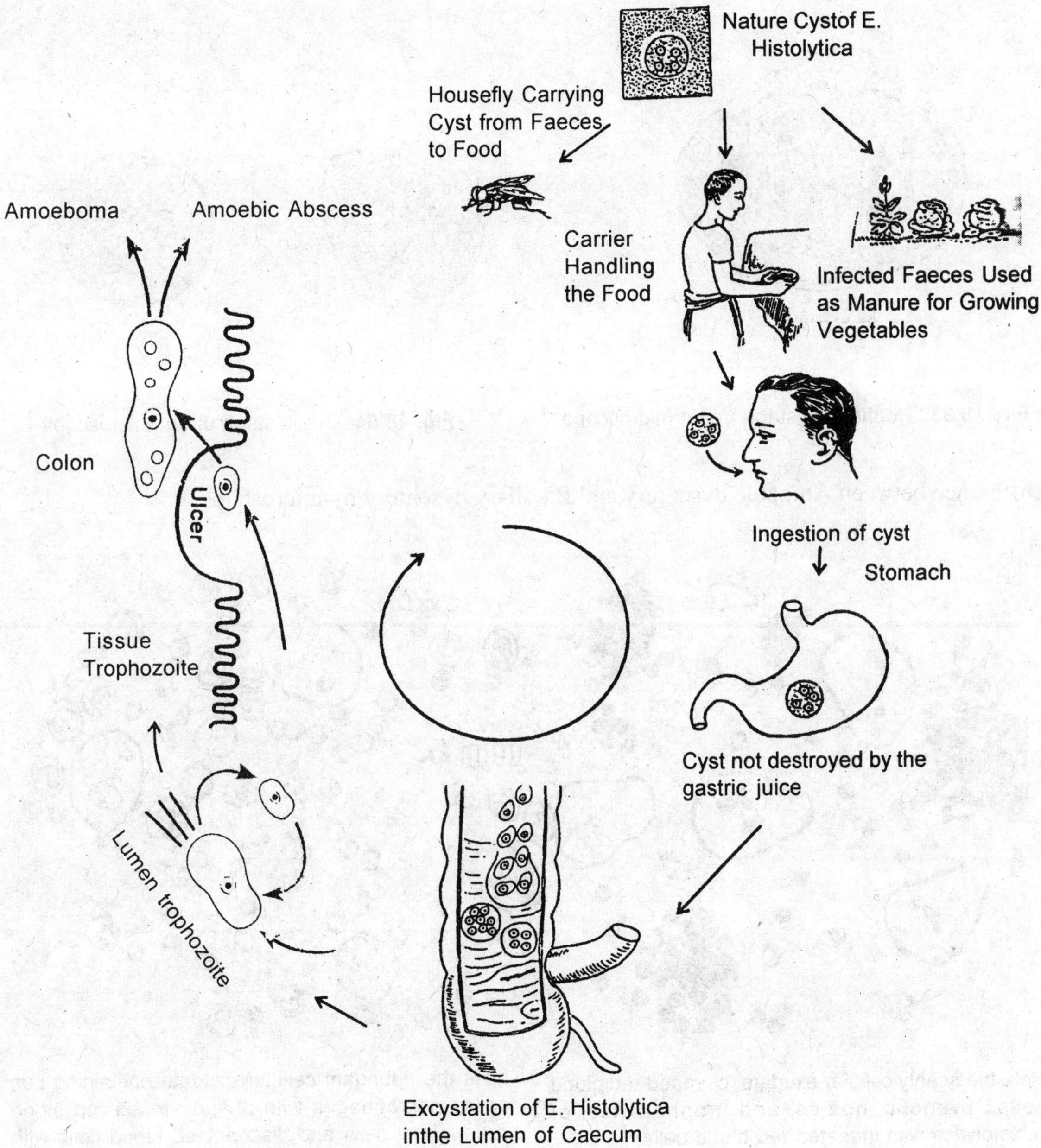

Fig. 18.82: Life cycle of *E. histolytica*

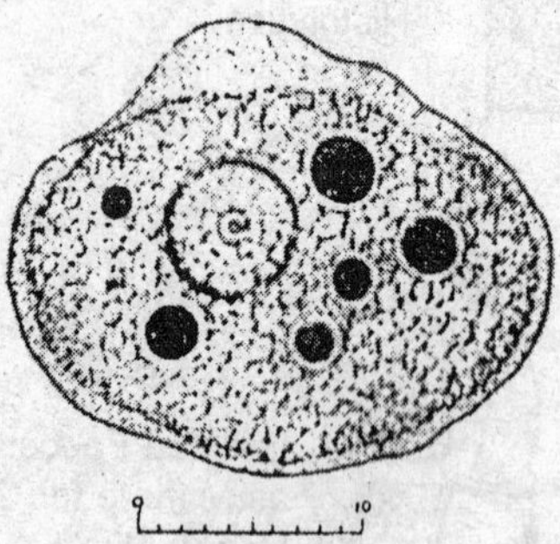

Fig. 18.83: Trophozoite stage under microscope

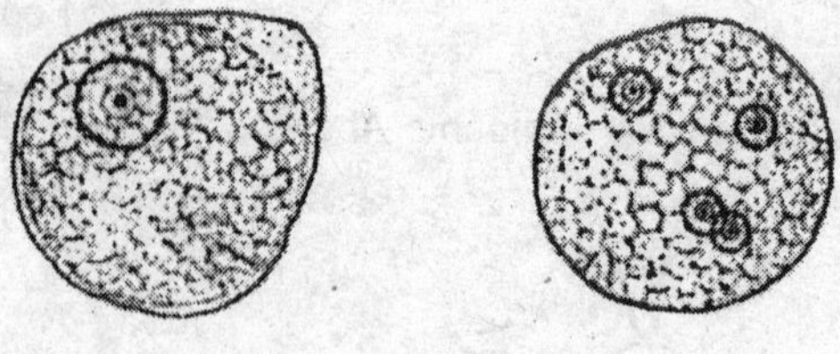

Fig. 18.84: Cystic stage under microscopy

Difference between Amoebic dysentery and Bacillary dysentery by microscope.

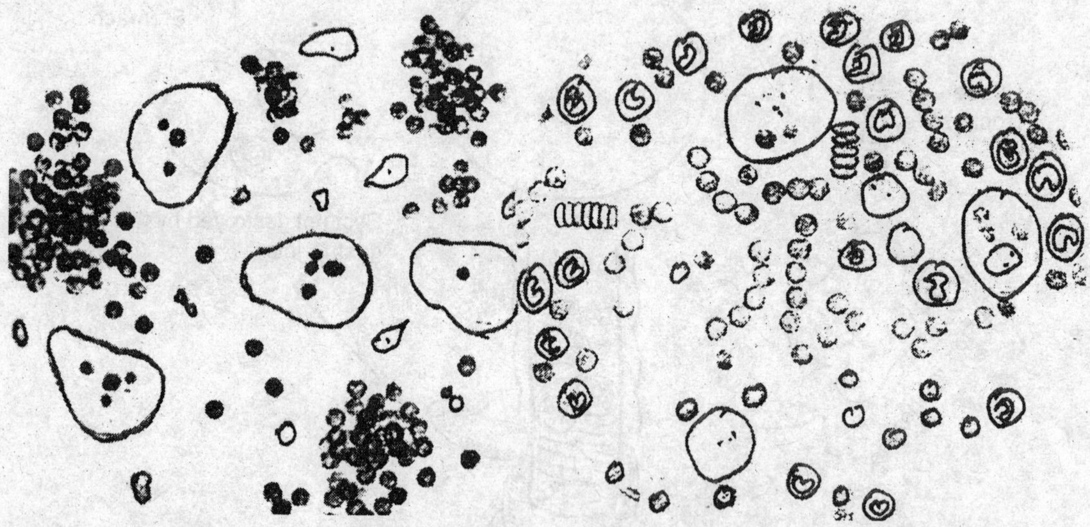

Note the scanty cellular exudate, clumped red blood cells, pyknotic bodies and trophoziutes of E.histolytica with ingested red blood cells

Amoebic dysentery

Note the abundant cellular exudate containing pus cells, macrophages with phagocytosed red blood cells, ghost cells and discrete red blood cells with occasional rouleaux formation

Bacillary dysentery

Fig. 18.85: Microscopy in amoebic and bacillary dysentery

symptoms, as an emergency, in a small proportion of cases.

Case Management

Intestinal amoebiasis responds very quickly to oral Metronidazole. The dose recommended is 800 mg 8 hourly for 5 days. (4 Tablets of 200 Grams at a dose). To eliminate cystic forms, Diloxanide furoate 500 mg orally 8 hourly for 10 days is used. Hepatic amoebiasis responds well with:

a. Metronidazole 800 mg 8 hourly for 5 days.
b. Tinidazole 2 G daily for 3 days.
c. Diloxanide furoate 500 mg 8 hourly for 10 days.
d. Aspiration if abscess is big.
e. Surgical drainage if rupture of abscess occurs.

Control and Prevention:
Early diagnosis and prompt treatment of cases as suggested in case management. There is no acceptable chemoprophylaxis for amoebiasis or mass treatment.

Safe disposal of human excreta by RCA latrine and good sewerage system, protected safe and wholesome water supply to the community, good behaviour in food hygiene, Health education on awareness of amoebiasis and personal hygiene prevents the disease to a great extent.

Giardiasis

Giardiasis is a common parasitic infection causing acute diarrhoea affecting most of the children, tourists and immunosuppressed individuals. This is commonly known as giardia lamblia and worldwide in its distribution. The parasite attaches to the duodenal mucosa and jejunal mucosa and causes inflammation. It is highly prevalent in developing countries with a prevalence rate of 32 to 35 percent. Age of the child is a risk factor; infant suffers more followed by 2-3 age group children. Only at breast feeding, infant up to 6 months usually escapes infection. Malnutrition precipitates Giardiasis. Agammaglobulinaemia predisposes infection where as HIV/AIDS do not seem to influence the infection. Outside the host cyst of G.lamblia survive longer which helps the continued transmission of the disease. Swimming pool sanitation can influence urban prevalence of Giardiasis. Contaminated surface water and man are known reservoir of this disease.

Acute Giardiasis manifests with diarrhoea as leading symptom and fever as least common symptom (Table 18.24).

Table 18.24: Leading symptoms – by proportion

	Leading symptoms on priority seen in Giardiasis
1.	Diarrhoea
2.	Weakness
3.	Weight less
4.	Abdominal pain
5.	Nausea
6.	Steatorrhoea
7.	Flatulence
8.	Vomiting
9.	Fever

Incubation period – 3 weeks.

Clinical Feature:
Diarrhoea, abdominal pain, weakness, nausea, anorexia and vomiting; on clinical examination abdominal distension and tenderness are common findings.

Life Cycle:
Ingestion of cyst is followed by multiplication of hatched out 2 Trophozoites in duodenum. Because of high acidity in duodenum, they can localize in gall bladder. In the time of unfavourable condition it enters large intestine to encyst. The secreted cyst is ingested by another person to continue its life cycle.

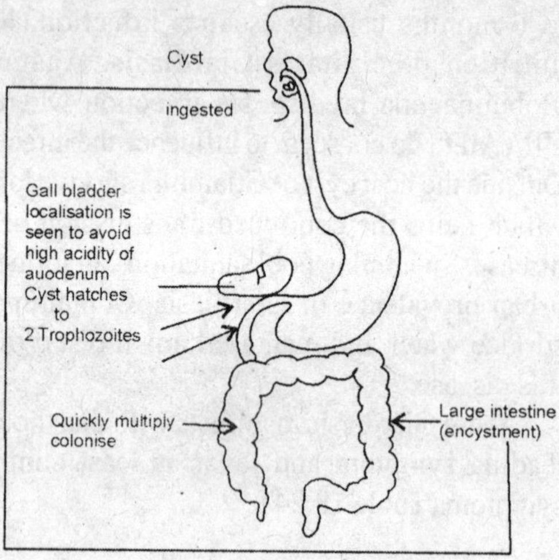

Fig. 18.86: Life cycle of G. lamblia

Laboratory Tests:

a. Microscopic examination of stool for cyst.

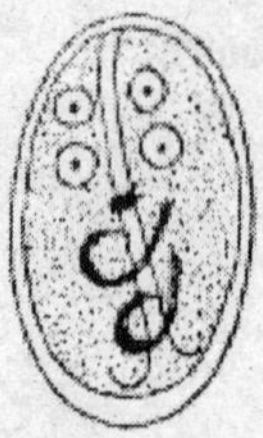

Fig. 18.87: Cyst of G.lamblia under microscope

b. Blood examination for eosinophilia.
c. Duodenal intubation and suction can show trophozoites.

Case Treatment:

a. Single dose of Tinidazole 2 grams.
b. Metronidazole 2 G. once daily for 3 days.
c. Metronidazole 400 mg 8 hourly for 10 days.

Prevention:

It is difficult to eliminate Giardiasis from environment. Contaminated surface water must be treated before it enters public water supply system. Personal hygiene helps to avoid faecal oral cycle.

HELMINTHIC INFECTION (INFESTATION)

Round Worm (Ascaris lumbricoides)

Roundworm is one of the most common and most widespread human intestinal infections. It is estimated that 1.3 billion people are infected at a given point of time in the world.

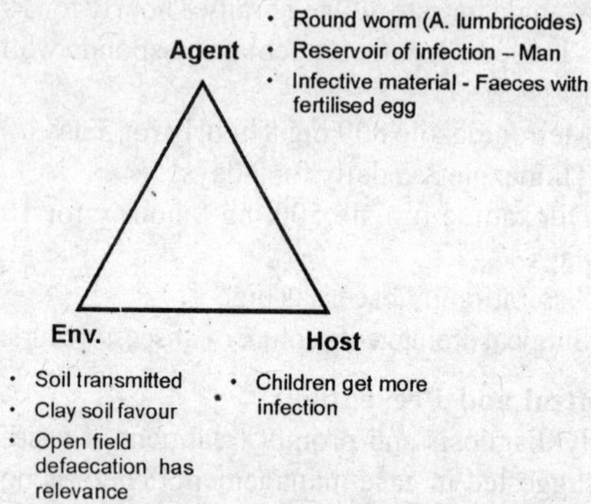

Fig. 18.88: Epidemiology of round worm

Mode of Transmission: Faeco-oral route when the infective eggs are swallowed with food. Raw foods convey infection readily. Water pollution also makes infection vulnerable.

Incubation Period is about 50 days. Course of larvae in man is showed in diagram.

Clinical Features:

Mainly gastrointestinal manifestation in the form of vague abdominal pain forms the main symptom. Extreme cases manifest as malnutrition. Migrating larvae produce (Ascaris pneumonia) fever, cough, dyspnoea, sputum examination show larvae. In 25% of cases urticarial rash and eosinophilia are seen. Due to circulating larvae, functional disorders of brain, heart and kidney are unusual manifestations.

Adult worm destroy nutrients and consume calories leading to subnutrition and malnutrition.

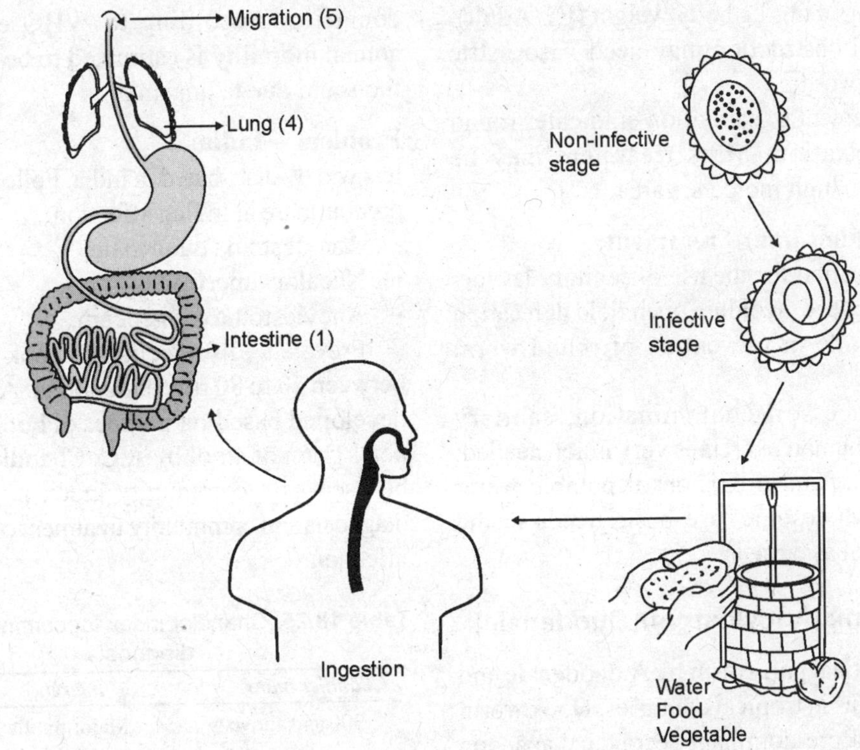

Fig.18.89: Life cycle of round worm

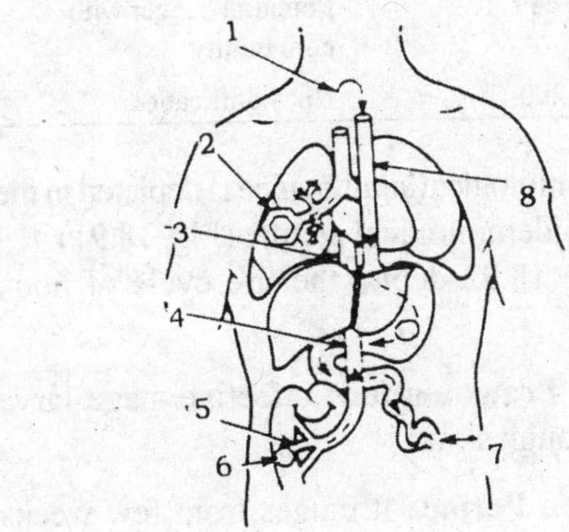

Fig. 18.90: *A. lumbricoides larva course in man* (1) Larva migrates to oesophagus; (2) Larva reach lung; (3) Larva reach inferior vena cava; (4) Larva enter portal vein; (5) Larva penetrate venule; (6) Larva reach intestine; (7) Worms in intestine; (8) Oesophagus

Even Vitamin A deficiency can also be seen, Ascarin in the body can also lead to oedema of the face, conjunctivitis, Urticaria and other toxic manifestations. Rarely, intussuception, obstruction and peritonitis (penetration through ulcers) are reported. Ectopic ascarisis can cause vomiting, suffocation, appendicitis, obstructive jaundice, pancreatitis and liver abscess.

Laboratory diagnosis is examination of ova by direct examination under microscope and concentration by floatation method. History of passing adult worms in the stool or vomitus and X-ray by barium examination are added pathognomonic investigations.

Specific Treatment:

a. Mebendazole 100 mg 12th hourly for 3 days.
b. Albendazole 400 mg as single dose.
c. Piperzine citrate 4 G. as a single dose.

d. Pyrentol 10 mg/kg body weight (IG. Adult).

Surgical obstruction may need nasogastric suction for worms.

Improvement of sanitation eradicates round worm infestation. Mass treatment may be advocated in high incidence area.

Primary (First line) Treatment:
Health education for the use of sanitary latrine, personal hygiene, avoiding open field defecation play main role in prevention of round worm infection.

To reduce soil contamination, sanitary disposal of human excreta is very much needed. Food hygiene and provision of potable water (safe and wholesome) are basic needs in the prevention of ascariasis.

Hook Worm: (Ancylostoma Duodenale)

It is an intestinal parasitism by A.duodenale and N. americanus in tropical countries. Hook worm anaemia is a pre-dominant secondary anaemia in the world. Heavy infection cause pulmonary eosinophilia. Average daily blood loss by one worm is estimated to be 0.15 ml for A. duodenale.

A phenomenon "Hypobiosis" where there is arrested development of migrating larvae is seen, which migrate to mammary gland and is secreted in milk (which can infect the infant). Veterinary experience has shown that Hypobiosis is common in dogs where all puppies are found infective (with dog hook worm).

Third stage larvae have the following anatomical differentiations:

a. Oral capsule is hardly visible and marked dorsally.
b. Tail is pointed.
c. Zone of closing cells leaves considerable space.

Problem – World:
It is eradicated in developed world. It is predominant in Tropical and sub tropical countries. According to WHO estimate the annual mortality is estimated to be about 65-70 thousand due to anaemia.

Problem – India:
It is widely distributed in India. Following species predominate in Indian infection:

- Ancylostoma duodenale
- Necator americanus
- Ancylostoma ceylanicum.

Prevalence of infection by hook worm range between 40 to 80 percent in India. An index was developed based on number of hook worm egg per 1 gram of stool by A.C. Chandler. This can be used as a community index in community diagnosis and community treatment of hookworm infection.

Table 18.25: Chandler index for community diagnosis

Chandler index	*Inference*
300 and above	Major public health problem
250 to 299	Minor public health problem
200 to 249	Potential danger with community
below 200	Not significant

Epidemiological significance is depicted in the triad of epidemiological picture (Fig. 18.91).

Figure 18.92 depict the life cycle of hook worm.

Mode of Transmission: Infective stage larva enters through skin.

Incubation Period: It ranges from few weeks to few months.

Clinical Feature: Ground Itch is common in early infection. Patient may come with presentation of dermatitis. Migration through lung is manifested with cough with blood stained sputum. Clinically there may be patchy consolidation.

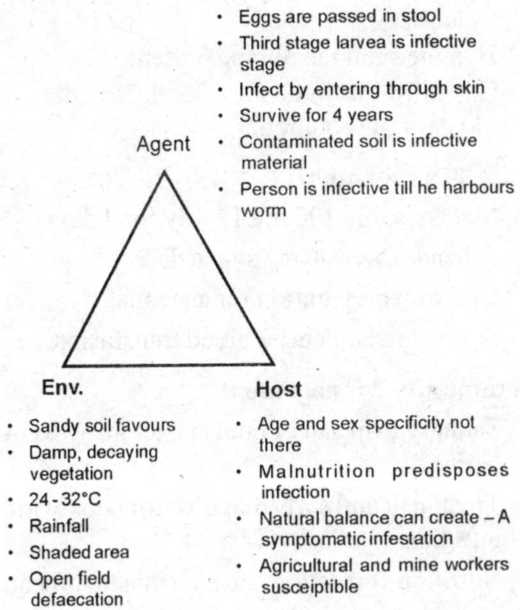

Fig. 18.91: Epidemiology of hookworm

Vomiting and epigastric pain are common in intestinal habitat phase. Loose motion may be subjective manifestations in some of the cases. Signs and symptoms of iron deficiency anaemia are very common in late phase of intestinal parasitism. Among under nutrition population, protein loosing enteropathy and hypoproteinaemia are observed. Iron deficiency anaemia can cause high output cardiac failure. Among children it effects growth and development. Creeping eruption by migrating larvae, bronchitis and bronchopneumonia produce specific clinical manifestations of respiratory systems.

Stool Examination

Following are special microscopic view of eggs of described hookworm and round worm.

- Round or oval shape

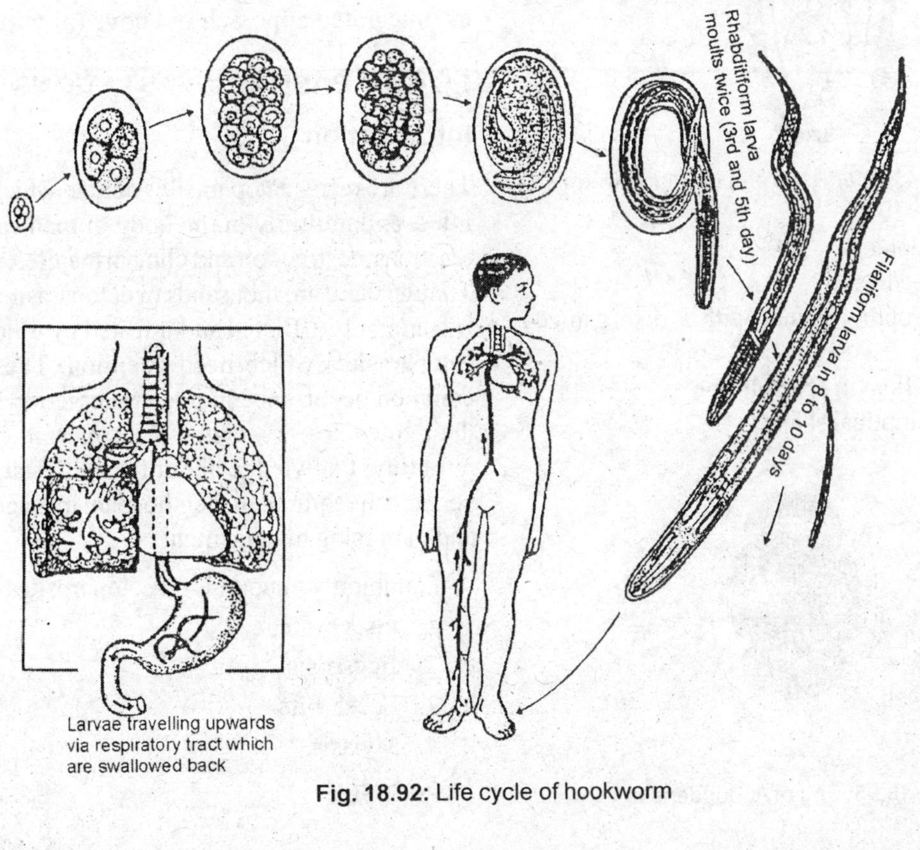

Fig. 18.92: Life cycle of hookworm

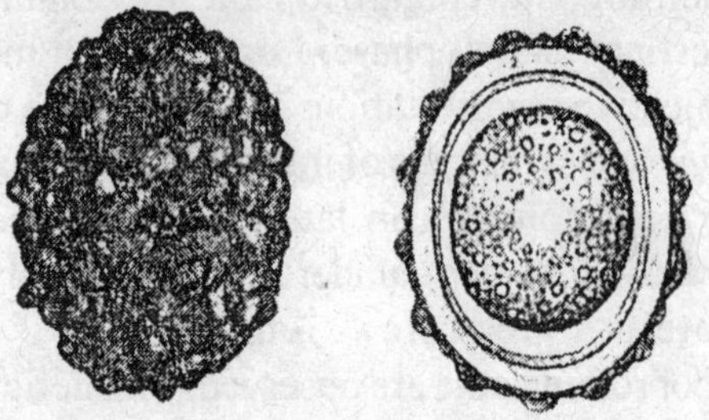

Fig. 18.93: Fertilised egg of round worm

- Golden brown in colour.
- Outer mammilation present.
- Large conspicuous unsegmented ovum.
- Floats in saturated solution of common salt.

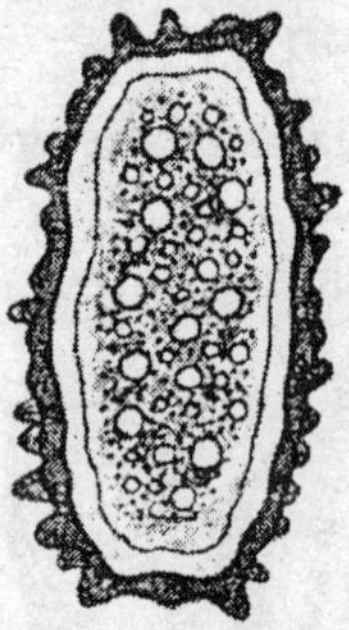

Fig. 18.94: Unfertilised egg of round worm

- Narrow, long.
- Bile stained.
- Small atrophied ovum with a disorganized shape.
- Does not float in salt solution.
- Oval or elliptical shape

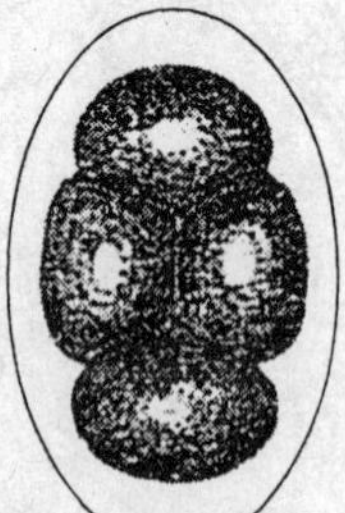

Fig. 18.95: Egg of A. duodenale

- Colourless.
- Hyaline shell membrane present.
- Contain 4 blastomeres.
- Floats in salt solution.

Case Management:

a. Mebendazole 100 mg 12 hrly for 3 days.
b. Albendazole 400 mg single dose.
c. Oral iron preparation for anaemia.
d. Severe anaemia need blood transfusion.

Community Management :

a. Sanitary disposal of human excreta by RCA latrine.
b. Treatment and early diagnosis of hookworm infection.
c. Nutrition correction and anaemia treatment.
d. Health education on use of chappal and not to walk barefoot in open field defecation area.
e. Integrated approach of above (a) to (d).

ECTOPARASITIC INFESTATIONS

Introduction

There are many ectoparasites of man which bite, infest and multiply in the body of man causing reactions, destruction and clinical manifestations. Though there are thousands of ectoparasites man is commonly afflicted and infested by following ectoparasites which need attention. These are common occurrence in hospital practice. Since their bites are associated with morbidity and mortality, knowledge about their infestation in very much required in their hospital management and in nursing management.

Commonly encountered ectoparasites are:

1. Insect bite.
2. Jiggarosis.
3. Leech bite.
4. Myiasis.
5. Scabies.

Insect Bite

Insect bite can cause dermatitis, eczema, troublesome chronic ulcers, and an irritant vesicular rash. Various biting midges and culicoides are seen attacking man in his surroundings. Very common hospital experiences are bee stings and wasp stings, which come with acute hypersensitive reactions.

Bee and Wasp Stings: Usually single sting produce mild reaction. In case of multiple stings severe hypersensitive reactions are expected. Because of anaphylaxis even deaths are expected. During anaphylactic reaction, muscular paralysis is seen which is curare like action on muscle end plates. Slightest disturbance near the hive of bee can cause hundreds and thousands become airborne and start attacking nearby men, cattle, and other animals. They also pursue the fleeing victim and attack them.

By the act of biting, sting of bee is torn. The attached poison gland continues to inject venom to the wound.

Some bees are stingless social bees, their biting does not produce reaction but people get scared because of their aggressive nature of attack.

Honeybee venom contains Histamine, acetylcholine and enzymes which are tolerable at small level. Wasp venom contains higher proportion of histamine and seratonin which are more active than that of honeybee venom.

Paper wasps nest under eaves of houses and people are likely to be exposed to their stings.

Clinical Features:
Sweating, skin colour change, dyspnoea and muscular weakness are commonly observed. At the biting site, reddish swellings and injuries are seen. This at a later stage becomes suppurated. In 20% of cases lymphangitis are observed. Sensitive cases will become ill and nervous for 8 to 10 days following bite.

Case Management:
Mild local reaction is very easily attended with ice pack application. In hospital or health centre, diluted vinegar or antihistaminic ointment is applied. Severe cases need injection of adrenaline.

Sting should be carefully removed and remaining venom is expressed from the gland with the help of forceps.

Jigger Flea Bite

It is caused by the intracutaneous attachment to man by Tunga penetrans, called "sand flea" or "jigger flea".

The fertilized female sand flea tries to penetrate crevices of skin. It attaches by its mouth parts and swells to size of pea. Within 10-12 days after infestation skin irritation starts, which is followed by inflammation and ulceration. Scratching helps in expulsion of eggs.

Clinical Features:
Any part of the body may be attacked; but always it infests below the ankle. Many such jiggers give the appearance of honey comb. By skin ulceration, the eggs are expelled out and the sore left out may become infected by bacteria including tetanus. Pus, ulceration, pain, itching are characteristic of sand flea infestation.

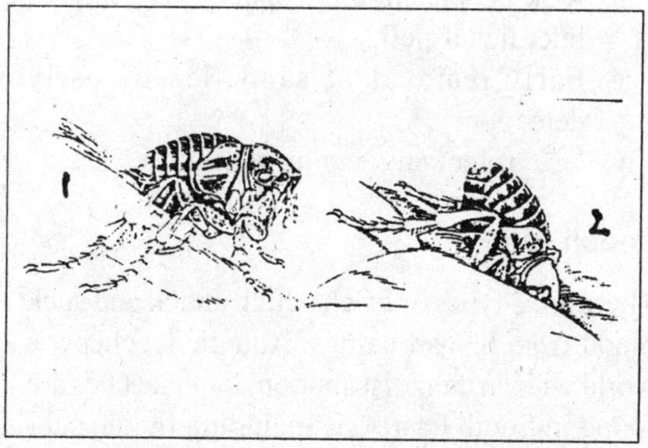

Fig. 18.96: (1) Sand flea female (2) Piercing and penetrating skin of man

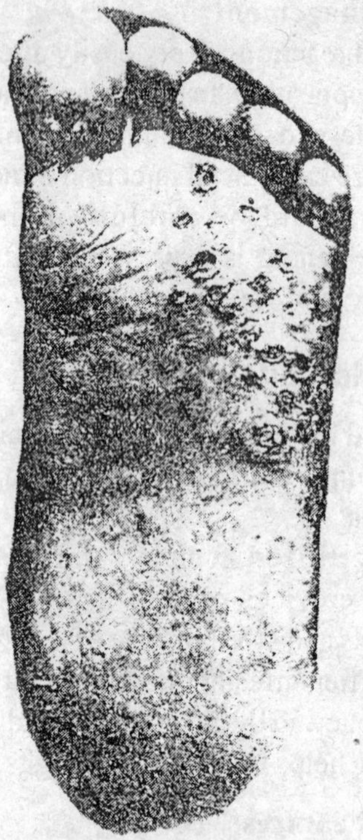

Fig. 18.97: Jiggers in the sole

Treatment:

With the help of sterile needle the sand flea is carefully removed without allowing bursting.

Prevention:

i. Affected area of soil is burnt off.
ii. Risk people should inspect their feet and interdigital cleft.
iii. Early removal of sand flea by early detection.
iv. Use of foot enveloping shoes.

Leech Bite

There are 2 types of leech which attack and suck blood from human beings. Aquatic leeches are world wide in their distribution. Land leeches are found in South East Asia including Indian sub-continent.

They are invertebrates with 3 jaws and 2 suckers. They attach by posterior sucker and allow their anterior end free. With sucking blood they present as dark bloated objects. Their bite produces triradiate wound. Land leech can attack any part of our body. Aquatic leeches have week jaws and get attached to human body orifices.

Clinical Feature:

Land leech make puncture, feed and is painless and bleeds even after leech has gone. Their attack causes anaemia. Aquatic leech will enter mouth, pharynx, larynx, vulva, vagina, urethra while bathing or drinking.

Treatment:

Land leech must be induced to get detached. Strong salt solution, alcohol, strong vinegars or heat will cause the release of land leech. In pharynx and mouth they are to be extracted by proper positioning; otherwise suffocation occurs. Laryngoscopic extraction when it is in larynx, Oesophagoscopy cocaine treatment when it is in oesophagus are advocated. In case of genitourinary tract, irrigation with strong salt solution is advocated.

Prevention:

i. Boots, trousers to prevent attack by leeches.
ii. Garments are treated with Dibutyl phthalate.
iii. Appropriate clothing at swimming.

Myiasis

Myiasis is a clinical condition caused by the attack of larvae of common housefly. They attack tissues, intestine or bladder. When maggots cause furuncle, attack and multiply in wound they cause creeping eruption. When they enter through natural orifice the manifestation depends on the body cavity attacked. If accidentally ingested, it can enter intestine. It is not "obligatory myiasis" since development of housefly larva in human tissue is not essential for their complete development. Housefly larva can be "facultative myiasis" because it attacks the wound when housefly laid their eggs in wound.

Wound Myiasis

Wound of a person which could be a chronic ulcer, a post operative wound or very commonly advanced cancer wound are produced by facultative parasite of Musca domestica (housefly) larva.

Lucilia group of fly maggots are seen used to cleanse wounds by removal of infected tissues. This practice is seen still appropriate for cases where antibiotics are not effective and where surgery is impractical.

Control and Prevention

Personal hygiene and environmental sanitation are best suited answers for the control and prevention of Myiasis due to housefly larva.

Scabies

Morphology, life cycle and other details are highlighted under Chapter 9.

Itchmite which is also called as scabies mite (Sarcoptes scabiei) causes human scabies.

It is transmitted by person to person contact, through bedding and through clothing. The infective agent is fertilized female. The itchmite female makes a permanent burrow in the horny layers of the skin (Fig. 18.98).

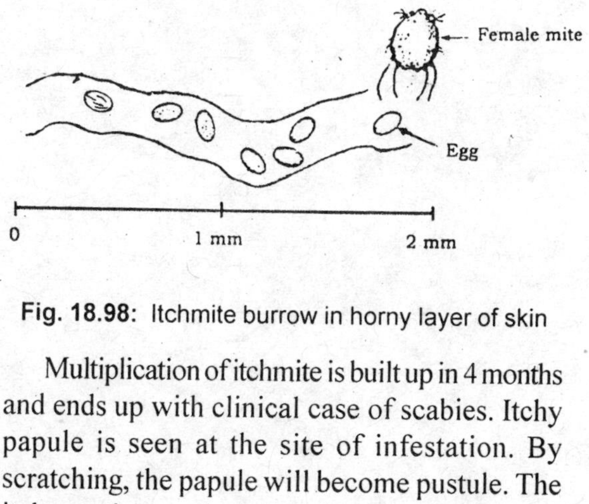

Fig. 18.98: Itchmite burrow in horny layer of skin

Multiplication of itchmite is built up in 4 months and ends up with clinical case of scabies. Itchy papule is seen at the site of infestation. By scratching, the papule will become pustule. The itchy erythematous rashes do not correspond to the site of infested area. Axilla, waist, inner (medial) thigh, back of legs and dorsum of webs of fingers are normal sites of infection. In developing countries infected scabies are common. Where beta hemolytic streptococci infection is profound, clinical case of nephritis among children will be seen.

Case Management and Nursing Care

All the members of the family of case are given simultaneous treatment. 20% emulsion of benzyl benzoate is applied from neck down after a bath and allowed to dry and clothing is put. The next day second bath and clothing wash are a must. The treatment is repeated on 6th day.

Secondary infection is treated by penicillin one course for 5 days.

Other alternative drugs are:

a. NBIN emulsion (1:15 water before use)
   - Benzyl benzoate 68%
   - DDT 6%
   - Benzocaine 12%
   - Polysorbate 14%
b. BHC – Malathion lotion
   - Malathion 0.5%
   - BHC 1%
c. Crotamiton daily application for 5days. It is suitable for infants since it is antipruritic.
d. Tetmasol 5% solution.

Control and Prevention

Personal hygiene and environmental sanitation can control and prevent scabies.

FURTHER REFERENCES

1. Prabhakara G.N. – Short textbook of PSM (JP).
2. WTO agreements and Public Health – A joint study
3. NICD Bulletin on Eradicating Guineaworm – Indian scenario.
4. Guidelines for National programmes, WHO – Treatment of TB.
5. WHO Research for action – Understanding and Controlling TB in India.

6. NACO National guidelines for clinical management of HIV/AIDS – Govt. of India.
7. Control of Communicable Disease in MAN – APHA, USA.
8. WHO Malaria – a Manual for C.H.W.
9. WHO – Prevention of Disabilities in Patient with Leprosy – A Practical Guide.
10. WHO D.H.F. – Diagnosis, Treatment, Prevention and Control.
11. N.H.D. of TB – WHO, William Harris.
12. Ball and Gray – Aids Infectious diseases (Churchill Livingstone).
13. G.O.I. – Nutritional care during Diarrhoea.
14. WHO – Treatment and Prevention of Dehydration in Diarrhoea.
15. Management of severe malaria – WHO.
16. NACO – Surveillance of S.T.D.
17. ICMR – Treatment of Diarrhoeal Diseases and Programme Management.
18. Chaterjee K. D. – Parasitology, Kolkata.
19. Manson's Tropical Diseases – G.C.Cook (ELBS).
20. WHO – The Management of A.R.I. in Children.
21. WHO – Lab. Techniques in Rabies.
22. Prabhakara G.N. – Manual of Lab. Technology (Paras).
23. G.O.I. – Report on the Third Modified Leprosy Elimination Campaign 2001-2002.
24. Prabhakara G.N.—Policies and Programmes of Health in India 2004 (Jaypee).
25. Prabhakara G N – Trends, Issues and Management in Nursing (PeePee).

19

Non Communicable Diseases

IMPORTANCE

Diseases which do not have specific agents as their cause and which are not communicable, have only risk associations, where vectors are unknown, which do not have specific incubation period, rather usually have latent period are called *Non Communicable Diseases.*

Common examples are metabolic disorders (Diabetes), Cardio vascular disorders (Coronary heart disease, Hypertension, Stroke, Rheumatic heart disease), Malignancy (cancers), Nervous disorders (Alzheimer's disease), musculoskeletal disorders (arthritis, gout) and other life style associated disorders.

They are increasing day by day and causing an upset in Health care and nursing care services. Diagnosis, Treatment and prevention are difficult because of their indefinite onset, long latent period, multiple factors associated and absence of the causative agent.

Epidemiological findings have shown that some of the risk factors are found responsible for the morbidity and mortality of non communicable diseases. They are:

- Nicotine use by different forms
- Alcohol use
- No preventive health services obtained
- Incorporated life style changes
- Occupational hazards
- Air pollution and water pollution
- Stress.

MAJOR N.C.D.'s

Blindness

Blindness is visual acuity of less than 3/60 Snellen chart or its equivalent. It is equal to finger counting at 3 meters. If it is 1/60 it is finger counting at 1 meter. Total blindness refers to no light perception.

Problem:

World: 180 million are visually disabled and 45 million are blind.

India: Cataract induced blindness has exceeded 3 million, about 2 million are waiting for corneal transplantation.

Major causes of blindness are:

a. Cataract
b. Glaucoma
c. Tracoma
d. Vitamin A deficiency
e. Corneal opacity

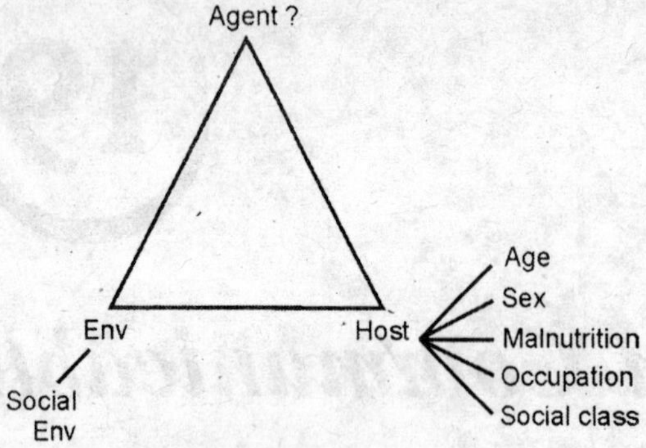

Fig. 19.1: Epidemiology of blindness

f. Refractive error
g. Other causes.

Intervention:

Primary	*Secondary*	*Tertiary*
• Foreign body removal	Cataract treatment	Corneal graft
• Infection control	Glaucoma treatment	Retinal surgery
• Vitamin prophylaxis		

Long-term Measures:

- Water supply
- Vitamin A supplementation
- Social upliftment.

Special Programmes:

i. Trachoma control: 1% ointment BD 5 days a month for 6 months. Blanket treatment to all below 10 years
ii. School eye health service
iii. Vit-A prophylaxis
2 lakh unit orally at six monthly intervals (9 months to 3 years age)
iv. Occupational eye care.

Accident

Accident is an unexpected event involving injury, disability or death. Common accidents are:

a. Vehicle accident
   - Road traffic
   - Aircraft
   - Railway
   - Sea traffic
b. Self inflicted accidents
c. Accidental falls
d. Industry accidents
e. Drowning
f. Poisoning
g. Fire accidents
h. Disaster accidents.

Problem: 9% of deaths at global level and 4% of death in Indian context. Traffic accident alone is killing more than 2 lakh per year.

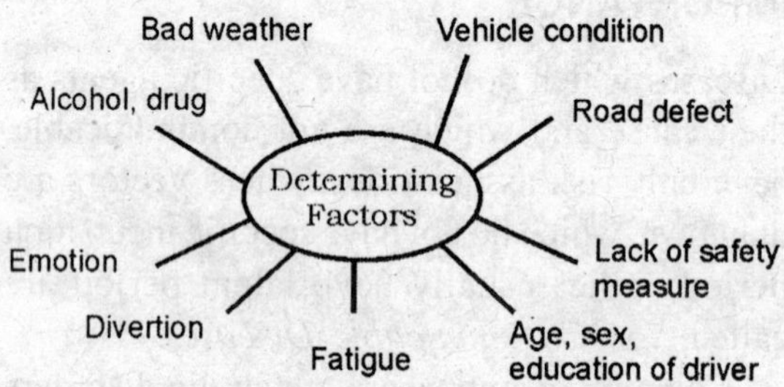

Fig. 19.2: Factors in accident

Prevention of Accidents:

- Development of basic reporting system
- Development of safety education to public
- License withholding to alcoholics and drug user
- Susceptible zones should have trauma care centres.
- Highway development programme
- Incorporation of new technology in vehicles
- Action force developed from fire force
- Safe storage of poisons
- Accident research
- Law enforcement for:
  - Fitness certificate to drivers
  - Seat belts
  - Helmets

- Factory safety
- Industry safety.

Diabetes

Diabetes mellitus is a metabolic disorder with various manifestations. They are Insulin dependent, non insulin dependent, malnutrition related, drug induced types in clinical practice. Impaired glucose (IGT) and Gestational diabetes (GDM) are other 2 variants of diabetes.

Problem:

World: 150 million are suffering from diabetes.

India: 19 million are suffering from diabetes.

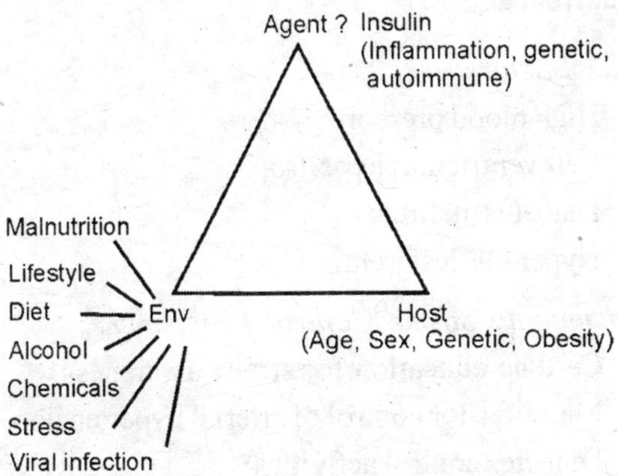

Fig. 19.3: Epidemiology of diabetes

Screening tests like urine sugar, RBS, PPBS are suggested to high risk group.

Prevention:

Population strategy primordial	*High risk strategy*	*Tertiary strategy*
Weight control Good balanced diet Physical exercise	Treatment, diet, drug, exercise Periodic examination Half yearly glycated Hb%	Case of blindness Kidney failure Gangrene of limb Coronary thrombosis

Cardiovascular Diseases

C.H.D. (Coronary Heart Disease)

It is due to inadequate blood supply to heart due to coronary artery obstruction.

Problem: It is exceedingly high in developed countries. In India 4 to 5% of people are showing clinical evidence of coronary artery obstruction.

Clinical Picture

- Angina pectoris
- Myocardial infarction
- Atrial and ventricular fibrillations
- Sudden death.

Risk Factors:

Modifiable	*Non modifiable*
Smoking	Age
Serum Cholesterol (LDL)	Sex
Diabetes	Genetic
Obesity	
Sedentary habit	
Stress condition	
Type A personality	

Role of Serum Cholesterol:

Elevation of serum cholesterol increases the risk of MI. LDL is directly associated with CHD. VLDL is associated with premature athero-sclerosis. The suggested Cholesterol/HDL ratio is 3.5 as an indicator of prevention. Recently apolipoproteins level is used in risk assessment of CHD.

Prevention:

Population strategy	*Others*
Smoking prohibition	High risk strategy
Maintain physical activity	Secondary prevention
Diet control	
Blood pressure control	
Life style change	

Hypertension

According to WHO, a systolic BP equal to or greater than 160mm Hg and a diastolic BP equal to or greater than 95 mmHg is treated as hypertension. There are two types: (a) Primary hypertension and (b) Secondary hypertension.

Problem:

World: 10–20% prevalence.

India: 5–6% prevalence.

WHO has noted that proportion of adequately treated for hypertension is only 10-12%. It is depicted by rule of half.

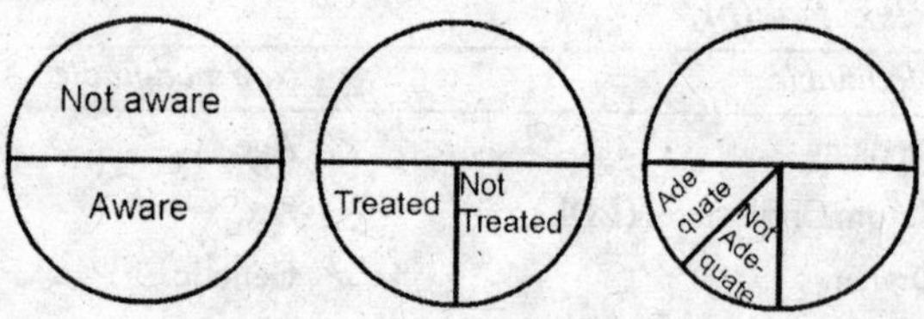

Fig. 19.4: Rule of halves

Risk Factors:

Modifiable	*Non-modifiable*
Overweight	Age
High salt, High fat, intake	Sex
Alcohol	Genetic
Physical activity	
Tension	
Stress	

Prevention:

Primary prevention	*Others*
Population strategy	
• Weight control	High risk strategy
• Strict diet	Secondary prevention
• Physical activity	
• Meditation	
• Awareness	
• Participation	

Stroke

Stroke is rapidly developed clinical sign of focal disturbance of cerebral function lasting more than 24 hours or leading to death with no apparent cause other than vascular origin.

Cerebral hemorrhage and cerebral thrombosis contribute to the major causes of stroke.

Problem: 2 per 1000 population per year.

Prestroke Warning:

Presence of microemboli causing sudden focal reversible neurological deficit which is less than 24 hours duration is called T.I.A. (Transient Ischemic Attack) It forms warning signal to recurrence.

Risk Factors:

- High blood pressure
- Left ventricular hypertrophy
- Diabetes mellitus
- Hyper cholesteremia.

Community Stroke Control Programme:

- Cardiac education for stroke awareness.
- Measures for control of arterial hypertension
- Diabetes control activities
- Elimination of smoking
- Training of health personnel for stroke control.

Rheumatic Heart Disease

It is one of the preventable heart diseases. If not treated properly, it becomes a crippling disease causing heart damage and disability.

Problem:

World: 6-33/10000 population

India: 2-6/10000 Population.

Diagnosis:

Community diagnostic tool is "Jones Criteria".

- 2 major criteria
- 1 major criteria + 2 minor criteria
- Throat culture
- A S O Antibody titre.

"Jones Criteria" according to WHO:

Major	*Minor*
• Carditis	• Fever
• Polyarthritis	• Arthralgia
• Chorea	• Past H/O Rheumatic Fever
• Erythema marginatum	• Abnormal ESR
• Subcutaneous nodule	• C-reactive protein
	• Leucocytosis
	• Prolonged PR interval (ECG)

Rheumatic Fever Prevention Chart:

Primary Level	*Secondary Level*
a. Benzathine penicillin IM single dose (Crystalline 3 lakh + Procaine penicillin 3 lakh + Benzathine penicillin 6 lakh)	a. Monthly injection of 6 lakh unit Benzathine penicillin for 5 years or till attain 18 years
b. Penicillin V oral 10 days 250 mg TDS	b. Early diagnosis and prompt treatment of Rheumatic fever
c. For penicillin allergy Erythromycin oral 10 days 40 mg / kg / QID	
d. Improve standard of living	
e. Improve environmental sanitation	
f. Decrease overcrowding	
g. Sore throat screening procedure	

Cancer

This non communicable disease is characterised by unlimited growth of tissues, invasion to organs, organs' failure and ultimately death. In clinical practice carcinoma, sarcoma, lymphoma, myeloma, leukaemia are major categories. Colloquial word for cancer is "Tumor". As per cited occurrence cancer can be primary or secondary in nature.

Problem:

World: 14% of death is by cancer.

India: Annual occurrence of cancer is 7 lakh, with 50% mortality.

Table 19.1: Common cancer in India

Sex	*Type cancer*
Men	Oral cancer Ca. pharynx Ca. oesophagus Ca. stomach Ca. lung
Women	Ca. Cervix Ca. Breast Oral Cancer Ca. Uterus

Attributed causes associated as under:

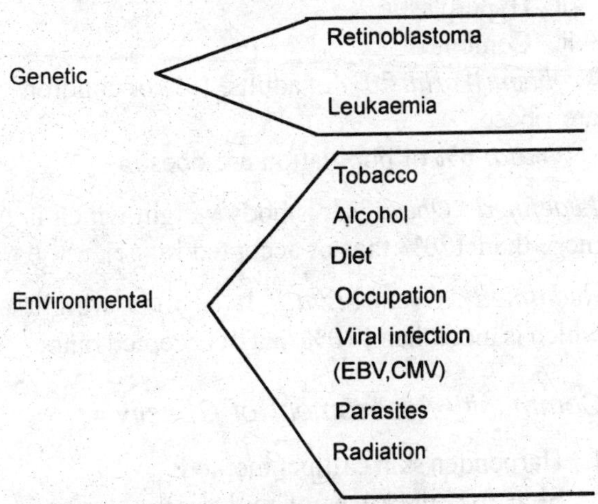

Fig. 19.5: Attributable causes for cancer

Cancer Control Approach:

Primary Prevention

- Tobacco
- Diet
- Alcohol
- Occupational environment
- Infection and cancer
- Sunlight

- Sexual and Reproductive factors.

Early Detection:

- Education for early diagnosis
- Screening for cancer.

Treatment for Cancer

- Chemotherapy
- Radiotherapy
- Surgical intervention.

Palliative care for pain relief.

Cancer control research.

Obesity

It is a pathological state of overweight for the given age, sex and height of an individual. A body mass index (Quetelet's index) of above 30 in men and above 28.6 in women indicates obesity.

Types of Obesity

i. Hypertrophic
ii. Hyperplastic
iii. Combined

Problem: World: 20% of adults, 10% of children are obese.

India: 6% of population are obese.

Redefined "Obese": It is body weight which is more than 120% that of accepted range.

Redefined "Overweight": It is body weight which is more than 110% that of accepted range.

Community Assessment of Obesity

1. Harpenden skin calliper method:
   Skin fold thickness of mid triceps, biceps, subscapular region, suprailiac region are obtained.
   Standard: Sum of measurement 40 mm in boys and 50 mm in girls are acceptable level.
2. Quetelet's index (B MI).

   It is found out by $\left(\frac{\text{Weight}}{\text{Height}^2}\right)$ popularly called Body Mass Index (BMI)

   Std. 18.5 – 24.99 – Normal

Over weight – Grade 1	25.0 – 29.99
Grade 2	30.0 – 39.99
Grade 3	> 40.0

3. Broca index is found out by height (cm) – 100 (gives weight)
4. Ponderal index is found out by $\left(\frac{\text{Height}}{\text{Weight}^3}\right)$
5. Corpulence index is found out by $\left(\frac{\text{Actual Weight}}{\text{Desired Weight}}\right)$ (acceptable level = 1.2)
6. Lorentz's index is

$$\text{Height} - 100 - \left(\frac{\text{Height} - 150}{4}\right) \text{ for men}$$

$$\text{Height} - 100 - \left(\frac{\text{Height} - 150}{2}\right) \text{ for women}$$

Health Problem of Obesity:

- Hypertension, diabetes, C.H.D.
- Vericose veins
- Hernia
- Arthritis
- Reduced life expectation.

Prevention:

- Diet
- Exercise
- Regulation over feeding behaviour.

Smoking, Alcohol, Substance Abuse

All the three are life associated; habit forming items are known to cause millions of premature deaths. World problem is increasing because of its higher incidence in (a) Developing countries (b) In females and (c) In young children.

The vicious cycle starts with psychic dependence, passes through physical dependence, addiction and tolerance.

Smoking habit with Bidi, Cigarette, Cigar, Chutta, Chilum, Hookha, Chewing and snuff –

all allow tar, carbonmonoxide and nicotine toxication. Cancer and ischemic conditions are significantly associated with nicotine intoxication. Country's Economy and health loss are known from smoking. Health education, no tobacco campaign and policy may help in reducing smoking induced disorders.

Alcohol and substance abuse (Drug abuse) are known to be related to (a) Availability (b) Social acceptance (c) Broken homes (d) Life style change (e) Modernization. Health aspects of alcohol and substance abuse (Drug abuse) are highlighted in Chapter 2.

Psychotherapy, Detoxication process and rehabilitation can, to a given extent, bring down these non communicable diseases.

FURTHER REFERENCES

1. Prabhakara G.N. – Short Text Book of PSM (JP)
2. W.H.O. – TRS no. 732, 727, 894.
3. W.H.O – Cancer pain relief.
4. W.H.O. – Workshop report on Diabetes (1998).
5. D.G.H.S. – Chronicle 1979.
6. Prabhakara G.N.—Policies and Programmes of Health in India 2004 (Jaypee).
7. Bulletin of Pan American Health Organisation 1987 vol 21 No.2.

20

School Health

IMPORTANCE

For raising health status of a Nation, School age group children are to be given special care. Being future generation, school children form an economic group of the country. It is categorised under personal Health services. Early days of Medical Examination is totally changed for a comprehensive school health services.

As per 2001 census 24.9% of Indian population (1,027,015,247) constitutes 256 million, who are of school age between 5 and 14 years of age. So health care and nursing care needs of 255,725,796 school children becomes a stupendous task unless a formulated national guideline is prepared.

School Health services are an important function of Primary Health Centre in India.

HISTORICAL DEVELOPMENT

1909	First school Medical examination at Baroda city.
1946	Bhore Committee recommends its importance.
1953	Secondary education committee emphasised need of examination and school feeding.
1960	G.O.I. Constituted a school health committee which suggested means of improving school health.
1961	The School Health Committee recommended School Health Committees at all levels (National, State, District, Block and village levels).
1995	Ministry of Welfare GOI introduced a comprehensive Bill called "Persons with disability (equal opportunities, protection of rights, full participation)"
1997-2002	9th Five Year Plan envisaged the progress of school health care.
2003-2007	Formal documents have been prepared and are waiting for clearance which include widened version of school health care.

HEALTH PROBLEMS IN SCHOOL CHILDREN

Main problems noticed are malnutrition and infectious diseases. Emphasis is laid on following illness among school children.

- Skin infection including scabies and louse infestation
- Dental caries

- Measles, mumps and chickenpox
- Round worm and hook worm infestations
- Vision alteration
- Hearing impairment
- A.R.I.
- Diarrhoea.

Role of nursing profession is in provision of comprehensive nursing care as educator, counsellor, organizer and co-coordinator. They include:

i. Health appraisal – General Examination and risk child identification.
ii. Treatment and follow up.
iii. Advice on healthful school environment.
   - Good floor space of more than 10 sq ft per school child and not more than 40 students in a class.
   - Proper sitting desk arrangement.
   - Door and window should be 25% of floor space.

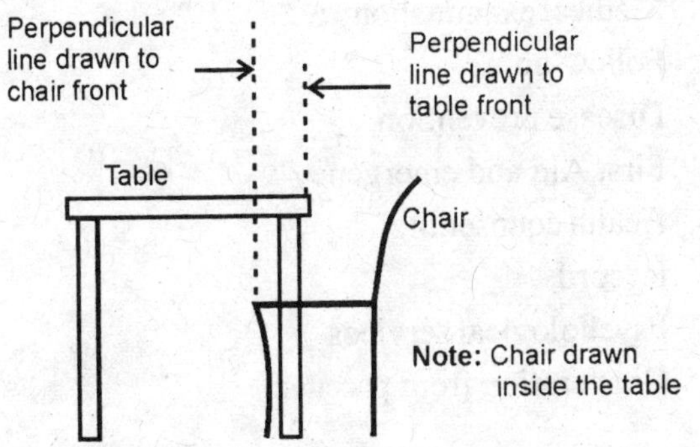

Fig. 20.1: Chair Table alignment for negative desk for sustained study

   - Good lighting.
   - Good protected water supply.
   - Urinals and Latrine at 1 per 60 and 1 per 100 respectively.

iv. Preventive immunisation like child T.T. as per schedule, cholera, typhoid at requirement.
v. *Nutrition:*
   - Arrangement of mid day meal programme providing 250 days of feeding with supplementary food which should provide.

75G	Cereals and millet
30G	Pulses
8G	Oil
30G	Leafy vegetables
30G	Non leafy vegetables

   - Broad principle of mid day meal is to supply 1/3 daily calorie and half of daily protein. They are prepared as home foods. It is advisable to adopt low cost meal. Range of calorie and protein can be adjusted to 350-570 calories and 13-32 grams protein per day.
   - It can be alternated with snack called "Meal Snack" days.

vi. *First Aid:* Teacher training for first Aid is a requisite.
vii. *Mental Health:* To maintain positive mental health and to overcome behavioral deviation.
viii. *Dental Health:* To control dental disease and defects.

Menu for North Indian School Children:

Menu	*Programme*	*Calorie*	*Protein*	*Cost (Rs.)*
1. Maize roti+ rape leaves + Butter milk	3 days a week	380	16	1.25
2. Bajra cooked + curry		430	15	1.60
3. Tandoori roti+ aalu chole		420	16	1.80
4. Missi roti+ curd		560	17	1.50
1. Aalu chole+ bread	2 days a week	370	14	1.80
2. Marunda+Khaman Dhokla		560	27	2.40

Menu for South Indian School Children:

Menu	Programme	Calorie	Protein	Cost (Rs.)
1. Rice + Sambar + Buttermilk	3 days	550	15	1.80
2. Pongal + Curry + Buttermilk	a	500	15	1.75
3. Veg Chapaties	week	500	21	1.60
4. Wheat pulse porridge + buttermilk		450	14	2.00
1. Sundal+ Buttermilk	2 days	36	13	1.75
2. Laddu+Buttermilk	a week	500	19	2.00

ix. *Eye Health:* For correction of refractive error, squint treatment, trachoma treatment and Vitamin A administration.

x. *Health Education:* On personal hygiene, health awareness, first aid.

xi. *Health Appraisal:* Teacher to be educated to note and to take action on:
- Skin rash
- Respiratory symptoms
- Neck rigidity
- Eye redness
- Diarrhoea
- Fever and chills
- Headache
- Vision defect
- Hearing defect
- Behaving rudely
- Flushed face
- Swollen face.

INITIATION OF SCHOOL HEALTH BY NURSE

- Know the set up of school (Administration)
- Establish rapport with teachers
- Make periodic visits to school
- Check physical facilities at school
- Arrange parent-Teacher counselling
- Arrange meetings for school improvement
- Arrange and help physical check up of children
- Take care to observe chronic defects among school children
- Help in their treatment and referral.

COMPONENTS OF SCHOOL HEALTH SERVICES

- Medical examination
- Follow-up
- Disease prevention
- First Aid and emergency
- Health counselling
- Records
- Psychological services
- Cooperation from parents.

SCHOOL HEALTH RECORDS

Along with cumulative card, health card should also be maintained for each student. That should contain the following:
- Identification data.
- Past health history
- Family history of any illness
- Findings of medical check-up
- Information on care given.

NURSING ROLE IN HANDICAP CHILDREN

Special attention is required for a school child which is handicapped because education of handicapped child is not an easy task. Physically, mentally and Socially handicapped children require special nursing care and a good interaction with parents and school management.

FURTHER REFERENCES

1. G.O.I. – Report of the School Health Committee.
2. Turner C.E. – School Health and Health Education (C.V. Mosby).
3. Report of Seminar on School Health Services held at Delhi.

21

Occupational Health

IMPORTANCE

Industrial revolution and progress in science and technology has brought in changes the occupational status. Gradually, for the past 50 years, these changes have become cognizant of the benefit of Nurse's professional skills in safeguarding health status of workers.

Primary health care of any occupation relay on ethical issues, Loyalty to worker-patient, confidentiality and reporting health risks. Treating the injured or ill require understanding of industrial hygiene which is renamed as *Occupational Health*.

DEFINITION

According to I.L.O., it is defined as "Occupational health is the field of science which aim at promotion and maintenance of highest degree of physical, mental and social well being of workers in all occupation, at prevention of departure from health at working condition.

ERGONOMICS

It is derived from Greek meaning work + Law. It is a recognised discipline for developing efficiency of man and machine.

Indian Picture:

Constitution of India has included the Directive Principles like: (a) Security of workers in an occupation. (b) Child labour (c) Humane condition of work. Many committee reports are available like.

- Adarkar Report
- Bhore Committee Report
- Thomas Bedford Committee Report
- Jones Committee Report.

Further India has taken steps for legal measures through:

- I.F.A.
- Coal Mines Labour Welfare Act
- E.S.I.S. Act.

The welfare of workers in any occupation is being taken care of through:

a. DG, Factory inspection and Advisory service and
b. Central Labour Institute.

There are many research centers on occupational health and I.C.M.R. has a division for effecting measures.

OCCUPATIONAL ENVIRONMENT

It is a sum of external conditions that influence

health status of workers. It can be represented by Figure 21.1:

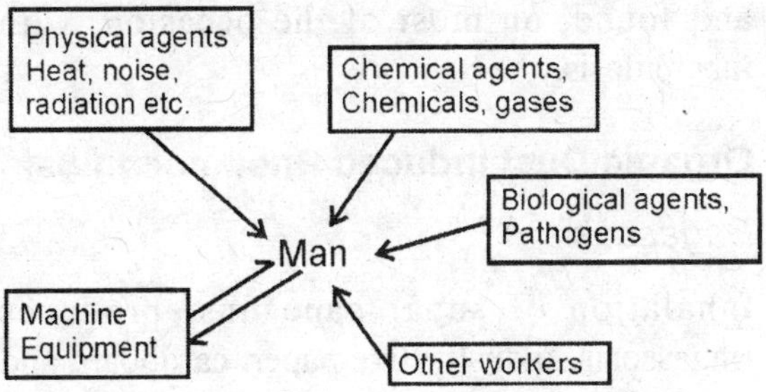

Fig. 21.1: Man in his working environment

Agents mentioned above may be adverse to health of a person in a working condition. Accidents due to fatigue, muscle joint impairment are common occurrence. Human relation with coworkers decides good working atmosphere.

HAZARDS IN OCCUPATION

Physical Hazards

Heat:	Burns, heat exhaustion, heat stroke, heat cramps, fatigue
Cold:	Chilblains, erythrocyanosis, Immersion foot, Frostbite
Light:	Eye strain, headache, eye fatigue, miner's nystagmus
Noise:	Hearing loss, nervousness, annoyance
Vibration:	White fingers by spasm, joint injury
U.V. Rays:	Welder's flash, conjuctivities
Radiation:	Cancer, depilation, sterility.

Chemical Hazards

Local – Dermatitis
Dusts – Inhalation and lung change
Gases – Fibrosis of lung, malignancy, poisoning.

Biological Hazards

- Anthrax
- Brucellosis
- Encephalitis
- Fungal infections
- Hydatid disease
- Leptospirosis
- Psittacosis
- Tetanus.

Mechanical Hazards

- Fall
- Crush injury
- Loss of vision
- Fracture
- Loss of organ.

Psychological Hazards

- Frustration
- Lack of Job satisfaction
- Emotional tension
- Depression
- Alcoholism
- Psychosomatic like headache, peptic ulcer.

PNEUMOCONIOSIS

Organic or Inorganic chemical dust (of size 0.5 to 3 micron in size) when inhaled over a period of time cause lung changes by inflammation followed by (with or without) infection leading to reduced ventilatory capacity called "Pneumoconiosis".

Common types of pneumoconiosis are described in the following section.

Inorganic Dust Induced Pneumoconiosis

Anthracosis

Coal dust inhalation over a period of 12 years cause simple pneumoconiosis. Later with the development of Progressive Massive Fibrosis (PMF) severe respiratory disability and premature death occurs. It is a notifiable disease.

Asbestosis

Silicates of magnesium are a fibrous material, which when inhaled gives rise to Asbestosis. It is associated with a serious cancer type Mesothelioma of pleura which kills the worker within 3 months. Sputum exam showing "Asbestos bodies" and X-ray showing ground glass appearance are established criteria of diagnosis.

Siderosis

Lead is common metal used in many industries like, battery, glass, ship building, printing, potteries, rubber etc. There are non occupational sources like gasoline use, lead paint on toys, water running through lead pipes etc.

Inorganic lead poisoning cause abdominal colic, constipation, loss of appetite, blue lines on gums, stippling of red blood cells, anaemia, wrist drop, foot drop etc.

Organic lead cause headache, loss of sleep, mental confusion and delirium.

Prevention of siderosis is by:

- Isolation.
- Personal protection.
- Good house keeping like cleaning of floor, bench, machine etc.
- Periodic examination of workers.
- Personal hygiene.
- Creation of Health awareness among workers.
- Availability of emergency nursing care like:
  - Saline purge
  - D – penicillamine
  - E.D.T.A.

Silicosis

Inhalation of silica in mining, ceramic industry, metal grinding, construction work, iron and steel industry cause premature death.

It produces nodular fibrosis, poor ventilatory capacity, X-ray show snow storm appearance and found, on most of the occasion, with tuberculosis.

Organic Dust Induced Pneumoconiosis

Bagassosis

Inhalation of sugar cane dust produces Bagassosis. Industry like paper, cardboard and rayon show a fungal growth (actinomycete) on Kernel of sugarcane which causes bronchiolitis changes. Reduced pulmonary ventilatory capacity, fibrosis, emphysema and bronchiectasis are common.

Dust control, personal protection and sprinkling 2% propionic acid on Kernel prevents Bagassosis.

Byssinosis

Inhalation of cotton fibre produces Byssinosis. Cotton industry show, among its workers chronic cough, progressive dyspnoea, chronic bronchitis and emphysema.

Containment of cotton dust and periodic examination of workers help in the control of Byssinosis.

Farmer's Lung

It is also called Hey fever since grain dust is inhaled which produce lung change causing fibrosis and corpulmonale. Fungal actinomycete causes lung changes. In the beginning it is manifested as allergy disorder and later as infective disorder.

Personal protection and health aware-ness help in the control of Farmer's lung.

Tobacossis

Nicotine in tobacco when inhaled constantly produce lung changes causing bronchitis, emphysema and bronchiectasis. It is associated with bronchogenic carcinoma.

Personal protection and periodic examination helps in the control of tobacossis.

CANCER AND OCCUPATION

Certain occupations are found associated with specific cancers. They are:

Blood Cancer: Workers in X-ray, workers in Isotopes, Benzol are prone to blood cancer.

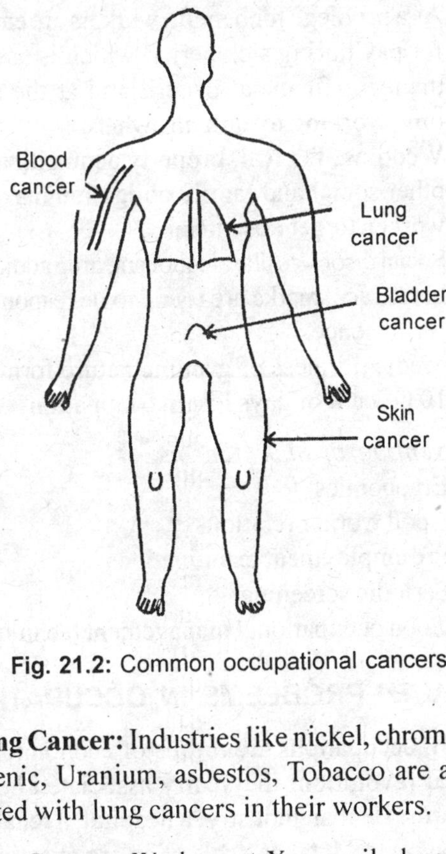

Fig. 21.2: Common occupational cancers

Lung Cancer: Industries like nickel, chromium, arsenic, Uranium, asbestos, Tobacco are associated with lung cancers in their workers.

Skin Cancer: Workers at X-ray, oil, dyes, gas workers, tar distillery and chimney sweeping are found to get skin cancer.

Urinary Bladder Cancer: Industries like rubber, aromatic amines, dyeing industry, electric cable, magenta and aniline affect this organ to develop cancer changes.

SKIN AND OCCUPATION

Dermatitis is known in all most all working placements where physical agents like heat, cold, moisture, friction, pressure, X-ray, chemical agents like acid, alkali, dye, solvents, phenols; Biological agents like Bacteria, parasite and plant products like dust of flower and vegetable dust comes in constant contact with skin.

Occupational dermatitis can be prevented by following measures:

- Preplacement examination
- Skin protection
- Personal hygiene.

X-RAY INFLUENCED HAZARDS

Occupations like Radiology, Radiodiagnosis, Radiotherapy, watch industry, radioactive ore, arc welding, foundry work etc. have effects of radiation which can cause following health hazards:

- Skin burn
- Chronic dermatitis
- Blood cancer
- Tumor development
- Genetic defects.

Personal protection and periodic examination prevent X-ray influenced hazards.

AGRICULTURE AND HEALTH HAZARDS

India is mainly rural and agriculture based which cover over 79% of population.

Now innumerable number of health hazards are observed in agriculture. They can be grouped as under:

Toxic hazard:

Insecticide poisoning.

Accidents:

Fall, fracture, snakebite, scorpion bite.

Zoonotic disease:

Man may get diseases of lower animals like anthrax, brucellosis, tuberculosis.

Soil contaminated:
Tetanus.
Physical environment:
Rain, hot sun.
Respiratory diseases:
By organic dust.

ACCIDENT AND OCCUPATION

Accidents are causes of production loss, human suffering and loss of worker's day in occupation. Human and environmental factors play vital role in occupational accidents.

Human Factors: Incapability of worker, vision impairment, hearing impairment, immature mind, fatigue, carelessness, emotion.

Environmental Factors: Poor light, unsafe machines, high temperature.

DIAGNOSIS OF ABSENTEEISM (SICKNESS ABSENTEEISM)

Employees are expected to come to work when scheduled to do so: but it is generally accepted that, at times, there may be valid reasons for workers not to attend.

Absence: Absenteeism and sick absence are common words for workers in their scheduled work when they are expected to attend, excluding overtime.

It is defined as absence from work attributed to sickness or injury and accepted as such by the employer or the social security system.

Diagnosis of absence is done by:

- Gross absence rate
- Sickness absence rate
- Unauthorized absence rate
- Absence frequency rate.

Gross absence rate should be below 5%.

If it is 10% it is serious as per standards.

Absence frequency rate of 0.5 per annum needs attention for improvement. 1.0 and above is serious as per standard.

Sickness absence rate if high and is above 4, this indicates a high degree of morbidity in working class and this points out to a medical rather than a managerial problem.

Unauthorized absence rate of spells longer than 14, require special attention as per standard.

Incidence: India is showing 15 to 20% sickness absenteeism as per findings from the National Productivity Council (NPC).

Causes of Sickness Absence:

- As a privilege for benefit, workers are entitled for pay during sick period which is used by them for financial benefit and at the same time working to earn elsewhere.
- Wedding, festival, property acquisition and other social and family obligation make the worker to get absented.
- Social disorders like alcoholism, drug addiction, horse race, matka are found to be responsible for absence.
- Medical illness of genuine nature form 8 to 10 percent of days lost in occupation.

Prevention of Sick Absence:

- Ergonomics
- Good worker relations
- Pre employment examinations
- Periodic screening
- Good occupational management techniques.

HEALTH PROBLEMS IN OCCUPATION

In all, occupations are means of economic and social revolution; they carry associated health hazards. Be it an industry, a hospital, a rehabilitation centre, it takes a role of an organisation to face inevitable health sets and upsets during the course of its working culture.

Main problems are enumerated below:

Housing – Shelter problem is increasing in vertically grown cities.

Water – Scarcity, pollution leading to water borne diseases.

Air	–	Toxic gases, dusts pollute the air causing allergy, asthma, chronic bronchitis.
Sewage	–	Poor sewage system leads to soil pollution, high parasitic and helminthic infestations.
Diseases	–	Tuberculosis, STD, and Malaria are raging due to overcrowding of cities.
Food	–	Typhoid, Hepatitis are becoming more conspicuous due to poor food sanitation.
Mental health	–	Psychoneurosis, behaviour disorders, delinquency are increasing due to altered, civilized, and urbanized ways of life.
Accidents	–	Congestion and vehicular traffic is leading to many highway traffic accidents leading to mortality and morbidity.
Social problems	–	Alcoholism, drug addiction gambling, prostitution, divorce, crime have increased in densely populated industrialised area.

SPECIFIC PROTECTION OF HEALTH OF WORKERS IN OCCUPATION

International Labour Organisation, through its subsidiary National Labour Organisations, is trying to uphold health protection measures as its aim in promotion and maintenance of the highest degree of physical, mental and social well being of workers in all occupation . They are summarized as under:

i. *Health Education:* Health awareness for personal hygiene, personal protection, good and healthy atmosphere of working condition are need of the day.

ii. *Mental Health:* Workers in any occupation require love, affection, recognition, job satisfaction, rewards and discipline. Nursing profession being highly skilled occupation require utmost attention in this regard.

iii. *Nutrition:* Balanced diet at reasonable rate to workers of an organisation is a must. This is compulsory as per legislative standards when number of employees exceed 250.

iv. *Medical Care:* Facility for diagnosis, treatment, hospitalization of affected workers is obligatory on the part of employer.

v. *Environmental Sanitation:* Any factory, industry, organisation require facility under this, which are prime requisite for health of workers. They are:
   - Protected water supply
   - Hygienic food
   - Separate toilet for male and female
   - One Latrine for every 25 workers
   - General cleanliness of Industry, Factory, Hospital, Nursing home or organisation
   - Floor space of 500 cub.ft per worker
   - Good lighting
   - Good cross ventilation
   - Anti fire measures
   - Good dust containment measures.

vi. *Special care of women* :
   - Maternity leave to expectant mothers.
   - M.C.H. services.
   - Crèche in factories, industries or organisation if more than 30 women are working which can take care of their children.

vii. Welfare schemes for small family norm.

PREVENTION OF OCCUPATIONAL DISEASES

They are grouped under 3 heads:

1. Medical
2. Engineering
3. Legislation.

Medical Measures

a. *Medical examination before appointment:* This is called Preplacement examination. The purpose is to place proper person to a given work placement, depending upon his ability and capability.

At the time of Medical examination the certifying doctor categories the worker according to his fitness for the work

– A	–	Fit for any work
+ B	–	Got remediable disease
++C	–	Not fit for employment fit for limited work
++D	–	Unfit for any work

If the person is suffering from diseases, he will not be taken to certain related risky occupation.

Table 21.1: Undesirable occupations for given disease

Diseases present)	*Industry where he is (If not appointed*
Asthma, skin disorders, kidney problem, pre-cancerous lesion	"Dyes" industry
Anaemia, Hypertension, Nephritis, Peptic ulcer	"Lead" involving occupations
Tuberculosis of Lung, Chronic Bronchitis with emphysema	'Silica' related occupation
Liver disease, Kidney	'Solvents' production units
disease, Dermatitis, Alcoholism	
Blood disorders	X-ray dept. Radium unit, Cobalt Therapy unit

b. *Periodic Examination:* Normally annual examination is recommended. In case of occupation where Radium, Dyes, Lead are used – it will be every month. In case of irritant chemicals, ionising radiation, High dose cobalt therapy, Investigations with radio active isotopes- daily examination at the end of shift is advocated.

c. *E.S.I. Hospitals:* In case of Factories, Industries and organisations, facility for medical check up, treatment and investigations are made available to workers.

d. *Notifications:* Notification of cases and suspected cases in occupational diseases are mandatory as per legal standards.

e. *Supervision of Working Environment:* Physician and Nurse should enlist the cooperation of safety engineers, psychologists and industrial hygienists for the health and welfare of workers in an occupation.

f. *Occupational Records:* Records on worker's health, disability or absence help in improving the best device for good working condition.

g. *Use of protective Devices:* Mask, glove, helmet, apron, shoes, Lead or cloth working white coat help in personnel protection in occupation.

Universal precaution is a typical example of personal protection of nursing profession from infectious diseases.

Special protective devices in AIDS cases, SARS cases are other examples.

Engineering Devices

a. Design of Factory, Industry, Hospital, Health centre should start from blue print stage.

b. *Good house keeping:* It includes general cleanliness, lighting, ventilation to eliminate occupational hazards.

Hospital waste management is an example of good house keeping in Nursing Care services.

c. *Containment:* To collect all dust and eliminate from working area is called containment of dust or agents.

d. *Dilution:* Developing green belt around Factory, Industry, Hospital or organisation maintain air purity and hazards due to atmospheric pollution can be reduced.
e. Engineering devices for personal protection are well known. Apron, glove, mask, helmet, sterile suit are examples.
f. *Monitoring:* Environmental monitoring for permissible limits and statistical monitoring for health criteria are required for positive occupational health.
g. *Research:* It is a podium for better understanding of health problem in occupational health.

Legislation

To govern the condition of a Factory, an industry, a hospital, a nursing home or an organisation and to safe guard the health and welfare of the worker, Laws are framed at National level and are amended from time to time.

The Factory Act 1948:
Since 1881 the rules and regulations were in force till the Act was promulgated.

Much revision took place and latest revision (amendment) was in 1987.

Scope: Any organisation which appoints 20 workers comes into its preview. (It is 10 when power is not used which is becoming rare). It includes contract labour also.

Health, safety, welfare: Provision of working environment, medical and nursing facility and provision of waste disposal are included in the provision. Agewise, sexwise limit is prescribed for effecting work in an occupation. "Safety Officers" for every 1000 workers is made mandatory. It describes special welfare measures like washing, first aid, lunchroom, and crèches. A canteen for every 250 workers, a crèche for every 30 women workers and a welfare officer for every 500 workers are recommended.

Child labour: Prohibits employment of children below 14 years of age.

Shift basis: It prescribes 48 hours of work per week which should be 8 to 9 hours per day.

Leave with pay: 1 day for every 20 days is advocated.

It is obligatory to notify specified occupational disease. Hazardous process should be viewed for service condition of employees.

E.S.I.S. 1948

Employees' State Insurance Act 1948 was amended recently in 1989.

Scope: It covers all establishments where 20 or more people are working. It includes shops, hotels, cinemas, transport service and newspaper establishments.

Administration: It is outlined in Figure 21.3.

Finance:

Employer	4.75%	of wage
Employee	1.75%	

Expenditure:	7/8 by corporation
	1/8 by states.

Benefits

Medical Benefit: Investigation, treatment, hospitalization, individual health care and family care of employee is taken care under this. ESI dispensaries are set up where more than 1000 workers are employed, a part time ESI dispensary where 750 workers are employed, through General Practitioners in other situation.

Doctor population ratio in ESI is 1: 585 at present.

ESI has a long-term goal of ESI hospitals at the rate of 4 beds per 1000 employees.

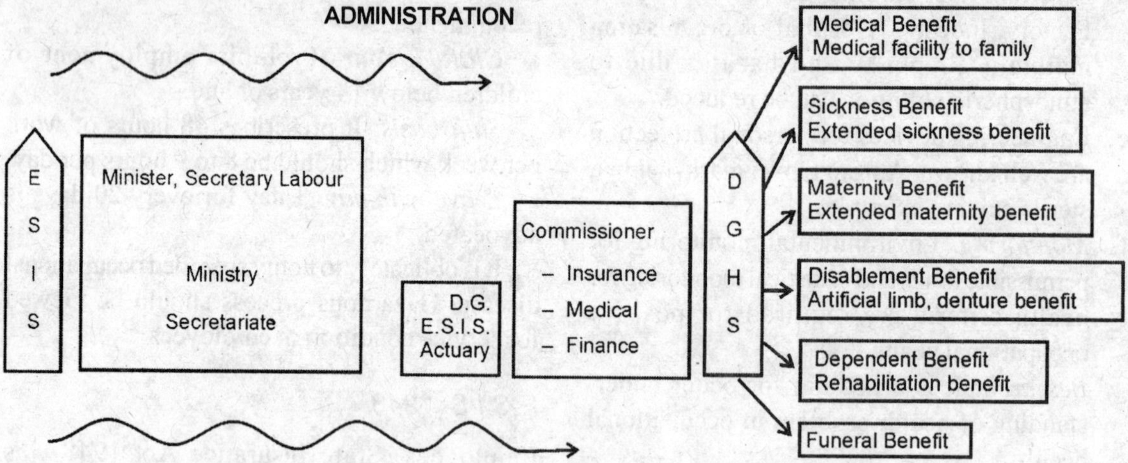

Fig. 21.3: Administration of E.S.I. Scheme

Under medical benefit, following additional facilities are provided:

- Dentures, spectacles, hearing aids, artificial limbs, Hernia belts, walking calipers.
- Surgical boots, spinal brace, jackets.

Per capita cost of medical benefit is Rs. 905 in the present situation.

Sickness Benefit: The benefit of 91 days wage per year is allowed. It pays 7/12 of wage of employee; certain long term illness are considered for allowing 309 days since chronic course of disease need long time. They are:

- Tuberculosis, Leprosy
- Cancer
- Paraplegia, hemiplegia
- C.C.F.
- M.I.
- Disc prolapse
- Retinal detachment
- Chronic renal failure
- Burns above 50% with infection.

Maternity Benefit: Twelve weeks for confinement, 6 weeks for miscarriage are allowed.

Disablement Benefit: 70% of wage for temporary disability and life pension (70%) for permanent disability.

Dependent Benefit: Dependents get 40% of standard benefit rate periodically. 70% of wages as pension in case of death of an employee.

Funeral Benefit: This is an amount of Rs. 2500.00 towards funeral expense.

Rehabilitation Allowance: At insurance of Rs. 10 per month by worker, medical treatment of disabled and members of family till life. About 3 lakh employees are covered under this.

Other Acts

The Mines Act, The Plantation Act, The Minimum Wages Act, The Maternity Benefit Act, etc.

Rajiv Gandhi Shramik Kalyan Yojna: This was launched in April 2005 which gave a vent for an unemployment allowance for an employee who looses his job (involuntarily due to factory closure, retrenchment, invalidity etc. Maximum period of 6 months benefit is allowed in this scheme as per standard benefit rate specified by ESI Rules.

OCCUPATIONAL HEALTH NURSE

In early days home nursing service for workers was given by industrial nurses. Nursing care at Hospital, Nursing homes, Health Centres, Physician or dentists office and Nursing education are predominant areas of placement of nurses. Now new area of interest for nursing care services are:

- School health
- Occupational health.

In developed countries nurses are employed in factories. This requires specialized knowledge and skill with proper training. U.K. and Canada are imparting advanced courses in occupational health nursing. Standing committees are giving service activities which are now under the banner of American Association of Occupational Health Nurses (AAOHN)

Apart from general nursing, special nurse management in performing lung function tests, audiograms and vision tests are the needs of nursing care.

Job description of occupation health nurse:

- Assist rehabilitation of employee at plant site.
- Conduct walk through inspection of plant from health point of view.
- Treating, educating employee.
- Attend safety meetings.
- Assist occupational physician in clinical examination.
- Maintaining records.
- Act as a liaison.
- Check over hazard data sheets.

FURTHER REFERENCES

1. I.L.O. – Volume I and II.
2. Call Zenz – Occupational Medicine (Year Book Med. Pub).
3. G.O.I – Indian Factory Act.
4. G.O.I – E.S.I.S.
5. ESI Samachar Dec 2005.

22 Mental Health, Mental Health Nursing, Community Psychiatry

IMPORTANCE

Apart from interpersonal relations, how person conducts himself in society to behave as normal regulated person form the basis of Mental Health. Starting from asylum, Jailing, coma therapy, electric shock and tranquility, present concept of management of mental patient has found revolutionary change.

In nursing care, a nurse has a duty of very many complicated issues which are as under:

- Mental illness of patient depicting many mental disorders.
- Working of a good practice in nursing care where psychology of nurse works a lot.
- Understanding of hospital and community where, role, status, morale, leadership work upon her.

INTRODUCTION

Concept of Normalcy, Abnormalcy

Mental health is poorly understood with regard to a person's normalcy and abnormalcy and prescribes the word mad or not mad. If a person is not found adjustable then he is termed mad, which is not the case. Degree of mental health varies and no one is hundred percent healthy; varying degrees of adjustments, understanding and ability to cope with emotional problems make a person Normal or Abnormal.

Criteria of Abnormal Behaviour

According to William C Menninges, the criteria of abnormal behaviour are:

- Always worrying
- Unable to concentrate
- Unhappy without justified cause
- Very often and very easily loose temperament
- Regular insomnia
- Depression which makes incapacitated to fight
- Routine life is not normal
- Unnecessarily getting frightened
- Total disparity with always right and always wrong
- Somatic incurable pains and aches.

Review of Defence Mechanism

For the first time Sigmund Freud identified "Ego Defence mechanism". These defence mechanism are automatic unconscious response that help a person reduce painful feelings associated problems. It helps in the following manner:

- Protects from anxiety.
- Insult is protected by self esteem
- Done or occurred at unconscious stage; it is a natural protective phenomenon.
- It acts by denying mistakes, denying true motives and denying actions or impulses.

Common Defence Mechanisms are:

Repression: Forgetting unacceptable idea. E.g., Under fits patient urinates which he can not recollect a month later.

Sublimitation: Diverting unacceptable feeling E.g., Unmarried is dedicated to career.

Reaction formation: Unconscious dealing for unacceptable desire. E.g., Afraid of surgery, patient jokes at it.

Dissociation: Unconscious removal of painful experience. E.g., Parents are charred to death in front of child and child cannot recollect it.

Conversion: Change feelings to emotions. E.g., Man does not want to marry gets fits (Common in hysteria).

Rationalisation: Give excuses (Unconsciously) E.g., A girl always seen seminude, when asked says that she can never find anything else to wear.

Projection: Shift the blame to others E.g., Poor dancer blames floor level.

Regression: Childish behaviour E.g., Anxious husband become completely dependant on wife, refusing to do even smallest thing for him.

Problem of Mental Disorder

General behaviour is changed – loss of appetite, refusal of food, hostile, angry, give up a job, restless, irreverent and incoherent talk and obsession.

Perception change: Illusion, hallucination.

Memory change: Amnesia.

Altered consciousness: Disorientation.

Emotional disturbance: Mood change, depression.

Motor activity change: Stupor, pathological imitations (ecopraxia), immobile positions (catalepsy).

Classification of Mental Disorders

I. Schizophrenia (Split Personality)

1. Schizophrenia (Simple)
   a. with +ve symptoms
   b. with –ve symptoms
2. Paranoid schizophrenia (delusion + Jealousy)
3. Hebephrenic schizophrenia (disorganised)
4. Catatonic schizophrenia (stupor or rigid)
5. Residual schizophrenia (eccentric)
6. Undifferentiated schizophrenia.

II. Maniac Depressive Psychosis (Excitement or depression)

1. Hypomania
2. Manic excitement.

III. Paranoia

1. Psychoneurosis
2. Character disorders.

THERAPEUTIC NURSE PATIENT RELATIONSHIP

Therapeutic relation starts with giving little possible attention "Talking of nursing the whole patient" which refers to body and mind is key to success for Physical and Emotional difficulties. Patient's new social attachment to ward may not be overlooked.

There is a need to perform many treatments in private in order to spare sensitive patients the distress of watching and being observed.

Nursing staff creates the feeling of relaxation (Optimism). Strain (or pessimism) is also possible in her nursing role.

In recent years the atmosphere in children ward and geriatric ward are receiving much attention. The pathetic loneliness of the aged when they are in bed is a handicap to recovery. Deafness, shortsightedness and inhibited movements make it too difficult to bridge the conventional distance of beds. Playrooms are used for each child patient advantage in case of paediatric ward.

In mental hospitals the therapeutic effect of group treatment where, use of patients' ability to help each other has been found immensely helpful.

The term "Therapeutic Community" was originally coined to describe how in a particular hospital for psychopathic, a community spirit developed which helped many patients to gain self respect, to cultivate their assets to the fullest degree and to gain control over their antisocial and aggressive tendencies.

Understanding of stages of motivation helps the approach in such important matters as toilet training, weaning, feeding, play, education etc., among child patients.

Psychoanalytical Model

Therapeutic nursing involves many activities that will improve health care. Following are the basis of an effective therapeutic nursing care. They are:

- Always sickness is associated with Psychological basis.
- Treatment by drugs, injections, operations alone are not sufficient.
- Sympathy, care, comfort are part of treatment of any illness.
- Emotional problems should be under-stood and should be taken care of.
- Nurse should understand that three factors influence any physical illness and they being:
  - The patient
  - The illness
  - The social environment hence, there is a need for holistic approach.
- Psychotherapy is required to patients, paramedical and medical service givers.
- Psychological comfort and care of relatives should be attended.

Behavioural Model:

Conscious mind has all awareness; subconscious mind comprises memories that can be brought out; whereas unconscious mind contains memories which can not be recalled. So psychoanalysis of behaviour is possible by (a) Free association and (b) Dream analysis.

The interacting systems according to Freud's Theory are (a) Id, (b) Ego and (c) Superego. They are primitive, reality based and controlled mind respectively.

i. *Inter personal Model:* Patient, nurse, and other health care personnel interaction.
ii. *Communication Model:* Social, spiritual and nursing skill interaction.
iii. *Nursing Model:* Work, intelligence, personality, remembering, forgetting, perceiving, interaction.
iv. *Medical Model*: True treatment part of a patient.
v. *Holistic Model:* Patient, illness and social environment interact here.

THE INDIVIDUAL WITH FUNCTIONAL PSYCHOTIC DISORDERS

Schizophrenia

Swiss Psychiatrist Eugen Bleuler coined the word Schizophrenia which is derived from Greek Schizo (split) phrenic (mind). It is a functional psychosis characterised by disturbances in thinking, emotion, violation and perception. Finally it leads to personality deterioration. Nearly 50% of mentally ill are Schizophrenic. It could be due to imbalance between interacting biological, psychological and social factors. Genetic basis is thought to be around 0.8%. Diagnosis is based on eliciting positive symptoms like Delusion, Hallucination, Aggression, Suspicion, Conceptual Disorganization: negative symptoms like apathy, social withdrawal, artificial gestures, and lack of spontaneity.

Treatment method include anti-psychotic drugs, ECT, Psychotherapy and health education.

The nursing management needs may vary from defining reality, handling patient control, strengthening the patient's self image and strengthening the inter personal relationships. The chronic patients need stimulation, occupational and recreation therapies.

Mood Disorder

Mood disorder (affective disorder) is an emotional state characterised by an ex-cessive swing of mood. Manic depressive psychosis (now called Bipolar disorder) is common manifestation of mood disorder. In India 1-6 percent of population suffers from mood disorder. Apart from heredity, imbalance of biogenic amines in the brain can cause depression. This may be associated with alcohol. Suicide is common among these patients. Management include hospitalization, drug therapy (Anti depressant) ECT and Psychotherapy.

Nursing care is required for good sleep, food intake, drug intake, safety measures and health education.

THE INDIVIDUAL WITH ORGANIC DISORDERS

Mental illness resulting from transient or permanent CNS dysfunction caused by brain pathology which may be acute or chronic (delirium or dementia) constitute organic mental disorders.

Differences between acute and chronic organic mental disorders are:

Acute (Delirium)	*Chronic (Dementia)*
Disorientation, anxiety	Disturbed memory
Drowsy	Alert
Illusion, hallucination common	Cerebral function is lost
Variable clinical course	Progressive
Reversible	Irreversible

Common Causes of Delirium:
Infection of brain, head injury, Ureamia, Pellagra, Drug toxicity due to atropine, cocaine and bromide.

Common Causes of Dementia:
- Degeneration of nerve (Alzheimer's)
- Infection (Syphilis, AIDS, Multiple sclerosis
- Toxic (alcohol, carbon monoxide and heavy metal poisoning)
- Metabolic (Hypothyroidism, chronic ureamia, pellagra)
- Tumors (Meningioma, Hydrocephalus)
- Trauma (Head injury).

Management of Organic Mental Disorders:

Treatment of delirium	*Treatment of dementia*
Diagnosis, treatment	Drug treatment (Papaverine), Piracetam lecithin
Sedation	Psychosocial management
Diet	Patients' safety
Rest	Restraint violent cases
Reassurance	Reassurance
Support	Educate for no' bed wetting
	Education of relatives

Toxin and poison need specific treatment by stopping drug, using antidote and reassurance.

Epilepsy:
Sudden loss of consciousness which is often accompanied by repeated jerky movements

called convulsions (Fits or Seizures). It may be primary or secondary epilepsy. In primary epilepsy cause is not known. Secondary epilepsy is caused by Tumor, brain haemorrhage, electrolytic imbalance and alcohol withdrawal. Grand Mal is major epilepsy characterised by aura, tonic phase, clonic phase and recovery phase; other types are focal epilepsy which show jerky movement of one part of body. One of the complications of epilepsy is status epilepticus which is an emergency. Diagnosis is done by history, investigation of blood for VDRL, Calcium and sugar, X-ray, EEG and CT scan of brain.

Management of epilepsy includes drug treatment by phenytion sodium, carbamazepine, sodium valproate, diazepam, pheonbarbitone. Nursing care during attack include maintaining calmness, clear the area, actions to prevent aspiration pneumonia and allowing for full rest. Status epilepticus need 10 mg slow IV diazepam.

Nursing care after attack includes health education, guidance and counselling.

THE INDIVIDUAL WITH PSYCHO NEUROTIC DISORDERS

They are less severe form of psycho-logical disorder where patients show either excessive or prolonged emotional reaction to any given stress. Symptoms are anxiety, fear, sadness, vague aches, pains and other bodily symptoms. Nearly 10% of population suffers from psycho-neurotic disorders.

Specific reaction, pattern; Basic and predominant feature of specific reaction are tension, fear, worry, during difficult situation. They are able to cope up with the situation and can overcome the tensions. If tension is intense it may disturb his normal function. There are no organic problem, no violation of basic social norm, no loss of orientation.

Anxiety

We are in the "era of anxiety", current conflict of civilization and rapid changes in urbanised life. It is an unpleasant emotion when a man seeks urgent relief. They are classified into 4 groups.

1. Generalised anxiety disorder
2. Panic disorder
3. Phobic disorder
4. Obsessive compulsive disorder.

1. *G.A.D.:* It is characterised by persistent anxiety expressed by Tachycardia, choking, dry mouth, dyspepsia, urinary frequency, body pain.
2. *Panic Disorder:* It is sudden attack of intense discomfort, fear, terror. Panic attack are horrifying and threatening which are without any warning. It is seen with intense anxiety and derealisation. Physical symptoms are Dizziness, Sweating, dyspnoea and G.I. disorders.
3. *Phobia Disorder:* It is an unreasonable fear of an object or situation. This is similar to acute anxiety. This can be a Simple Phobia (Specific to one item), Agora Phobia (fear of being alone) and Social Phobia (fear and avoiding situation).
4. *Obsessive Compulsive Disorder (OCD):* It is persistent and uncontrolled thoughts and irrational beliefs that cause an individual to perform compulsive rituals that interferes with his daily life.

   Important categories of obsession are:

   a. Dirt and contamination
   b. Aggression
   c. Orderliness of inanimate objects
   d. Sex and
   e. Religion.

It is believed to be due to deficiency of serotonin a neurotransmitter which plays an important role in causing O.C.D.

Dissociative Disorders (Hysteria)

Hysteria, a common type of neurosis cause hysterical personality which may be Dissociative disorder or conversion disorder. In dissociate disorder he separates from original self and acts in a new manner. In conversion hysteria pain, paralysis, fits and aphonia are common which is due to increased stress, repeated ideas and maladaptive coping methods.

Multiple personality: The existence within individual of two or more distinct personalities, one of which is dominant at a particular time. The original personality is not aware of this. It is associated with psychological stress and tends to become chronic.

Nursing Care in Psychoneurotic Disorders

i. *Anxiety Disorders:*
   - Health education on psychological problems
   - Simple relaxation exercises
   - Encourage to take care of his/her own activities
   - Comfort and safety.

ii. *Hysteria:*
   - Problem identification
   - Assurance of relatives
   - Attention and sympathy
   - Encourage independence.

iii. *Dissociative Disorders:*
   - Reassurance
   - Avoid exposing patient to memory recollection
   - Expose patient to stimuli that represent pleasant experience.

THE INDIVIDUAL WITH PSYCHO PHYSIOLOGICAL DISORDERS (PSYCHOSOMATIC)

They are group of disorders in which emotional factors have a demonstrable role in the aetiology. They are stress related disorders.

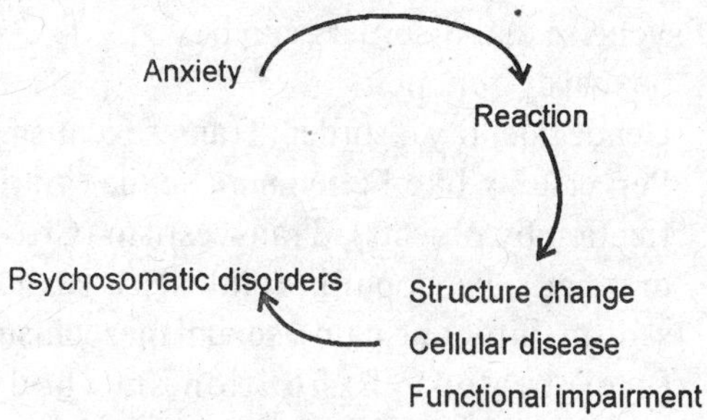

Fig. 22.1: Progression path of psychosomatic disorders

Common disorders seen are:
- High B.P.
- Asthma
- Peptic ulcer
- Ulcerative colitis
- Irritable bowel syndrome
- Arthritis
- Headache
- Eczema
- Diabetes
- Anorexia nervosa
- Obesity
- Psychogenic pain.

Common causes could be response to emotion, personality traits, family pattern, prolonged stress.

Management includes symptomatic treatment. Nursing care includes:
- Good therapeutic relationship
- Encourage patient to discuss his problem
- Create a feeling of acceptance
- Encourage family participation in therapy.
- Teach relaxation exercises.

THE INDIVIDUAL WITH CHARACTERISTICS DISORDERS

Sexual Disorders

It is difficult to define it because the disorder is decided by social norms and customs which vary in different countries and cultures. We have certain normal sexual behaviour.

Psycho sexual disorders can be:

i. Sexual dysfunction
ii. Gender identity disorder (Trans-sexualism)
iii. Perversions like Fetichism (Sexual gratification by objects), Transvestism (Cross dressing), Paedophilia (childsex), sexual sadism (inflicting pain), sexual masochism (seek beaten), Exhibitionism (body exposure) voyeurism (peep undressing).

Alcohol and Substance Dependence

Alcohol withdrawal delirium occurs in 5% of alcoholic who stop alcohol. Correction of dehydration, electrolytic imbalance and control of fits are to be attended along with careful monitoring of vital signs.

Opioids, antipsychotic drugs show in-voluntary muscle contractions ending with stiff neck, stiff mouth, elevated eyeball.

Care has to be managed as inpatient along with the special nursing care of psychiatric emergencies.

Sociopath Reaction

Antisocial, cruel minded personality needs attention of safety, security and its management is similar to psychiatric emergency.

CHILDHOOD DISORDERS

Proportion of childhood mental disorders can be gauged by the fact that they constitute 38 to 40% of our population which comes to about 390 million at present as per 2001 census.

Common causes of disorders are Biological cause (hereditary, illness); Psychological cause (broken homes) and Social cause (poverty).

Common illnesses are:

- Mental retardation
- Autism (driven to fantasy)
- Conduct disorders
- Specific development disorders
- Personality developmental disorders
- Hyperkinetic disorders
- Tics
- Mannerism.

Basic responsibility of a nurse should be based on recognising child on following features:

- Child behaviour not appropriate to age.
- Child behaviour leads to disability.
- It is against social expectation.

Apart from carrying out instructions for Therapy, a nurse should:

- Obtain detail of problem.
- Explain parents.
- Assurance to parents.
- Play therapy.

MODERN THERAPY

In mentally ill health person treatment is not specific since it varies from person to person. Nurse being closer with patient, has important role in therapy. Her action, attitude and skills to help patient to deal with his problems are themselves an essential part of his treatment.

a. *Physical Therapy:* It includes drug treatment, ECT, Psychosurgery.
b. *Psycho Pharmacology:* This includes psychotherapy of individual, group, family.
c. *Hypnosis:* By altered state of consciousness induced by conditioning and skilled use of suggestions.
d. *Play Therapy:* Very helpful for young and the old. Diversion by play can get over tension and anxiety.
e. *Activity Therapy:* There are specific therapy like occupational, Music, dance, psychodrama, recreation and psychosocial therapies.

CRISIS SITUATION

It is also called crisis intervention which is a type of brief psychological method of treatment for the person who is in an emotional crisis. Crisis is a sudden event in one's life that disturbs the mental equilibrium during which the usual coping mechanism fails.

Grief is a crisis which normally does not require intervention. Reassurance, suggestion and environmental manipulation are found sufficient. In some cases it may require psychotropic medication

Suicide is an emergency crisis which needs one or two sessions of treatment. If necessary hospitalization may be necessary. It is possible to prevent suicide by behavioural therapy and relaxation therapy.

Grief and Bereavement

Introduction: This course on loss, grief, and bereavement is adapted from the summary written for health professionals. The passage from the final stage of life to the death of a loved one is different for everyone. This summary describes loss, grief, and bereavement; the stages of grief; and methods for coping with grief. This summary also includes sections on children and grief.

Grief is the normal process of reacting to the loss.

Phases of Grief: The process of bereavement may be described as having 4 phases:

1. **Shock and numbness:** Family members find it difficult to believe the death; they feel stunned and numb.
2. **Yearning and searching:** Survivors experience separation anxiety and cannot accept the reality of the loss. They try to find and bring back the lost person and feel ongoing frustration and disappointment when this is not possible.
3. **Disorganization and despair:** Family members feel depressed and find it difficult to plan for the future. They are easily distracted and have difficulty concentrating and focusing.
4. **Reorganization**

   Bereavement is the period after a loss during which grief is experienced and mourning occurs.

   Mourning is the process by which people adapt to a loss.

Treatment: Most of the support that people receive after a loss comes from friends and family. Doctors and nurses may also be a source of support.

LEGAL ASPECT OF MENTAL HEALTH NURSING

Law is involved in many situations which compel us to focus our attention on this aspect. Legal aspects of Mental health are:

i. Civil responsibility
ii. Criminal responsibility
iii. Admission procedure
iv. Discharge procedure.

Above conditions occur among people (a) Who harm themselves or harm the society, (b) Those who cannot take care of themselves or their family, (c) Those who turn dangerous if they act upon society, and (d) In the matter of divorce.

Civil Responsibility

Mentally ill person cannot make will (Testamentary incapacity). Marriage with mentally ill is declared null and void.

Mentally ill person cannot give witness and cannot (a) Transfer or sell property (b) Stand for election (c) Enter into business.

Criminal Responsibility

According to section 84 of IPC.
"Nothing is an offense which is done by a person, who at the time of doing it, by reason of unsoundness of mind, is incapable of knowing the nature of act, or that he is doing what is either wrong or contrary to law"

Mentally ill is exempted from punishment for a crime.

Admission Procedure

It is governed by Mental Health Act 1987. It is done on:

- Voluntary admission (major)
- Admission by parents, relatives
- When mentally cannot express (90 days admission allowed)
- Reception order from Magistrate which can be done by petition and Medical certificate
- Reception by a police commissioner
- Judicial enquiry
- Criminals
  The prisoners Act III 1900 (convicts)
  Sec 330 of CPC (Under trial)
  Sec 335 of CPC (Guilty insane)
- Military person
  Sec 144 of the A.F. Act, 1950
  Sec 145 of the Army Act, 1950
  Sec 143, 144 of the Navy Act, 1957.

Discharge Procedure

- Voluntary admission within 24 hours.
- Sec 335 CPC by criminal committee when improvement.
- Sec 330 Act III sent back to Jail when improvement.

The Indian Lunacy Act 1912

It has been the governing Act for many years in India. It is being replaced by original Mental Health Act for the reason of incorporation of human rights of the mentally ill.

The Mental Health Act 1987

In India, it governs the welfare of mentally ill. It controls the treatment procedure of mentally ill. It takes care of human right aspect and property also. The Lunatic is replaced with mentally ill and asylum is replaced by Psychiatric hospital.

COMMUNITY PSYCHIATRY

It is a branch of psychiatry that develops and maintains organised programmes for the prevention, promotion and rehabilitation of mentally ill person.

In a defined population, care given through health workers and community Health guide for a continuous care and integrated with regular health service is called community mental health care.

Primary Prevention:

- Elimination of causative agent.
- Reducing risk factors.
- Enhancing man's resistance.
- Reducing stress.
- Counselling (Student, marriage, sex and genetic).
- Mental health education.

Secondary Prevention:

- Population screening
- Crisis intervention service centres are established.
- Health awareness for early diagnosis.

Tertiary Prevention:

- Rehabilitation after defects noticed.

The Nurse in Mental Health Nursing

It is now a well established fact that it is not just diagnosis and treatment, but requires promotion and preservation of good mental health. There are many areas where Mental Health nursing play vital role. They are:

- Early diagnosis, prompt treatment
- Rehabilitation
- Group psychotherapy
- Individual psychotherapy
- Mental health education
- Use of psychoactive drugs
- Follow-up services.

National Mental Health Programme

Government of India has launched National Mental Health Programme during VII Five Year Plan with the objectives of:

- Ensuring availability of service.
- Make Mental health service accessible.
- Its application in General health care.
- To promote community participation.
- To help for self help.

Now, it is under the shade of comprehensive mental health programme where mentally ill is treated with common man in community health activity.

FURTHER REFERENCES

1. Psychiatric Nursing 5th Edition –Topalis, Mathem (CV Mosby).
2. Mental Health Manual – NIMHANS.
3. Mental Health, community psychiatry – NIMHANS (Mimeographed).
4. Prabhakara G.N.—Sociology for Nurses (Peepee) reprint 2005.

23

Leadership

IMPORTANCE

Achieving able and effective nursing role by a nurse need an achievement by "Self" and an achievement through "others" As a leader in her group nurse has to maintain the cohesion of the nursing group and guide her group to achieve highest level of achievement. Another aspect of her leadership, external to her nursing group is that, she has to represent nursing profession and has to represent as nurses' spokeswoman for uplifting the nursing organisation. She has to gather information and resources that are necessary to facilitate the work of nursing group. Nurse will be representing this in the community and other agencies in the field.

THEORY OF SELF

This theory advocates dictating the terms and getting work done by authority called "Authoritarian Attitude". This is also called Autocratic leadership where all authority is vested in the leader himself or herself. This theory of self-command overcomes the tendency of staff to find ways to keep away from working. Regardless of approach, all nursing staff performs their duties under strictly controlled conditions. This self concept of leadership has an authoritarian attitude in dealing with other staff nurses. The actions and decisions are influenced by nurses' assumptions about human nature. This theory is postulated by Douglas McGregor as a style of leadership.

Therapeutic use of self has wide application in nursing care, in overcoming impediments. For example: (Let us presume certain human nature)

a. Workforce has inherent dislike for work and will avoid if they can. This makes the leader to emphasise productivity. Leader by using authoritarian style overcomes the tendency of work force to escape from work.

b. Workforce dislike work, wants to get away but nursing code can suspend them from work, can punish with disallowing one increment etc.; so staff automatically does routine job with the fear that they may be suspended.

c. Workforce prefers to be directed, avoid responsibility and want secured harmless working condition. This makes the leader to be authoritarian in dealing with their staff.

UNDERSTANDING OF OTHERS (IN LEADERSHIP)

There are many patterns a leader may adopt to understand others and to get work done by them. They are:

a. *Telling:* The leader makes a plan, announces decision, and follows through.
b. *Selling:* The leader makes a plan, persuade others to assist him in implementing the plan.
c. *Consulting:* The leader asks the group to make a plan from subordinates, tests the essential parts of the plan with them and is responsive to their inputs.
d. *Joining:* The leader encourages the subordinates to begin making plan, but joins with them later.

Nurses as leaders tend to do better when using the pattern of leadership that is more natural for them. But a leader should also understand that subordinates have different personalities, varied problems and situation. Such diverse group calls for a variety of leadership pattern.

Thus telling, selling, consulting and joining are known as: "group dynamics". This attitude where organizational or professional prestige is given importance over the leadership or activity performance is called "group morale". Group morale is one of the influencing characters that builds group dynamics and understanding of others.

CHARACTERISTICS OF LEADERSHIP

Most people realise that much is expected of an individual in a leadership role. Many character TRAITS have been studied in an effort to determine the qualities that were common to the largest number of successful leaders.

In most situations, leaders have to be chosen, trained and appointed although this does not have to preclude emergence of spontaneous leaders. Ward sisters must be chosen; it cannot be left to the group to select someone to lead a nursing team. A good ward sister makes it possible to allow individual nurses to assume leadership for a special purpose; for example in planning a nursing project or in organizing the Nightingale day; The matron of a hospital is an appointed leader. She discovers large variety of nursing activities. Delegation of responsibility is a part of good leadership. Use of position has given rise to 3 types of characteristics.

1. Autocratic
2. Democratic
3. Laissez-faire

In Autocratic type, all authority is vested in leader herself. In Democratic type, responsibility is delegated. In Laissez –faire type, there is no demarcation of authority and responsibility.

Leadership depends on its success on the channels of communication which are available in a system or organisation (Fig. 23.1).

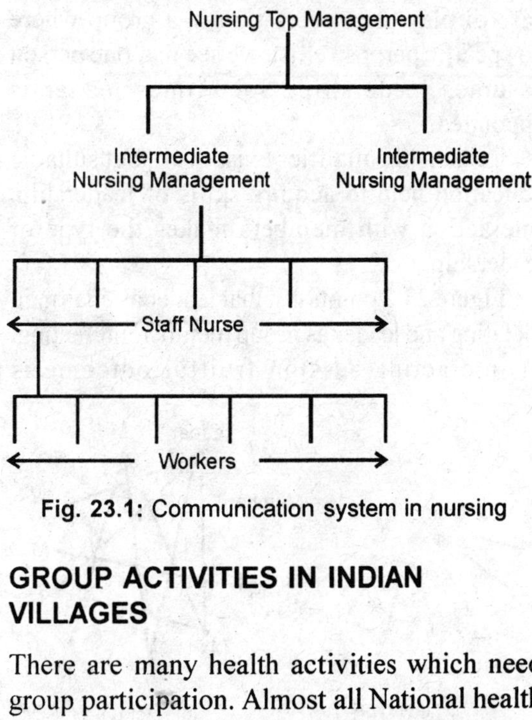

Fig. 23.1: Communication system in nursing

GROUP ACTIVITIES IN INDIAN VILLAGES

There are many health activities which need group participation. Almost all National health programmes are carried out as group activity and hence their understanding is a requirement for an effective health programme.

Immunisation of children, a Tubectomy camp, an O.T.C. camp (Orientation Training Camp to village leader for health awareness) a school health checkup programme, a cancer screening programme, a blood donation camp are examples of group activities. Following are basics in group activities.

- Need people's involvement.
- Need people's participation.
- Need to work through community leaders
- Village leaders are to be trained before a health activity.
- Social acceptance is required.
- It needs interdepartmental co-ordination (Inter sectoral coordination).

LEADERSHIP

Whenever nursing profession embark on a joint project, some form of leadership is required. In case of play or conversation in a group where no specific purpose exist, we see that one person assumes leadership. Sometimes leader is appointed.

Leadership qualities exist in all, but suitable education help to acquire skills of leadership. Interaction with members makes the type of leadership.

Figure 23.2 points out that leader as chairman dictating and leader as group member interacting. In interacting session fruitful outcome is expected mainly because of involvement and sharing responsibility.

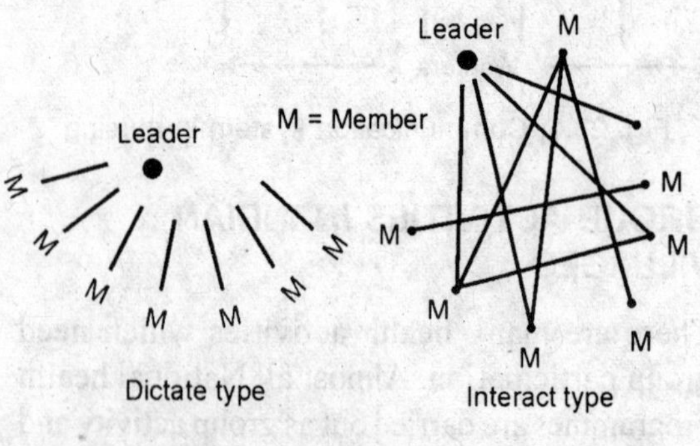

Fig. 23.2: Leader – Member in dictate and interact forms

Leader seated high away from others clearly demarcate a barrier, which is an obstacle to the function of a leader.

There are advantages and disadvantages in both type of leadership. Most committee procedure is formal and all remarks are addressed to the chair. Committee is meant to settle issues efficiently and fairly rapidly after preliminary discussion has already taken place. Hospital with large staff and complex problems may need both types of leadership on different occasions. Both need practice for successful use.

LEADERSHIP TRAITS

Research conducted by social scientists has shown that leadership is made up of a number of traits and that there is no single type of personality that can be labeled as a leadership type. Certain traits, if are on pronounced degree, they can understand the need and desire of a group. Trait help in gaining group confidence.

Most common traits are:

- Intelligence
- Self confidence
- Formal education
- Adaptability
- Emotional stability
- Enthusiasm
- Conceptual ability
- Human relations skills.

Now traits can be learnt by trail and error and can be made suitable to a given group.

FUNCTIONS OF LEADER

- Finding out human behaviour in a social interaction or in a group activity.
- Taking decision for practical approach.
- Plan, organise and direct the efforts of others.
- Relate social actions for human benefits.

LEADERSHIP DEVELOPMENT

Leadership development is a developed style, is an appropriation, and is dependable on workers and situation. It is not a static, but goes on modifying according to season, people and situation.

When workers (staff) are insecure in position and in an unstructured situation, the leadership developed will be an authoritative or a directive type. The best for all seasons is participatory type.

An effective leader is the pride of a group. This is one thumb-rule test one can apply in assessing one's own leadership effectiveness.

Nurse as a Leader

What is the best way to lead nurses by a nurse? There can be no readymade answer to this question. Much will depend on what the nurse is like and what is the situation. Team leadership has to take 3 factors into account:

1. Nurses' personality.
2. What jobs have to be done by the nurse.
3. Personal and professional maturity of other nurses in the group.

Realising the importance of above factors, we can recommend the nurse leader to use participative leadership as long as it suits her personality. It is better for her to remember that she should be firm when occasion arises, and should understand the need of more freedom on other occasions.

FURTHER REFERENCES

1. Public Health Administration – Hanlon.
2. Prabhakara G.N. – Write up on leadership training on nurses (Mimeograph).

24

Guidance and Counselling

GUIDANCE

Guidance is helping a way for an approach in health and disease. It is a transitional unit in the process of education. The education spiral includes various steps and stages, which, sometimes, involve one another.

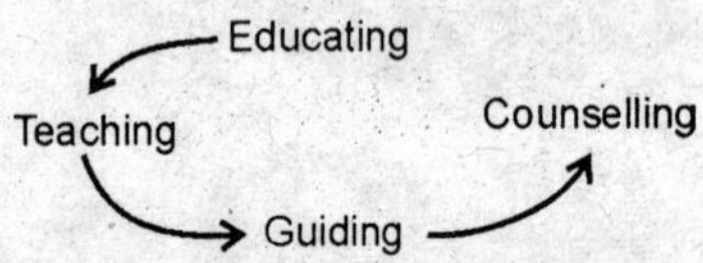

Fig. 24.1: Knowledge – awareness spiral

Guidance includes activities varying all the way from informing individual, his family or his community what they should do or what they should know. Guidance gives encouragement and support that provide a setting within which an individual, when healthy or when sick, can think through their problems with somebody's direction.

Guidance persuades an individual or his family to do something; it helps in recognition of what they needed and help in their action that is necessary for family decision.

Purpose and philosophy of Guidance lies in stimulating a conviction that people want to help

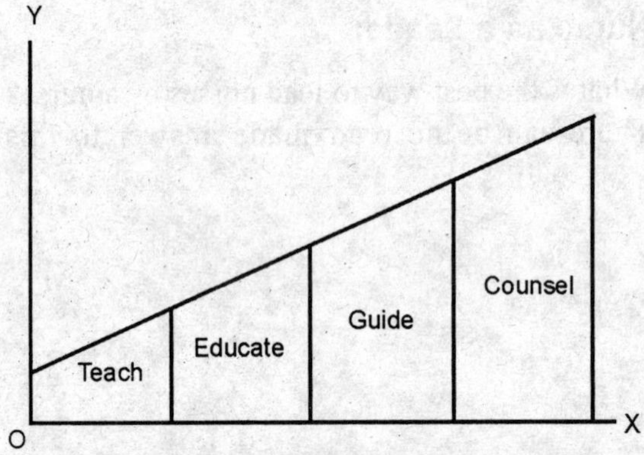

Fig. 24.2: Level of doing in guidance

themselves, which helps in convincing people towards a goal and building up confidence in doing so.

Trend in Guidance Movement

Trend in guidance depends on recognition and acceptance for a need in the society. Illness especially when associated with incapacity, may offer a threat to guidance by a nurse. The nurse can contribute to the patient's satisfaction through an acceptance with reference to his values and beliefs. Non judgment attitude is associated with rejection of guidance, even if done forcefully.

Fear as a compensatory behaviour can be a media for strong response to guidance. A young woman who has many fears associated with her pregnancy always finds a reason for not going to hospital and may show disinterest. Guidance in the pretext of maternal death, foetal death guides her to a doctor as a strong response to guidance.

Guilt or shame is another factor that influences the trend of guidance movement. In nursing care following life situation explains the role of guidance.

- Unmarried girl who is pregnant prefers not to go to a hospital for a follow up.
- Tuberculosis patient feels his condition is due to past sin committed.
- Mentally ill may feel a stigma attached to illness.
- STD or AIDS patient refuses to bring contacts for examination.

In above circumstances GUIDANCE is needed for fruitful action and for building up a positive attitude. This is followed by counselling which clarifies their doubt and help them to react for an effective nursing care.

Difference between Guidance and Counselling

Table 24.1: Difference between guidance and counselling

Guidance	*Counselling*
By any body	By trained person
At emergency situation of illness or problem	In the course of illness or problem
Position of person giving guidance is not important	Position of person giving counselling is important
It is not one time phenomenon	It is continuous process
It is not a before and after process	It is a before and after process (e.g. pretest and post test counselling)
Thinking and action are not associated with guidance	Thinking and action are associate with counselling

Organisation of Guidance Services:

Types

Conventional Guidance: It is the generational experiences that motivate guidance as a responsibility. Father guiding his son in education process, Mother guiding daughter in personal hygiene at menses are typical examples.

Approximate Guidance: Suitable and feasible guidance makes the guidance appropriate by situation, time and orderly consideration. A nurse gives appropriate guidance to an intern in doing a Lumbar Puncture.

Feature

When facing a problem, confidence built on the personality who gives guidance, relationship of person giving guidance and emotional state of individual allow either accepting or rejecting the guidance for individual benefit or family benefit.

Guidance Committee

In a society, all our movements are guided by recognised elders who can guide them for reaching a goal. Formulation of committee consisting of accepted members in any of the following can form guidance committee:

- Religious leaders.
- Parents and teachers in school.
- Village leaders in a PHC area.
- Local respectable members of a community to look into a hospital as visiting members.
- Members in a town planning situation.
- Members in cooperative sectors.

COUNSELLING

In nursing, counselling is considered as the application of the professional nursing relationship and of professional knowledge and skill for the purpose of increasing the competence of individual or families in defining and acting upon their own health problems.

Counselling is an interaction or phenomenon of Telling – Explaining – Directing. Counselling provides information, directs in matters where an individual or family needs facts and skill to proceed. The counsellor is nurse where she stands as an expert. In telling, explaining and directing the nurse needs to organise and present materials in accordance with the present knowledge of the family and in such a way that the facts are clearly understood and acceptable.

Elements of Counselling

a. Establishing professional relationship.
b. Motivating individual or family.
c. Telling, explaining and directing the action.
d. Releasing the family potential and guiding family for self help.
e. Anticipating and combating impediments to care.
f. Evaluating results.

Present Status of Counselling

Though good counseling assists people to make informed decisions, cope better with their health conditions, lead more positive life and prevent further occurrence of problems, there is little value placed on counselling in Indian community. It receives little financial support. Fragmentation has occurred and there is no designated place or designated time for sessions. Though, there are trained counsellors available, but nurses and caregivers are often in ideal position to provide counselling advice and support. When nurses are busy, emotional caring and support are often overlooked or sometimes nurses are in a dilemma as to how to provide counselling and emotional support.

Counselling is concerned with individual, couple, family and group. It provides psychological support and strengthens the responsibility of people.

Characteristics

It is a face to face communication by which one can help a person to make decisions and act on them. It helps in preventing recurrence of problem and provides psychological support. It is aimed at problem solving. It helps a person to understand:

- His need
- His strength
- His limitations
- His resources.

Counselling brings about changes through a supportive relationship aiming to make the client independent through interpersonal contact along with an opportunity to ask questions and to meet frequently needed help without fail.

Functions of Counselling

i. It helps to prevent recurrence of problem.
ii. In disease context it prevents transmission to others.
iii. It modifies high risk behaviour.
iv. Counselling is key for health promotion.
v. It allows individual to develop specific protective ways against health problem.
vi. It gives emotional and psychological support.

COUNSELLOR

He is to get the client and make the client comfortable by creating a sense of confidence. He should listen carefully and not interrupt at talking. He should elicit more information from client, along with providing information on issues for which client has come. Counsellor is for helping to reach decision, for reassurance and encouragement for better communication.

Cumulative record and Anecdotal record gives information and selection criteria of a test in counselling. Following are some of the virtues to be developed by counsellor.

- Willingness to listen
- Empathy
- Understanding patient's dignity
- Good communication skill
- Non-judgemental attitude
- Maintenance of confidentiality
- Boosting their self confidence
- Improving relationship
- Providing encouragement.

PRINCIPLES IN COUNSELLING

Principles involved in counselling are:

- Rapport
- Acceptance
- Accessibility
- Consistency
- Accuracy
- Confidentiality.

PURPOSE OF COUNSELLING

Purpose depends on what problem (health) is encountered or what illness is encountered by the client who is going to get counselling. For example in case of HIV, the purpose of counselling can be mentioned as under:

As HIV is progressive (HIV is a viral and sexually transmitted disease) it is necessary that counselling should be undertaken regularly to understand what the client is going through due to the various changes occurring within him and those around him. The counsellor should also provide to the client the necessary information regarding where he will be able to get medical support, community resources and what changes he can make in his life style to cope with emerging needs.

FEATURES OF COUNSELLING

A counselling can end up with "good counselling" or "bad counselling". Taking an optimistic approach to counselling by a trained person, we can describe the features of "good counselling". They include following features:

1. Counsellor, client make comfortable in a set situation.
2. Counsellor greets the client.
3. Confidence of client is obtained and assurance for confidentiality is given.
4. Problems are listened carefully.
5. There is no interference by counsellor at talking by client.
6. More information is elicited
7. Arrangement of many sessions is planned.
8. Information is provided to client on whom he has come for counselling.
9. Client is helped by the counsellor in decision taking.
10. Time to time assurance is given at counselling, when follow – up is done on health condition.
11. Client is encouraged to communicate the problem to his/her parents, brothers, sisters and kin without hesitation.
12. Discussion with spouse or other members of the family may be of help.

PROCESS OF COUNSELLING

The process of counselling is an activity which follows 4 stages during its conceptual transformation. They are:

A. Facing the problem.
B. Building family confidence in its ability to handle the problem.
C. Modifying destructive emotional states.
D. Securing forward movement in thinking and action.

During the process of counselling, stages which a person passes through is expressed through face and reaction (Fig. 24.3).

INTERVIEW

During counselling, the counsellor uses following methods of face to face interaction.

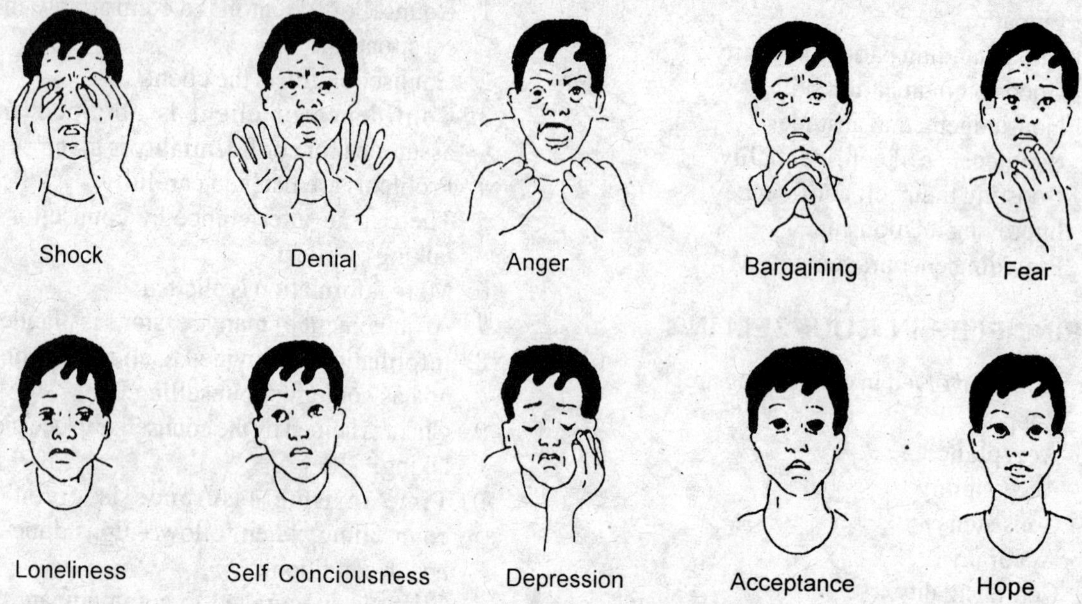

Fig. 24.3: Stages in the process of counselling

Directive Type of Interview

Here specific direction and guidance is given to the client at counselling to take decisions on health situation.

Example: A single test of HIV positive patient is given counselling. He is told that single +ve result does not mean HIV infection and that three tests of antibodies based on different antigen methods are to test +ve. Here he is directed for the action.

Non Directive Type of Interview:

When a patient is HIV –ve, and when he is guided by counselling for the development of avoiding high risk behaviour, it is a counselling but not directive in nature.

ETHICAL STATES OF COUNSELLING

Counselling of healthy, sick, disabled, old, AIDS patient etc., has both legal and ethical issues to the forefront. Most of the health problems are social problems; apart from medical problem, it has to carry ethical component in its process. There have been allegations of human rights violation across the globe. For example HIV infected persons are discriminated. Ethical issue stands to safeguard HIV/AIDS patients that they should have the same rights as normal persons to ensure that they are not discriminated in their communities. Even this holds good with a case of leprosy or tuberculosis.

Following are the principles that guide the nursing profession and the client for a better counselling action:

- Compassion
- Confidentiality
- Distributive justice
- Element of informed consent
- Availability of information
- No discrimination
- Respect for client and counsellor

- Act responsibly towards problem
- Well being of beneficence.

GENERAL FUNCTION OF GROUP GUIDANCE

Group guidance help in realising family potential or group potential to help themselves as contrasted to helping them. In group guidance, the nurse's primary tools are not her technical skills and know how, but the relationship she has established with the group. Nurse's position as a recognised expert and at the same time friendly, nonjudgmental supporter, makes the nurse a significant factor in group guidance.

GROUP COUNSELLING

Following are requirement for a group counselling:

a. The setting.
b. Group acceptance and group concept of a given problem.
c. Building self confidence to whole members.
d. It should modify destructive emotional states of the group.
e. Counselling should attack fear component of a group.
f. Group inhibition which is a strong impediment to desirable action is to be tackled.
g. Nurse should effect counselling within the maturity limit of the group, realising that group will respect the counsellor.
h. Superstitious or fallacious beliefs may have to be tackled in a group counselling.

APPLICATION OF COUNSELLING

In Patient

- Health promotion
- Specific protection
- Psychological support
- Preventing recurrence.

In Staff

- Development of social interaction
- Building confidence
- Good communication skill development
- Understanding risk and cause of problem.

Students

- Learning opportunity
- Learning group interaction
- Learning natural history of disease
- Learning support activities
- Get to know feeling of client
- Get to know communication.

REHABILITATION COUNSELLING

Counselling given for all treated cases and whenever rehabilitation is required, is called Rehabilitation Counselling. The main aim is to get attainment of highest level of functional ability. Mental therapy after diagnosis, surgery, prosthetic fixation form rehabilitation counselling. Common examples of rehabilitation counselling are:

1. Counselling for an artificial limb to polio affected lame child (for restoration of function of walking).
2. Counselling to burnt out case of leprosy to do garden work and earn livelihood (Restore capacity to earn).
3. Counselling of a client who has a son suffering from tuberculosis and wife HIV +ve for family rehabilitation (to restore social relation).
4. Counselling of a middle aged man who met with an accident and lost both upper limbs who has come for psychotherapy (to restore personal capability, confidence).

The Comprehensive School Counselling Program

This is a sequential, developmental program designed to benefit all students in preparation for their futures. Such a program includes a curriculum organized around three areas essential for students' growth and development: Academic Development, Career Development and Personal/Social Development.

This attracts a positive attitude toward self as a unique and worthy person and develops responsible social skills and an understanding and appreciation of being a contributing member of society.

The Guidance Curriculum for a Comprehensive School Counselling Program is student centred and teacher friendly. Counsellors should use it as a blueprint for collaboratively building a sequential and developmentally appropriate school counselling program.

Nursing Careers Centres

The Centre is responsible for:

- The Processing of Mature applications to the Pre-Registration Honours Degree Programmes.
- The Promotion and Marketing of Nursing.
- The Provision of Information to Registered Nurses and Midwives.

FURTHER REFERENCES

1. Kuppuswamy – Introduction to social psychology (Asia pub).
2. Crow and Crow – Introduction to guidance.
3. Freeman – Public Health Nursing Practice (WB Saunders).
4. WHO – Fact sheets on HIV/ AIDS for nurses.

25

Nursing Component

INTRODUCTION

As early as 1937, the American nurses Association defined nursing (professional) as: "A blend of intellectual attainment, attitudes and mental skills based on the principles of scientific medicine acquired by means of a prescribed course in a school of nursing affiliated to a hospital, recognised by the state and practiced in conjunction with curative and preventive medicine by an individual licensed to do so by the state."

Nurse in her nursing profession recognises and understands the fundamental needs of a healthy person, a sick person and who knows how these needs can best be met. She possesses body of scientific nursing knowledge which is based on science and technology. She will apply this knowledge to an individual and the community. She discerns her area of work with the work of other health professionals.

The term professional nurse is given to those who are graduate as per Nursing Council of India guidelines and affiliated to University of health sciences.

NURSING AS A PROFESSION

It is an emerging profession with a distinguishing feature of Artistic way of use of nursing technique. It has a legal aspect caring for bodily and mental comforts of a patient by remedial and non remedial means under the supervision of a licensed physician. The characteristics of nursing profession are:

- Mental and physical health
- Alertness
- Technical competence
- Dependability
- Ability to inspire confidence
- Resourcefulness
- Poise
- Consideration for others
- Cooperation
- Agreeableness
- Nursing culture
- Work satisfaction
- Professionally responsible.

Her ability to understand and adjust to other people is the greatest influencing factor in the success of nursing profession.

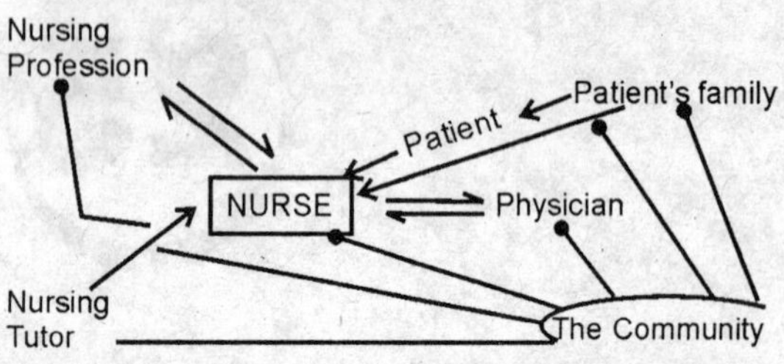

Fig. 25.1: Professional responsibility of nurse

Figure 25.1 illustrates the professional responsibility of nurse.

CHANGING CONCEPT OF HEALTH CARE DELIVERY

Medical treatment had a narrow limit giving diagnosis and specific treatment at individual level in a dispensary. It was literally dispensing the patient than managing. Examining and giving treatment do not complete health care. It extends beyond the limit of medical care to adequate food, housing, basic sanitation, healthy lifestyle, protection against environmental hazards and diseases.

Thus, concept of health care is now a service provided to individual or community by agents of health service or health professionals for the purpose of promoting, maintaining, monitoring or restoring health.

Medical care and nursing care given to an individual in a hospital set up. Health care and public health nursing care inclusive of "domiciliary care to inpatient hospital care".

Health is a public right. It is the responsibility of Government to provide health care.

Health Care Delivery of Community Health

a. *Comprehensive Health Care:* It denotes provision of integrated preventive, curative and promotional health services from womb to tomb to all residing in a defined geographical area.

b. *Basic Health Service:* It is a network of coordinated, peripheral and intermediate health units capable of performing effectively a selected group of functions essential to the health of an area and assuring the availability of competent professional and auxiliary to perform these functions. It is called total patient care under nursing component.

MULTIDISCIPLINARY APPROACH

Now it is understood that one discipline cannot provide health care to the community.

In addition to health sector all related sectors and aspects of national and community development, in particular Agriculture, animal husbandry, food industry, education, housing, public works and communication are to join and give health care through multidisciplinary approach (Fig. 25.2).

TEAM NURSING

Very few activities in nursing are carried out in isolation. Most of nursing work is to be done in Team Nursing. History helps to explain the elusive boundaries between various fields of

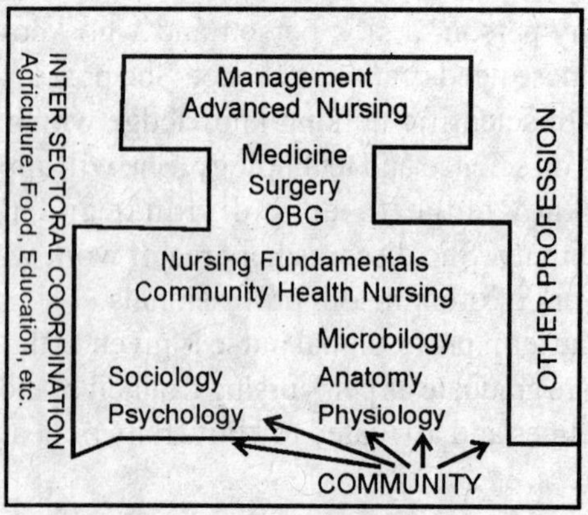

Fig. 25.2: Multidisciplinary approach in health care

medical, health and nursing practice. Centuries ago a doctor and a nurse used to be treatment givers. With the expansion of scientific knowledge, diagnostic and therapeutic approaches have multiplied and specialization in nursing is seen. Thus in a team we see additional members like medical social workers, nutritionist, physical therapist, occupational therapist, clinical psychologist, rehabilitation officers, vocation officers, health educators, medical clerks, laboratory technicians, anaesthetists and many more.

In a set up of health centre nurse has to work with medical officer of Health, LMO, X-ray technician, Health supervisor male, Health supervisor female, MPW male, MPW female, Trained Dais, Health educator and many more.

For the total programme, team work is mandatory because Job responsibilities are laid down at hospital, at centre and at home visiting. Thus group dynamic has become a process for the spirit of team nursing.

In team nursing, quality of leadership, element of supervision and able administrative efficiency are called for.

INTER PERSONAL RELATIONS AND COMMUNICATION

The effect of patients on each other has received relatively little attention. A patient to be alone is not found beneficial. Nurses and doctors often talk and behave as if each patient were being treated as an isolated separate individual. They ignore the influence of patients on each other and the influence of nurse on each other. Nursing the whole patient "refers to the patient's body and mind, his physical and emotional difficulties."

A nurse has her own social background; her family. Social commitments are similar to that of a patient and a doctor. Patient's anxiety may be overlooked. Nurse's new social obligations to patients, doctor, administrators may be overlooked.

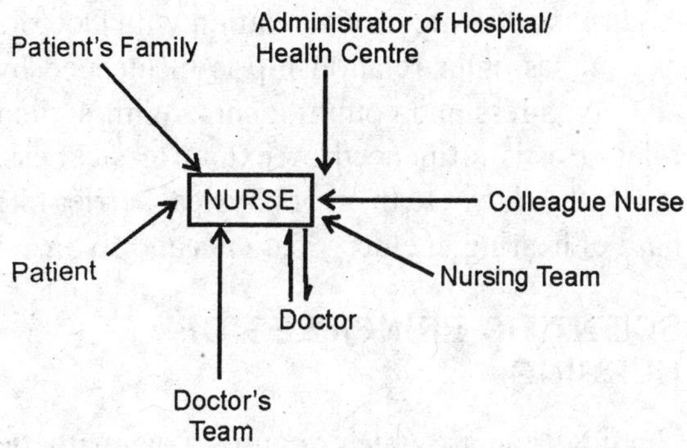

Fig. 25.3: Inter personal relation in professional nursing

The element of inter personal relations and communications are highlighted in respective chapters sociology and health education.

Senior nursing faculty showing concern for junior nursing faculty for her understanding, learning and attaining skill in working competence is a very crucial element in introducing quality in nursing profession. Learning by doing is a fact in nursing profession.

A good doctor – nurse relationship, nurse – patient relationship and nurse-nurse relationship are 3 broad basic ruling in an efficient nursing care service.

When group morale is high nursing group tend to be active and productive. It concerns itself with its main purpose. Group rules are generally accepted and there are few problems of rule enforcement.

When group morale is low, the group as a whole behaves in a very similar way as some neurotically ill people behave. The group resorts to a variety of defense mechanism which may be successful in keeping it intact but interfere with productive function of the nursing group. Misunderstandings often occur where nurses are not cordial with each other.

So good culture and good communication is a theme of high quality nursing component.

In case of professional relation with Doctors and nurses, inter relationship is influenced by anxiety, stress and commitments. With patient relation it is influenced by extent of sickness, sympathy shown to them or physical barrier like hard of hearing in elderly patients and so on.

SCIENTIFIC PRINCIPLES OF NURSING

Nursing is an art which requires a sympathetic heart and willing hands. The chief purpose of nursing today is to help the individual to attain or maintain health. Nurse has dual responsibility; one is concerned with relieving suffering in relation to caring for the sick; the other is placed upon preventive and educational aspects. Along with attendant, she is a teacher of health also.

Skills to be learnt by a nurse are:

- Skills in dealing with and influencing people
- Skills in observing
- Skill in manual dexterity needed in certain techniques
- Skill in operating types of machines used in giving nursing care.

Scientific principles in nursing can be classified under following heads:

1. **Principles related to meeting the need of patients:**
   - Safe and comfortable environment for patient
   - Bed making
   - Admission procedures
   - Observation and charting
   - After receipt of instructions in ward rounds, sound planning of nursing care
   - Discharge procedures.
2. **Principles of daily fundamental care:**
   - Comfort position
   - Care of the skin
   - Care of nails
   - Care of hair
   - Care of mouth
   - Food requirement in terms of balanced diet or therapeutic adaptation of normal diet
   - Elimination and treatment of large intestine
   - Elimination and treatment of bladder.
3. **Principles to vital signs:**
   - Temperature recording, treatment
   - Pulse and BP recording
   - Respiration and nursing treatment of respiratory tract.
4. **Principles of drug administration:**
   - Oral medicine
   - Injections
   - Infusions
   - Transfusions
   - Radiation (X-ray, Cobalt).
5. **Therapeutic measures and diagnosis test:**
   - Heat application and withdrawal
   - Treatment of vaginal canal
   - Treatment of eye
   - Treatment of ear, nose, throat
   - Treatment of stomach
   - Diagnosis tests.
6. **General principles to meet the need of special patients:**
   - Communicable diseases
   - Surgery and post surgery
   - Wound bandaging and care
   - Chronic ill patient
   - Care of dying and dead.

PROBLEM SOLVING AND PLANNING IN NURSING CARE

In spite of learning by texts, journals and ward exposure, case management is not that easy because the patient treated and patient to be treated show large variation. The case management need appropriate, timely and on the spot decisions. To get prepared for this type of odd situation, planning in nursing care, considering each patient as a unique problem is very much essential.

Definition, purpose, components and design are similar to the one discussed under nursing research (Chapter 5).

Data Collection

Details about present illness, diagnostic test with results and ward instructions are taken note in the case sheet. They give the idea of curable disease, incurable disease, only nursing care needed and therapy and counselling needed etc.

Assessment of Case

The assessment of case is guided by the knowledge gained by the nurse and practical skills learnt. The given case is categorized as acutely ill, chronically ill, apparently healthy, needs selective treatment or need emergency treatment.

Accordingly contacting duty physician for early needful is made possible.

Analysis of the Problem

Depending on discussion with physician, nursing care analysis is carried on for final analysis of the given situation. Senior Tutor, Matron and Nursing Superintendent are available for consultation. Critical appraisal of the situation is done with head nurse for identification of main or chief problem which need immediate attention.

Identification of Patient Problem

Collection of data, case assessment and critical analysis of situation are done to make sure of arriving at the main problem of the case. Identification of patient problem by physician, social worker, dietician and area therapist allow the nursing staff to point out problem solving in nursing component.

Planning for Nursing Care

There might have been a systematic protocol for all diseases/problems/cases. But there is a need of modifying and suiting that to the given situation. This is the area which is to be tackled by scientific approach by the attending nurse for an effective nursing care.

Implementation of Interventions

The possible intervention to be implemented may be medical, surgical, midwifery, general or specific in nature. Invasive interventions are undertaken with informed consent, under supervision of a senior staff. In case of health personnel bringing about intervention, it can be assisted by nursing staff.

Evaluation

Implementation of intervention by health professional or nursing professional need to be evaluated by monitoring the vital signs and progress observed in the patient. There is no harm in taking second opinion in the matter.

MAN – THE RECIPIENT OF CARE

Man is a biopsychosocial being and understanding him in his environment is utmost important for an effective treatment. Apart from health need, other aspects of needs (human needs) are to be contemplated in diagnosis, therapy and rehabilitation of a given patient. Following different situations (personalities) are encountered that need elucidation.

Infancy

He is completely a helpless patient. He has only reflex and no activity can be carried out. He is totally dependent for everything. Breast feeding by mother is an added compliment which the nursing component should look for. Another point of consideration is to look into growth and development at hospital admission. Because the infant has no speech, no thought in terms of adult concepts, it must be assumed that her early experiences are recalled in the realm of feeling.

Early Childhood

A great deal of success in case management depends on the mother's skill in giving hand with nursing care. Again growth, development and importance of breast feeding are to be considered in analysis of the case. Toilet training, family closeness, play therapy are to be included in the nursing component of health and nursing care.

School Age Child

School age children always want to conform. They do not know what is expected of them. They have to be informed and even if they know would have forgotten. Hence, they need to be reminded and this could help in correcting their behaviour.

Adolescence

The transformation from childhood to adulthood is the adolescence stage. There is instability and immaturity in emotional and social behaviour. They suffer from identity crisis. They are rebellious in their attitude. Nursing component has to understand and accept the above group of patients in their background. This will go a long way in offering nursing care effectively and efficiently.

Adult

It is possible to widen the scope for emotion and to feel strongly about patient's feeling and causes as well as about people.

Old Age

Eye sight and hearing loss should be remembered in this category of patient for an appropriate action through nursing component. Loneliness, worries, anxiety are to be taken note in problem evaluation. Recently Geriatrics nursing is becoming a specialty.

ILLNESS AND SICK ROLE

Illness is an unwelcome intrusion: some may regard this as a challenge : many people's attitude to illness is much less constructive, and many nursing problems arise because sick people often behave not as adults but as if they were much younger. Under stress they revert to earlier pattern of behaviour (Regress). It is not uncommon for people to adopt this attitude of guilt and shame towards their own suffering. It is interesting to note that word *pain* has come from Greek word *Poine* which means penalty. Some of the diseases attract negative attitude by the attending health professional. STD, HIV, AIDS, leprosy and tuberculosis are such examples.

Some patients turn to God and desire comfort from such action.

Whatever people suffer from, at treatment, patient (sick) must give up oneself and submit to the authority of nursing. In some respect sick resembles that of a child who needs attention from his/her mother.

Nursing component should visualize "attention seeking" behaviour of patient.

COPING STRATEGIES BY THE SICK

Hostility

Hostile attitude of the sick is a deterrent to all nursing care unless it is tackled in the beginning itself. Non cooperative, non submissive takes away nurse's energy in diagnosis, treatment and rehabilitation. Sympathy, understanding and taking the help of members of his family are available weapons in such cases. Only in case of life saving situations force can be used with ward boys which in no way is inhuman.

Manipulation

In communication, in progress response and in nursing examination, patient may show manipulated tactics. Manipulation is highly dangerous because of its influence in problem solving through data collection, analysis and assessment. Second opinion, re-examination and repeat assessment are available means to over come manipulation.

Loneliness

This is natural in case of geriatric patients. In them it is reversible with available means of concern, sympathy, constant hearing and psychotherapy. There are selected group of patients who are basically introvert who are not to be confused with loneliness. Good interaction, assurance and building confidentially help in overcoming loneliness due to introvert nature.

REHABILITATION ASPECT IN NURSING COMPONENT

Definition

The rehabilitation aspect of nursing is coordinated and combined efforts of medical, social, educational and vocational measures to give the patient good functional ability.

Principles

Rehabilitation aspect of nursing include element of social integration. Secondary nursing component should include multidisciplinary approach involving physiotherapy, occupational therapy, speech therapy, psychotherapy, educating, social welfare work, vocational guidance and placement services.

The main nursing aim in rehabilitation are:

- Restoration of function (medical)
- Restore capacity of earn (vocational)
- Restore social relation (social)
- Restore confidence (psychological).

Process

Illness and disability has a threat to economic security and involve more suffering than pain connected with illness. Worry over finance, disrupted family relation, unemployment, loss of organ etc., not only delay recovery but also healing of organic lesion.

Nursing component should have a sufficient knowledge of the community resources to enable them to advice the patient and his family.

Their burden will be lightened if specialists in social work and vocational guidance are participating in patient's care.

Team required for rehabilitation aspect is:

- Orthopaedician
- Physiotherapist
- Occupational Therapist
- Speech Therapist
- Audiologist
- Psychologist
- Psychosocial counsellor (MSW)
- Social worker (MSW)
- Government administrators.

Nursing responsibility as a professional is a wider activity in collaboration with team suggested above. She follows instructions, monitors rehabilitation, records the progress of action, and submits report of progress to concerned specialties of rehabilitation team.

Since nursing element is a chemical bond in each act of rehabilitation be it physical, vocational, social or psychological no specific marking can be done as to nursing responsibility. Nurse initiates, implements, monitors, reports and dismisses and thus is a key person in nursing rehabilitations.

Nursing Informatics as Nursing Component

Registered nurses should serve by her contribution to the society through evolving health care system. Basic, essential nursing information is required by nurses, employers, researchers, educators, policy makers, and clients so that informed decisions can be made about nursing role in the changing health care system.

Nursing has evolved significantly over the past few decades, with many of the changes being driven by advances in information and communication technology (ICT). ICT has permeated all aspects of society, including health care and affects all members of the interdisciplinary health team. Since nurses are the largest group of health care providers, discipline-specific competencies in the use of ICT and other technologies are imperative. This realization has catalyzed the steady development of nursing informatics.

E-nursing strategy includes:

1. Advocating for nurses' access to ICT.
2. Supporting continuing competence.
3. Advocating nurses in decision-making about information technology and information systems.

The e-nursing strategy will help in accessibility to work environment, competency on ICT skill development, and participation word processing, graphical design, using databases, desk-top publishing, spreadsheets, using the Internet, web page design, multimedia design and the use of Nursing Information Systems (NIS) are some examples.

Nursing Informatics has developed as a component of nursing, administration, and research. Nursing students find value in these learning activities in upgrading their knowledge of science and practice of Nursing Informatics.

FURTHER REFERENCES

1. Prabhakara G.N. – "Essential Medical Education" (Mehta Publication).
2. Bertha Harmer and Virginia Henderson – Textbook of principles and practice of nursing (MacMillan)
3. Altschul A. – AIDS to psychology for nurses (Bailliere, Tindal, CO).
4. Mc Clain and Gragg – Scientific principles in Nursing (C.V. Mosby).
5. WHO – TRS 419 and 668.
6. Prabhakara G N - Trends Issues and Management in Nursing (Peepee).

26

Supervision

Supervision and Leadership are closely related. Supervision requires leadership. Leadership does not necessarily have to involve supervision.

According to Carter McNamara, supervision is the activity carried out by supervisors to oversee the productivity and progress of employees who report directly to the supervisors.

For example

First-level supervisors supervise entry-level employees. Depending on the size of the organization, middle-managers supervise first-level supervisors; chief executives supervise middle-managers, etc. Supervision is a management activity and supervisors have a management role in the organization.

IMPORTANCE

Effective supervision is the key to the success of nursing care in a hospital, a centre or in an Institution. However competent a nurse may be individually, she will not be effective in nursing care unless she can make nursing team work successfully.

In all walks of nursing profession, diagnosis, treatment, transfusion, preparation for surgery, surgical procedure, post-operative set up etc.; even with little negligence on the part of supervision, we expect high morbidity or even mortality. Supervision does not stop short of nursing profession but also encroach upon Medical, Surgical, Obstetric and Gynaecological activities. Nursing supervision guides them and helps them in their work.

The ability to understand other staff and to engage them in productive work to further health programme is what distinguishes a nurse as a successful supervisor.

Counselling Supervision

Working under supervision means that a nurse uses the services of another nurse to review their work with patients, their professional development, and often their personal development as well. Supervision is a professional service, rather than a managerial role, and for nurses who work in institutions, supervision and management will normally be entirely separate. The supervisor acts not as a 'boss', but as a consultant.

Function of Supervision

According to Alfred Kadushin functions are summarised as under:

Administrative

The promotion and maintenance of good standards of work, co-ordination of practice with policies of administration, the assurance of an efficient and smooth-running office.

Educational

The educational development of each individual worker on the staff in a manner calculated to evoke her fully to realize her possibilities of usefulness.

Supportive

The maintenance of harmonious working relationships, the cultivation of esprit de corps.

DEFINITION

The supervision is a teaching learning process. It is defined as "an art or a process by which designated individual or group of individuals oversee the work of others and establish controls to improve the work as well as the worker".

The concept of supervision is to guide and help the subordinates in their duties, work and activities.

Main components of supervision are training, guidance, demonstration, counselling of an individual and checking.

Supervision is done at all levels of nursing care. Matron, head nurse, staff nurse are all at supervision when nursing care starts on their shift.

But at national health programme and schemes, middle level personnel are mainly responsible for supervision. Medical officers (L.M.O.) and Health Assistant Female (Female Supervisors) are designated as supervisors of health activities of R.C.H. at P.H.C. and sub-centre level.

OBJECTIVES OF SUPERVISION

- To meet predetermined work objectives
- To promote effectiveness of workers
- To promote morale and motivation among workers
- To promote team work
- To bridge the gap between personal goal and organizational goal.

PRINCIPLES OF SUPERVISION

1. No undue pressure for achievement
2. Autonomy to subordinate preferred
3. Supervisor should have competence
4. Subordinate should receive training
5. Decision making is encouraged
6. Free communication is required
7. No overburdening to staff
8. Good leadership by supervisor
9. Suitable climate for work
10. Give guidance.

COMMON SUPERVISORY METHODS

- Individual conference
- Group conference
- Staff meeting
- Training sessions
- Review of records
- Evaluation sessions
- Direct observation.

Supervision is done by surprise as well as by previous appointment. Direct supervision is to observe subordinates concurrently how they are working. Indirect supervision is to go after the subordinates have performed and check in the hospital or in the community as to what has been done. Reviewing records and reports are indirect supervision.

EFFECTIVE SUPERVISION

For effective supervision, the supervisor must have certain skills, knowledge and attitudes. Effective supervision provides direction and guidance. Good supervisors guide subordinates in the work and also help in solving their problems and difficulties.

Role of Supervisors

Supervision of a group of employees often includes:

1. Check the skills for problem solving and decision making.
2. They organise nursing team in routine and special tasks.
3. They observe role of nurse in assignment given.
4. Recruit new nurses.
5. Give orientation or training.
6. Periodic check for performance in nursing practice.
7. Help in policy making and internal regulations.

Effective Delegation

The hallmark of good supervision is effective delegation. Delegation is when supervisors give responsibility and authority to subordinates to complete a task, and let the subordinates figure out how the task can be accomplished. Effective delegation develops people who are ultimately more fulfilled and productive. Nurses become more fulfilled and productive themselves as they learn to count on their staffs and are freed up to attend to more strategic issues.

In order to do good and effective supervision, supervisors must be given proper training. They should be able to understand human relations and supervise in a cordial manner rather than in an authoritarian fashion.

Skills

Supervisors should have the capability and tact to deal with their subordinate staff in a friendly and polite manner and yet be firm when the occasion demands.

Knowledge

Supervisors should know all nursing skills, all nursing care and all about a programme activity and procedure. They should be in a position to demonstrate to their staff how each activity is performed and performance can be improved. A good supervisor is generally expected to do better than what subordinates can do.

Leadership

A good nursing leader supervisor should display the following characteristics:

- Coexistence with subordinates.
- Assumption of responsibility.
- Impartial and fair attitude.
- Capacity to understand feelings.
- Capacity to understand problems.
- Ability to take decision.
- Willingness of personal sacrifices to assist subordinates.

Supervisory Checklists

Technical supervision is best handled with checklist designed according to Medical care service and health care services being offered. They can be clinical, maternal, child or community health. It is a systematic approach to good supervision which reminds the supervisor about activities to be monitored.

Adaptive Supervision

Supervision involves an evaluative, long-term relationship between a "more senior member of a profession" and "a more junior member or members of that same profession". The supportive and educative process of supervision is aimed toward assisting supervisees in their application of knowledge.

Supervisory Styles

They are differentiated by the degree of support and direction given by the supervisor to the supervisee, based upon supervisee readiness. The four styles are labeled (1) Mentor and Supporter (2) Mentor and Teacher (3) Colleague and Delegator and (4) Director of Technicality.

Sample 1: Sample checklist of pre-operative preparation

Case :	Bathing	Yes / No
Name :	Grooming	Shaving of parts OK / not satisfactory.
Code :	Feeding	stopped 12 hours back/ 24 hours back. IV fluid Yes / No.
	Elimination	Bladder Bowel
	Pre-sedation	Yes/No Dose correct/not correct
	Preparation for post operative care.	Done / partial /none

Sample 2: Sample Check list for Supervision by Health supervisor female at P.H.C. area

TRAINEE	TRAINER	
	Mentor and Supporter Mentor and Teacher	**More support and Less direction**
Willingness Readiness Ability Confidence	Colleagues and Delegator Director of Technicality	**Less support and More direction**

Fig. 26.1: Styles in adaptive supervision

Activities and skills	*to be monitored*	*Note*	*Date of visit*
1.			
2.			
3.			
4.			
5.			

Above are only sample format, one has to develop suiting to the requirement.

FURTHER REFERENCES

1. G.O.I. – Management Training Modules.
2. Mcclain, Gragg – Scientific Principles in Nursing (C.V. Morby).
3. A.Altschul – Aids to Psychology for Nurses (Nurses Aids Series).
4. Trends, Issues and Management in Nursing by Dr G.N. Prabhakara (Peepee).

27

Nursing Education and Health Education

NURSING EDUCATION

Introduction

Nursing education like any other education has the aim to guide the nursing student in evolving dynamism through which she shapes herself as a nurse with knowledge, strength of judgement and moral virtues. To achieve this aim of nursing education, she should acquire knowledge, skill and communication through self discipline and self control. This is possible by teaching learning situation created in an atmosphere of spirit, zeal and regulated ordinance. In nursing education, principles are thought of as broad unchanging truths applicable in a practical way. They suggest and furnish the guidance of action of procedure. Principles of nursing education designate the fundamentals in which methods may be used to indicate an orderly way and an orderly procedure for their specific application in a particular teaching-learning situation.

A Social Change

Nurse in nursing education is a young girl adolescent whose needs to correspond to the needs of that group. She wishes to be accepted as a nurse yet share with others a common human nature. It is idealism, new social change, showing a role of sacrifice and all these tend to lead to a strong motivation for the study of nursing. The nursing teacher, who is in her adulthood, is faced with the necessity of making decisions about teaching and coordination. Even there may be parental limitations in Indian context and will have an influence on the social change.

Philosophy of Nursing Education

Nursing education characterise modern educational thought and clinical nursing as well as other phases of life. In order to acquire an acceptable philosophy of nursing education, student should comprehend the meaning of philosophy. Greek word "phileo" and "sophia" meaning to love and wisdom gives an idea of searching for wisdom. Philosophy illuminates the knowledge by means of interpreting knowledge and its ultimate causes. Science establishes the facts; philosophy interprets them with universal reasons.

Nursing education is deliberate and systematic influence exerted by mature nursing profession upon the immature through instruction, discipline and harmonious development of all aspects of nursing student. They are physical, social, intellectual, aesthetic and spiritual for community uses.

Philosophy and education are so closely connected that one without the other is meaningless. Many bonds like natural bonds, logical bonds, social bonds, cultural bonds and religious bonds are interwoven together. Four philosophies of nursing education are:

Supernaturalism

It is based on theology and philosophy. Basis is in a personal god who can help in attaining destiny. It recognises the social nature of man whose nature determines that he live in society, serve in society and the patient (who is near to god). Patients who are "objectives" near to God are made an "objective knowledge" or reality, to harmoniously order for social purpose.

Experimentalism

It teaches that everything is changing continually including man, mortality, democracy and education. According to this philosophy experience is *the only reality.*

Neorealism

This theory excludes theology and philosophy as source of knowledge and truth. This looks to science as its primary source.

Idealism

This philosophy is similar to supernaturalism in that it stresses the importance of the spiritual aspects of life. It stresses the progress towards the ideal, help to attain self realisation or becoming what he is intended to be. It includes objectives for the individual and society.

Committee

National nursing council, board of studies of affiliated universities, respective nursing institutions have committees which from time to time formulate and stipulate ordinance, syllabus and curriculum for nursing education.

Current Trend

Current trend is towards preservation of human life and betterment of health. She learns curative, preventive and rehabilitative care. It does not stop at hospital, but extends to family, community and society. Nursing care involves *whole patient,* (Body, Mind and Spirit), stresses health education, ministration to sick involves total environment, gives services to family and community.

Current trend is defined to have:

- Technical competency based on scientific knowledge and clinical skill.
- Knowledge and skill in human relations.
- Social understanding.
- Health knowledge and teaching skill.
- Realisation of professional responsibility.

Curriculum

Concept

The curriculum of a nursing school or college should be based on the following:

i. Nursing school/college aims, objectives and needs.
ii. Educational principles accepted.
iii. Level of students admitted.
iv. Needs, purpose and interests of nursing students.
v. Resources available at local, regional and national level.
vi. Present trend of nursing education.
vii. Society needs.
viii. Socioeconomic conditions of the community.

Above 8 factors influence the selection of educational objectives underlying curriculum. Study and research of essential learning experiences contribute in planning the curriculum in nursing education.

Planning

Curriculum derived from Latin mean "a course to be run for reaching a goal" (currere = to run). It is the sum total of effort to help and influence teaching learning activities in:

- Class room
- Seminar hall
- Laboratory
- Campus
- Playground
- Extra curriculum activities.

Planning of curriculum includes the following:

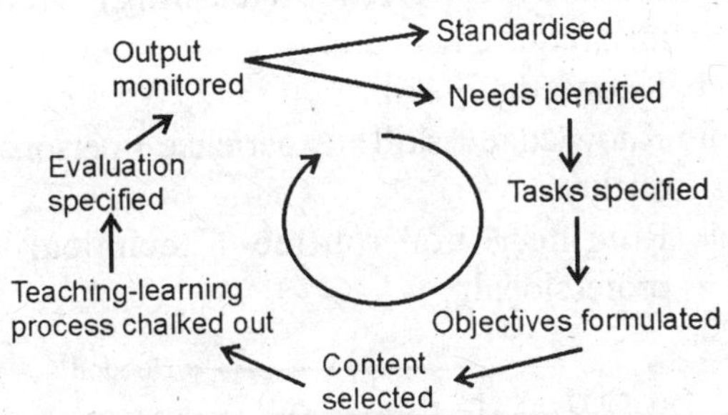

Fig. 27.1: Planning cycle of curriculum

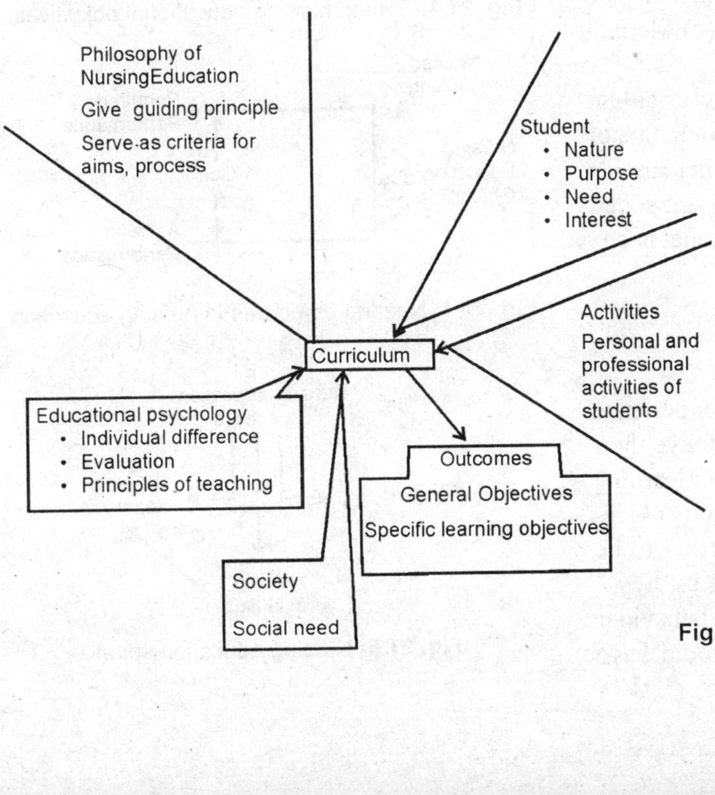

Fig. 27.2: Curriculum development factors

Fig. 27.1 presents demarcated steps in the form of curriculum planning. There are 6 major factors which produce curriculum. They are:

a. Philosophy of nursing education
b. Student
c. Activity
d. Outcomes
e. Society and
f. Educational psychology.

i. *Step 1:* Philosophy of nursing is vital factor for a purpose. And the purpose of education is to bring about changes in the behaviour of nursing student. The type of change to be brought out is the problem of education. Philosophy makes the curriculum, which can be – *Subject oriented*, where course offers for successful completion of course depending on completion of discipline.
   - It can be *activity based* – where it takes into account of all learning through cognitive domain, psychomotor domain and an affective domain.

- It can be *experience based* – Hospital based or community based which is self directed study where problems are tackled under teacher supervision.
- It can be *Core pattern* – it allows teacher and student to know the required knowledge and skill. Nursing education delineates the area of "*must know*", "*need to know*" and "*desirable to know*" at different stages.

ii. *Step 2*: Selecting learning experience to visualise what students are expected to do and learn for acquiring professional competence. The gradation of experience also is to be jotted down in the process.

iii. *Step 3*: Organise learning experience which serve the identified need and maturity level of learner group. This helps in acquiring anticipated knowledge and skills. They are given in the form of time table.

iii. *Step 4*: It includes evaluation of curriculum. Teaching – Learning is evaluated in terms of concurrent evaluation and terminal evaluation. Specifications of evaluation include (a) Nature (b) Frequency and (c) Method of evaluation.

iii. *Step 5*: The standardisation of curriculum forms the fifth step. This is an outcome of "monitored output" in curriculum planning cycle. Changes are allowed to suit social need, community need and national need.

Organisation

Learning Experience

The curriculum includes all learning experience planned and guided by faculty to achieve their stated objectives. The source of data for learning experience also helps in framing learning objectives. For example, a diabetic patient is to be taught self administration of insulin by hypodermic route. Here a change in patient behaviour is expected. Nurse in her studies would have read about hypodermic injections. She would have studied the underlying principle of hypodermic injection; she even knows how to give hypodermic injection. But these do not provide the learner an opportunity to learn the skill of teaching a patient on injection. Therefore, learning experiences must be selected in relation to the desired objectives.

Educational Objectives in Nursing Education

Objectives shape a permanent change in behaviour by experience (learning). Here redefined requirement are:

i. Knowledge + skill.
ii. Knowledge + skill + experience + personal quality.
iii. Routine + non routine + technical + professional.

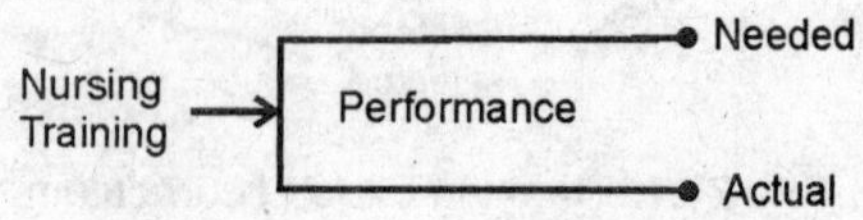

Fig. 27.3: Setting nursing educational objectives

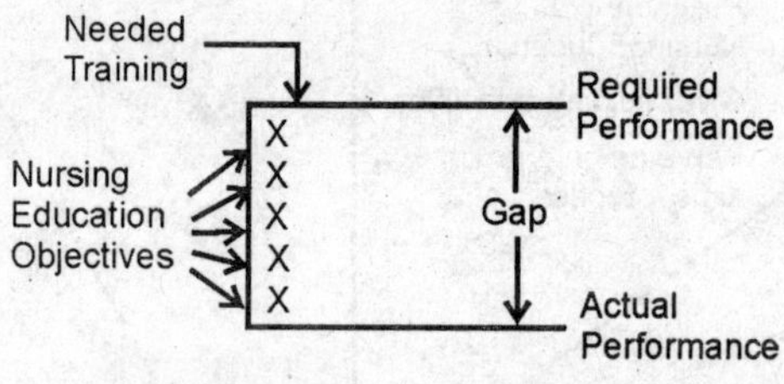

Fig. 27.4: Needed objectives in nursing education

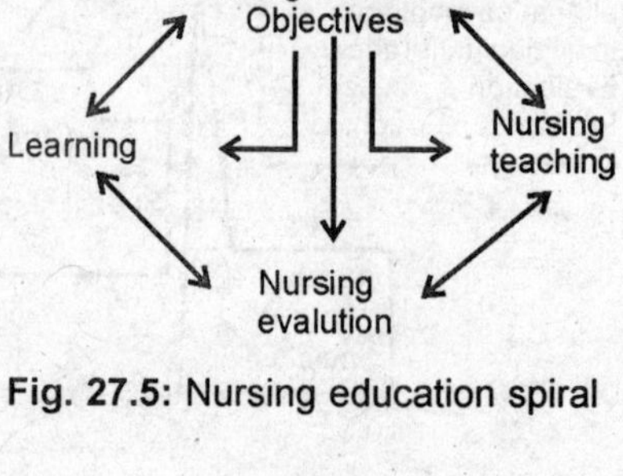

Fig. 27.5: Nursing education spiral

Nursing educational objective refers to:

A. *Knowledge (Cognitive domain)*
   E.g. Nurse would be able to define diabetes mellitus.

B. *Skills (Psychomotor domain)*
   E.g. Nurse prepares and starts I.V. fluid to a patient.

C. *Attitude (Affective domain)*
   E.g. Nurse gives clear picture of cause of leprosy and how it is a social disease (to a patient).

A few examples of each area are tabulated below:

Table 27.1: Examples of three nursing educational domain

Intellectual skill (Cognitive)	*Practical skill (Psychomotor)*	*Communication skill (Affective)*
Describe	Demonstrate group discussion	Participate
Explain	Inject	Appreciate art
Identity	Insert	Help patient
Infer	Palpate	Accept culture
Distinguish	Manipulate	Show concern

Course Plan

Course plan is to prepare the nurse who after training is able to plan for and give complete unified nursing care and health guidance to patient, his family and his community.

The course in the beginning should have basic sciences like physics, chemistry, social science like psychology, sociology, human basics like anatomy, physiology and nursing fundamentals. Succeeding year it is followed by advanced applied nursing, medical, surgical, mental health and paediatrics. Later the course should adopt more skilled midwifery and professional training. At the end, clearing with learning by doing, observed skills, assisted skills and performed skills. Course recommendation by Indian Nursing Council is given in appendix (Appendix – I).

Lesson Plan

For carrying out lesson through different teaching methods one has to think, write down the steps, sketch the events, outline the content and stipulate course of action which constitute *lesson plan.*

Lesson plan in nursing education is required all along different set up of nursing teaching. They can be in:

- A classroom
- O.P.D.
- I.P.D.
- O.T.
- Ward
- Kitchen
- Matron chamber
- Injection room
- I.C.U.
- I.C.C.U.
- Dressing room etc.

Normal duration of lesson can be:

- 1 hour theory
- 2 hours practical
- 40 min tutorial
- 45 min group discussion
- 1-½ hour case clinic
- 6 hours field visit etc.

Approaches to Lesson Plan are:

System Model Approach (of RCE Mysore):

Input ——→	Process ——→	Output
• Objective	• Methods	• Success
• Method	• Media	• Failure
	• Experience	• Assessment

Fig. 27.6: System model approach

Bloom's Approach

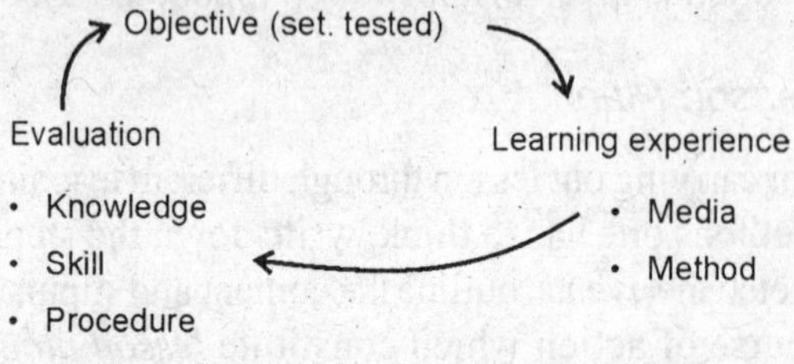

Fig. 27.7: Bloom's Evaluation approach

Herbart's Approach

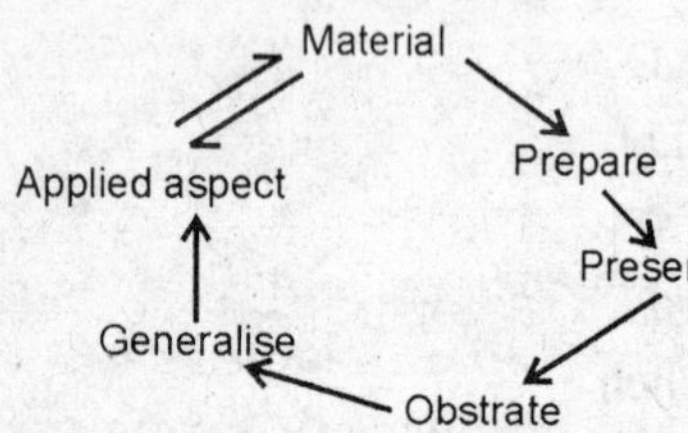

Fig. 27.8: Herbart's approach of presentation

Morrison's Approach:

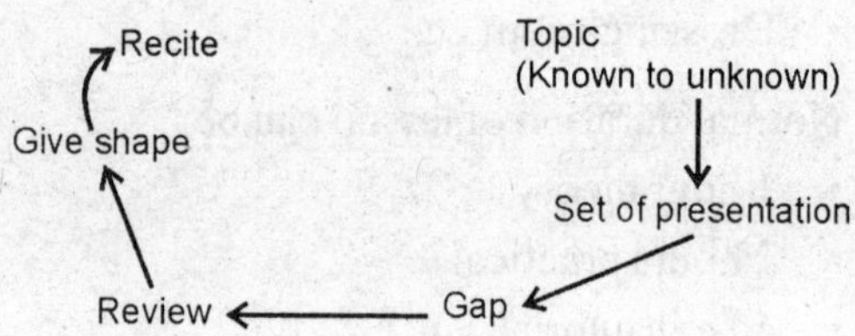

Fig. 27.9: Morrison's approach of units

Model of Lesson Plan

Teacher: Tutor Date

Class: III B.Sc Nursing Time: 60 min.

Topic: Epidemiology and control of ARI.

Objective:

At the end of the class, the nursing student should be able to describe epidemiology and control of ARI.

Specific Learning Objective:

1. Definition of ARI
2. Clinical feature, type, complication
3. Triad of epidemiology
4. Common pathogen
5. High risk children
6. Case management plan
7. Control
8. Conclusion.

Set induction:

Emphasis on morbidity, mortality and National ARI control programme.

Master Schedule:

This is a master time table and class-wise time table prepared by principal of nursing school / college incorporating syllabus, course and objectives (general and specific).

Clinical Components

Case Study

Nursing case study include sickroom, Bed making, Patient toilet, observation of the sick, injection, surgical technique, diet, medicines, special conditions and bandaging.

Further clinical component include care of old, long term patient, special drug, special treatment, shock, blood transfusion, nursing of special diseases and child birth management.

Project Method

Clinical study of nursing case is learned through project method. Nursing students use their activities and produce tangible results.

The Problem Solving Methods

This is a clinical component of learning which is highlighted under nursing research (Chapter 5).

Duration	–	1 hour
Evaluation	–	By short answer questions
Follow up assignment	–	Nurse students to collect common pathogens of ARI in their paediatric ward.

Lesson plan "ARI"

Sl. No.	Time	Content	Method/Media
1.	5 min	Clinical conditions involving respiratory tract infections—Virus, Bacteria	• Blackboard Narration
2.	10 min	• Cough, fever, ear discharge, fast breathing • Stridor at rest, drowsiness, fits, cyanosis • URI - Sinusitis, Pharyngitis, ASOM Tonsillitis, Epiglossitis, laryngitis • L.R.I.—Broncho pneumonia, Bronchitis, Asthma • Complications – Emphysema Pneumonia lung abscess, Collapse of lung	• Slide • O.H.P. • Explanation
3.	5 min	Common pathogens Virus, bacteria	• Chart • O.H.P. • Narration • Illustration
4.	10 min	Agent – virus, bacteria Host – age, sex, immunity Env.- Physical, Biological, Social	• Chart • O.H.P • Narration
5.	5 min	High risk children, preterm, small for date, new born, malnutrition with measles	• O.H.P • Narration
6.	20 min	Case management Mild (home care), Moderate (antibiotic, homecare) Severe (Referral, Admission, Assessment)	• Explanation • Nursing Chart • Case sheet
7.	5 min	Control - health education (nutrition, breast feeding, immunisation) • Risk child identification • Avoid trigger factor	• Derivation
8.	10 min	Conclusion Mortality, morbidity, ARI control programme	• Narrate • Blackboard

In all the above 3 approaches nursing student uses her knowledge (Theory) and apply it at practical learning. Here nursing education allows self involvement of both tutors and students. Further many units of clinical component will allow rotatory posting and learning on rotation.

Educational Strategies

Educational strategies incorporate two main components (1) Teaching and (2) Learning. Traditionally nursing tutor has dominated with active role in nursing education and what tutor does forms teacher's objective or teaching objectives. Now focus is drawn on nursing students who are learners and they are to know, what they should be able to do are focused under learning objectives. So the learning experience is nothing but teaching-learning (T-L) experience which forms the basic strategy in nursing education.

Teaching

By teaching, tutor encourages nursing students:

- To think
- To feel

Which form 3 major component of experience. So sister-Tutor acts as (i) Manager (ii) Communicator (iii) Self learner (iv) research worker (v) and a role model.

Learning

By learning, nursing students will have a relatively permanent change in their behaviour. It can be in their thinking, in their feeling and in their practical doing. The Education Strategy can adopt any one of the following mode of learning. They are called "Theory of Learning".

Conditioning Theory

This is a response to stimuli. It is a spontaneous action of learned behaviours.

E.g. When a patient collapses, nurse quickly allows patient to lay down, exam the pulse, decides it could be due to heart attack, gives morphine injection and call on duty doctor at once.

Connectionism Theory

This is strengthening bonds between response and stimuli in a learning behaviour. Here law of readiness and belonging act forcibly.

E.g. A student has a fall resulting in limb fracture. Her colleagues with readiness and belonging attend *to her for emergency need.*

Field Theory

E.g. In home visiting under public health nursing, sudden realisation of true relationship of situation is emphasised.

Model Theory

E.g. Seen, done, repeated in a mannequin is a true experience of this theory.

Effective Teaching

Teaching is effective when it follows democratic style of leadership which involves delegation and several role plays by students. Good communication for sharing thought and feelings are essential. Choosing relevant information, aware of recent advancement can help a sister Tutor to facilitate learning by nursing students effectively and efficiently.

Nursing Teacher who has a scientific attitude, willing to generate new idea is a role model for Research work. She can effectively facilitate T-L process, if as a role model can help nursing students to acquire desirable skills and attitudes.

Methods of Teaching

Lecture

Lecture is a careful presentation of facts with organised thought and ideas by a qualified sister Tutor. It is a common method. Effective Lecture can be delivered if Sister Tutor informs the students what she is going to say, then say it clearly and then repeat what she has said.

Table 27.2: Advantage and disadvantage of lecture

Advantage	*Disadvantage*
Live	Low reception
Personal means	Do not stimulate
Economical	Concentration doubtful
Gives latest	Self learning possible
Can give clarification	Slow learners have difficulty
Big batch is taught	

A lecture should have a purpose, sequence, organised material and proper delivery.

Active lecturing, microteaching, mini-teaching and classroom interaction and analysis help to improve lecturing.

Demonstration

Here nursing tutor performs some operations to demonstrate skills which are watched by student nurses. It is a second stage learning. Tutor discusses the theory and later demonstrates.

Role Play

It is acting out of a situation. Group of nursing students can learn attitude, empathy and self awareness.

Group Discussion

It is a face to face interaction between Tutor and nursing students of batch of 20. It is informal and democratic which allow good interaction. There are variations in group discussion like, (a) controlled discussion (b) Buzz session (c) Free group discussion (d) Syndicate session (e) Brain storming (f) T-group session.

Table 27.3: Advantage and disadvantage of group discussion

Advantage	*Disadvantage*
Nursing students participate	Big group useless
Students gain new insight	Needs good preparation
Allow synthesis of ideas	Some times mechanical
	Time factor

Seminar

Seminar does not have audience. It leads to in-depth study. It engages students in advanced study of a subject. It needs suitable resource Tutor.

Symposium

It is a large group of T-L process. It contains series of prepared talks given by 2-5 nursing experts on many aspects of one nursing Topic under a chairperson. Audience will be passive in symposium. It helps in logical presentation. Many speakers create interest.

Panel

It is a large group method of T-L process, with one moderator (a senior nursing professor) and 4-6 nursing teachers and holds an orderly and logical conversation on one topic. This allows exploring a problem from all angles.

Micro Project

It is a plan of activity by a nurse student, sometimes a batch of nurses, involving in identification of problems during T-L process and appropriate solution to those problems.

E.g., 10 nurses prepare MCQ Question bank on public health nursing.

Problem Solving

It is a learning approach where nursing students tackle (in groups) to solve a given problem under supervision of a tutor. Problem solving gives good opportunity for cognitive psychological approach. The problem is given on a patient in a ward, on a problem in one ward or on a given situation in a classroom. Tutor should be dynamic and should facilitate discussion.

E.g.

1. A child of 5 years is admitted to paediatrics with the complaint of tiredness, passing discoloured urine, swelling around eye. There is no family history of tuberculosis, hypertension or diabetes. On examination:
   - No temperature
   - Pulse 100 per minute regular good volume
   - R R 20 per minute
   - B.P. 110/80 mm Hg
   - No clubbing, no lymphadenopathy
   - Pitting oedema limb +.

   Suggest emergency investigation and immediate nursing care and case management.
2. A case, adult female 43 years is listed to O.T for hysterectomy. Discuss preparation, procedure and after care services.
3. You are given an instruction to give 2 bottles of blood for a case of severe anaemia as preoperative preparation. Outline your approach step by step. What special precaution you take in blood transfusion?

Questioning

This is a common T-L process in classroom, wards, OT, and Fields. Appropriateness, allowing for clarification and learning by sister-tutor makes questioning a best practicable method.

Laboratory Work

It is an active learning process which is limited to a small group. It allows the evaluation of all 3 domains of learning viz; knowledge, skills and communication.

Programmed Instruction

Practical, bedside nursing teaching and field work are traditionally programmed instructions. It gives a good quality of scientific thinking.

Recently computer programme instruction with tutorial mode, case simulation mode and nursing care mode are effectively used in T-L process. It has the following advantages: (a) It will be very interesting (b) There will not be any mistakes (c) It permits good interaction. (d) Student can take her own time to learn and hence, is useful for slow learners.

Simulation

It is imitating at teaching learning process. Patient case management can be simulated in Teaching Learning. Of late, computer simulation has simplified the issue. Senior student as patient and junior student as nurse can simulate in a nursing care management. Mannequin for CPR is a good example of simulation.

Assignment

It is called individual task given to a nurse student. It is a variation of project. A problem given in a class, problem given for home work, a topic given for presentation, a skill allotted which is to be performed in a ward are common examples of Assignment.

Media

Scope

To achieve educational objectives of different domains, nursing education needs T-L media. They are means of communication of nursing subjects. Only oral talk does not make class effective and fruitful. Use of media can stimulate, allow concentration and make teaching effective and fruitful.

Classification

Non projected	*Projected*
Blackboard	O.H.P.
Display board	Slide projector
Charts	Episcope (opaque direct projector)
Models	T.V.
Photos	Multimedia

Another type of classification is.

Visual	*Audio*	*A.V.*
Blackboard	Public address system	Video tape
O.H.P.	Audiotape	TV
Chart	Radio	Multimedia
Slide projector		
Model photos		
Display board		

Common Projected Media

O.H.P

It is a projected visual aid in a class, even can be used in day light. Darkening of room is not necessary. Tutor has to prepare transparency before hand. Even Xerox copy on O.H.P. sheet is excellent and eye to eye contact is possible. On the spot drawing can be done. Each OHP sheet is used for one message without over-crowding.

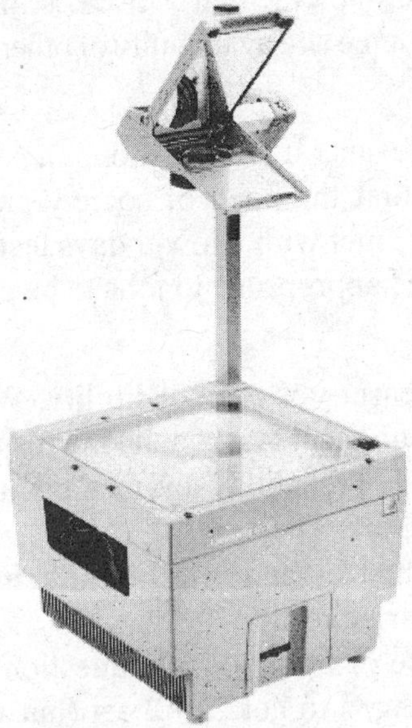

Fig. 27.10: O.H.P.

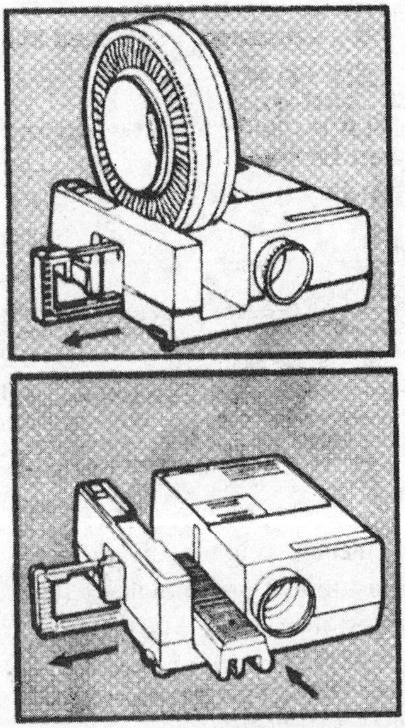

Fig. 27.11: Slide projector

Slide Projector

Prepared slides projected as visual aid help good retention among learners.

Each slide should have 5-6 lines. Each line should be less than 30 letters. Format shape can be horizontal or rectangular.

Slide projector needs darkening of classroom. There will no eye contact at teaching. Now, computer generated slides are taking an advancement over traditional simple prepared slides.

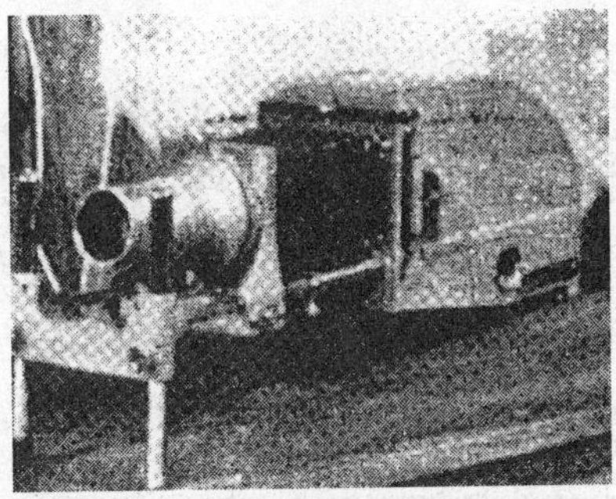

Fig. 27.12: Epidiascope

Episcope/Epidiascope

It is an opaque direct projector of a diagram, picture, data from a book, journal etc. Easy handling and no preparation hallmark is its advantage.

Non Projected Media

Blackboard

It is very common but now is available in different colours like white board, green board etc. It is cheap and helps students to make their notes. Teacher has to write key words and step by step concepts.

Fig. 27.13: Blackboard

Limitations of black board are:
- No eye contact while writing
- Teacher needs skill to use black board
- Written item cannot be preserved.

Evaluation

Definition

Evaluation is a process to determine the achievement of predetermined educational objectives. It needs an appropriate instrument to measure the achievement.

Purpose

1. Placement testing for selection.
2. Pre-test to test pre-knowledge.
3. Post test to test after T-L process.
4. Terminal for award of degree.

Formative evaluation:
This helps to know how much and how well a student nurse has learnt. It serves as a feedback.

Summative evaluation:
This helps an organisation to evaluate whether a student nurse is fit to get her degree or not. This is by a single score like pass or fail.

Criteria of Evaluation

Most important criteria of evaluation are as under:

Objectivity
This criterion answers us the question – Will the result is same with II and III evaluation? Recently MCQ are formulated, modified essay questions are framed, OSCE (Objective structured clinical examination) and OSPE (Objective structured practical examination) are framed for a better evaluation.

Feasibility
It pertains to planning for an evaluation which is feasible. It answers our question "can the evaluation be implemented"? It takes into account time, resource and availability of other test forms.

Relevance
Is this relevant? If this question is answered then we feel that the need of society and need of nation are met with. Now-a-days tests are to be conducted appropriate to jobs to be performed.

Reliability
It is a measure of reproducibility. When same test or equivalent test is done the result must be the same. For reliability few methods are adopted by evaluators. They are:

a. Repeated test and re-testing after interval and comparing result.
b. In case of MCQ of 100 questions they are rearranged to get 2 or 3 set (but with same questions) by altering the sequence of questions.
c. Reliability by using Kudar-Richardson formula which should give above 0.8 for summative evaluation.

Validity
It refers to both test and instrument. Validity checks whether content is valid? Whether criteria are valid? And whether construction is valid?

E.g. "What are the steps of bed making"? It is not a valid question.

"Make and demonstrate an unoccupied bed." This is more valid than earlier statement.

Technique and Tools of Evaluation

In nursing education, following techniques and tools are used in nursing evaluation:
- Essay type of questions
- Short essay type of questions
- Short answer type of questions
- M.C.Q.
- Nursing case management problems
- Viva voce examination
- Modified essay question

- Clinical nursing examination
- O.S.C.E.
- O.S.P.E.

All the above evaluation procedures are followed under 3 major headings viz; Theory examination, Practical Examination and Oral Examination.

Question Bank

Recently OSCE and OSPE have given rise to an opportunity of developing a bank with stored questions for an unbiased set and reset at nursing education evaluation.

HEALTH EDUCATION (IEC)

Definition

According to the National conference on preventive medicine in U.S.A. the definition of Health education is:

"A process that informs motivates and helps people to adopt and maintain healthy practices and lifestyles, advocates environmental changes as needed to facilitate this goal and conducts professional training and research to the same end."

Purpose of Health Education

i. To encourage people to adopt and sustain health promoting lifestyles and practices.
ii. To promote the proper use of health services available to them.
iii. To provide knowledge to develop positive attitude and to practice on rational decisions to solve their problems.
iv. To stimulate self reliance and community participation for achieving health development.

In reality health education gives an opportunity to make realistic improvements in the quality of life.

Approaches to Health Education

a. **Regulation:** By Government Acts, Amendments and Rules the behaviour of man can be managed hence it is called regulatory approach.
Compulsory helmet to 2 wheelers.
E.g. Child Marriage Restraint Act
Regulatory approach is not appropriate because health education do not carry force or law.

b. **Service:** By giving service, people can be made to inculcate the habit of changing their behaviour.
E.g., Free health care to mothers and children to make them to accept small family norm.
   - Sanitary latrine is provided free of cost under basic health service to reduce faecal borne disease.

Here the draw back is that people do not accept or use unless they feel that there is a felt need of the situation.

c. **Health Education:** New attitude and new habit for healthy life by creating health awareness is a task which takes longer time to achieve. It depends on mass media and social organisation. Stopping smoking, using filtered water or planning one child for their family etc., need an autonomy of person on their lives. Planned learning experience and motivation by satisfied people can take us a long way under this approach.

d. **Primary Health Care Approach:** Active involvement and community participation, a new approach of first contact care by the people is taking a boost as a good approach in health education.

Principles of Health Education

i. Trustworthy and credible message must be given.
ii. It should be related to the interest of the people.

Table 27.4: Difference between health education and health propaganda

	Health education	*Health propaganda*
Knowledge	Acquired	Instilled
Skill	Acquired	Instilled
Animal instinct	Taken away	Put to action
Action	Think and Act	By reflex act
Emotion	No	Yes
Reasoning	Yes	No
Attitude	Positive	Negative

iii. People's participation should be encouraged.
iv. Use of motivation is a requisite.
v. Health education must be given in an understandable language and to the level of I.Q. of people.
vi. Repeated efforts are needed.
vii. Learning by doing encourage positive outlook.
viii. Awareness must be from known to unknown at health education.
ix. Good human relation is mandatory.
x. The person giving H E should be a model.
xi. Command and respect help health education. Leaders of village, religion, politics etc. can help us in conveying health message.

Methods of Health Education

I. Individual
- Contact
- Home visiting
- Postal

II. Group
- Lecture
- Demonstration
- Group discussion
- Panel
- Symposia
- Workshop
- Conference
- Seminar
- Role play

III. Mass
- Museum
- Poster
- Newspaper
- Radio
- T.V.
- Folk method
- Internet

Individual Method

When a nurse individually contacts a patient in ward and / or in home visiting, she will be in a position to discuss, argue and persuade the patient to change his/her behaviour in the interest of patient's health status. However there is limitation in the above method since the size of the population needing counselling being such that they cannot be reached individually by the nursing community.

Group Methods

Lecture: It must be combined with AV aids like flip chart, Flannel graph, model, specimen and charts. 20 minutes talk followed by discussion is preferred.

*Demonstration:*It is of great value in environmental sanitation like hand pump, sanitary latrine, ORS packet use etc., It arouses interest and makes "seeing is believing".

Group discussion: It is face to face interaction of a small group on health education. A group leader has to lead this. A well conducted discussion is found effective; however one person may dominate as there may be a shy group. Deviation causes the group discussion irrelevant. OTC (Orientation training camp) of village leaders is example.

*Panel discussion:*A given topic discussed by 4 to 8 members who are experts in the field.

Symposium: It is a series of speeches on a selected topic by experts.

Workshop: Series of meeting about 3-4 with emphasis on individual work. Here resource persons help in conducting workshop.

Conference: It is held at District, state, National or International level, for a given duration making use of group method of education using media.

Seminar: Seminar contain large component of material for a day or two on a given topic or on selected group of topics. Report prepared is also circulated later as material of reference and awareness.

Role play: Sociodrama like mono acting on Family planning, street play on HIV/AIDS etc., getting popular methods of propagating the messages.

Mass Media

T.V. Radio, Newspaper, Internet, printed material, posters, health exhibition and folk media like *Harikatha, Yakshagana*, puppet show, drama etc., are made use of in creating health awareness through mass media. All these are called Media of health education.

Planning and Management of Health Education

Since health education has to be carried out within the context of socio-cultural, political and socioeconomic conditions, planner should take care in:

- Programming
- Planning
- Implementation
- Evaluation and, its administration.

Step in Organisation of Health Education

1. Information on health problem is collected
2. Problem is properly identified
3. Priorities in the process are decided
4. Goals and objectives are set
5. Resources are mobilised
6. Possible solution to the problem are kept ready
7. Plan of action as to who is giving H E? On what aspect is giving? and when is that done.
8. Actual H E session
9. Monitoring and evaluating
10. Reorganising by noted flaws.

Administration

It can be represented as under:

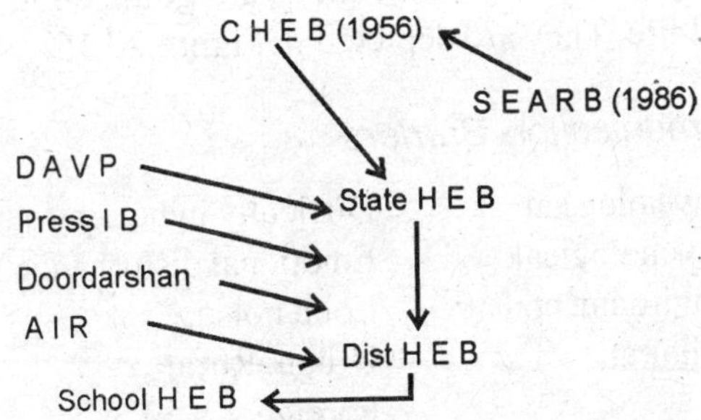

Fig. 27.14: Administration of health education in India

Note:

CHEB	–	Central Health Education Bureau
SEARB	–	South East Asia Regional Bureau
DAVP	–	Directorate of Advertising and Visual Publicity
PIB	–	Press Information Bureau
AIR	–	All India Radio.

Content of Nursing Health Education

- Human biology
- Better nutrition
- Personal hygiene
- Family health

- Mental health
- Health programmes
- Disease control
- Others (relevant to local area).

Communication

"It is a two way process of exchanging and shaping ideas, feelings and message."

Communication can be for:

- Acquiring knowledge
- Learning skills
- Develop good attitude.

Components of communication are represented as under:

Day to day communications are going on in social life. They are depicted in Figure 27.15.

Communication Barriers

1. Physiological – Difficulty in hearing
2. Psychological – Emotional disturbance
3. Environmental – Loud noise.
4. Cultural
   – Urban: Rural
   – Foreign: Local (National)
   – Positive: Negative attitude

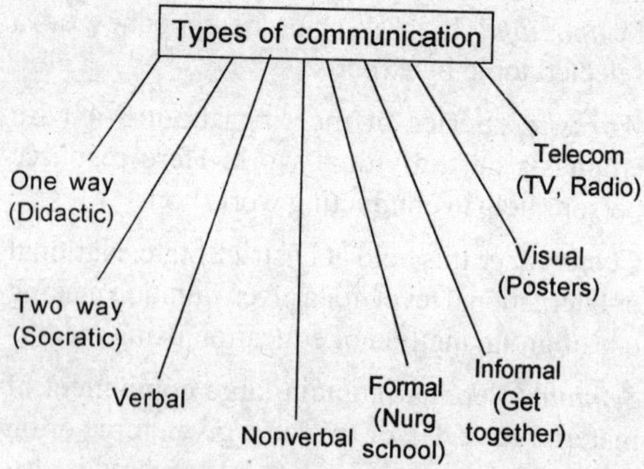

Fig. 27.16: Types of communication

Need of Communication

- To inform other
- To educate the group (formal and non-formal)
- To motivate people
- To persuade people
- To give counselling
- To raise morales of a group
- For health development
- To organise a programme.

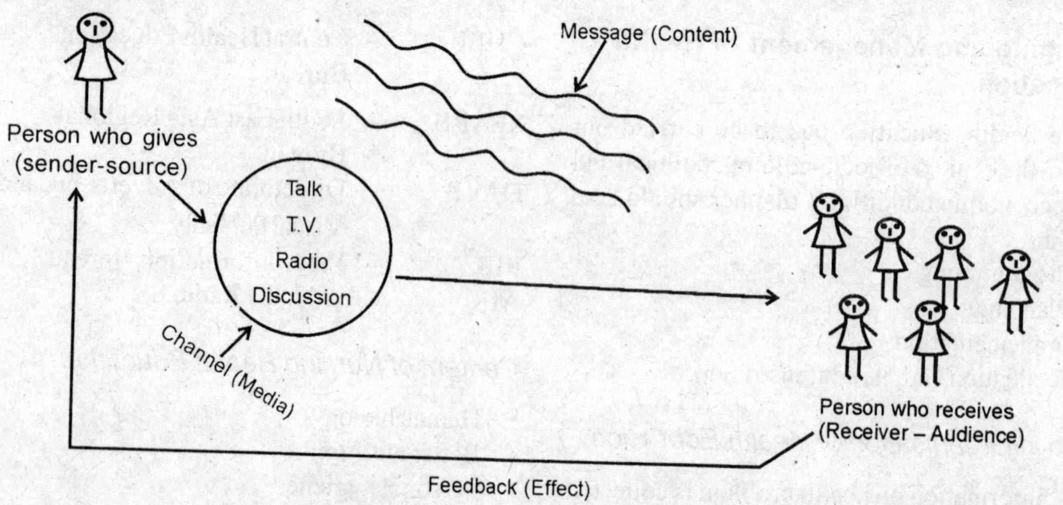

Fig. 27.15: Components of communication

Special Areas

There are 5 areas which have widened their coverage, need special mention. They are:

a. AIDS education
b. Cancer education
c. Nutrition education and
d. Population education
e. Sex education.

AIDS Education

An educational programme which provide a study of AIDS situation for a better development of responsible attitude towards HIV/AIDS.

Content:

- Making life – saving choices
- Guidelines for prevention of AIDS
- Nature of AIDS
- Transmission of AIDS
- Risk factors in AIDS
- National AIDS situation.

There is a requirement of high political commitment for AIDS control. Educational goals for AIDS control should be self awareness on benefits of living in simple and self cultured to be disseminated. Available treatment for AIDS facilities and clinics are explained.

Cancer Education

An educational programme which provide a study of cancer situation for a better development of responsible attitude towards cancer control.

Content:

- Warning signs of cancer
- Risk factors
- National cancer situation
- Political commitment for cancer centres
- Educational goal of cancer centres
- Benefits of simple living
- Economics of smoking
- Economics of alcoholism
- Occupational aspects of cancer
- Carcinogens in atmosphere
- Cancer screening programmes
- Available treatment for cancer.

Nutrition Education

This is aimed at providing a study of nutritional situation for a better development of responsible attitude towards better nutrition and better health.

Content:

- Malnutrition
- National nutritional status
- Political commitment for better nutrition
- Food hygiene
- Special group requirement
- PFA Acts
- National programme on nutrition
- Balanced diet
- Nutritional assessment
- Nutrition and health.

Population Education (Extension Education)

An educational programme which provides a situation for a better development of responsible attitude towards population growth.

Content:

- National demographic situation
- National political commitment to population growth
- Educational goal for population growth
- Benefit of small family norm
- Economics of population growth
- Sociology of population growth
- Statistics of population growth
- Levels of living by population growth
- Effects of population explosion.

Sex Education

Sex education is described as "sexuality education", which means that it encompasses education about all aspects of sexuality, including information about reproduction, and information about aspects of one's sexuality including: body image, sexual orientation, values, decision making, communication, relationships, sexually transmitted infections (STIs) and how to avoid them, and birth control methods.

Reproduction under sex education includes fertilisation, conception, embryo development, fetus development and labour.

Sex education may be taught informally, such as when someone receives information from a conversation with a teacher, parents or friends. Formal sex education occurs when schools offer sex education.

The existence of HIV/AIDS has given a new sense of urgency to the topic of sex education. Planned Parenthood considers that broad sex education programs have global benefits, such as controlling the risk of over population and the advancement of women's right.

Morality of Sex Education

One approach to sex education is to view it as necessary to reduce risk behaviours such as unprotected sex, and equip individuals to make informed decisions about their personal sexual activity.

Many religions teach that sexual behavior outside of marriage is immoral, so their adherents feel that this morality should be taught as part of sex education. Other religious conservatives believe that sexual knowledge is unavoidable.

At School and Colleges:

Teachers are being issued with new guidelines to encourage them to teach sex education around relationships rather than biology.

Schools have, in the past, received criticism for teaching sex education in biology lessons and failing to educate pupils on relationships. The new guidance aims to redress that balance.

Key Stage 1 (aged 7)	*Key Stage 2 (aged 11)*	*Key Stage 3 (aged14)*	*Key Stage 4 (aged 16)*
Children can recognise the effect of their behaviour on other people, and can cooperate with others. They can identify and respect differences and similarities between people, and can explain different ways that family and friends should care for one another (For example telling a friend that they like them, showing concern for a family member who is unwell).	They can discuss some of the bodily and emotional changes at puberty, and can demonstrate some ways of dealing with these in a positive way. They can demonstrate how to look after and save money. Children can make choices about how to develop healthy lifestyles (For example by knowing the importance of a healthy diet and regular exercise). They can identify some factors that affect emotional health and wellbeing (For example exercise or dealing with emotions).	Pupils can recognise some strong emotions and identify ways of managing these emotions positively (For example talking with a friend or teacher about their feelings on divorce or falling in love).	Pupils can discuss relationships, feelings and emotions, and can analyse ways of managing these in connection with family events (For example the arrival of a new baby or parental separation). They can explain the importance of different relationships and associated responsibilities, including those of marriage, parenthood and family life.

The guidance on sex education has been issued along with detailed advice for schools on how to teach pupils about managing their health and finances. Along with existing guidance on avoiding drugs and alcohol, the documents form the new suggested teaching package for personal, social and health education.

The guidance on sex and relationship education deals with families, puberty and physical changes. Young people receive appropriate information and are helped to develop the skills they need to develop healthy relationships and protect their sexual health.

FURTHER REFERENCES

1. Prabhakara G.N. – "Essential Medical Education" (Mehta Pub).
2. Heidgercein – Teaching and learning in school of nursing (J B Lippincott).
3. Bloom – Taxonomy of educational objectives (David McKay).
4. Cyril Bibby – Health Education.
5. Prabhakara G.N. – Short text book of PSM (JP).
6. Prabhakara G.N. – Short text book of PG Orientation course (JP).
7. Prabhakara G.N.– Trends, Issues and Management in Nursing (Peepee).

28

Family Care, Domicilary Care and Home Visiting

FAMILY CARE

Family is the unit of society or community and here maximum interaction occurs within the family and outside the family. Studying individual or a patient from his family background, managing the case at family within available resources make an effective care called Family Care.

Family care needs a good nurse-family relationship. Nurse needs her public health training to treat common illness at family. Integration of Indian systems of medicine, if requested by the family, is to be considered as priority based health care. Family care involves recording system of family composition, size and type of family and pattern of family health.

Family care skills are to be developed by the nurse to attend to illness or health from family background which is surmounted with belief, culture and values. Making the members of the family to accept and to develop positive attitude towards family care is the task of nursing care under family care.

DOMICILIARY CARE

Family care has evolved into comprehensive care and it is made accessible through domiciliary care. Domiciliary care is that given to people in their homes. This was not known earlier and now is an organised controlled practice in health care services.

Domiciliary care was (earlier) the responsibility of churches. Florence Nightingale revolutionized and took the nursing task to people in their living atmosphere (to their door step). As a friend and advisor, nurse gives domiciliary care in the following specific situations:

- Mother craft
- Pregnancy, delivery, childcare
- Tuberculosis treatment.
- Leprosy nursing
- Mental illness
- S.T.D. care
- Malaria surveillance and treatment.

HOME VISITING

In public health nursing, nurse visits home to give advice which will promote mental and physical well being of all the members of the family and reinforce the stability of the home. Thus the objectives of nursing care are:

- To carry out nursing care at home

- To prevent diseases among members
- To promote health of all members.

Principles of Home Visiting:

- It should be a need based visit.
- Family information is made available before hand for appropriate action.
- Family problems are identified.
- Technical skill learnt and nursing procedure known are to be put into action.
- Make sure of scientific base in creating health awareness among members at home.
- Nursing approach should build a sense of confidence.
- Kind and courteous at care.

Home Visit Planning:
This is to be planned with available resources and on the available information on families. Map of the area, approaching roads, family folders if available, individual health cards will help in initiating home visit.

Needs are identified for home visit. They include pregnant woman, lactating mothers, a child, a sick or a family problem.

During initial home visits, introducing her, building up confidence and clarification of their doubts mark the success of home visiting.

Nursing bag is carried for primary care and treatment of minor illness. There are 2 nursing bags one for delivery and the other for general nursing. The content of delivery kit and nursing bag are given in the appendix.

Home visit will be incomplete without follow up of cases. Achievement of home visiting can be assessed by many available methods.

Bag Technique

Canvas, leather or light metal bag is used. This is stitched in such a way that it can be carried either by hand or over shoulders. It should have an outer packet to keep a note book, measuring tape, newspaper sheet, towel, soap and a nail brush.

Bag Usage Technique

Since the bag is used for many home visiting, it must be kept clean. When a home visit is made the bag is placed over a newspaper, hands are washed before opening the bag, only required are removed for the given nursing procedure, used ones are washed and carried in an other bag for future Sterilisation. After nursing care, soiled dressings are burnt; newspaper is folded with used side inside and kept in outer packet of bag.

Care of Nursing Equipments

- Bag – Metal bag to be washed with soap and water canvas bag to be washed and dried.
- Rubber goods – Sterilised by boiling for 10 minutes; but disposal gloves are disposed by sanitary method.
- Thermometer – Soaked in antiseptic lotion.
- Glass bottles – Sterilised in boiled water.
- Enamel or steel items – 20 minutes boiling.
- Cord ligature – Pre-sterilised pack is available; otherwise thread is boiled for 20 minutes; It is handled with sterile forceps and scrubbed hands.
- Eye drops – Opened ones are used within 10 days. Later to be discarded and a new one is to be procured.
- Dry dressing and swabs – Autoclaved material is carried and used ones are disposed by burning.
- Instruments – Sterilisation procedure learnt is followed.
- Weighing machine, B. P. apparatus and Foetoscope or stethoscope are handled properly.

Precautions in Bag Technique

- No personal material are kept in the nursing bag.
- No meddling of the content without hand wash.
- Open only when required.
- Used items are not put into nursing bag.
- It is kept on a stool or box or a paper at home visiting.

Referral at Home Visiting

Cases are categorized into:
- Fatal condition
- Serious condition
- Minor condition.

One has to think and take decision in fatal case because if the same cannot be saved even with treatment with referral, it may be a waste of energy and sometimes may be against the will of members of the family. Serious condition may be serviced with first aid and immediate referral by transport. The attempt may be life saving. Minor ailments can allow delay in referral.

A referral card should have following information:

Name, address of patient Complaint Treatment given Name and designation of persons referring To where reference made Date and time of referral

Recording System

In public health practice recording system is to be updated at health centre after each home visiting. Records help in early action, minimize repetition, help in follow up or progress.

Type of records may be:
- Village record
- Family folders
- Individual health records
- MCH (RCH) cards
- Immunisation card
- Growth chart
- TB treatment card
- Leprosy treatment card
- School health record
- Records of vital events (Birth, Death, Marriage)
- OPD record
- IPD discharge slip
- Daily log book
- Monthly reports.

Recording system should have data in complete form. It is preferred to be in structured format (which minimize clerical work). They are kept confidential.

Recording system may have following types:
- Folder type
- File type
- Envelop type
- Card type
- Book type.

Health Education at Home Visits

Nurse play greater role in educating, informing and motivating the members of the family at home visit. Selection of appropriate content, use of appropriate method are required for an effective health education.

EXTENSION OF HOME VISITING – A NEW CONCEPT OF PUBLIC HEALTH NURSING

Home Care

"***Home care***" and "***Home health care***" are phrases that are used interchangeably to mean any type of care given to a person in their own home. Both phrases are used interchangeably regardless of whether the person requires skilled care or not.

Home care aims to make it possible for people to remain at home rather than use residential, long-term, or institutional-based nursing care. Home care providers render services in the client's own home. These services may include some combination of professional health care services and life assistance services.

Professional home health services could include medical or psychological assessment, wound care, medication teaching, pain management, disease education and management, physical therapy, speech therapy, occupational therapy.

Nurse acts as nurse practitioner in giving primary health care, required nursing care or home care services.

Nursing (Homes)

Recent upsurge of nursing homes expect over 60 percent of health care activities by a trained nurse. The nursing component of a nursing home is catered at all levels viz., reception, advice, counselling, ward duty, follow up of instructions, case preparation, O.T assistance, Dressing, maintenance of ICU, ICCU etc.

R.C.H. Nursing

The nursing component includes conducting home deliveries and after nursing care. It includes new born care also.

School Health Nursing

It includes health check up, health teaching, dental health, first aid, recording system and referral care.

Public Health Nursing

Public health in Health and F W service has these designated posts and it includes family care at health and in sickness. R.C.H. care, immunisation, psychosocial counselling and carrying out P.H.C. function in the service area.

Industrial Nursing

As highlighted earlier, nursing care is a requisite in factories where more than 500 workers are employed. In the background of industrial set up care of sick, injured, first aid, safety, crèche, rehabilitation and nursing administration are the main nursing care activities.

Rehabilitation Centres

Nursing component in diagnosis, surgical correction, prosthesis provision, orthopaedic appliances are demanding nursing care services in rehabilitation centres.

Mental Health Nursing

Community psychiatry and community mental health demand the services of nursing profession. Nursing component in diagnosis, drug administration, guidance, counselling, body care, personal hygiene of mentally ill demands the call for nursing care without which there cannot be comprehensive mental health care.

Geriatric Nursing

It is in hospital, health centre, old age home or elderly in their home call for nursing care which itself is 90% of total health care of the elderly. Along with clinical rehabilitation staff home visiting is demanded by the community.

THE HOME HELP SERVICE

With widening of dimension of nursing component through midwifery, home nursing and health visiting, adequate domestic help in the home is a created demand of urban family life. Nursing component is accepting shopping, cooking, washing and keeping house clean apart from regular nursing care on mutually agreeable terms.

Hospital deliveries, hospital admission in chronically ill, post operative cases of spouse are demanding home help services.

The aim in providing all these facilities is to ensure sufficient support so that medical and nursing care in the home is a practical possibility.

FURTHER REFERENCES

1. Priest – Modern Textbook of Personal and Communal Health for Nurse (Heineman).
2. Prabhakara G.N. – Trends, Issues Management in Nursing (Peepee).

29

Nursing Administration and Public Health Administration

NURSING ADMINISTRATION

Introduction

Significance, Meaning, Nature

The field of administration consists of two essential parts.

One: Administrative organisation which describe structure, personnel and resources

Two: Administrative management which directs health personnel, Finance control and operations.

Nursing administration arranges the professional group into working group for efficiency and to obtain desired result from group action. Here we see that nursing administration as an arrangement of personnel for facilitating the accomplishment of some agreed upon purpose through the allocation of function and responsibilities. It is the relating of the efforts and capacities of individuals and groups engaged upon a common task in such a way as to secure the desired objectives with the least friction and with the most satisfaction for those for whom the task is done and those engaged in the enterprise.

Scope

The perimeters of acceptable areas of administration are moving at a rapid rate. Now we started looking at man in his total environment. Personal health services are being directed by Government policy. Administrative activities involve the following areas:

- Infectious diseases, communicable diseases, non communicable diseases and contagious diseases.
- Dietary deficiencies
- Behavioural disorders
- Mental illness
- Allergic disorders
- RCH activities
- Equitable distribution of health care
- Resource management
- Screening programmes
- Graduation nursing education
- Vital record data collection
- Health education activities
- Research activities
- Insect, vector, rodent control
- Environment pollution control
- Supervision of food and water.

Philosophy

Administration is mainly for gaining material benefit for the health of the community. This depends on dedication and enthusiasm of personnel involved in the team. Able administration can prove the result through an enhanced life expectation, reduction in morbidity and mortality due to sickness and improvement in standard of living.

For analytic purpose the able administration is for public health, which is the science and art of preventive disease, prolonging life, promoting health and efficiency through an organised effort for:

- The development of the social machinery to insure everyone a standard of living adequate for the maintenance of health.
- The organisation of medical and nursing services for the early diagnosis and preventive treatment of diseases.
- The education of the individual regarding personal and environment hygiene.
- Control of infection, contagious, communicable and non communicable diseases.
- And better sanitation of our environment.

The above items are organised for the benefit of people and enable every citizen to realize his birthright of health and longevity.

Approaches

i. Biomedical approach through knowledge of science and technology. Great discoveries of diseases can be diagnosed and discoveries of drugs can be given for therapeutic management.
ii. Ecological approach through perfecting the environment for disease control.
iii. Holistic approach which recognises the strength of social, economical, political and environmental influences. They are tackled through multisectoral management.

Human Factors in Public and Private Administration:

Human are composite of a society or a compromise of various strengths and weakness, interests, prejudices, abilities and feelings. They share common need and common interests. They are dependent upon one another within the groups for sustenance, education, inspiration, economic welfare and entertainment as well as many other needs. Different groups are needed for different purposes. In administration human factors that need consideration are:

- Religious, social and nationality of group.
- Economic and social groups which determine the extent of participation.
- Family as a powerful social cohesion.

Ignoring these factors usually guarantees failure of administration. As a next factor, the culture of society which determine how a person thinks, feels and acts is a human factor determining administration. Public health activities and programmes are influenced by the cultural pattern of the society.

Administration and Management

Administration

Administration is "getting things done" whereas management is the purposeful and effective use of resources viz., manpower, money and material. Administration and management fulfill the predetermined objective.

They are common words used in nursing administration for getting "nursing care" and an able management by using nursing manpower, material and finance. Here health care and nursing care delivery are catered to the community through modern management methods and techniques.

Administration and management are both art and science for using them as weapon for:

- Preventing diseases.
- Prolonging life.
- Promoting health and efficiency through organised effort.

Elements of Administration

To perform functions effectively through administration, administrators require adequate knowledge of application of all facts of administrative practice. Gulick has indicated the component function or activities involved in administration through an acronym "POSDCORB" Their meaning is explained as under:

Planning the things that need to be done.

Organising the formal structure of the agency.

Staffing the agency.

Directing the work of the agency and making decisions relating there to.

Coordinating all staff activities

Reporting to the executive and through him to those to whom he is responsible.

Budgeting and all other aspects of fiscal management and control.

Litchfield has characterised the administrative process as a cycle which can be represented as under:

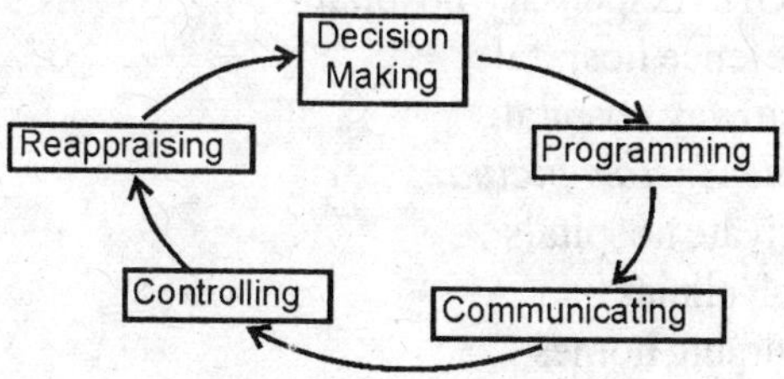

Fig. 29.1: Litchfield administrative cycle

The Scalar Principle

This consists of the administrative arrangement of the functional groups or functional units in steps as a scale. This can be represented as a "Scalar principle of nursing administration".

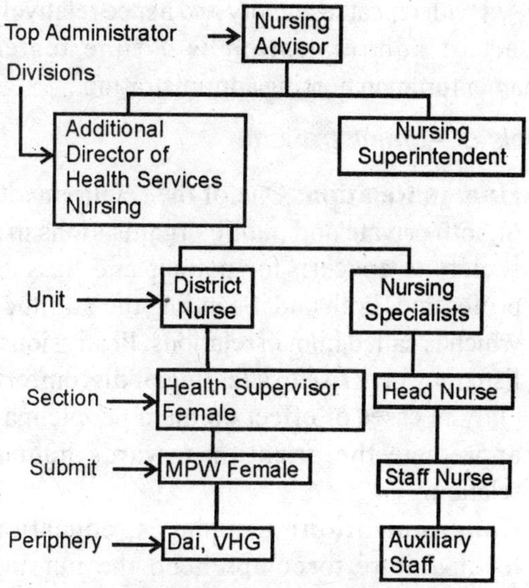

Fig. 29.2: The scalar process

Review of Leadership

It is the sum total of activity a supervisor or nursing administrator does in the nursing institution. It influences the reactions of the members of the work group. Nursing administrator should have the following qualities:

- Insight into human behaviour.
- Decision making ability in nursing care.
- Ability to plan, organise and direct efforts of others.
- Ability to relate to others on a face to face basis.

Qualities of leadership include intelligence, self confidence, formal education, adaptability, emotional stability, enthusiasm, conceptual ability and human relation skills.

Pattern of leadership like telling, selling consulting and joining are highlighted in Chapter 27.

Uses of Creativity

Creativity is a sensitizing art which influence the organizational capability. It allows new innovative method or an invention in the field of public health. Both monotonous and ambiguous methods get diluted with repeated activity and hence relatively an art of administration is a time tested ornamentorum in nursing administration.

Tools of Administration

a. **Human Relation:** One of the requirements of both private and public organisations in a society is concern for patient and nursing professions both understanding their attitude which is called human relations. Professionalism may give rise to a feeling of discomfort. Only in cases of effect on them people may appreciate the attention towards human relation.

b. **Communication:** Languages, education level, failure to comprehend the nursing instructions, fear and anxiety over supervisor are found to be an obstacle for communication. Outward and downward communication of knowledge is a foundation of good nursing care system.

c. **Coordinating:** It is a leadership quality that makes the administration and management effective. Flaws and loopholes are override by coordinating the activity in a stipulated manner and on time.

d. **Supervision:** It is a process by which designated nursing administrators over-see the work of other nursing staff and establish controls to improve the work as well as the worker.

e. **Decision making:** This is a major tool of administration. This, is no doubt, a final step of administration would have taken sufficient time, effort and cost. Present trend is to make decision with the help of senior faculty and with team spirit. It should look into acceptability as for as practicability is concerned.

Health Administration and Hospital

Health care institution works on socioeconomic and political framework of society. The word HOSPES is a root word for hospital (even for Hotel and Hospice) which originally was shelter of the homeless and for entertainment of travellers. In modern times, however, the chief function of the hospital has been the care and treatment of the sick. Hospital of the future would extend the care of the sick with in its walls to the nursing supervision and nursing care of the sick within a given district served by the hospital. They have OPD, IPD, care of the ambulatory, sick on emergency and now concept of home care programme for the sick extending from the hospital is seen. Responsibility of the hospital is fixed for the realisation of community health programmes. Physician, nurse, dietician, social worker, physiotherapist, administrators are taught in hospital. The education of health workers and health professionals are prime concern. Research and its application within the hospital is time tested and doubtless.

Classification of Hospitals

Public Health Sector include:

- Primary health centres
- Community health centres
- Civil hospitals (District)
- Speciality hospitals
- Teaching hospitals (attached to colleagues)
- ESI hospital
- CGHS dispensary/hospital
- Defence hospital
- Railway hospital.

Private Sector Include:

- Private hospitals
- Polyclinics
- Nursing homes
- Private dispensaries.

Indigenous Systems of Medicine:

- Ayurveda hospitals
- Sidda hospitals
- Unani hospitals
- Tibbi dispensaries
- Homeopathy dispensaries.

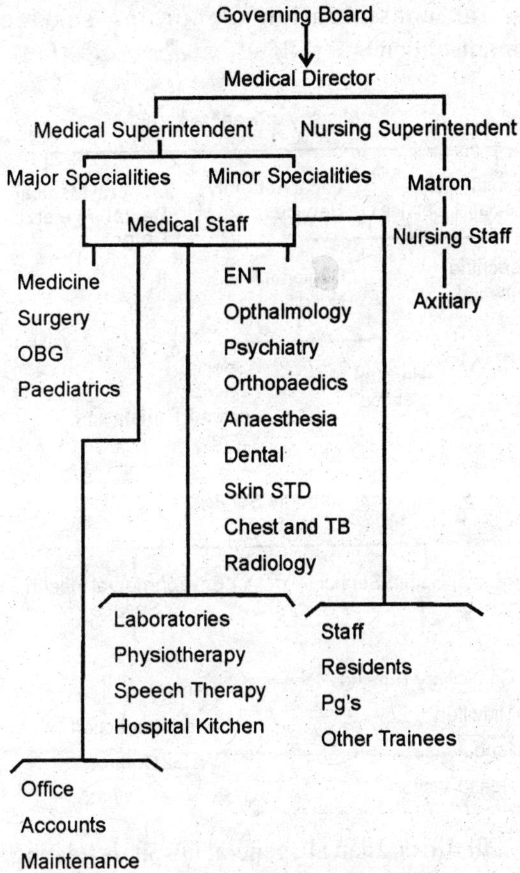

Fig. 29.3: Organisation of a hospital

Classification thus depends on type of service, ownership and quality of service given.

Standardisation of Hospitals

Hospital construction, organisation and practice that serve as standards have been recommend from time to time. Hospital administrators, physicians, nurses, dieticians and other health workers have to thrive hard for establishing standards. Minimum standards for hospitals can classify them under fully approved, provisionally approved or not approved. This formulation depends on the nature of hospital administration by the existing administrators.

Evaluation of hospital is done by periodic assessment and medical auditing. It is reflected on Mortality rate and hospital bed occupancy.

Organisation of Hospital

In all most all hospitals a visiting Board of Directors, who direct the administrators are present.

Usual pattern consists of certain specified units, departments and sections which can be represented as in Figure 29.3.

Functions of a hospital is unique in human service through medical care, nursing care, surgical intervention, emergency care, preventive care and rehabilitation care for the community.

Students may pay a fee to hospital for its use as a practice field or the hospital may pay the student for his service during learning period. If a student is a paid member, hospital can demand a reasonable high standard of performance and conformity to hospital regulations.

Nursing Service Administration

Care of the sick was carried out in different ways in olden days. Early period prior to 1800 did not specifically mention the hospital as we see today. There was no record of skilled nursing care though many religious foundations had set up treatment centres. Many such centres were closed when dissolution of the monasteries took place. Nurse trained for services on record, is available only after 1860.

Prior to 1948 voluntary hospitals and municipal hospitals existed. With the National Health Service act, hospitals came under the control of minister of health and were answerable to parliament for the administration of service.

Even then MCH, school, domiciliary and ambulance service were by local authorities.

The Minister of Health has advisors as chief medical officers, chief nursing officer and professional assistants. A general structure seen for the consideration of nursing service administration is as follows:

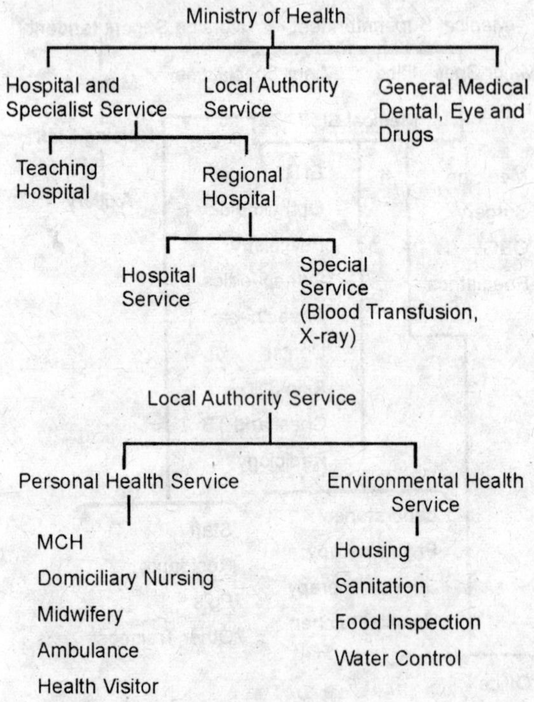

Till fifties, all in all, general hospitals treating all general and varied cases, sanitaria treating tuberculosis were of highest order. Some of the types of hospitals recently visible are:

- General hospital
- Children hospital
- Maternity hospital
- Infectious disease hospital
- Orthopaedic hospital
- Hospital for chronic sick
- Hospital for nervous disorders
- Hospital for plastic surgery.

Within each hospital there is medical, nursing and auxiliary staff.

At the top of the nursing staff, is the matron who is responsible for the nursing care of all the patients and in training programmes of hospitals. She is responsible for training student nurses according to the requirements of the general nursing council. Matron is assisted by deputy Matron, sister tutor, assistant matron and various administrative sisters.

The actual immediate care of the patients is delegated to the ward sisters and department sisters. Each ward is with student nurse, assistant nurse, pupil assistant nurse, nursing auxiliaries and lay assistants. Domestic workers are also available. It is the task of ward sister to make this group into a team all working together for patient care. The efficiency of the staff of any ward and the atmosphere of happiness within ward depends on team spirit which enables everyone to work together and not for any individual gain. By becoming member of nursing team, the pattern of nursing care is seen being given to patient. Each duty has its place in the whole scheme which is highlighted in Chapters 25 and 29.

The auxiliary staff includes the specialist in the various branches of treatment that are included in the patient care. They are coordinated by ward sister for their therapy like physiotherapy occupational therapy, radiotherapy, pharmacy and diet.

Technique

Nursing service administration can be efficiently handled by the following nursing administrative techniques.

MBO (Management by Objectives)

For different nursing service, different objectives are set with its own plan of action on short term basis. Main aim of MBO is to achieve good result in nursing administration.

Cost Benefit Analysis: The economic benefit of a nursing service is compared with the cost of that nursing service. It may sound usual to think on economic basis. If the benefit is doubtful, an alternative can be selected. However in nursing care it is not money that matters but the relief and service that counts. Hence, many of the occasions applying cost benefit analysis in nursing service administration becomes vague.

Cost Effective Analysis: It is a promising tool in nursing service administration. The benefit is expressed in terms of results achieved. Life saved from sepsis, infection, illness can be counted.

Cost Accounting: How money is spent in each act of nursing is recorded. Permitting costs for given purpose is analysed. It helps in cost control and control of unnecessary waste in nursing service administration.

Input Out Analysis: Here input like nursing manpower, money, material, time spent and output like lives saved, transfusion done, first aid provided, injections given etc. are accounted. Here we can analysis "X" input has yielded "Y" output and correct the fallacies in nursing service administration.

Model: A concept of management in nursing is prepared. Say a case preparation for surgery, surgical nursing at OT, post surgery nursing in post operative ward till dismissal is jotted. The model contains a decision on each phase. Service administration in nursing profession if has given a good result in this model type of MBO.

System Analysis:

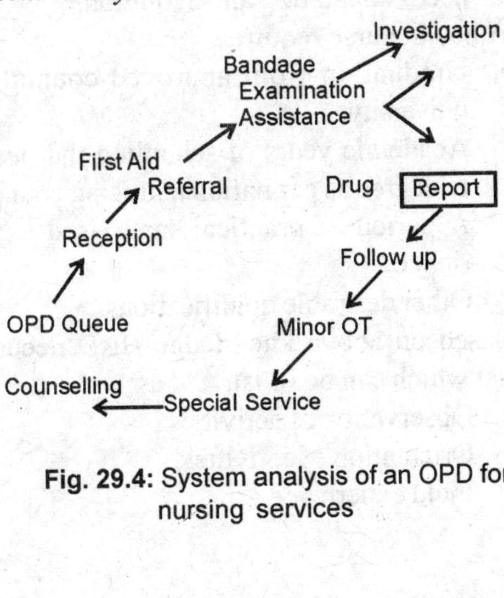

Fig. 29.4: System analysis of an OPD for nursing services

System analysis (Fig. 29.4) in OPD work, ward work, hospital supply system, information system, a community health service system or any nursing system is prepared. They help in decision making and for appropriate action to be taken in nursing care. Any system will have sub system for analysis (Fig. 29.5).

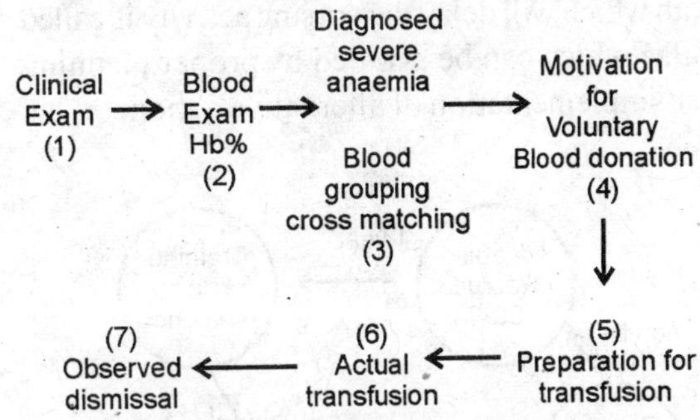

Fig. 29.5: Seven subunit system analysis of blood transfusion system analysis

Evaluation Technique

There are 2 network evaluation techniques that are used in nursing service administration. They are PERT and CPM.

PERT (Programme Evaluation and Review Technique): This helps in detailed planning and in comprehensive supervision. It is made by

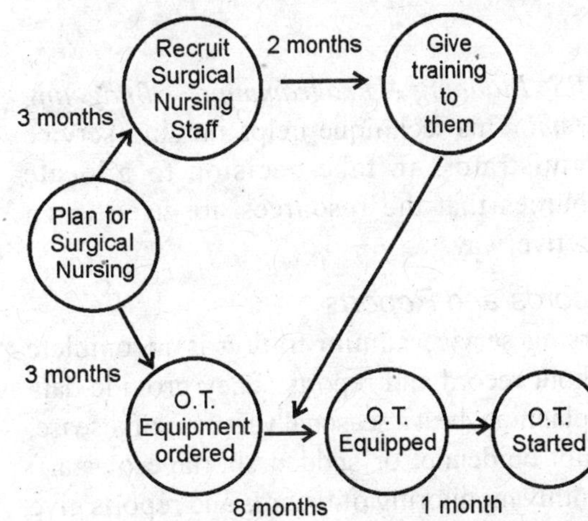

Fig. 29.6: Network analysis of surgical nursing for O.T. functioning in the hospital

sequence arranged logically with arrow marks for steps and timings.

PERT helps in planning, scheduling, monitoring, communication problem identification, gives progress report, and thus, is a good evaluating method in nursing service administration.

C.P.M. (Critical Path Method): The longest path which will delay the nursing activity is called CPM which can be avoided by proper planning and implementation of alternative action.

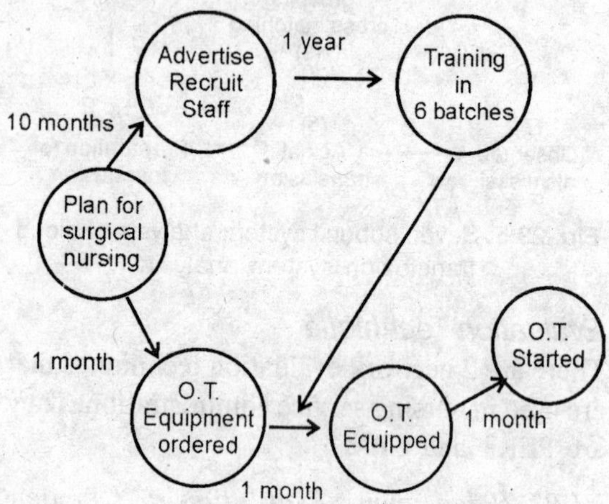

Fig. 29.7: Critical path in recruiting and training staff is shown in PERT

PPBS (Planning – Programming – Budgeting System: This technique helps nursing service administrators to take decision to allocate resources that the resources are used in an effective way.

Records and Reports

Nursing service administration is incomplete without record and reports. They provide data for planning, be it a seasonal variation of disease, abrupt epidemic, or sudden shortage of staff. Monthly monitoring of records and reports give a good picture for effecting the required nursing administration.

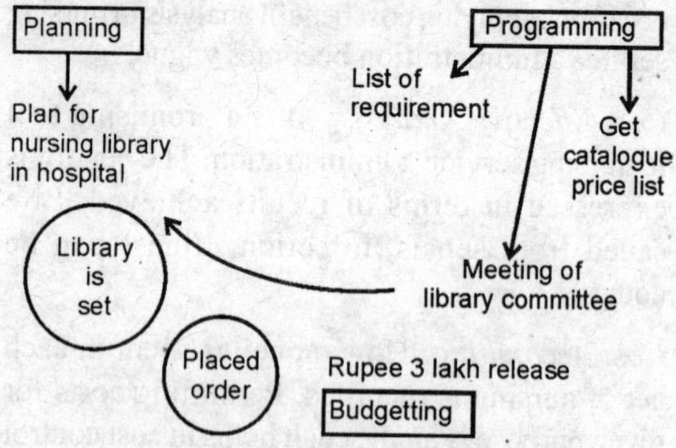

Fig. 29.8: PPBS for a nursing library

Functions of Nursing Service Administration

Human Resource Management

A force of well trained nurses is the prime requisite of nursing service. Nursing profession is covering a huge area of health care and now special nursing has added an additional requirement of manpower. The decision on HRD (nursing) depends on Government policy and financial resources available. Nursing profession is unique in certain characteristics like knowledge to care the sick, skill to nurse, public and social responsibility and service. A complex spectrum of ability and function is required for nursing type of personnel. Activities of nursing are changing which needs adaptation and evolution.

A health nurse requires:

- Graduation from approved council or university.
- Academic years of schooling that leads to degree as per national nursing council.
- A period of practical supervised experience.
- Other desirable qualifications.

Based on above knowledge HRD needs a format which can be illustrated as:

1. Observation of activities
2. Orientation of activities
3. Field experience

4. Apprenticeship
5. In-service training.

HRD need adherence to national minimum standards, specified from time to time.

As per 2001 census for the population of 1,027,015,247 the requirement of nurses is 2,06,000 (as per suggested norm) we cannot get qualified nurse even to cover 50% of minimal norm. But getting unqualified nurse may not be a problem because; estimated nurse population exceeds 3 lakh which include all unqualified nurses also.

Table 29.1: Suggested norms for nursing services

Nurse (Bed side nursing)	1 for 2500 population
Nurse (No bed side nursing)	1 for 5000 population
Health worker female	1 for 5000 population 1 for 3000 population (Tribal and Hilly area)
Trained Dai (Trained TBA)	1 for each village
Health assistant female	1 for 30,000 population (20,000 in Tribal, Hilly area)

As per estimate we have following public health nursing manpower at the end of Tenth Five Year Plan period.

ANM	– 506,925 (133194 during current plan)
Health assistant female	– 17,371
Nurse midwife	– 865,135 (28930 during current plan)
Nurse: Population ratio	– 0.8 / 1000 population (2004 estimate)
Midwife: Population ratio	– 0.47 / 1000 population (2004 estimate)

Requirement and Employment

Merit system principle for recruitment and selecting capable individuals to fill up nursing professions is followed in civil service.

Compensation, Tenure and Promotion

Equal pay for equal work allow compensation plan. The factors involved in determining tenure and promotion are essentially the same that determine the granting of step increase in compensation.

The Executive and his Personnel

Nursing administrative management is essentially a question of the organisation of manpower, material, resource and strategy for the accomplishment of a desired goal. This is impossible unless administrator has successfully organised herself to understand the cause of problems in day to day work. It requires curiosity, imagination, integrative ability and good judgment.

Delegation of Powers

Nursing service functions most effectively when a capable administrator, rather than attempting to control and supervise intimately each of the various activities that make up the total nursing care programme, is able to delegate control and supervision to responsible subordinates.

Morale and Discipline

In nursing profession there are code of conduct, rules and regulations to be followed. If they are to be effective, they must be few, simple, readily understandable and inflexible.

Effectively includable items are hours of work, length of lunch period, handling of certain records and correspondence, holiday, leave, etc.

But real difficulty begins with the professional behaviour of all her subordinates.

Conditions of Work

The conditions of work depend on incentive scale available.

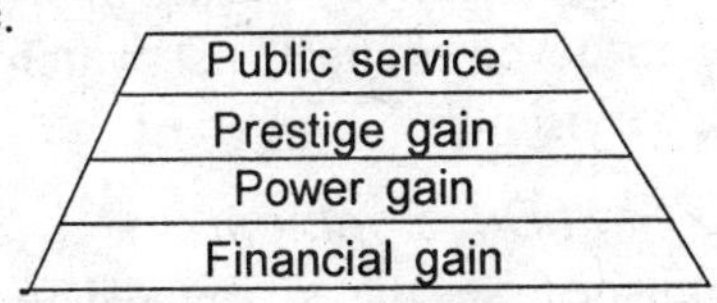

Fig. 29.9: Personnel incentive scale according to Dimock

Hence the influencing factors are job appeal, overtime, leaves, inservice training and retirement benefit system.

To conclude the functions of nursing service administration, nursing service should consider human resource management techniques. Nursing staffing should have specified recruitment, selection, induction, confirmation, probation and termination. Nursing service should consider the personnel policies like:

- Staff computation
- Job analysis
- Job specifications
- Job description
- Staff assignment

Examples of job description of health nurse are given in appendix.

Supervision of Nursing Service

All categories of nursing staff have the opportunity of supervision to oversee the work of others, to control subordinates and to see that improvement of work is done. It is advocated to the supervisors to be friendly and polite and yet be firm when the occasion demands. Senior nursing staff should have good knowledge of the activity and procedure because supervising staff is expected to do better that what subordinate can do.

The element of nursing supervision should have (a) Coexistence (b) impartiality and (c) understanding problems of subordinates.

Staff meeting, record review, direct observation and periodic evaluation help in good and appropriate supervision of nursing staff.

In nursing, for activity of staff supervision it is better to develop check list which help in proper supervision.

Nursing Staff Development

It is a requisite to see that all round development of nursing staff is advocated for an effective nursing services, since nursing care has become vast, special nursing requires update of knowledge and skill. If this component is forgotten, the nursing service is downgraded and achievement of nursing care goal will be lowered.

Following staff development programmes are advocated from time to time for an effective use of nursing manpower. They are:

- In-service education
- Continued education
- Specific orientation courses
- Specific skill training.

Welfare of Nursing Staff

It is one of the secret areas of management which holds the crown of nursing; that is welfare available to nursing staff.

Working Condition

It must be a friendly and homely atmosphere. Rigid actions are unwanted in genuine cases, minimum physical facilities like sitting arrangement, recreation arrangement, toilet facilities, working lunch or snack at affordable rates etc.

Safety

Safety procedures are adopted in nursing care procedures. First aid and immediate nursing provisions are made available; Nurses are amenable for physical attack and mental abuse which are to be safeguarded.

Health

Free or reimbursable facility for medical care, leave allowance for the period of illness or maternity are basic health facilities that are called for.

Salaries

It is to be compensated as wage for the work. Compensation and incentive which provide basic financial need make a nurse to be punctual, attentive and prompt in her discharging duties.

Benefits

Leave, privilege of medical benefits, compensation, tenure and promotions are considered the professional benefit for financial gain, power gain, prestige gain and public service.

Recreation

Holiday compensatory leave; get together, recreation facility during off days, facility for indoor games is suggested recreation facilities under staff welfare scheme.

Material Management

In day to day hospital practice or in the health centre practice material of constant use is to be managed well. They are:

Drugs

Substances used in patient care. They are in the form of tablet, capsule, solution, ointment, injection, I V infusion etc.

Medical Supplies

Items used along with drugs to provide curative, preventive and rehabilitative services. They are cotton roll, bandage, needle, syringe, suture material, infusion set etc.

Non Medical Supplies

Non medical items used in providing nursing care services. They are linen, clothing, supplies, stationary supplies etc.

Equipment

They are movable items used by nursing profession which are for long term use. They are refrigerator, beds, table, desk, sterilizer, weighing machine, B.P. apparatus, clinical thermometer etc.

Facility

They are nonmovable items like dining room, latrine, dressing room, fencing for protection etc.

Inventory Management

Right drug supply, the equipment is at the right place, at the right time, and in the right quantity in order that nurse delivers nursing care. Without material supply nursing staff gets frustrated and patient community lacks confidence in nursing service.

Good material management involves the following procedures:

a. Regular and systematic inventory by nursing staff.
b. Daily indenting according to actual need by sending request indent.
c. Indent is received and checked with request indent.
d. Material supply received is stored properly and are protected from misuse.
e. Procedure is followed for use for patient care.

Regular replenishment of drugs, medical supplies and non medical supplies are done. Regular and proper use and preventive maintenance is advocated. Preventive maintenance is checking equipment and facilities regularly to keep them in good condition.

In material management no over-stocking or under stocking is advised. Over-stocking is not a

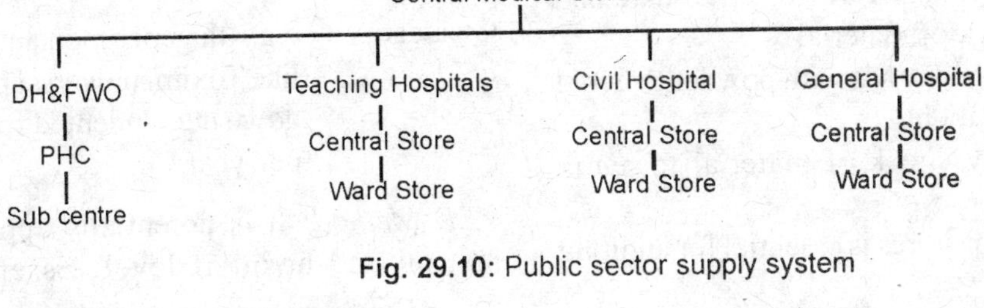

Fig. 29.10: Public sector supply system

proper material management which causes losses from pilferage and waste due to spoilage. Under stocking is also poor material management because it causes shortage and hardship.

Policy and Procedure in Material Management

Within the country many variations are seen from state to state and hospital to hospital. In private sector, bulk purchase and a central store is maintained which supply on daily basis. In public sector procurement of supplies is made by central medical stores.

As a part of ward management, a nurse should know the concept of inventory control, proper indenting procedure, maintaining proper register and taking timely action towards replenishing stock.

Material management includes the proper store of drugs, medical items in a place protecting from temperature, humidity and rainfall. Facilities and equipment should be kept in good working condition.

Guidelines to nursing staff for an effective nursing administration under material management are:

- Have an idea about past 3 year requirement sought for
- Estimate present requirement
- List the item with particulars
- Indent early allowing for appropriate time lag from the date of previous indent
- Proper bottling, accounting and labelling are necessary for good drug management
- Organise the material in the store, label them, and keep an index of available item in the store. Make a tally card for up-to-date and accurate stock of material
- Preserve rubber goods with powder to avoid their deterioration
- Have weekly check of material to avoid rusting
- Accounting of stores is essential for auditing
- Train the subordinate staff for proper use and handling of supplies and equipment
- Always keep a track on the date of expiry of medicaments
- Prompt reporting of loss, theft or damage help in replacement or condemnation
- Non consumable goods should have the following information:
  a. Date of purchase
  b. Source of procurement
  c. Cost at the time of purchase
  d. Cost of maintenance if under repair
  e. Reason for condemnation, if to be condemned.

Inventory control methods in material management in nursing service administration are:

Intuitive Method: As per requirement, commonly required are indented, stocked and followed. This is simple and appropriate method for ward management.

Perpetual Inventory Method: It is useful at main store level. At hospital, nursing staff must be diligent in record keeping.

ABC Analysis: High priority items under A and least required under C are indented and adjusted to budgeting which help in continuous supply. This is useful at hospital level.

Example: If 3 lakh is budget for 1 year for hospital for drugs

A category – e.g. APC, aspirin, paracetamol, sulpha, piperizine etc., indented for 2 lakh per year.

B category – e.g. Dressing, antibiotics etc indented for 75,000 per year.

C category – e.g. 4th generation antibiotics like Toxim, universal precaution gown etc., indented for 25,000 per year.

VED Method: It is potentially appropriate at matron and hospital level. Essential, very essential categorisation at indent, supply and inventory are done.

Two Bin Method: This method is appropriate for ward management. Two portions one for immediate utility and the other for next requirement are kept. When first bin completes and second bin is used. Quick provision for indent is made to see that no shortage or hardship is caused.

Nursing service administration requires Material Requirement Planning (MRP) which can be independent Demand or dependent demand. Sometimes Just In Time (JIT) planning also is suitable for unusual and rare nursing acts and performances

Financial Management

This system in nursing service includes law, policy, regulation, procedure and proforma related to the receipt and expense of money during patient care and patient management. Main idea is to protect misuse and waste.

Senior nursing staff should know what a budget is. Knowledge of procedure and deadline can make input possible and no lapse of allocated budget. There are 2 types of money recognised in financial management.

Invisible Money (Budgetary Allocation)

It is for drugs, staff, transport etc., where actual money does not pass the hands, but spent through allocations. For example: There are 10 wards in a civil hospital where 84 staffs are working. These wards has a budget of 5 lakh rupees for drugs and medical items and 16 lakhs 8 thousand budget for staff salary. When the budget is released to the civil hospital, the supply is automatically done and salary is spent. In this way the civil hospital spends 5 lakh for drugs and Rs. 16,08,000 for salary without any money passing through the hospital.

Visible Money or Cash (Imprest Amount)

It is provided to meet unforeseen emergencies. Nursing staff is authorized to spend imprest money and then replenish the amount spent. But imprest is replenished against an original receipt in order to prevent misuse of funds. Each time when imprest money is spent, it must be recorded on a cash voucher. Each cash voucher is numbered and must have a receipt attached to it from the person who has sold the goods to the hospital.

In financial management funds allocation are done under head of account, like:

213 Cabinet (Non plan)
280 Medical (Non plan)
281 Medical Plan
281 Family welfare – Plan
282 Public Health – Plan
282 Public health – Plan
299 Hills – Non Plan
288 *Samajik suraksha* and *kalyan* (Non plan)
289 Relief in natural calamities (Non plan)

There are specified forms, vouchers, receipts, registers that are to be used in financial management. Nursing staff on administration should know about them which are possible by the existing compulsory departmental examination in "Accounts Higher" which is the requisite qualification for an administrative post in nursing service.

Nursing Management of Unit/Ward/Dept

Nursing management requires certain qualities in a nurse which are time tested and remunerative from humanitarian angle. They are:

- Patience, sympathy, understanding
- Gentleness and willingness
- Reliability
- Resourcefulness
- Power of observation.

Rules to be Observed in Cleaning:

i. All should be cleaned before start of a nursing act.
ii. Clean duster, rubber, brushes and clean water must be used.
iii. Sweeping should be before dusting except in high dusting of walls.
iv. A damp duster is preferred for furniture.
v. Corner and edges should not be forgotten.
vi. Cleaning must be done with little disturbance.
vii. All rubbish collection and disposal must be done twice a day.
viii. Check for forbidden articles by the patient.
ix. Tiles, floors are scrubbed with yellow soap and water.
x. Everyday cleaning with dry cloth of electric lights is a requirement.
xi. Metal fittings are periodically checked for proper cleaning.

i. **Treatment and Preparation Room:** For safe aseptic practice surgical dressings are done in an annex, one annex for "Clean" preparation of sterilisation procedure, another for "septic" treatment.

ii. **Ward Bath and Sanitary Annexes:** Soap and water are used for washing. For bowl and mug hot soap water containing 1: 80 Lysol is used. The dressing piles need crude phenol (1:10).

iii. **Ward/Unit Kitchen:** Basic principles of kitchen sanitation are followed.

iv. **Bedpan and Urinals:** Automatic bedpan washers in which bed pans are enclosed for flushing with hot and cold water are used.

Sputum mug is boiled for 5 minutes; sodium bicarbonate solution (1:160) is added before taking sputum mug to patient.

Water closet are sprinkled with chlorinated soda and left for 30 minutes. The brush used for water closet is disinfected with Jeyes fluid (1:40).

Care of bedspreads and beddings are followed as per hospital disinfection procedure. Bed mackintoshes, air rings and beds are mopped with 1:20 phenol or 1:30 Lysol before wash.

Ward linen has to follow procedures adopted by hospital infection control committee as per guidelines for nursing procedures so that care of soiled linen is taken to prevent cross infection.

Stain Removal Procedures

Blood—Use of peroxide of Hydrogen or ammonia and rinse later.
Ink—Rubbing a paste of salt and lemon juice and a wash.
Ball pen ink is removed by methylated spirit.
Tea coffee cocoa—Use of a bleaching agent and a rinse.
Fruit stain—Rub with salt and wash.
Rust mark—Salt and lemon juice and exposure to sun light.
Iodine mark—Apply ammonia, rinse and wash.
Skin ointment, paste liniment—They are resistant to removal.
Laundry has special methods.

Duties of a Nurse

To the Patient

Apart from earlier detailing, chief factors to be looked into are:

- Rest
- Toilet
- Diet
- Excretion of waste material
- Mental outlook.

To the Doctor

Carrying out instruction and written report avoids risk of omissions:

- Temperature, pulse, respiration
- Action of bowl, nature and composition of stool
- Type, amount of urine
- Nature of sleep

- Appetite, type of food taken
- Report of any pain, relief given
- Report of vomiting, nature
- Report of cough, nature
- Medicines administered
- Chart of fluid intake and fluid output.

To Herself

Nurse has to use rules of personal hygiene to maintain her health and for service efficiency:

- Cleanliness
- Clothing
- Food
- Rest, exercise

Nursing Education Administration

This is governed by standards laid down by National nursing council and ordinance of affiliated universities.

Minimum Staff Under Nursing Education

(for 50 admissions per year)

Principal 1
Vice principal 1
Tutors/ Instructors 15
External guest lecturers as needed

Office:

Steno 1
UDC + Cash account 1
LDC + Type work 1
Librarian 1
Asst librarian 1
Lab attendant 1
Chowkidar 4
Driver 1
Cleaner 1
Peon 3
Sweeper 3
Duplicator operator 1

Physical Facilities

Classroom 4
Laboratory 1
Auditorium 1
Library 1
Examination hall 1
Office 1
Common room 1
Record room 1
Store room 1
A.V. room 1
Facility for water and toilet.

Clinical Facility

- Field practice area with accommodation, transport, security
- Hospital 150 Beds
  Nursing Superintendent 1
  Deputy Superintendent 1
  Asst. Superintendent 2
  1:1 to 1:3 Ratio staff nurses
  1:13 to 1:120 Ratio staff to OPD
- Hostel
- Bedroom, Bath, Recreation, Visitor room, Kitchen, Pantry, Wash, Accommodation, Crèche, Canteen, Transport
  No. of Teaching hours – appendix enclosed. (Appendix 1)

Regarding policies of nursing education, evaluation tools, records and service utilisation, they are detailed in Chapter 27.

Medico Legal Aspect of Nursing

In the course of nursing service, nurse is responsible for voluntary consent of patients which is absolutely essential. This means that the patient should have legal capacity to give consent, should be able to exercise free power of choice without the intervention of any element of force, fraud, deceit, duress, over-reaching or other ulterior form of coercion.

The nurse on duty has the responsibility for ascertaining the quality of the consent, which may not be delegated to another with impunity.

Code of Ethics framed under section 33 of IMC act 1956 is to be followed in principle and practice. They include character of nurse and the nursing responsibility. It is unethical to enter into a contract of "no cure no payment". A nurse shall not solicit or receive any gift.

Duties of the nurse to patient are:

- Obligations to the sick.
- Patience, delicacy and secrecy.
- No exaggeration of prognosis.
- No neglect of patient when once undertaken the case.

Regarding nursing profession, nurse is given an oath for (Nightingale oath):

- Upholding the honour of nursing profession
- Be a member of nursing society.
- Safeguard the nursing profession.
- Avoid exposure to unethical conduct.

Nursing ethical code obligates her to engage for an obstetric case management to give nursing care to mother and child and on no account be refused.

Nursing Council of India

Every qualified nurse should enroll herself under NCI to practice nursing. NCI desires to bring to the notice of registered nurses on certain statement upon offences and form of professional misconduct which may be brought before the appropriate nursing council for disciplinary action.

General and specific ethical and legal aspects are followed for Assisted Reproductive Technologies in India which are available in consultative documents of ICMR.

Nursing Ethics: It is a code of moral behaviour, loyalty behaviour, trustworthiness and reliability.

Professional Ethics: It is etiquette, the code of manners or the ceremonial observed in certain circumstances.

Legal Issues in Specialty Area: They are detailed and available as documents to nursing professions to follow in the fields of:

a. Medicine
b. Surgery
c. OBG
d. Psychiatry and
e. Community health nursing.

COPRA (Consumer Protection Act)

One who purchases health service and nursing service for his/her use is called consumer. The user of nursing service with permission is also a consumer as per legal terminology.

Nursing service given should be free from defects, deficiencies and free from unfair practices. Receipt, bills and cash memo against all services are compulsory as per the Act. Consumer can demand good services in exchange of money. The Consumer Protection Act (COPRA) 1986 ensures rights covering all nursing services in Government hospitals, private hospitals. Nursing homes, private clinic, cooperative clinics and consultation centres.

Consumer court set-up under COPRA at National, State and District level provide simple, expensive and speedy redressal of consumer disputes including excess price charged. Complaints can be made for compensation on plain paper without court fee and without a lawyer.

District forum can be approached for compensation up to 5 lakhs, the state commission should be approached if it is between 5-20 lakhs and the national commission if it exceeds 20 lakhs. The department of consumer affairs under the central ministry of Government of India is in charge of the above.

Following factors are taken note of under COPRA:

- Consumer health awareness.
- Existing constraints in the infrastructure.
- Misuse by the consumer.
- Safeguard of nursing service providers.

PUBLIC HEALTH ADMINISTRATION

Health for All (HFA)

Member countries of WHO has defined HFA as under:

"Attainment of a level of health that will enable every individual to lead to socially and economically productive life."

India developed its policies, strategies and plan of action to launch H.F.A. under its own norms and indicators. WHO has established 12 global indicators as the basic point of reference to assess the progress towards HFA. Two major goals that all member countries have adopted are (a) Life expectancy of 60 years and (b) IMR 50 per 1000 live births.

In India, the laid down goals for HFA are:

i. Attaining IMR below 60 per 1000LB
ii. Rise in expectation of life to 64 years
iii. To reduce CDR to 9 per 1000 MYP
iv. To reduce CBR to 21 per 1000 MYP
v. To achieve NRR of 1
vi. To provide potable water to the entire rural population.

Health Related Millennium Development Goals in India

The goals in the area of development and poverty eradication are called **Millennium Development Goals** to tackle ill health, gender inequality, lack of education, access to clean water and environmental degradation. Main goals that are to be considered are:

Goal No.	*Goal*
1	Eradicate extreme poverty and hunger
4	Reduce child mortality
5	Improve maternal health
6	Combat HIV/AIDS, malaria and other diseases
7	Ensure environmental sustainability
8	Develop global partnership for development

Primary Health Care

The Alma Ata has defined Primary Health Care as under:

"Primary health care is essential health care made universally accessible to individuals and acceptable to them, through their full participation and at a cost the community and country can afford."

Elements of Primary Health Care

i. Health education on health problems and their control
ii. Promotion of food supply and proper nutrition
iii. Safe and wholesome water and basic sanitation
iv. M.C.H. and F.P. (RCH)
v. Immunisation against major diseases (UIP)
vi. Prevention and control of locally epidemic diseases
vii. Appropriate treatment of common diseases and injuries
viii. Provision of essential drugs.

Principles of Primary Health Care are:

i. Equitable distribution
ii. Community participation
iii. Intersectoral coordination
iv. Appropriate technology.

Community Health Nursing

Definition

A public health nurse is professionally equipped with additional qualification to serve the community. WHO has defined public health nursing as under:

"Public health nursing combines the skills of nursing, Public health and some phases of social assistance and functions as a part of the total public health programme for the promotion of health, the improvement of conditions in the social and physical environment, the prevention of illness and disability and rehabilitation. It is concerned for the most part with the care of well families and with non hospitalized sick persons and their families, with groups of people and with health problems that affect the community as a whole."

History and Development of nursing in India is highlighted in Chapter 1.

Principles

The nurse who is engaged to serve the community has to follow the following nursing principles:

i. **Appraisal of Community Health:**
Already existed base line data of the community under a primary health centre will give background picture of the community. It reflects Demographic, Socio-economic, Morbidity and Mortality characteristics of the community. Nurse has to establish contact with the community through village leaders to appraise health status of members of the family. Family being the unit of observation, the problem study, centres round the family.

ii. **Identification of Health Problem:**
Survey, surveillance and screening help to identify health problem in the community, survey information, PHC records individual health assessment of the family, mortality data, fertility data give clues to identify existing problem. The problem can be sickness, deaths, poverty, malnutrition or social problems.

iii. **Identification of Cause of Health Problem:**
This is a community assessment to find out the cause of problem. Individual health examination, social interaction with members of the family give the clue to the source of infection, cause of poverty, cause of malnutrition or root cause of social problems.

iv. **Setting Priority for Public Health Intervention:**
Priority is fixed based on Home visiting findings which determines:
a. Frequency of occurrence of problem.
b. Seriousness of problem for the individual and for the family.
c. Urgency with which the problem is to be tackled; and
d. Practicability or feasibility of control of the problem.
A scoring system may be used for fixing the priority

v. **Planning:**
After identifying the health problem, course of action to be taken by the Team of PHC is identified. Setting the objectives, defining solutions to the problems and procurement of material for case management is undertaken.

vi. **Programming:**
Planning schedule is programmed in such a way that who, when, where, and how the public health measures are adopted is deployed.

vii. **Implementation:**
It is the stage of intervention where the activities are carried out. This includes tasks, procedure and practical skill to be applied by public health nurse.

viii. **Evaluation:**
This is an assessment of how far the implemented intervention was useful. Evaluation gives a feedback that can help in programme modification. Evaluation is a tool for making a public health action effective.

Qualities

i. **Patient Sympathy and Understanding:**
In order to be able to help the community

in her adjustment to pain, frustrations and limitations of illness. She must exercise tact in her social interaction with the members of the family and must show tolerance towards their likes and dislikes.

ii. **Gentleness and Willingness:**
In carrying out of all nursing duties however trivial it may be exercising self control and remaining calm and gracious at all the time is required.

iii. **Reliability:**
All instructions given by MOH to her must be carried out correctly and conscientiously. She must observe honestly in deed and word.

iv. **Resourcefulness:**
So that she may act immediately in any emergency using her commonsense to protect the family from ill effects.

v. **Loyalty to the MOH:**
Upholding his authority at all times and never allowing anything to be said or done that may undermine the confidence of the community and family on the health staff.

vi. **Power of Observation:**
So that she may report accurately any changes in the health of the community, and may also anticipate and fulfill the community requirements at her earliest.

Functions

Public health nurse has to be member of health team and should be able to make decision, have management skill to help all national health programmes. Main functions of Public Health Nurse are:

i. **Public Health Administration:**
Within the jurisdiction of PHC and attached sub centres she has to plan, implement and evaluate public health nursing services. She provides direction and leadership to her subordinates. Day to day assignment, supervision and monthly meetings are her administrative functions.

ii. **Health Communications:**
Ability to communicate and maintain good working relationship with team members is one aspect. The other aspect is creating awareness among individual, family, community on health and disease as well as availability of services.

iii. **Nursing Service:**
She provides comprehensive nursing care services to the population covered under PHC area. Under specific nursing care she is responsible for the care of pregnant women, Deliveries, Lactating mothers, care of the new born, infant, Toddler, preschool children and school children. Her area includes nutrition and family planning.

iv. **Training Activities:**
Training of Health workers female, MPW (Female), Dais, community health guides on RCH activities and on the functions of national health programmes.

v. **Research:**
With her knowledge of sociology, psychology, family pattern and local health problems, she is able to postulate cause hypothesis and can prove the hypothesis through community research activity.

Aspect of Community Health Nursing

Family health and personal health dealt in terms of RCH, FP and school health form main aspect of community health nursing. They are dealt in detail under Chapters 28, 11, 6 and 20 respectively.

National Health Problems

Both health status and health problems need community diagnosis for their identification. In any health planning, the requirement of health status and health problems determine action plan.

Data required for the community diagnosis of health problem are morbidity, mortality, demography, environmental aspect, socio-economic aspects, sociocultural aspects, Health service available and level of community participation.

Health problem of India can be grouped under 5 categories.

1. Population problem
2. Health care system
3. Environmental sanitation problem
4. Nutritional problem
5. Communicable disease problem

Sub components of these health problems are depicted in the Figures 29.11:

National Health Programme

Various ongoing health programmes are depicted in Figure 29.12 and in relation to the health problems depicted in Figure 29.13. Accordingly they are grouped under following categories:

1. For population problem
   A. National FWP programme
   B. I.P.P. (India Population Project)
   C. P.P.C. (Post Partum Programme)
2. For health care problem
   A. H.F.A. (Health for All)
   B. Primary Health care
3. For Environmental Sanitation Problem
   A. N.W.S. and S.P (National water supply and sanitation programme)

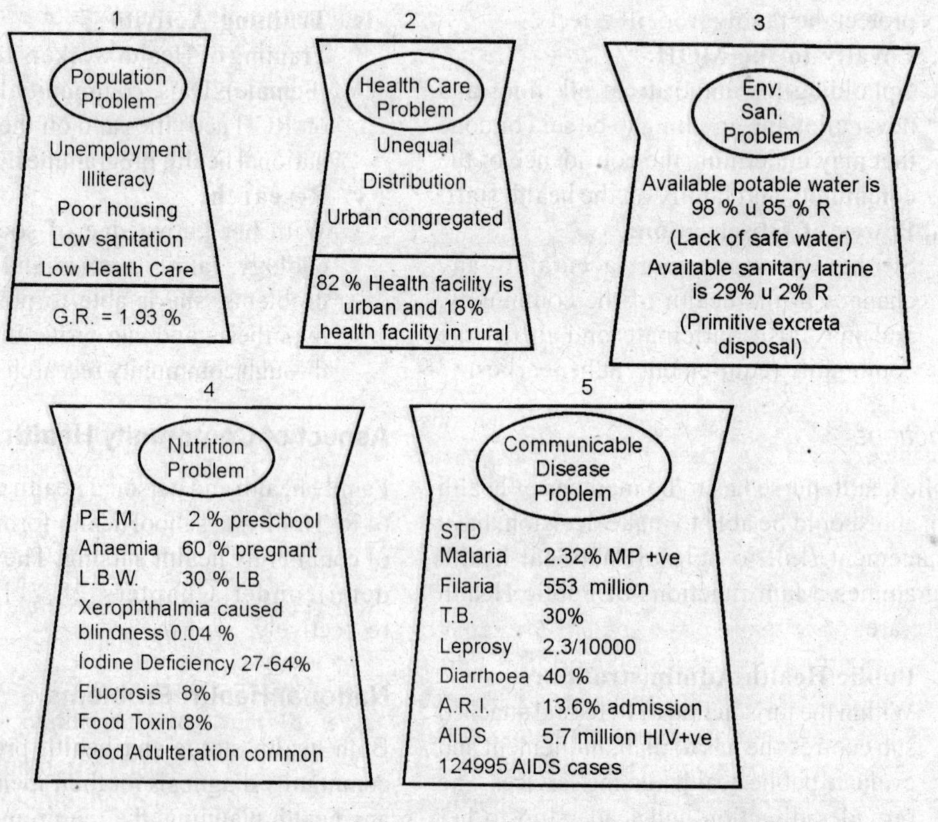

Fig. 29.11: Health problems

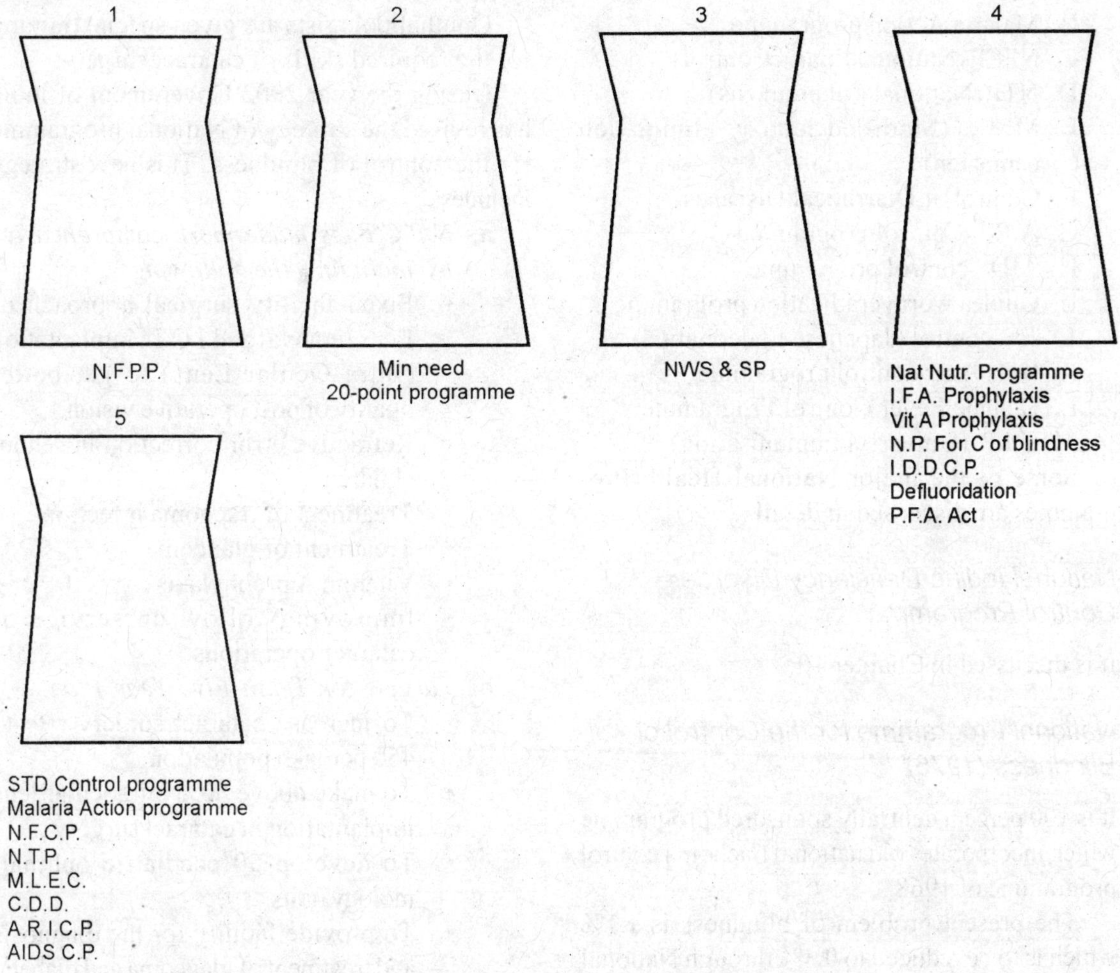

Fig. 29.12: Health programmes

   B. Accelerated Rural W.S. Programme (Rural water supply)

4. For Nutrition Problem
   A. A.N.P. (Applied Nutrition Programme)
   B. S.N.P. (Special Nutrition Programme)
   C. B.N.P. (Balwadi Nutrition Programme)
   D. Mid day meal school programme
   E. Vitamin A Prophylaxis Programme
   F. I.F.A. (NNAPP) (Iron Folic Acid Supplementation Programme) (National Nutritional Anaemia Prophylaxis Programme)
   G. N.I.D.D.C.P. (National Iodine Deficiency Disorder Control Programme)
   H. I.C.D.S. (Integrated Child Development Service Scheme)
   I. I.P.P. (India Population project)
   J. Defluoridation of water
   K. P.F.A. Act (Prevention of Food Adulteration Act)
   L. National Programme for Control of Blindness
5. For communicable diseases problem
   A. S.T.D. Control programme

B. Malaria Action programme
C. NFCP (National Filaria Control)
D. NTP (National Tuberculosis)
E. MLEC (Modified leprosy elimination campaign)
F. Control of Diarrhoeal Diseases
G. A.R.I. Control programme
H. AIDS control programme
I. Guinea worm eradication programme
J. J.E. control (Japanese Encephalitis)
K. Kala Azar control programme
L. Dengue Fever Control Programme
M. U.I.P. (Universal Immunisation).

Some of the major National Health Programmes are discussed in detail.

National Iodine Deficiency Disorder Control Programme

It is discussed in Chapter 10.

National Programme for the Control of Blindness (1976)

It is 100 percent centrally sponsored programme which incorporates old national trachoma control programme of 1968.

The present problem of blindness is 1.1% which is to be reduced to 0.3% through National level programme.

Chalked out programme contained:

- Establishment of regional institute of ophthalmology
- Upgrading medical colleges hospitals
- Upgrading district hospitals
- Development of mobile ophthalmic units
- Recruitment of ophthalmic manpower
- Provision of ophthalmic services

By improving physical, technical and managerial capabilities of teaching hospitals. District hospitals, community health centres, PHC's and NGO institutions, it is possible to provide high quality cataract treatment either by camp approach or by hospital approach.

Ophthalmologists are given special training for the required skills of cataract surgery.

During the year 2002 Government of India has revised the strategy of National programme for the control of blindness. This new strategy includes:

a. *N.P.C.B. is made more comprehensive by including the following:*
   - Fixed facility surgical approach of Lens removal and I.O.L. implantation (Intra Ocular Lens) to get better quality of post operative vision.
   - Refractive error correction in school children
   - Treatment of trachoma infection
   - Treatment of glaucoma
   - Vitamin A prophylaxis
   - Improving follow up service of cataract operations.

b. *Targets for Tenth Five Year Plan:*
   - To increase cataract surgery rate to 450 per lakh population
   - To make above 80% intraocular lens implantation in cataract surgery
   - To develop 50 paediatric ophthalmology units
   - To provide facility for the diagnosis and treatment of glaucoma and diabetic retinopathy
   - Setting up 20000 rural vision centres
   - To develop 25 operational eye bank network
   - To develop manpower and facility for eye care.

c. *Vision 2020: The Right to Sight*
   Planned to develop four tier structure which include:

20 Centres of Excellence ...	Tertiary eye care services
200 Training Centres ...	Tertiary eye care services
2000 Service Centres....	Secondary eye care services

20000 Vision Centres ... Primary eye care services

Committed to attend target diseases like cataract, refractive errors, childhood blindness, corneal blindness, glaucoma, diabetic retinopathy.

National STD Control Programme

STD control programme started in 1946. Sex related disease (STD) relies on health seeking behaviour of patient. Diagnosis and treatment of STD is done at five regional STD referral centres and 735 District hospital and STD Clinics across the country. Since HIV/AIDS more easily gets transmitted in presence of STD, both are linked together for an effective control. Hence HIV/AIDS control includes diagnosis and treatment of STD as a recently drawn strategy.

STD clinics carry out clinical, laboratory and epidemiological components under STD control.

Case reporting by STD/ AIDS created awareness and involvement of General practitioners in STD control.

Contact tracing, cluster testing and special group screening help in case finding. Medical social worker will help in Guidance, Counselling and Motivating for full treatment.

Condom promotion as prophylaxis against STD is advocated.

Health education for creating awareness about source, transmission and impact in the community is very important because of health seeking behaviour of patients with STD.

Others measures include:

- Control of prostitution
- Control of drug abuse and alcoholism
- Rehabilitation of C.S.W. (Commercial Sex Workers)
- Family health awareness campaign.

Now, it is linked to HIV/AIDS Control Programme.

Syndrome Approach:

This is a method of management and control of STD's where diagnosis and treatment is based on a group of symptoms and signs (See Appendix VII). Treatment is targeted towards all diseases that could cause that syndrome. It allows diagnosis without extensive laboratory test and treatment with a single visit.

National AIDS Control Programme

It was launched in 1987. In the year 1992 NACO (National AIDS Control Organisation was set up to monitor the components of the programme. Government of India launched 100 percent centrally sponsored project in all states and union territories.

In 1999 Phase II Programme was initiated to reduce the spread of HIV and to build up country's capacity to respond to HIV/AIDS. During 2004 following initiatives were undertaken:

Preventive steps in high risk population like targeted interventions STD treatment, Condom Programme, Multisectoral collaboration and Public Private Partnership.

Preventive steps in low risk population like Holistic IEC, Social Mobilisation, Safe blood, Voluntary counselling and testing, AIDS vaccine initiative and sensitising youth and adolescents.

Care at low cost and support like Prevention of parent to child transmission, Management of HIV-TB coinfection, Treatment of opportunistic infections, Piloting ART and Post exposure prophylaxis.

Collaboration by intersectoral collaboration like Involvement of ministries and departments, Workplace interventions, Public Private Partnership, Partnership with other stakeholders and Involvement of PLHA.

Capacity building with institutional strengthening like Programme management, Surveillance, AIDS vaccine initiatives, Operations research and Training.

Capacity building with evidence based planning like Annual sentinel surveillance, AIDS case detection, Mapping of high risk groups and Behavioural surveillance.

During 2002 Government of India approved the National AIDS Prevention and Control Policy which included the following:

- Blood safety programme
- Counselling and HIV testing
- STD control programme
- Condom promotion
- HIV surveillance
- HIV sentinel surveillance and behavioural surveillance
- Targeted interventions
- School AIDS education programme
- I E C and social mobilisation
- Family health awareness campaign
- Prevention of HIV transmission from mother to child
- Anti retroviral treatment
- National AIDS helpline.

Tenth Five Year Plan has the following targets:

- 80% high risk coverage through targeted intervention
- 90% school college coverage by health education
- 80% awareness in public
- Blood transmission is reduced to less than 1%
- Establishing one VTCC in every district
- Adopting measures to prevent mother to child transmission
- Aiming at zero level prevalence.

National AIDS Day (1st December of every year) Theme to implement HIV/AIDS control programme, since 2000 AD:

2000 - AIDS : Men make a difference
2001 - I care Do You?
2002 - Stigma and Discrimination
2003 - Stigma and Discrimination
2004 - Women, Girls, HIV and AIDS
2005 - Stop AIDS: Keep the promise
2006 - Stop AIDS: Keep the promise–Accountability
2007 - Stop AIDS: Keep the promise–Leadership.

National Antimalaria Programme

National Malaria Control Programme (NMCP) was started in 1953 with DDT spray twice a year. By 1958 the successful result made the programme to eradication called (NMEP) National Malaria Eradication Programme. In 1971Urban Malaria scheme was started covering 181 cities and towns. There was reappearance (resurgence) of malaria in 1976 due to many reasons like (a) Operational defect (b) Technical defect (c) Administrative defect etc., In 1977 M.P.O. (Modified Plan of Operation) was launched which was mainly based on API Zones (Annual Parasite Index).

During all these period Active Surveillance were done, where health workers visited houses, collected blood smear of fever cases and gave treatment. In passive surveillance fever cases come to hospitals and health centres. Health workers are given targets of smear collection in the field.

Two main indicators used in malaria effective control are:

$$\text{API} = \frac{\text{Confirmed cases during 1 year}}{\text{Population under Surveillance}} \times 100$$

(annual parasite incidence)

$$\text{ABER} = \frac{\text{No. of slides examined}}{\text{Population}} \times 100$$

(annual blood examination rate)

In 1978 malaria control through primary health care was approved. Because of increase in malaria, in 1994 Malaria Action Programme was initiated.

Later in 1997 World Bank gave support for Enhanced Malaria Control Project.

In 1998, by roll back malaria programme, the health system got strengthened.

From 1999 malaria control is going on under "National Anti-Malaria Programme."

Intensified Malaria Control Project was launched in 2005 with the assistance from Global Fund for AIDS, TB and Malaria.

Anti Malaria Month campaign is observed every year in June in India to enhance level of awareness and encourage community participation.

Tenth Five Year Plan has set goals for malaria control as under:

Annual Blood Examination Rate over 10%

Annual Parasite Index 1.3 or less

Reducing morbidity and mortality by 25% by the end of 2007 and to 50% by the end of 2010.

Main activities for malaria control are as under:

In areas with A.P.I. above 2:

- Pyrethroids spray 2 rounds at 6 week interval
- Entomological assessment (Mosquito examination)
- Active and Passive Surveillance
- Treatment of Malaria case

In Areas with API below 2:

- Spraying – Focal sprays around severe malaria cases.
- Surveillance both active and passive.
- Radical treatment of detected cases.
- Blood smear follow up for 12 months (every month) from positive cases.
- Epidemiological investigation.

Surveillance

This is scrutiny of fever cases, systematic data collection and evaluation of field investigations and using specific parameters for evaluation.

Detection of malaria parasite by blood smear test and providing facilities for proper treatment through active and passive surveillance.

Active surveillance is carried out by health workers visiting the community, taking MP smear and providing Presumptive and Radical treatment.

Passive surveillance is carried out on patients attending health centres or hospitals at hospital or centre and providing treatment.

DDC and FTDs (Drug Distribution Centres and Fever Treatment Depots):

They are run by voluntary workers from the community and we have about 357000 such centres in the country. DDC dispense antimalarial tablets as per NMEP schedule. FTD collect blood smear and dispense antimalarial tablets.

P.T. (Presumptive Treatment):

All fever cases are presumed as malaria and presumptive treatment is given soon after taking blood smear (also refer page 309).

R.T. (Radical Treatment):

If blood smear is positive, Radical treatment is given (also refer page 309).

National Filaria Control Programme

It was started in 1955. Now it is estimated that 420 million people are exposed to the risk of infection in India. In 1978 this programme was combined with malaria control because of uniformity in control measure and for proper effective use of resources. Main activities include antilarval measures and filaria treatment.

At present, there are 206 filaria control units, 27 survey units and 199 filaria clinics functioning.

WHO recommendation is followed in endemic areas:

"Annual single dose therapy with DEC along with NFCP strategy."

N.I.C.D. Delhi is conducting training and research on filaria control.

Revised Filaria Control Strategy:
Annual single dose mass drug therapy with DEC with albandazole for 5 years is used as strategy. It targets to eliminate lymphatic filariasis by 2015. Home based morbidity management and hydrocoelectomy in hospitals are taken up. Mass Drug Administration is scheduled in 243 districts covering 525 million population.

National Tuberculosis Programme

In 1962 with the establishment of N.T.I. (National Tuberculosis Institute) at Bangalore, the control programme was launched with a long term and short term objectives.

Long term – To make Tuberculosis no more a public health problem by check at no new case occurrence and reducing prevalence rate to below 1%.

Short term – Diagnosis and Treatment
B.C.G. Vaccination
As an integrated health service.

D.T.C. (District TB Centre) is the nucleus of the programme. Out of existing 600 TB clinics 390 are upgraded to D.T.C to undertake the control in a District. Planning, Organising and implementing D.T.P. through all hospitals, centres and dispensaries, covering rural, suburban and urban areas are the functions of DTC.

In India there are 609 districts and among them 446 districts have D.T.C. In available TB clinics about 47,600 beds for TB patients is made available. For training and Demonstration N.T.I. Bangalore and T.C.C. Chennai (TB chemotherapy centre) are well known.

Activities of D.T.C.

a. Case finding – Detection of cases by sputum examination M.M.R. (Mass miniature Radiography) and Tuberculin Test.
b. Treatment is offered by domiciliary care by motivation and treatment.

Table 29.2: Structure and function of D.T.C.

D.T.C.
Covers (Average) 50 health institutions

Staff	*Function*
1 D.T.O.	1. Case finding
1 M.O.	M.M.R.
2 Lab technicians	Tuberculin test
2 Health visitors	Sputum exam
1 X-ray technician	2. Record maintenance
1 Team leader	3. Treatment by
(Non medical)	R.N.T.C.P. (Dots method)
1 Statistician	4. B.C.G. vaccination
1 Pharmacist	5. Preventive treatment
	6. Rehabilitation
	7. Surveillance

In 1992 National TB control was revised with following strategies:

a. To achieve 85% cure rate of infectious cases by directly observed treatment.
b. To achieve 70% detection rate by quality sputum microscopy.
c. To involve NGO for I.E.C. activities.

RNTCP (Revised National Tuberculosis Control Programme)

All tuberculosis patients receive free treatment under DOTS which is community treatment. Under supervision M.P.W. of P.H.C. and local voluntary workers like Teacher, Anganwadi worker, Dai, Ex-patient, social workers help in DOTS. Other workers are DOT agent. They receive Rs. 150. honorarium per patient after completing treatment. The success of DOT depends on Accountability, good drug supply. Directly observed treatment by health workers, good quality sputum microscopy and political commitment.

The drugs are supplied in blister packs, separately for intensive phase and continuation phase. They are kept ready in boxes for supply to patients for a full course of treatment. One day's medication in each pack for intensive phase and one week's medication in each pack for continuation phase are kept in boxes.

DRS (Drug Resistance Surveillance)

A new protocol for DRS is developed in 2005 to survey drug resistance by a network of investigators. It has culture and sensitivity laboratories.

DOTS –Plus

This is developed to tackle drug resistance cases under RNTCP. We have internationally recommended DOTS-Plus sites, guidelines which have access for testing and treatment. Here second line of drug regiment is used with a logistics system and standardised information system.

Detailed drug regimen and specifications are dealt in Chapter 18.

World TB Day

Every year on March 24th, TB Day is celebrated to build public awareness. Following are the World TB Day Themes since 2000 AD:

2000 - Forging new partnerships to stop TB
2001 - DOTS: TB cure for all
2002 - Stop TB, flight poverty
2003 - DOTs cured me – It will cure you too
2004 - Every breath counts – Stop TB now
2005 - Frontline TB Care Providers: Heroes in the fight against TB
2006 - Action for Life: Towards a world free of TB
2007 - TB anywhere is TB everywhere
2008 - I am stopping TB.

Modified Leprosy Elimination Campaign

It started in 1955 with case detection and DDS Drug treatment on ambulatory basis. In 1980 Government felt the possibility of eradication. Since 1983 N.L.E.P. with a goal of eradication by reducing case load to below 1 per 10,000 population was considered.

N.L.E.P. contained:

- Population survey
- School survey
- Contact examination
- Voluntary referral
- Multi Drug Regimen (MDT)
- Health education
- Rehabilitation.

For the control and eradication we have about 800 leprosy control units and about 6000 SET centres (Survey Education Treatment) and 1440 SAEL/LEC Projects.

Table 29.3: Difference between LCU and SET centres

LCU	*Set Centre*
1. M.O.	1. Paramedical worker cover 20 to 25 thousand population
2. Non medical supervisor	
20 Paramedical workers	
Cover 4 to 5 lakh population	
Urban Leprosy Centre Cover 50,000 Population	

Since 1997 M.L.E.C was launched with training to Medical Officers, health workers and volunteers. Two main activities included are:

- House to house search for case.
- Health awareness on leprosy.

This M.L.E.C had an objective of elimination of leprosy by 2005 in the world. Research activities are going on in Agra, Chingelput, Orissa, Chhatisgarh and West Bengal, International organisation like SIDA, DANIDA, WHO, Damien Foundation are providing assistance in M.L.E.C.

National Action Plan for 2006-07 under NLEP:

This was launched in April 2005 to continue our efforts for elimination, to maintain the gains achieved and to provide quality leprosy services. This incorporated decentralization, integration of services, disability care, IEC activities and training.

During Tenth Five Year Plan, Government of India intended to bring prevalence rate of leprosy to less than 1 case per 10000 population with specified strategies such as horizontal integration of programme, redeployment of leprosy workers, training programmes, re-constructive surgeries, rehabilitation and involvement of NGOs.

W.H.O has announced global strategy for further reducing leprosy through activities during 2006 -2010; by malaria mortality rate reduction of 50% by 2010 and an additional 10% by 2012.

C.D.D. (Control of Diarrhoeal Disease)

This was started in 1978 to reduce deaths and defects occurring due to diarrhoea. Upto 1985, emphasis was on case management. After 1985 O.R.T. was emphasised and knowledge on home available fluids were disseminated. Later in 1992 it got incorporated under CSSM. Presently CDD is taken care of by R.C.H. programme from 1997 which is detailed in Chapter 11.

U.I.P. (Universal Immunisation Programme)

Most powerful and cost effective weapon of disease control is U.I.P. In 1974 E.P.I. (Expanded Programme on Immunisation) was initiated to prevent 6 vaccine preventable disease viz., Diphtheria, whooping cough, Tetanus, Poliomyelitis, Tuberculosis and measles. The word expansion meant for extension of services, extension of coverage and extension of vaccines. U.I.P. is assisted mainly by UNICEF. In 1985 E.P.I. was remained as U.C.I. (Universal Child Immunisation). Since 1985 this is done with the name U.I.P. where universal coverage mean to cover all aspects of immunisation activity i.e. Research development and delivery.

Additional force of coverage of U.I.P. has been by I.P.P.I. (Intensive pulse polio immunisation) U.M.C. (Urban Measles Campaign) and N.N.T.E. (Neonatal Tetanus Elimination).

Incidentally U.I.P. is a part of C.S.S.M. (from 1992) and is a part of R.C.H. (from 1997).

NRHM (National Rural Health Mission)

This was launched by Government of India on 5.4.2005 with the objective of improving rural health care delivery system. AYUSH (Ayurveda, Yoga, Unani, Siddha and Homoeopathy) are brought to the mainstream of health care. NRHM has created ASHA (Accredited Social Health Activist) for the implementation of activities. This works by integrating many health programmes in the country including RCH II.

ASHA, a resident woman 25-45 year age, 8th standard education, good communication skills and leadership qualities. She works for 1000 population.She gives health education, gives counseling, mobilize the community for health care, works with gram panchayat, accompany pregnant to hospital, treats primary ailments. She takes care of DOTS, ORS, IFA OC, delivery kits. She will be guided by Anganwadi worker and ANM of the area.

Monitoring and evaluation are done under NRHM.

NRHM initiates strengthening sub-centre, PHCs, Community Health Centres, creates the cadre of ASHA. District Health Mission as it is called core unit of planning and implementation is the district. This has set Public Private Partnership to programme better in the community.

This has schedule for implementation of its major components from 2005 to 2008.

Goals of NRHM

- Bringing IMR to 30/1000 LB.
- Bringing MMR to 1/1000 LB.
- Malaria mortality rate reduction.
- Kalaazar mortality rate reduction.
- Dengue mortality rate reduction.
- JE mortality rate reduction by 2012.
- Cataract operations 46 lakh per year, by 2012.
- Filaria elimination by 2015
- TB DOTS service with 85% cure rate
- Upgrading community health centres
- Engaging ASHA in all states
  Training community level worker and drug kit to them
- Health Day activities in Anganwadies
- Generic drugs for common ailments at sub centre and hospital level
- Good quality health care
- Good RCH services
- Provisions of household toilets
- Good outreach services.

Home Visiting

This is dealt in detail in Chapter 28.

Health and Social Services in India

Health Planning Reports

A number of committees starting from pre-independence have given a few recommendations for the health development and social development. A brief review of major committee reports need highlighting.

Bhore Committee 1946

Under the leadership of Sir Joseph Bhore the committee made recommendation for the future development of the country. We have 4 volumes of committee report:

Volume I - Survey report of health survey and development committee.

Volume II - Recommendations report of health survey and development committee.

Volume III - Appendices report of health survey and development committee.

Volume IV - Summary report of health survey and development committee.

The committee quotes:

"If the nation's health is to be built, the health programme should be developed on a foundation of preventive health work and that such activities should proceed side by side with those concerned with the treatment of patients".

II Recommended:

a. Integration of prevention and cure at all levels.
b. P.H.C. Development
   Short term – Rural P.H.C per 40,000 population with 2 MOH, 4 PHN, one nurse, 4 ANM, 4 Dais, 2 SI, 2 HA, One pharmacist and 15 class IV employees.
   Long term – Called 3 million plans
   Rural P.H.C per 20,000 with 75 Beds.
c. 3-month Rural posting to house surgeons
   It is a major document which has provided health planning in India.

Mudaliar Committee 1962

This is called "Health survey and planning committee". This studied the progress of Bhore committee report and made certain recommendation for health service expansion. They are:

- District hospital must be strengthened with specialized posting.
- Regional (Divisional) level office to supervise 2 to 3 district health and F.W. officers.
- Each P.H.C. should cover 40,000 population.
- P.H.C. should provide quality health care.

- Integration of medical service and health service.
- Development of all India medical service similar to I.A.S. cadre.

Kartar Singh Committee 1973

It is called "Committee on multi purpose worker under health and F.P."

Main recommendations made by the committee are:

- A.N.M. are redesignated as M.P.W. (F)
- B.H.W. Malaria surveillance worker, H.E. Assistant, F.P. Assistant are redesignated as M.P.W. (M)
- In the beginning where malaria and smallpox were under control, multipurpose worker (M&F) scheme were to be initiated and later to other areas
- P.H.C. should have 50,000 population
- Each P.H.C. should have 16 sub centres each with 3000 population
- Each sub centre should have M.P.W (M) and M.P.W. (F)
- Health Supervisor (M) should supervise 3-4 M.P.W (M)
- Health supervisor (F) should supervise 3-4 female M.P.W.
- MOH of PHC should control all M.P.W. (M) and M.P.W. (F) in the PHC area.

Kartar Singh Committee report is a milestone in the history of public health nursing service administration.

Srivastav Committee 1975

This is called "Group on Medical Education and Support Manpower." Its main recommendations are:

- Each Health Assistant should supervise 2 MPW (M) and 2 MPW (F) and each MPW should cover an area of 5000 population.
- HA (F) and MPW (F) should be located in sub centre.
- For simple promotive, preventive and curative service a band of para professionals like school teacher, post master, gram sevak or a literate youth are created.
- Between P.H.C and community 2 cadre of health workers are created viz., H.A.'s and MPW's.
- Development of referral service involving civil hospitals, teaching hospitals etc.

Based recommendation, Rural Health Scheme was initiated in 1977 to provide primary health care in the community. Involvement of medical colleges, training of MPWs were major events after this committee report.

H.F.A. by 2000 A.D.– Report

As per WHO resolution 1977 HFA is for attainment by all the highest possible level of health along with productive life and good social life. It implies the removal of obstacle to ill health. It is a revolutionary and historic concept by WHO.

In 1978 Government of India developed a workable report by a committee for a National health policy.

The report is the response of WHO call for H.F.A. and Alma Ata declaration which earmarked the following goals:

- I.M.R. reduction to below 60
- Rising life expectation to 64
- Reducing crude death rate to 9
- Reducing crude birth rate to 21
- To achieve N.N.R. of one
- To provide potable water to entire rural community.

The report implementation is seen through Five Year Plan, Annual plan, Minimum need and 20-point programmes.

Health Service Organisation

Structure, functioning and essentiality of health system in India are unique. Centre makes health policy; states run health care independent of centre (Fig. 29.13).

Table 29.4: Health system in India

I District ( )		
D.H. & F.W.O. Zilla Parishad P.H.C. ( ) Sub centre ( )	District Hospital ( )	City corporation Health authorities
II State	( ) + U.T. ( )	
State Ministry	Directorate	Direct control
III centre	(G.O.I.)	
Union Ministry	D.G.H.S. (Director General of Health Services)	C.C.H. (Central Council of Health) (Chairman and Members)
Union function	- International Health Regulation - Drug standard	Policy of Health Legislation
Concurrent function	- Medical store - P.G., Training - Med. Research - C.G.H.S. - C.H.E.B. - Medical Library	- Grant in Aid - Cooperation with state

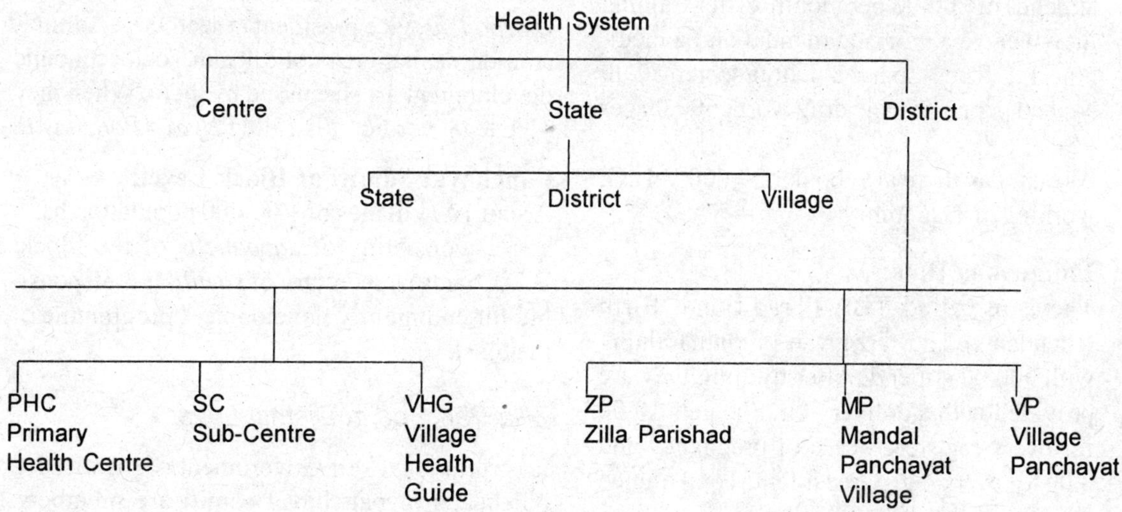

Fig. 29.13: 3 Tier system of heath care in India

2001 first stage census drafted 20 million households, 6.5 lakh villages, 5500 towns and cities which function on 3-Tier system of health care.

Decentralised State Administration

Village

To make health accessible and available, policy was made for the following:

a. **Village Health Guide (V.H.G.):**
He is a literate volunteer who can secure people's participation. Scheme of V.H.G came in 1977. They are chosen from the community. They act as a link between P.H.C. and Public. Criteria in their selection are:
   - Local residents
   - Able to read and write (6th std)
   - Acceptable to community
   - Should spare 2-3 hours per day for community work.

   They undergo training for 3 months (with stipend) of 200.00 per month. After training they receive a working manual and a medicine kit. They spare 2-3 hours, get 50.00 stipend per month and drug worth 600.00 per year.
   As on today there are about 3,23,000 V.H.G. working in the country.

b. **Indigenous Dais:**
They are called TBA (Traditional Birth Attendants). They are given 1 month training with 300.00 stipend. After training they are provided with a delivery kit. She gets 10.00 for every registered case of pregnancy and 3.00 for every registered infant. Total trained Dais are about 7,00,000 in India.

c. **Anganwadi Worker:**
Under I.C.D.S. an AWW is selected from the community. She undergoes training for 4 months. She is paid Rs. 250.00 per month honorarium for her service (Rs. 400/- when State Government Assistance is present). She helps in health check up, immunisation, supplementary nutrition, health education, non formal education and referral services.

Sub Centre – It is an out post attached to a P.H.C. covering a population of 5000. One MPW (M) and one MPW (F) are posted to work under a sub centre. Mainly RCH, Immunisation and F.P. are emphasised. Government is trying to give facility for I.U.D. insertion and urine examination for albumin and sugar. Health Assistant Female Supervises the activity of MPW (F).

Panchayat Raj System

It is a 3 tier health system at 3 levels. They are:
- Panchayat village level
- Panchayat samiti at block level
- Zilla parishad at district level.

***Panchayat* at Village Level:**
Gram panchayat is an executive organ responsible for village development. It has a president (*Sarpanch*), vice president, a secretary. Administration, sanitation, public health, socioeconomic development are discussed by them. When they give legal verdict it is called *Nyaya Panchayat*.

Panchayat Samiti at Block Level:
About 100 villages of 1,00,000 population has a *samiti* consisting of *sarpanchs* of the block. B.D.O. acts as secretary of *samiti*. It is responsible for community development programme of the block.

Zilla Parishad at District Level

It is rural local self Government of the district. All heads of panchayat samiti are members. Deputy Commissioner (Collector) is a non voting member. It will have above 60 members. Health services, Family planning service of the district come under *Zilla Parishad*.

Rural Health Services

It contains 3 levels cadre of health centres namely community health centre, primary health centre and sub centre.

Community Health Centre

Each C.H.C. covers 1,20,000 population in a community development block. It has 30 beds, specialists in Medicine, Surgery, OBG and Paediatrics. It will have X-ray and lab facilities. There are 3910 community health centres in the country.

Staff:

1 Community Health Officer (Medical or non medical)
4 Medical officers
7 Nurse midwifes
1 Dresser
1 Pharmacist
1 Lab technician
1 X-ray technician
2 Ward boys
1 Dhobi
3 Sweepers
1 Mali
1 Chowkidar
1 Aaya
1 Peon.

C.H.C. refers cases to state level hospital or medical college hospitals (Teaching hospitals).

Primary Health Centre

It is an outcome of Bhore Committee Report. P.H.C. provides integrated health services. We have about 23,000 PHC in the country. There are 23236 PHCs in the country.

Staff: (at PHC level which cover 30,000 population)

1 M.O.
1 Pharmacist
1 Nurse midwife
1 H.W. (F)
1 B.E.E.
1 H.A. (M)
1 H.A. (F)
1 U.D.C.
1 L.D.C.
1 Lab technician
1 Driver
4 Class IV employees.

Functions:

- Medical care
- Reproductive and child health
- Family welfare planning
- Water supply and sanitation
- Control of communicable diseases
- Collection of vital statistics
- Health education
- Carry out national health programmes
- Referral service
- Training of health assistants, health workers, health guides and local dais
- Basic laboratory services

  P.H.C. is equipped with the following:
  - Tubectomy
  - Vasectomy
  - M.T.P.
  - Minor O.T. procedures.

Government has proposed and brought to the action that each medical college to adopt 3 primary health centres for re-orientation of medical education.

Sub Centre

It covers a population of 5,000 and has following staff:

M.P.W. (M) – 1
M.P.W. (F) – 1
Voluntary health guide – 1

The function is the same as P.H.C. but restricted to the population it covers viz., 5,000 population. There are 144988 sub centres in the country.

Community Development Programme (CDP)

Community development is a process designed to create conditions of economic and social progress for the whole community with its active participation and the fullest possible reliance upon the community's initiative. Here people are united for their development.

C.D.P. was launched in 1952 for the all round development of Rural areas. It is an organised programme by community development blocks, each covering 1,20,000 population. There are about 6100 community development blocks in the country.

It envisages following programmes:

a. Improvement of agriculture
b. Improvement of communication
c. Education
d. Health
e. Sanitation
f. Housing.

The community development block will work for intensive development for 5 years followed by continued work in second phase of 5 years. It is mainly centrally sponsored programme. By its programme, it is tackling rural poverty and unemployment.

National Planning and Policy

Government of India set up a commission for assessment of human resource, capital and material of the country for drafting the development plans. It is called "Planning Commission". It was further developed with many divisions in 1957.

The structure of planning commission:

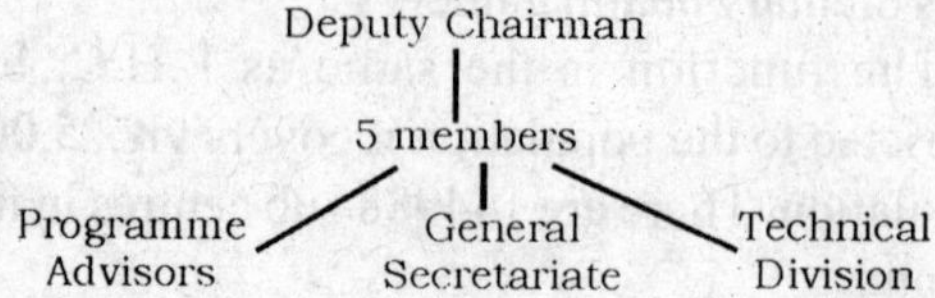

Functions are:

- Projections for future 25 years development
- Make recommendations to Government:
- On problems
- On policies
- On economic development.

Present State: District is unit for district planning by planning commission. It has given importance to developmental planning in health sector.

1. Water and sanitation
2. control of communicable disease
3. Medical education, training and research
4. Medical care through
    - Hospitals
    - Dispensaries
    - PHC's
5. Public health service
6. Family planning
7. Indigenous systems of medicines.

Depending on felt need of the people and technical feasibility, changes are brought out from time to time. The coordinating body between central Government and State Government is *A Bureau of Planning* which was formed in 1965. They are implemented at village level through district planning.

Five Year Plans

Planning commission which gave importance to health programmes has proposed five year plans to rebuild rural India, to lay foundation of industrial progress and to secure balanced development of all parts of the country viz., 28 states and 7 union territories. The broad objectives of health programme during five year plans are:

- Control and eradication of major diseases
- Establishing P.H.C and Subcentre for basic health services
- Population control (FWP)
- Development of health manpower

Five Year Plan Outlay:

First 5 year plan	1951-56
Second 5 year plan	1956-61
Third 5 year plan	1961-66
Annual plan	1966-67
Annual plan	1967-68
Annual plan	1968-69
Fourth 5 year plan	1969-74
Fifth 5 year plan	1974-1979
Annual plan	1979-80
Sixth 5 year plan	1980-85
Seventh 5 year plan	1985-90
Annual plan	1990-91
Annual plan	1991-92
Eight 5 year plan	1992-97
Ninth 5 year plan	1997-2002
Tenth 5 year plan	2002-2007

During 10th 5 year plan district level surveillance for diseases was strengthened, appropriate systems for emergency, disaster and accidents were implemented, screening of nutritional deficiencies was implemented, growth rate reduction policy was targeted and emphasis on RTI/STD surveillance was given.

Following is the achievement of 10th Five Year Plan (2007):

Village health guides trained	3,23,000
H.W. male	73,300
H.W. Female	1,34,000
Health visitors	50,393
A.N.M. (MPW (F))	5,06,925
Nurses	8,65,135
Doctors	7,67,500
Dental colleges	205
Medical colleges	242
Total beds	9,14,543
Community Health centre	3,910
P.H.C.	23,236
Sub centres	1,46,026

Social Welfare Services

This is highlighted in Chapter 11.

Voluntary Organisation

This is highlighted in Chapter 31.

Special Community Health Services

Community health service is comprehensive health care for giving medical care of the sick and community preventive care for health promotion. Primary health care or first contact care at family help in diagnosis and treatment of a case, side by side carrying out functions of P.H.C which are undertaken and designed for community health service.

R.C.H. activity covering perinatal, antenatal, natal and postnatal services and child care services are main area taking about 50% of health care services. They include two more main aspects of family planning and conducting home deliveries.

Immunisation for the prevention of preventable diseases is a full scale health care service.

Assessment of social, environmental and nutritional needs of the community and directing the attention of social workers to such need is an aspect of nursing care service in public health.

Some of the nurses are appointed as district public health nurse to plan, implement and evaluate nursing activities in the district.

Following are the special community health nursing services apart from regular hospital and health centre health care services etc.

Industrial Nursing Service

There is provision for appointment of nursing staff in factories where more than 500 workers are working. The area of nursing in industrial setting is discussed in Chapter 21. They include care of sick, care of injured, preplacement examinations, periodic examinations, sanitation or good house keeping in industry, first aid, industrial safety, organisation of crèches, counselling, guidance and rehabilitation.

Tuberculosis Nursing Services

Hospital, dispensary, PHC, sub centre – all are functionaries for tuberculosis control programme. Clinical examination, Radiological diagnosis, sputum examination, contact examination followed by directly observed therapy to patient under R.N.T.C.P. is specified as a special community health service.

When patient is provided with short course chemotherapy, the drug is administered under direct supervision (DOTS): DOTS is a Community Based Tuberculosis Treatment which combines the benefit of supervised treatment and the benefit of community based care and support.

Domiciliary care of nursing care, guidance, counselling, DOTS, follow up, contact tracing are added job responsibilities of a health worker.

Leprosy Nursing Services

Leprosy being a social disease and as an elimination campaign has many components of community health services. Training of health workers for diagnosis, treatment, nursing and rehabilitation is first line of action in M.L.E.C.

Secondly, house to house visit for the search of case to detect new leprosy cases is done on a scheduled activity at community.

Thirdly, creating awareness about leprosy by health education, clarification and clearing misconceptions for the social acceptance of cured cases.

Major community health service is the rehabilitation of a patient who is a burnt out case, for his self reliance and self support. This vocational rehabilitation forms major service under special community health services.

Leprosy hospitals and rehabilitation centres where complicated cases are admitted with tropical ulcer, wound, burns, skin lesions etc., which need daily or many times a day care for nursing and treatment.

Health Team

At district level, CHC level, PHC level or sub centre level, working health group complement each other. They share a common goal. After training, all possess ability and skills to manage any community health problem.

Health team has set objectives formulated by health and family welfare services and postulated by the felt need of the community. Health team follows certain rules, procedures and legal obligations in delivering health goods to the community.

Health team by their organised effort; plan, implement and evaluate health activity and health programmes is based on set of objectives. Team with their mutual cooperation and with the help of community participation renders care, prevention and promotion of health to the sick, disability and handicaps.

Health team of a community centre, of a primary health centre and a sub centre are listed above under rural health services.

M.O.H. of P.H.C. is the leader who supervises and administers the health activities. The job description of HS (F) MPW (F) Dais are given in appendix.

District Public Health Nurse

District Public Health Nurse will have the placement as district level nursing officer attached to district health and family welfare. All district public health nursing activities are coordinated, supervised and monitored by the public health nurse. At directorate level assistant director of health and family welfare services (nursing) will guide her from technical point of view. All P.H.C., sub centres, F.W. centres and all national health programmes in the district will come under her care.

Duties

General:

- Plan, develop and direct all district community health nursing activities.
- Take part in all district level meetings.
- Will convey the district need to D.H. and F.W.O. and Z.P. in terms of general and special community nursing care services.
- Take part in district level H and F.W. planning.
- Guide district manpower in training activities.

Administration:

- Help in policy decision matters of the district.
- Make recommendations regarding selection, appointment, Leave, Transfer, continued education and promotion of nursing staff of the district.
- She does the needed job of material management for the district and its related budgetary planning.
- Does evaluation of activity progress of nursing staff of the district.
- Submit monthly reports and annual reports of the district.

Supervisory:

She does the job of supervision in district public health nursing activities; bring out modifications and alterations for an effective work output in the district.

Education:

- Continued nursing education
- Orientation training programme
- Dais training programmes
- M.P.W. (F) training programme
- A.W.W. training programme
- Training of student nurse in Rural Field training centres.

Multi Purpose Health Workers

The committee on "MPW under H & FW" was recommended by Kartar Singh committee 1973, that there is a need of integrated health activity by a band of multi purpose workers. Thus MPW (M) are redesignated BHW, malaria surveillance worker, vaccinator, health education assistant, FP health assistants. The M.P.W. (F) are redesignated nurse midwives.

One M.P.W. (M) and one M.P.W. (F) are posted to sub centres which cover a population of 5000. They are given the assistance of voluntary workers.

These MPW's are supervised by health assistant male and health assistant female (Who are redesignated male and female health supervisors).

In spite of training and recruitment, MPW manpower is not fulfilling the norms suggested by planning commission.

MPW (F) is given 6 weeks training for the transformation of unipurpose state to multi purpose work. The new entrants of MPW (F) have to undergo 18 months training and should be a matriculate. Her job responsibility is given in appendix.

MPW (M) is given 8 weeks of training for his transformation from unipurpose job.

MPW (M) and MPW (F) form a health team of the sub centre to carry out comprehensive health care services.

Health assistant female are either recruited afresh or promoted ANM's after promotional training. Existing LHV training schools are used to give promotional training of 6 months. New entrants will have to undergo 2 years training.

Human Sexually

This is given in detail in Chapter 12.

Nursing Personnel

Nursing personnel are group of auxiliary health workers who go to form members of health team in sub centre, in PHC, in community health centre, in civil hospital and in teaching hospital. Accordingly categories of nursing personnel fall under following groups:

- Nursing advisor to central Government.
- Nursing specialist under CHS scheme.
- Nursing tutors in nursing education.
- Nursing administrators like nursing superintendent, matron, district public health nurse.
- Senior nursing staff like head nurse, health supervisor female.
- Junior nursing staff like staff nurse, ward nurse, MPW (F).
- Student trainees.

Following table provide the achievement in 9th five year and present estimate 2003 with regard to nursing personnel:

Table 29.5: Nursing personnel

2002-2007		*2008 (Estimate)*	
Nurse	865,135	Nurse	9,04,000
MPW (F) (ANM)	506,525	H.S (F)	49,010
Health visitor HS (F)	50,393	MPW (F)	6,09,000
Health worker (F) MPW (F)	133,194	TBA	4,17,000
Dais TBA/CHG	3,23,000		

Nurse Population Ratio:

The norm suggested is 1 per 5000 population. Taking all available figures it seems nurse population ratio norm is reached. But when qualified nurse proportion is taken there is still need for the further manpower development in India.

Presently there is a need for promotional training programmes and continued nursing education programmes to update the vast developing nursing education from general nursing care to special nursing care.

Management of PHC

This topic is highlighted under rural health services above.

Study of the Community

Study of the community is needed for community diagnosis and community treatment. Study of the community can be by:

- Community survey
- Community screening
- Community surveillance.

Community survey can be:

- Demographic survey
- Socioeconomic survey
- Sociocultural survey
- Morbidity survey
- Mortality survey
- Fertility survey
- Epidemiological survey for incidence, prevalence
- Research survey on a specific project
- Specific disease survey
- Environmental survey
- K.A.P. survey.

At P.H.C. basic information is available which is obtained by base line health survey done at the beginning. Annual re-survey is done to update the community information which is required for progress report and future year goal fixation.

Community survey is done by personal interview, proforma filling, structured questionnaire entry, case studies, family schedule, individual health records, MCH cards, child cards, tuberculosis treatment card, leprosy treatment card, and beneficiary enrollment survey forms.

Content of community survey:

a. Physical and geographic characteristics like boundary, road, rivers, schools, civil amenities.
b. Demographic characteristics like population, age, sex, race, religion, ethnic group, language.

c. Socioeconomic characteristics like occupation, income, family pattern, belongings, socioeconomic class.
d. Sociocultural characteristics like culture, tradition, taboo, belief.
e. K.A.P. characteristics on knowledge, Attitude and practices.
f. Target group survey like school age, elderly, reproductive age, lame, blind, deaf, handicapped.
g. Environmental characteristics like housing, refuse disposal, sewage disposal, water supply, vectors.
h. Characteristics of health service utilisation.

Data thus obtained through house to house survey, records, reports, personal enquiry is very useful in planning, implementing and evaluation of community health programmes through community diagnosis and community treatment.

Activities of Dai

It is detailed in RCH and appendix.

Job Responsibilities of H.A. Female MPW (F)

They are highlighted under R.C.H. and preventive obstetrics as well as appendix.

Ward Management

It is given in detail in chapter on job responsibility (Chapter 32).

FURTHER REFERENCES

1. N.A.C.O. – Training module on the surveillance of STD.
2. Walter W. M. Holland – Oxford, Textbook of Public Health, Vol 1,2,3,4 (Oxford).
3. Theodore H. Julchinsky. The New Public Health (Academic Press).
4. John J. Hanlon – Principles of Public Health Administration (C. V. Mosby).
5. Report of the Health Survey and Development Committee:
   4 volumes, (Govt. of India Press Delhi), (Govt. of India Press Simla), (Govt. of India Press Kolkata)
6. Prabhakara G.N. Short Textbook P & M (JP).
7. Prabhakara G.N. Short text book of professional medical ethics (Paras).
8. Prabhakara, G.N. Policies and Programmes of Health in India (JP).
9. Bulletin on Rural Health Statistics in India G.O.I. 2006.
10. Prabhakara G.N.– Trends, Issues and Management in Nursing (Peepee).

30

International Health

IMPORTANCE

The boom in science and technology during the last century has resulted in all-round socio-economic development of transport, Communication, education, Industry, trade and commerce around the globe. This has brought people closer with cross culture, around the world. Cutting across distances and culture, people travel long distances for the purpose of trade, commerce and education. This kind of a situation has thrown challenges on international health status. In this event, infections and communicable diseases, which were earlier restricted to selected countries are becoming global problems.

In the early centuries in order to avoid spread of such infections and communicable diseases, all ships, crew travellers and cargoes were to be detained for about 40 days at the dock, thus putting hardships to travellers, but with little benefit. This early practice "Quarantine" later become an international health measure against major diseases like cholera, yellow fever, plague, Relapsing fever etc.

HISTORY

First Sanitary Conference was held in Paris in 1851. In this conference participant countries wanted to bring out standards of quarantine. However, this first International Sanitary Conference failed in its purpose. With the same purpose Pan American Sanitary Bureau set up in 1902, later produced a code popularly called "The Pan American Sanitary Code". This got new names, in the coming years to PASO (Pan American Sanitary Organisation) and PAHO (Pan American Health Organisation). In the same decade, during 1907 Paris office was created (office International d' Hygiene Publique) which shifted its responsibility to WHO in 1950.

First World War gave an arena for an organisation of League of Nations in 1923 which got dissolved after 16 years (1939) but continued to publish weekly epidemiological reports.

During second world war (1943) U.N.R.R.A. (United Nations Relief Rehabilitation Administration) was set up which lost its shape when WHO was born in 1945.

Major International Health Organisations

W.H.O.

On April 7, 1948, WHO came into force as an international organisation under United Nations.

Each year WHO Day is celebrated on 7th April and a theme is selected to focus on International actions. Themes of current century are:

2000 – Safe blood starts with me – Blood saves lives.
2001 – Stop exclusion – dare to care.
2002 – Move for health.
2003 – Shape the future of life–Healthy environments for children.
2004 – Road safety is no accident.
2005 – Make every mother and child count
2006 – Working together for health
2007 – Invest in health, build a safer future.
2008 – Protecting health from climate change

WHO has given definition for health; has its own constitution, own governing bodies, own membership and budget. Alma Ata conference in primary health care and health for all by 2000 made good impact on global health care system.

WHO has about 200 country membership and has following functions which are being carried out successfully:

- Collaboration with all other International and National organisations.
- Literature and Information on Health and disease are released to the world.
- Stimulates all Research for human benefit.
- Reports, records, ICD are made available as Health statistics.
- Taken up Family Health as a major project.
- Environmental health activities like water for all, environmental health monitoring and Development of environmental health criteria are undertaken.
- Promotes and supports comprehensive health programmes.

Structure

It is depicted in the following diagram:

S.E.A.R.O.

The South East Asia Regional office in New Delhi is a Regional Office with the membership of 11 countries (India, Indonesia, Bangladesh,

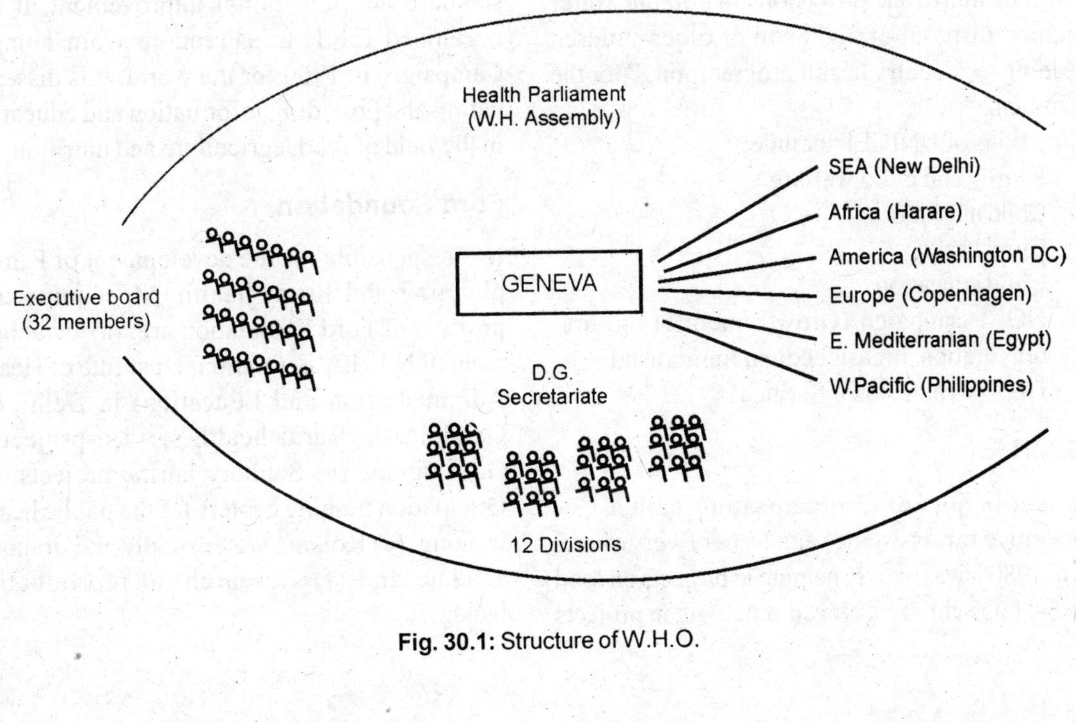

Fig. 30.1: Structure of W.H.O.

Myanmar, Korea, Thailand, Nepal, Srilanka, Bhutan, Mongolia and Maldives). Following are the major functions of this Regional Office:

- Control of communicable diseases
- Health laboratory services
- Health statistics
- Rural health services
- R.C.H. services
- Nursing education, training, care
- Environmental health
- Health education
- Nutrition
- Mental health
- Dental health
- Medical rehabilitation
- Drug control
- Medical education.

U.N.I.C.E.F.

It was established in 1946 and now is called U.N.I.C.F. [E = emergency is removed] (United Nations International Children Fund). This works with other international organisations in covering R.C.H., nutrition, provision of potable water supply, disposal of night soil of older children leading to "country health programming" for the children.

Functions of UNICEF include:

- Family and child welfare
- Child nutrition
- Child health
- Child education
- GOBI campaign (Growth monitoring, oral rehydration, breast feeding, Immunisation)
- UBS (Urban Basic Service).

C.A.R.E.

It is a major relief organisation called Co-operative for Assistance and Relief Everywhere. Till 1980 it was mainly helping in projects on food to 6-11 age children. Now it is helping in projects like I.C.D.S. Anaemia control, Adolescent Girls project and associated R.C.H. projects

Colombo Plan

It is a co-operative economic development plan mooted in 1950 as an out come of the meeting at Colombo. Industrial development and agricultural development are aimed at the plan. Major outcome in India are, establishment of A.I.I.M.S. in Delhi and cobalt therapy units in medical colleges.

D.A.N.I.D.A.

It is assistance by Government of Denmark for the prevention of Blindness, for the veterinary health (Dairy Development) and for higher studies in MSC ophthalmology for developing countries.

F.A.O.

It looks after several areas of world co-operation since 1945 for efficient farming, raising living standard and nutritional improvement. It has organised F.F.H.C. (Freedom from Hunger Campaign) in 1960 for the world. It is disseminating and providing information and education in the field of food, agriculture and nutrition.

Ford Foundation

It is responsible for the development of Family planning and Rural health. Most important projects of Ford Foundation are: (a) Establishment of N.I.H.A.E. (National Institute of Health Administration and Education) in Delhi, (b) Gandhigram Rural health service project at Gandhigram, (c) Sanitary latrine projects, (d) Orientation training centers for the public health training, (e) Kolkata water supply and drainage scheme and (f) Research on reproductive biology.

International Red Cross

It is a product of appeal by A Swiss, Dunant, for relief to help the wounded in times of war by means of volunteers. Initiated in 1859, formed a committee in 1864. Now Red Cross symbol denote its services anywhere for wounded, co-ordinated through 90 countries.

I.L.O.

Since working and living conditions of working population needed attention, International Labour Organisation was formed in 1919. It looks into social justice, improving labour conditions through social stability and health and welfare. Standard working conditions were formulated to the working force and I.L.O. is collaborating this all over the world.

Rockefellers Foundation

International famous philanthropist John D Rockefeller founded this in 1913 to promote the well being of mankind at global net. Public Health and Medical Education are two pillars of foundation, on which other advancement like life science, social science, humanities and agriculture science developed. Establishment of A.I.I.H. and P.H. (All India Institute of Hygiene and Public Health) at Kolkata, NIV (National Institute of Virology) at Pune and several field demonstration centers hallmark the focused attention of Foundation.

SIDA (The Swedish International Development Agency)

By procurement of X-ray unit, microscopes, anti TB drugs, SIDA is supporting Tuberculosis control all over the globe.

U.S.A.I.D.

It is an extended U.S. aid to many countries since 1961. United States agency for international development is helping to improve nursing education in developing countries. Other areas of U.S.A.I.D. assistance are: (a) Malaria (b) Health education (c) Family planning (d) Water supply and sanitation.

U.N.F.P.A.

The United Nations Fund for population activities is helping countries for the development of national capability for the manufacture of contraceptives and developing population education programmes.

U.N.D.P.

United Nations Development Programme in short UNDP is existing since 1966 to help poor nations to develop their own resources in social and economic areas. Assistance is offered in the development of agriculture, industry, education, science, health and social welfare of developing countries through aid from UNDP for their development.

World Bank

It is a specialized agency of UN; through Board of Governors, World Bank is helping developing countries to raise their living standards. I.P.P., Roadways, Power, Water, World food and population control are assisted wholly by World Bank.

FURTHER REFERENCES

1. W.H.O.- Work of WHO (Report).
2. Unicef – Current policies and working.
3. US information service – Fact sheet.
4. Prabhakara G.N. – Trends, Issues and Management in Nursing (Peepee).

31

Voluntary Health Agencies in India

INTRODUCTION

Promoting the health and welfare of the people has been the motto by some as individual or as a group is known from Vedic period. This needs a dynamic group and a good social interaction on the part of the group. Nurse as a member of community Health team need orientation and information on such agencies which are helping human community by their welfare programmes. It is voluntary agencies that have pioneered the health development in any country. They have missionary zeal and an organisation by itself consisting of an administrative body, a committee to raise funds through membership and all actions are through voluntary basis.

According to Gunn and Platt, Voluntary Health Agencies have certain characteristics. They are enumerated as under:

- They are organised.
- Have an autonomous board.
- Holds meeting.
- Collect fund.
- Conduct public health programme.
- Create health awareness.
- Help in policy making.
- They are small enough to reach any place.

FUNCTIONS

Services by Voluntary Health Agencies (Functions):

It can be represented in a diagram to depict its vast encroachment in the welfare of the people (Fig. 31.1). If there are any new ways of approach or ways of doing, it is always by a voluntary health organisation.

Pioneering health service activity and legislation on matters of health have always been from voluntary health agencies.

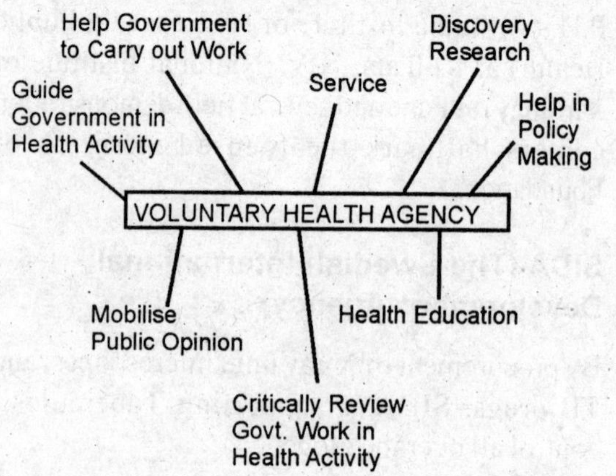

Fig. 31.1: Functions of a voluntary health agency

HISTORY

Group activity to help fellowmen has been in existence over many centuries in the world. Historic events depicting charity, welfare and free shelters for the poor are described in books. Such welfare activities were indirectly meant to help keeping the mankind healthy and to defend him in calamities.

During provincial administration, provincial health care was indirectly maintained in Royal rulings. Individual volunteers used to submit their services for the mankind.

In India, at the beginning of past century voluntary service worked for rehabilitation of war raged community. Leper's rehabilitation and women help by Gram Sevikas have been recorded.

After independence, India has seen well developed network of voluntary health associations which functioned for the welfare of mankind. Major agencies which are worth mentioning are under following heads.

1. *Relief Operation*
   - Indian Red Cross Society
   - Bharath Sevak Samaj
   - All India Blind Relief Society
2. *Specific Disease Control*
   - Hind Kusht Nivaran Sangh
   - Tuberculosis Association of India
   - Indian Cancer Society
3. *R.C.H.*
   - Indian Council of Child Welfare
   - The Kasturba Memorial Fund
   - F.P.A.I.
   - All India Women's Conference
4. *Professional Bodies*
   - The Trained Nurses' Association
   - I.M.A.
   - Indian Dental Association
   - General Practitioners' Association
5. *Social welfare*
   - Central Social Welfare Board
   - State social welfare Board

General functions of voluntary health agencies in India:

- Medical relief
- Initiation of measures according to their objectives
- Supplementing Government effort
- Development of manpower, media and methods for health education
- Evaluation of health activities in India.

AGENCIES

Trained Nurses Association of India

Before 1946 trained birth attendants used to gather in a forum which never made any group activities. When Delhi and Vellore started graduation, nursing care took a different direction to establish themselves as an organised group. By 1952 we could see an organised effort of grouping among trained nurses but without any registered body. Of late, various specialized courses are being made available such as community health nursing, midwifery, operating assistant and rehabilitation nursing. By sixties an organised group called Trained Nurses Association has formed with the objective of involvement into community welfare activities such as:

- Nursing care of children
- Nursing care of elderly
- Blood donation campaign and camps
- First aid facility
- Vocational rehabilitation
- Relief work with Red Cross, I.M.A. and General Practitioners.

India Red Cross Society

There are many branches across the country executing relief work during earthquake, floods, drought and disease epidemics. It is providing assistance to fetch milk and medical supplies to many hospitals, R.C.H. centers, orphanages. The primary obligation of the Red Cross is to take care of wounded, sick or injured armed forces. For permanent disabled ex-servicemen Red Cross has initiated "Red Cross Homes".

Recently, great attention of Indian Red Cross has fallen on First Aid, Blood donation (voluntary) and Family planning clinic which can bring Medical relief and social relief to the society.

General Practitioners' Association

Thousands of branches are doing yeomen service in bringing medical relief to vulnerable groups. It has its members from all systems of medicine Allopathy, ayurveda, unani, Homeopathy, siddha and other Indian systems of medicine. Over hundreds of health check up camps, health awareness camps, blood donation camps, screening camps are conducted every year thus providing access to health and welfare to common man.

All India Women's Conference

Started in 1976, is running ANC clinics, PNC clinic, child guidance clinics, adult education centers, milk distribution centers and Family Planning clinics.

All India Blind Relief Society

Started in 1946, is associated with eye camps for identification of preventable blindness and conducting cataract surgery camps with post operative follow-ups and free spectacles for refractory corrections. Recently AIBRS has introduced cataract surgery with I.O.L. implantation which otherwise is not affordable by a common man.

Bharat Sevak Samaj

Started in 1952 it is helping people to achieve health by their own effort and actions. Village sanitation is given priority by BSS workers.

Central Social Welfare Board

Under Ministry of Education, this Board is formed as an autonomous organisation. It is identifying voluntary welfare organisations and rendering financial aid to them for welfare activities. Running Balwadies, Mother Crafts, Play centers and women self employment assistance are its other added popular schemes.

Hind Kusht Nivarana Sangh (HKNS)

It started in 1950 with its headquarters in Delhi. Financial assistance to leprosy homes, health education by posters and training of physiotherapists are main activities of HKNS.

Indian Council for Child Welfare

It started in 1952. It has network of State Councils in India. Its main objectives are to provide social and economic security to child by legislative means through right of the child.

I.M.A.

It is a professional body which is guiding Medical Council of India. I.M.A. is helping in setting up Quality Standards in professional education in medical profession and Health Science profession. It is also involved in organising relief camps and medical relief during natural calamities. It coordinates with Indian Red Cross Society.

The Kasturba Memorial Fund

It started in 1944. It aims at helping rural women through Gram Sevikas.

Tuberculosis Association of India (TAI)

It started in 1939 and has many branches in India. It mobilises fund through "TB seal campaign", trains medical and paramedical in chemotherapy. There are many leading tuberculosis Institutions in India which are run by T.A.I.

FURTHER REFERENCES

1. Gunn and Platt: Voluntary health agencies (Ronald Press).
2. Leavell and Clark: Preventive medicine for Doctors in his community (Mc Graw Hill).
3. CHEB document on voluntary health organisation (G.O.I.).
4. Prabhakara GN–Trends, Issues and Management in Nursing (Peepee).

32

Job Responsibility

INTRODUCTION

Health care is now a team work. The team includes professional and auxiliary health personnel who are needed to give health care. Nursing care is nearly 50% of health care in the context of care, control and prevention.

Health committees have reported the desired nurse population ratio of 1:5000. But national average of Nurse Population ratio as per estimate 2001 is 1.02 per 5000 (2,10,000 Nurse for 1,027,015,247 population).

Health Manpower requirement of Nurse, Health Assistant Female, MPW female and trained Dais are fulcrum for the Indian Health Scheme.

AREA

Major areas of Nursing care include three areas as under:

1. *Maintaining the Individuality of Man:*
   A patient is an individual member of society who has rights, privileges and immunities which should be respected regardless of his race, creed, social or economic status and personal fears and needs which usually are exaggerated by his illness.
2. *Maintaining Physiologic Functions in Man:*
   The human body requires that certain physiologic activities be maintained if the body is to function effectively.
3. *Protecting Man Against External Causes of Illness:*
   Appropriate precautionary measures will help or eliminate physical, chemical or biologic factors in the environment which cause disease in man.

DAILY NURSING ROUTINE

The nursing care of each patient should be planned to meet the needs of individual patient physically, mentally and spiritually in the best possible way. His likes, dislikes and habits are to be respected.

Bed making, bed pan services are privilege of the nurse. She should supervise the disinfection of body discharges which are infective in nature.

Indian habit of using water for cleansing after urination and defecation is allowed since patient is accustomed to it. A check over instructions before ward rounds is a routine. Recording of vital rates like pulse, BP, respiration are common added routines in the sick.

Ward Management

Unit of a hospital which hosts the sick for Medical care and Nursing care form a ward in the hospital.

According to WHO the hospital is "an integral part of a social and medical organisation, the function of which is to provide for the population the complete health care, both curative and preventive and whose out-patient services reach out to the family and its home workers and for bio-social research".

Expected functions of professional care are:

- Care of the sick
- Care of the injured
- Prevention of diseases
- Promotion of health
- Diagnosis
- Treatment
- Rehabilitation
- Vocational training
- Nursing education
- Research.

Nursing Management includes:

- Division of work starting from nursing superintendent, matron, Dept sister, charge nurse, staff nurse, ANM, clerk, ward aides, cleaning staff.
- Division of work starting from principle senior sister tutor, junior sister tutor at nursing college level.
- Authority and responsibility in nursing duties.
- Discipline as per nursing code.
- Unity of command from one source.
- Unity of direction of work or activity.
- Subordinate coordination.
- Adequate remuneration.

Nursing skills at Hospitals and Health Centres are:

- Conceptual skills
- Human relation skill
- Technical skill.

Nursing Ward Management is summarized by following diagram:

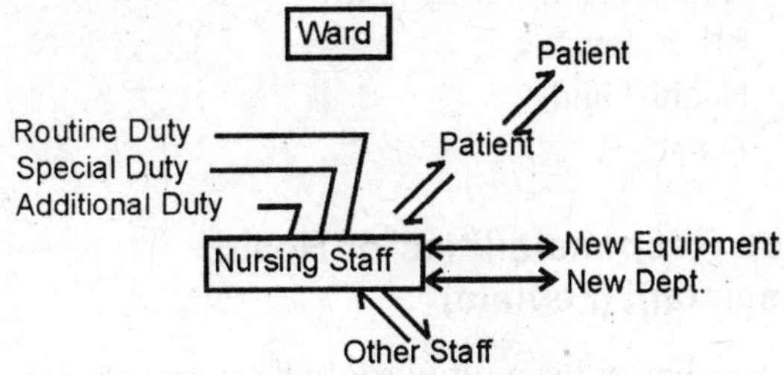

Fig. 32.1: Ward management

SPECIAL ROUTINE

In hospital procedures following are special routines that are to be attended in Nursing care services:

i. Employing techniques for infection prevention and control.
ii. Using proper positioning, mobilization and transferring techniques.
iii. Managing female reproductive procedures and immediate care of the newborn.
iv. Managing G.I. procedure.
v. Managing Respiratory procedures.
vi. Managing cardiovascular procedures.
vii. Managing Renal – Urinary procedures.
viii. Managing musculoskeletal procedures.
ix. Managing Neurosensory procedures.

ADDITIONAL ROUTINE

- Family health counselling.
- Inspection, survey of home, farm, school, industry plant, playground.
- Managerial responsibilities.
- Education and supervision of other workers
- Participation in research activity.

JOB RESPONSIBILITIES

Job responsibilities of nursing profession which constitute comprehensive health care for the following staff are enumerated in the following pages:

1. Health Assistant Female
2. MPW Female
3. Health Guide
4. *Dais.*

Job Responsibilities of Health Assistant (Female)

Note: Under the multipurpose workers scheme, a health assistant (female) is expected to cover a population of 20,000 in which there are four sub-centres, each with one health worker (female). However, in future she may cover one PHC with six sub-centres having 5,000 population each.

The health assistant (female) will carry out the following functions:

1. Supervision and Guidance

1. Supervise and guide the health worker (female) in the delivery of health care services to the community.
2. Strengthen the knowledge and skills of the health worker (female).
3. Help the health worker (female) in improving her skills in working in the community.
4. Help and guide the health worker (female) in planning and organising her programme of activities.
5. Visit each sub-centre at least once a week on a fixed day to observe and guide the health worker (female) in her day to day activities.
6. Assess periodically the progress of work of the health worker (female) and submit an assessment report to the medical officer of the primary health centre.
7. Carry out supervisory home visits in the area of the health worker (female).

2. Teamwork

1. Help the health worker to work as part of the health team.
2. Coordinate her activities with those of the health assistant (male) and other health personnel including the dais.
3. Coordinate the health activities in her area with the activities of workers of other departments and agencies, and attend meetings at block level.
4. Conduct regular staff meetings with the health workers in coordination with the health assistant (male).
5. Attend staff meetings at the primary health centre.
6. Assist the medical officers of the primary health centre in the organisation of the different health services in the area.
7. Participate as a member of the health team in mass camps and campaigns in health programmes.

3. Supplies, Equipment and Maintenance of Sub-centre

1. In collaboration with the health assistant (male), check at regular intervals the stores available at the sub-centre and help in the procurement of supplies and equipment.
2. Check that the drugs at the sub-centre are properly stored and that the equipment is well maintained.
3. Ensure that the health worker (female) maintains her general kit and midwifery kit in the proper way.
4. Ensure that the sub-centre is kept clean and is properly maintained.

4. Records and Reports

1. Scrutiny of the maintenance of records by the health worker (female) and guide her in their proper maintenance.
2. Maintain the prescribed records and prepare the necessary reports.
3. Review reports received from the health workers (female), consolidate them and submit periodical reports to the medical officer of the primary health centre.

5. Training

1. Organize and conduct training for dais with the assistance of the health worker (female).

6. Maternal and Child Health

1. Conduct weekly MCH clinics at each sub-centre with the assistance of the health worker (female).
2. Respond to calls from the health worker (female) and trained dais, and from the health worker (male) in the twilight area and render necessary help.

7. Family Welfare and Medical Termination of Pregnancy

1. Conduct weekly welfare clinics (along with the MCH clinics) at each sub-centre with the assistance of the health worker (female)
2. Personally motivate resistant cases for family planning.
3. Provide information on the availability of services for medical termination of pregnancy and refer suitable cases to the approved institutions.
4. Guide the health worker (female) in establishing female depot holders for distribution of conventional contraceptives and train the depot holders with the assistance of the health worker (female).

8. Nutrition

1. Identify cases of malnutrition among infants and young children (zero to five years), give the necessary treatment and advice and refer serious cases to the primary health centre.

9. Immunization

1. Supervise the immunization of all pregnant women, and infants (zero to one year).

10. Primary Medical Care

1. Provide treatment for minor ailments, provide first-aid for accidents and emergencies and refer cases beyond her competence to the primary health centre or nearest hospital.
2. Attend to cases referred by the health workers and refer cases beyond her competence to the primary health centre or nearest hospital.

11. Health Education

1. Carry out educational activities for MCH, family planning, nutrition and immunization with the assistance of the health worker (female).
2. Arrange group meetings with leaders and involve them in spreading the message for various health programmes.
3. Organize and conduct training of women leaders with the assistance of health worker (female).
4. Organize and utilize mahila mandals, teachers and other women in the community in the family welfare programmes.

Job Responsibilities of Health Worker (Female)

Note: Under the multipurpose workers scheme, a health worker (female) is expected to cover a population of 5,000. (At present, however, she is expected to cover a population of 10,000 of which about 4,000 will be her intensive area, she will be responsible for all the activities listed and in the twilight area for maternal and child health activities only on request).

She will carry out the following functions:

1. Maternal and Child Health

1. Register and provide care to pregnant women throughout the period of pregnancy.
2. Test urine of pregnant women for albumin and sugar and estimate haemoglobin level during her home visits and at the clinic.
3. Refer cases of abnormal pregnancy and cases with medical and gynaecological problems to the health assistant (female) or the primary health centre.

4. Conduct about 50 per cent of total deliveries in her intensive area and whenever called in the twilight area.
5. Supervise deliveries conducted by dais and assist them whenever called in.
6. Refer cases of difficult labour and newborns with abnormalities and help them to get institutional care and provide follow-up care to patients referred to or discharged from hospital.
7. Make at least three postnatal visits for each delivery conducted in the intensive area and render advice regarding care of the mother and care and feeding of the newborn.
8. Assess the growth and development of the infant and take any necessary action.
9. Help the medical officer and health assistant (female) in conducting MCH and family planning clinics at the sub-centre.
10. Educate mothers individually and in groups for better family health including MCH family planning, nutrition, immunization, control of communicable diseases, personal and environmental hygiene and care of minor ailments.

2. Family Planning

1. Utilize the information from the Eligible Couple Register for the family planning programme.
2. Spread the message of family planning to the couples and motivate them for family planning individually and in groups
3. Distribute conventional contraceptive to the couples, provide facilities and help the prospective acceptors in getting family planning services, if necessary by accompanying them or arranging for the dais to accompany them to hospital.
4. Provide follow-up services to female planning adopters identify side–effects for a given treatment on the spot for side-effects and minor complaints and refer those cases that need attention by the physician to the PHC/hospital.
5. Establish female depot holders; help the health assistant (female) in training them, and providing a continuous supply of conventional contraceptives to the depot holders.
6. Build rapport with acceptors, village leaders, dais and others and utilize them for promoting family welfare programmes.
7. Identify women leaders and help the health assistant (female) to train them.
8. Participate in mahila mandal / meetings and utilize such gathering for educating women in family welfare programmes.

3. Medical Termination of Pregnancy

1. Identify the women requiring help for medical termination of pregnancy and refer them to the nearest approved institution.
2. Educate the community of the availability of services for medical termination of pregnancy.

4.Nutrition

1. Identify cases of malnutrition among infants and young children (0 to 5 years) give the necessary treatment and advice and refer serious cases to the PHC.
2. Distribute iron and folic acid tablets as prescribed to pregnant and nursing mothers, infants and young children (0 to 5 years) and family planning acceptors.
3. Administer vitamin 'A' solution as prescribed to children from 1 to 5 years.
4. Educate the community about nutritious diet for mothers and children.

5. Communicable Disease

1. Identify cases of notifiable diseases, i.e. cholera, plague, poliomyelitis and persons with continued fever or prolonged cough, or spitting of blood, which she comes across during her

home visits and notify the health worker (male) about them.

6. Immunization

1. Immunize pregnant women with tetanus toxoid.
2. Administer BCG vaccination to all newborn infants, and DPT vaccination, oral poliomyelitis vaccine (where available) and BCG vaccine (if not given at birth) to all infants (0 to 1 year).

7. *Dai* Training

1. List *Dais* in the intensive and twilight areas and involve them in promoting family welfare.
2. Help the health assistant (female) in the training programme of dais (also refer to 1.5 regarding supervision of dais).

8. Vital Events

1. Record births and deaths occurring in the intensive area in the births and deaths register and report them to the health worker (male).

9. Record Keeping

1. Register (a) pregnant women from three months of pregnancy onwards; (b) infants zero to one year of age; and (c) women aged 15 to 44 years through systematic home visits in the intensive area and at the clinic.
2. Maintain the prenatal and maternity records and child care records.
3. Assist the health worker (male) in preparing the Eligible Couple Register and maintaining it up-to-date.
4. Prepare and submit the prescribed periodical reports in time to the health assistant (female).
5. Prepare and maintain maps and charts for her area and utilize them for planning her work.

10. Primary Medical Care

1. Provide treatment for minor ailments, provide first-aid for accidents and emergencies and refer cases beyond her competence to the primary health centre or nearest hospital.

11. Team Activities

1. Attend and participate in staff meeting at primary health centre/ community development block or both.
2. Coordinate her activities with the health worker (male) and other health workers including the health guides and dais.
3. Meet with the health assistant (female) each week and seek her advice and guidance whenever necessary.
4. Maintain the cleanliness of the sub-centre.
5. Participate as a member of the team in camps and campaigns.

Activities of Health Guide

Note: A health guide will be expected to cover the population of a village or, if the village is a large one, a population of about 1,000. He/she will receive technical guidance from the health worker (male/female).

After training, the health guide will be able to carry out the following activities.

1. Malaria

1. Identify fever cases.
2. Make thick and thin blood films of all fever cases.
3. Send the slides for laboratory examination.
4. Administer presumptive treatment to fever cases.
5. Keep a record of the persons given presumptive treatment.
6. Inform the health worker (male) of the names and addresses of cases from whom blood slides have been taken.
7. Assist health worker (male) and the spraying teams in spraying and larvicidal operations.
8. Educate the community on how to prevent malaria.

2. Communicable Diseases

1. Inform the health worker (male) immediately an epidemic occurs in his/her area.

2. Take immediate precautions to limit the spread of disease.
3. Educate the community about the prevention and control of communicable diseases.

3. Environmental Sanitation and Personal Hygiene

1. Chlorinate drinking water sources at regular intervals.
2. Keep a record of the number of wells chlorinated.
3. Assist the health worker (male) in arranging for the construction of the following:
   - Soakage pits
   - Kitchen gardens
   - Compost pits
   - Sanitary latrines
   - Smokeless chulhas
4. Educate the community about the following:
   - Safe drinking water
   - Hygienic methods of disposal of liquid waste
   - Hygienic methods of disposal of solid waste
   - Home sanitation
   - Kitchen gardens
   - Advantages and use of sanitary latrines
   - Advantages of smokeless chulhas
   - Food hygiene
   - Control of insects, rodents and stray dogs
5. Educate the community about the importance of personal hygiene.

4. Immunization

1. Assist the health worker (male/female) in arranging for immunization.
2. Educate the community about immunization against diphtheria, whooping cough, tetanus, tuberculosis, poliomyelitis, measles, cholera and typhoid.

5. Family Planning

1. Spread the message of family planning to the couples in his/her area and educate them about the desirability of the small family norm.
2. Educate the people about the available methods of family planning.
3. Act as a depot holder, distribute nirodh to the couples and maintain the necessary records of nirodh distributed.
4. Inform the health worker (male/female) of those couples who are willing to accept a family planning method so that he/she can make necessary arrangements.
5. Educate the community about the availability of services for medical termination of pregnancy (MTP).

6. Maternal and Child Care

1. Advise pregnant women to consult the health worker (female) or the trained Dai for prenatal, natal and postnatal care.
2. Advise pregnant women to get immunized against tetanus.
3. Educate the community about the availability of maternal and child care services and encourage them to utilize the facilities.
4. Educate the community about how to keep mothers and children healthy.

7. Nutrition

1. Identify cases with signs and symptoms of malnutrition among pre-school children (one to five years) and refer them to the health worker (male/female).
2. Identify cases with signs and symptoms of anaemia in pregnant and nursing women and children and refer them to health worker (male/female) for treatment.
3. Assist health worker (male/female) in administering vitamin – A solution as prescribed to children from one to five years of age (9 months to 3 years under RCH).
4. Teach families about the importance of breast feeding and the introduction of supplementary weaning foods.

5. Educate the community about nutritious diet for mothers and children.

8. Vital Events

1. Report all births and deaths in his/her area to the health worker (male).
2. Educate the community about the importance of registering all births and deaths.

9. First-Aid in Emergencies

1. Give emergency first-aid for the following conditions, refer these cases to the primary health centre as necessary and inform the health worker (male/female)
   - Drowning
   - Electric shock
   - Heat stroke
   - Snake bite
   - Scorpion sting
   - Insect sting
   - Dog bite
   - Accidents.
2. Carry out procedures in dealing with accidents.
3. Keep a record of first-aid given to each patient.

10. Treatment of Minor Ailments

1. Give simple treatment for the following signs and symptoms and refer cases beyond his/her competence to the sub-centre or primary health centre:
   - Fever
   - Headache
   - Backache and pain in the joint
   - Cough and cold
   - Diarrhoea
   - Vomiting
   - Pain in the abdomen
   - Constipation
   - Toothache
   - Earache
   - Sore eyes
   - Boils, abscesses and ulcers
   - Scabies and ringworm.
2. Keep a record of the treatment given to each patient.

11. Mental Health

1. Recognise signs and symptoms of mental illness and refer these cases to health worker (male/female).
2. Give immediate assistance in emergencies associated with mental illness.
3. Educate the community about mental illness.

Activities of *Dai*

The *Dai* is an important person in her village. She serves as a link between the families in her village and the health worker (female)/ANM. These are some of the things she can do to improve maternal and child health in her village:

1. She should contact every pregnant woman in her area and see that she is registered at the sub-centre or primary health centre.
2. She should attend the weekly prenatal clinic and assist the health worker (female)/ ANM.
3. She should try to ensure that every pregnant woman in her area attends the prenatal clinic at least three times, i.e. after the third month to confirm pregnancy, during the seventh month, and during the ninth month.
4. She should try to ensure that every pregnant woman is immunized against tetanus (two doses—the last dose at least one month before the delivery and the first dose one month before the last).
5. She should try to ensure that every pregnant woman takes iron and folic acid tablets as prescribed.
6. If any abnormal pregnancy is detected she should show the case immediately to the health worker (female)/ANM or health assistant (female)/LHV or refer the case to PHC.

7. She should ensure that preparations for delivery are made either at home or at the PHC or hospital.
8. If she finds any abnormality during labour she must seek medical aid without delay.
9. When she receives a call for delivery:
   - She should take her kit with her.
   - She should watch the progress of labour carefully.
   - She should allow labour to progress normally without any unnecessary interference.
   - She should observe aseptic techniques while conducting the delivery.
10. She should see that her kit is always replenished, clean, and ready for use during a delivery.
11. She should make the mother and baby comfortable and attend to the nutrition of both.
12. She should instruct the mother and the relatives as to when she should be called immediately, e.g. in case the mother has excessive bleeding or there is bleeding from the baby's cord.
13. In the postnatal period if she finds any complications in the mother, e.g. fever or foul lochia, or in the baby, e.g. cord infection or jaundice she should immediately inform the health worker (female)/ANM or refer the mother or baby to the PHC.
14. She should try to ensure that all infants in her area are immunized with BCG, DPT, measles and poliomyelitis vaccine.
15. She should motivate the eligible couples in her area to use a contraceptive method or to undergo sterilization.
16. She should distribute nirodh, foam tablets, and jelly to those couples who require these contraceptives.
17. She should report all births and deaths in her area to the health worker (male) or health worker (female)/ANM.

FURTHER REFERENCES

1. Pamela L Swearingen – Atlas of Nursing Procedure (Addison Wesley).
2. St. John, Ambulance Association – Nursing.
3. Elinor V Fuerst, Lu Verne Wolff – Fundamentals of Nursing (J.B. Lippincott).
4. Freeman – P.H. Nursing practice (W.B. Saunders).
5. NIHFW – Management Trg. Modules.
6. Prabhakara G.N. – Trends, Issues and Management in Nursing (Peepee).

Appendices

Appendix 1: Number of hours of teaching as per Indian Nursing Council Recommendation (Hours)

Year	Subject	Hours			
First year	Anatomy, Physiology	80			
	Microbiology	30	130		
	Physics, Chemistry	20			
	Psychology	60		565	
			90		
	Sociology	30			
	Nutrition	30			
	Hygiene	40			
			180		
	Health Education	10			
	Com. Health Nursing	100			
	Nursing fundamental		165		1165
Second year	Medical, Surgical		240		
	Psychiatry, Mental		30		
	Paediatrics		50	350	
	Advanced Nursing			30	
Third year	Midwifery		100		
	Com. Health nursing		100	250	
	Professional Training		30		
	Management		20		

42 week (250 days) per year totalling 4500 hours.

Appendix 2: Nightingale Pledge

"I solemnly pledge before God and in the presence of this assembly to pass my life in purity and to practice my profession faithfully. I will abstain from whatever is deleterious and mischievous and will not take or knowingly administer any harmful drug. I will do in all my power to maintain and elevate the standard of my profession and will hold in confidence all personal matters committed to my keeping and all my family affairs coming to my knowledge in the practice of my calling. With loyalty I will endeavour to aid the physician in his work, and devote myself to the welfare of those committed to my care."

Appendix 3: Permissible Error and Confidence Interval for Sample Size Determination

Confidence interval	*Error/Accuracy*	*Distance of S.E*
99 %	1 %	2.57
98 %	2 %	2.32
97 %	3 %	2.17
96 %	4 %	2.05
95 %	5 %	1.96
94 %	6 %	1.88
93 %	7 %	1.81
92 %	8 %	1.75
91 %	9 %	1.69
90 %	10 %	1.6448
80 %	20 %	1.2816
70 %	30 %	1.03
60 %	40 %	0.8416
50 %	50 %	0.6745

Appendix 4: Cumulative Distribution of Chi-Square

D.F	***Probability of a greater value***						
	0.5	*0.25*	*0.1*	*0.05*	*0.01*	*0.005*	*0.001*
1	0.45	1.32	2.71	3.84	6.63	7.88	10.83
2	1.39	2.77	4.61	5.99	9.21	10.60	13.82
3	2.37	4.11	6.25	7.81	11.34	12.84	16.27
4	3.36	5.39	7.78	9.49	13.28	14.86	18.47
5	4.35	6.63	9.24	11.07	15.09	16.75	20.51
6	5.35	7.84	10.64	12.59	16.81	18.55	22.46
7	6.35	9.04	12.02	14.07	18.48	20.28	24.32
8	7.34	10.22	13.36	15.51	20.09	21.96	26.13
9	8.34	11.39	14.68	16.92	21.67	23.59	27.88
10	9.34	12.55	15.99	18.31	23.21	25.19	29.59
15	14.34	18.25	22.31	25.00	30.58	32.80	37.70
20	19.34	23.83	28.41	31.41	37.57	40.00	45.32
25	24.34	29.34	34.38	37.65	44.31	46.93	52.62
50	49.33	56.33	63.17	67.50	76.15	79.49	–
100	99.33	109.14	118.50	124.34	135.81	140.17	–

Appendix 5: Short Table of Areas of Normal Curve

Z	*1-P*	*P*
0.0	0.0000	1.0000
0.1	0.0979	0.9203
0.5	0.3829	0.6771
1.0	0.6827	0.3173
1.5	0.8664	0.1336
1.64	0.9000	0.1000
1.96	0.9500	0.0500
2.0	0.9545	0.0455
2.5	0.9876	0.0124
2.58	0.9901	0.0099
3.9	0.9999	0.0001

General tips for statistical inference:
If Z calculated is more than 2, it is significant (P - 0.05)
If Z calculated is more than 3, it is highly significant (P - 0.001)

Appendix 6: The Distribution of t (Two Tailed Tests)

D.F	*Probability of a larger value, sign ignored*					
	0.5	*0.1*	*0.05*	*0.01*	*0.005*	*0.001*
1	1.000	6.314	12.706	63.657	–	–
2	0.816	2.920	4.303	9.925	14.089	31.598
3	0.765	2.353	3.182	5.841	7.453	12.941
4	0.741	2.132	2.776	4.604	5.598	8.610
5	0.727	2.015	2.571	4.032	4.773	6.859
6	0.718	1.943	2.447	3.707	4.317	5.959
7	0.711	1.895	2.365	3.499	4.029	5.405
8	0.706	1.860	2.306	3.355	3.832	5.041
9	0.703	1.833	2.262	3.250	3.690	4.781
10	0.700	1.812	2.228	3.169	3.581	4.587
15	0.691	1.753	2.131	2.947	3.286	4.073
20	0.687	1.725	2.086	2.845	3.153	3.850
25	0.684	1.708	2.060	2.787	3.078	3.725
50	0.680	1.676	2.008	2.678	2.937	3.496
100	0.677	1.661	1.982	2.625	2.871	3.390

Appendix 7A: Lower Abdominal Pain in the Female (PID)

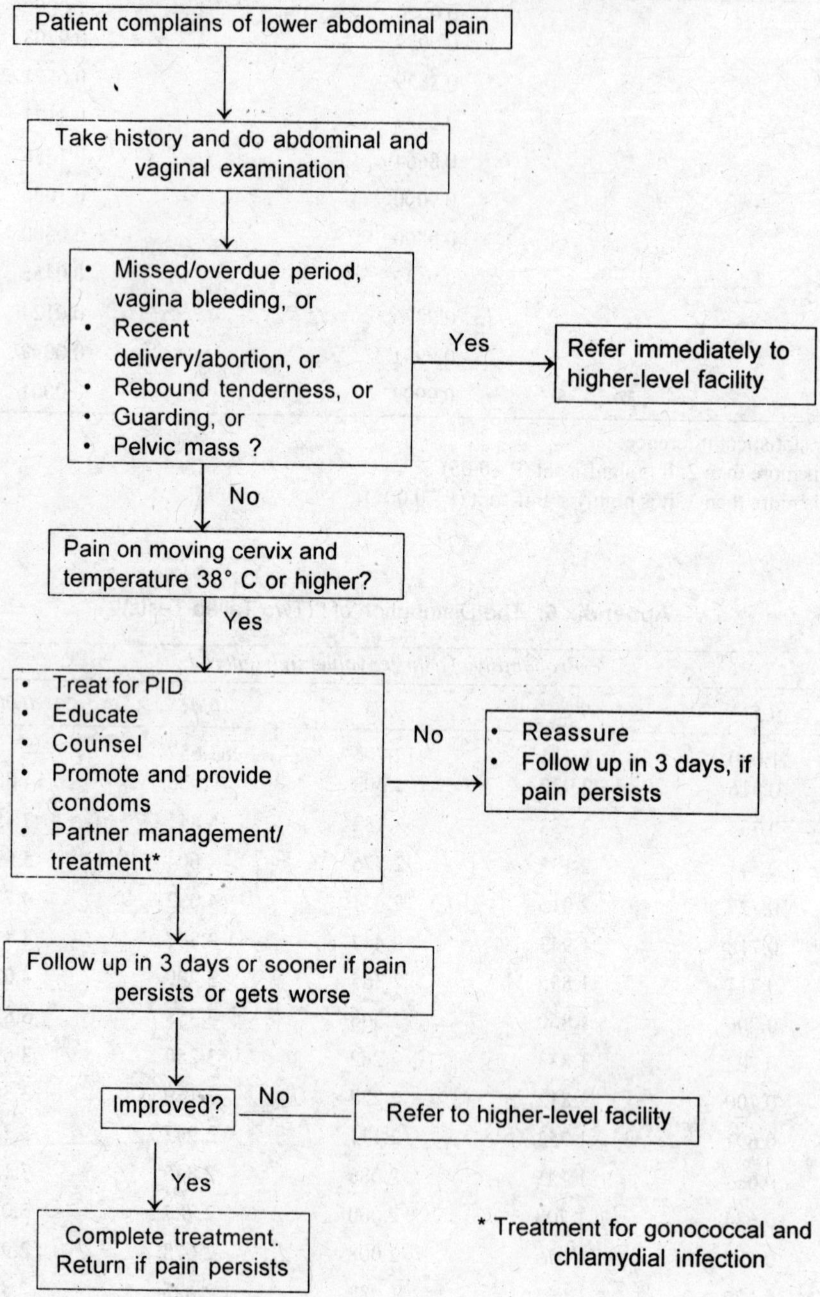

* Treatment for gonococcal and chlamydial infection

Appendix 7B: Urethral Discharge

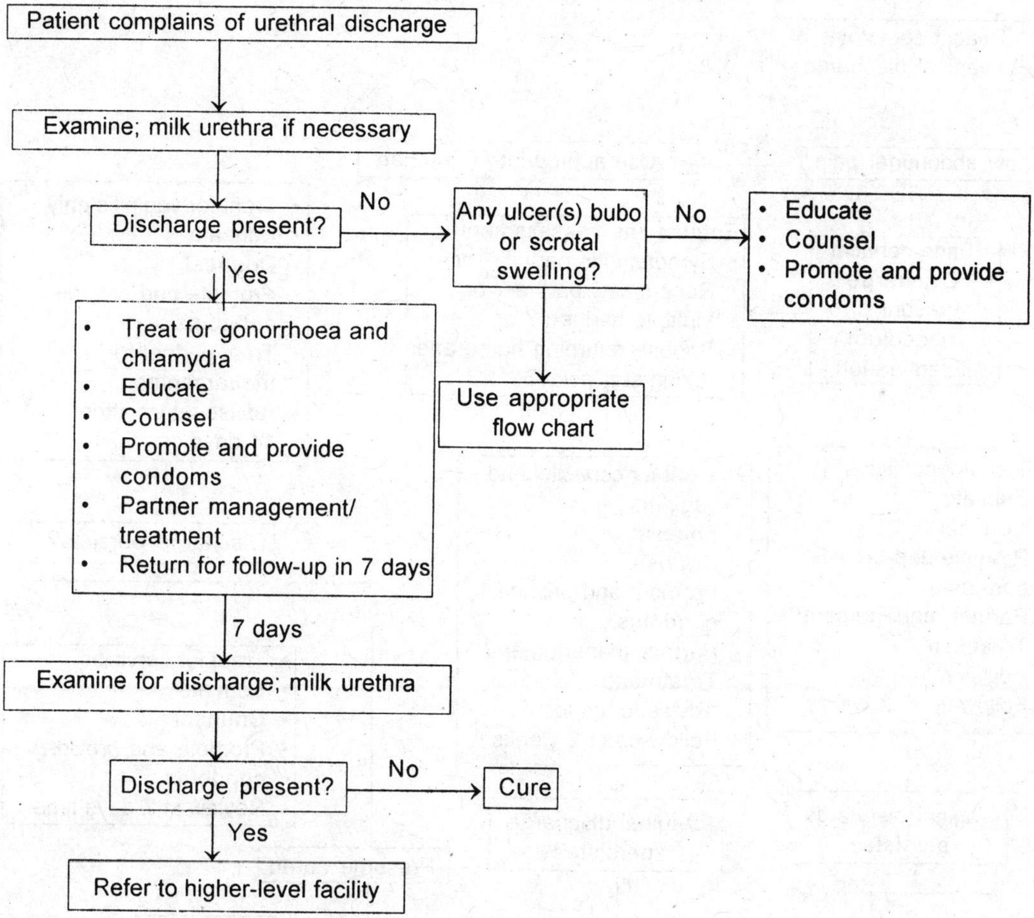

Appendix 7C: Vaginal Discharge
(With Speculum Examination)

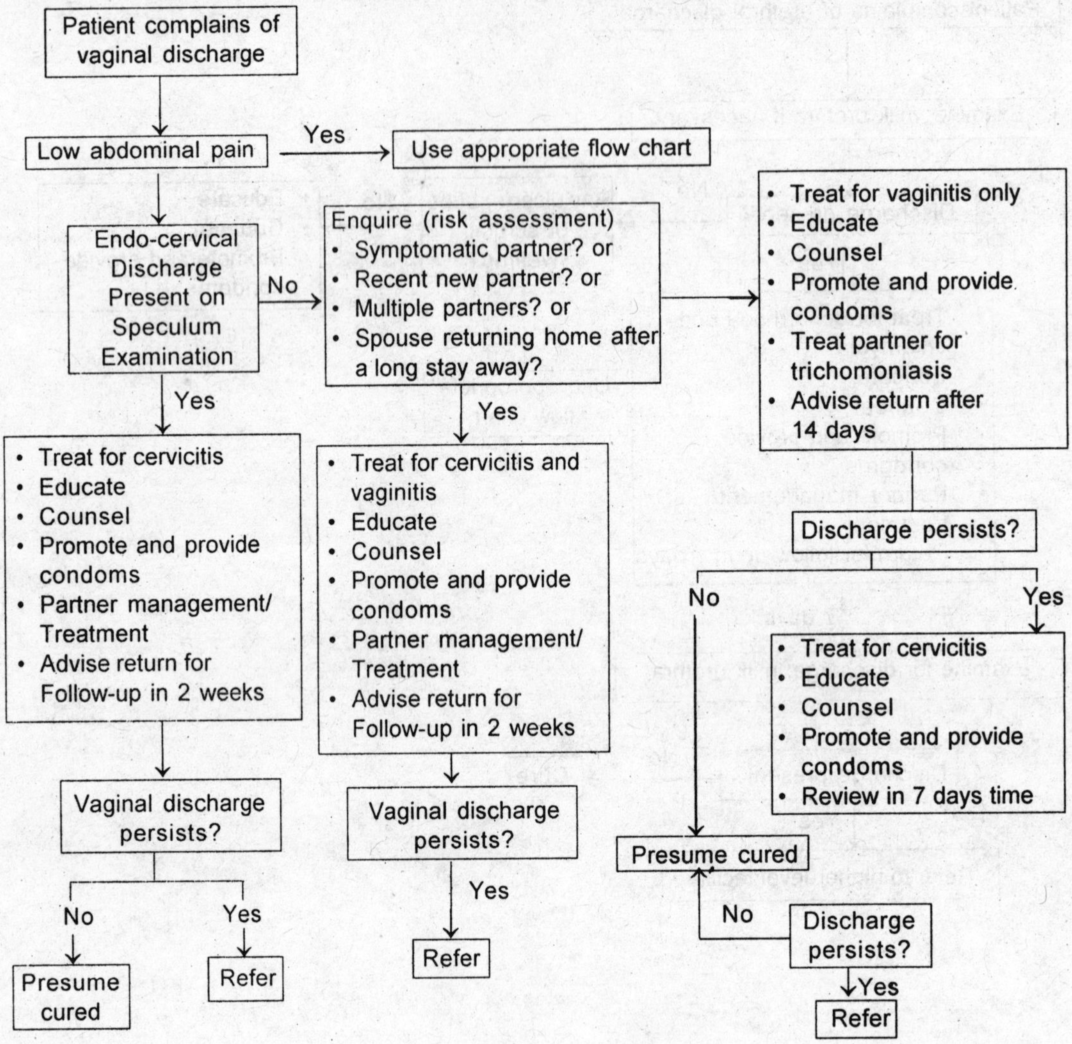

Appendix 7D: Vaginal Discharge

(No Speculum Examination)

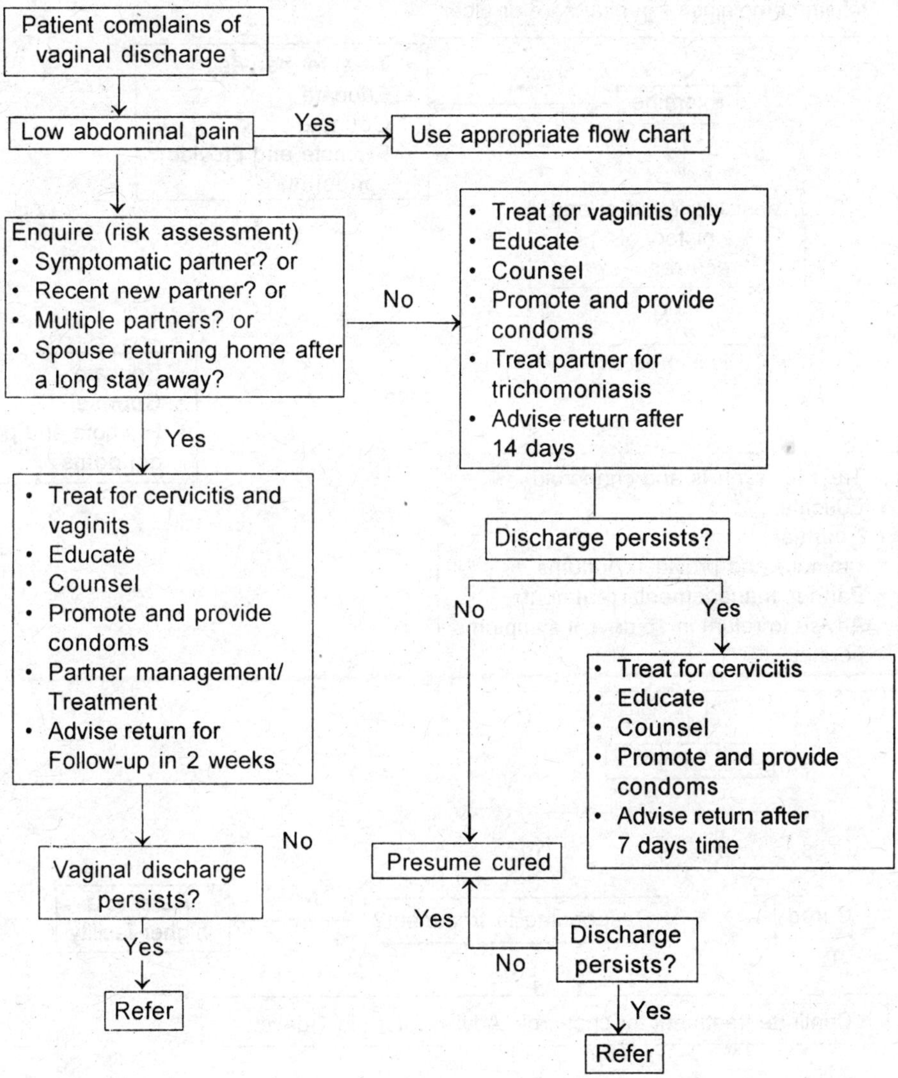

Appendix 7E: Genital Ulcers

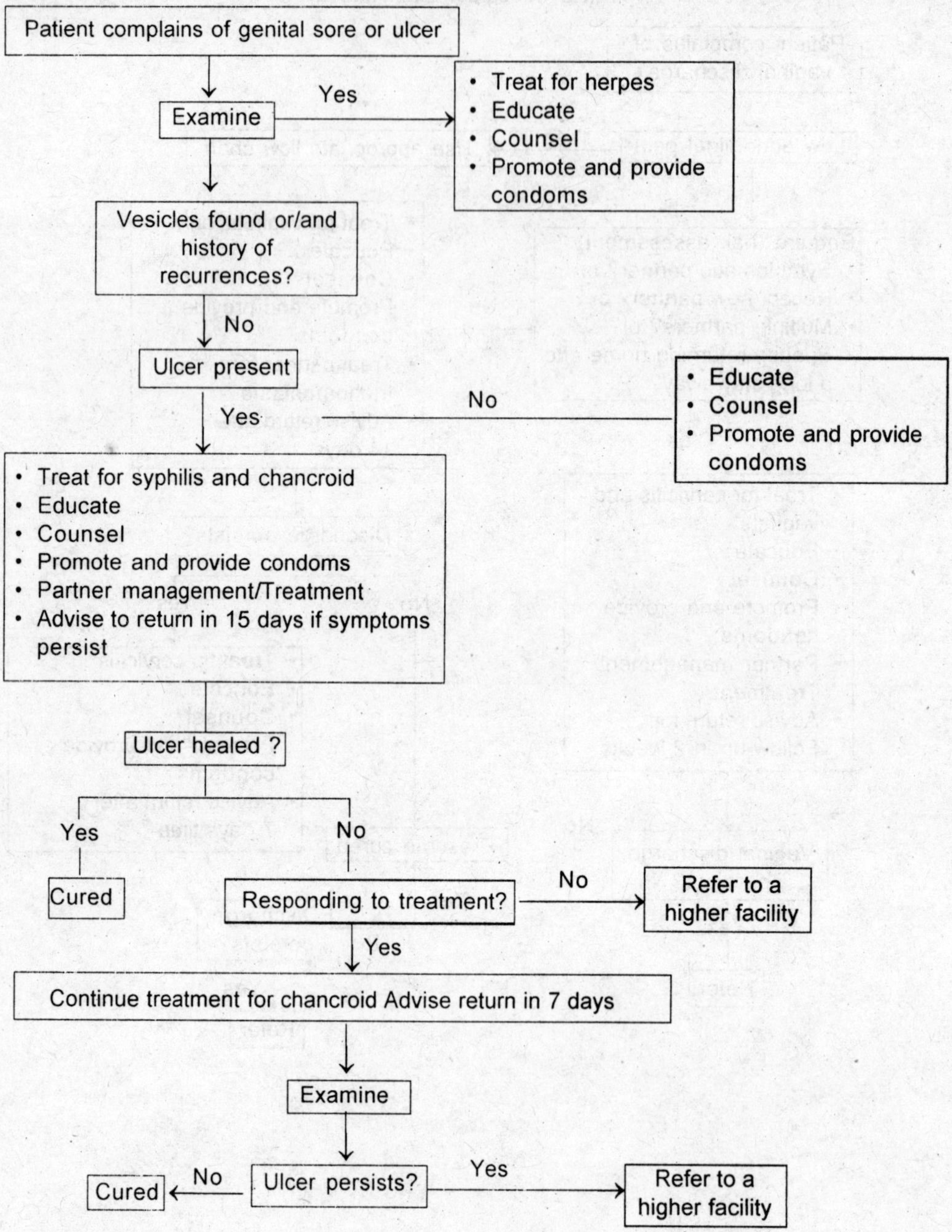

Appendix 7D: Vaginal Discharge

(No Speculum Examination)

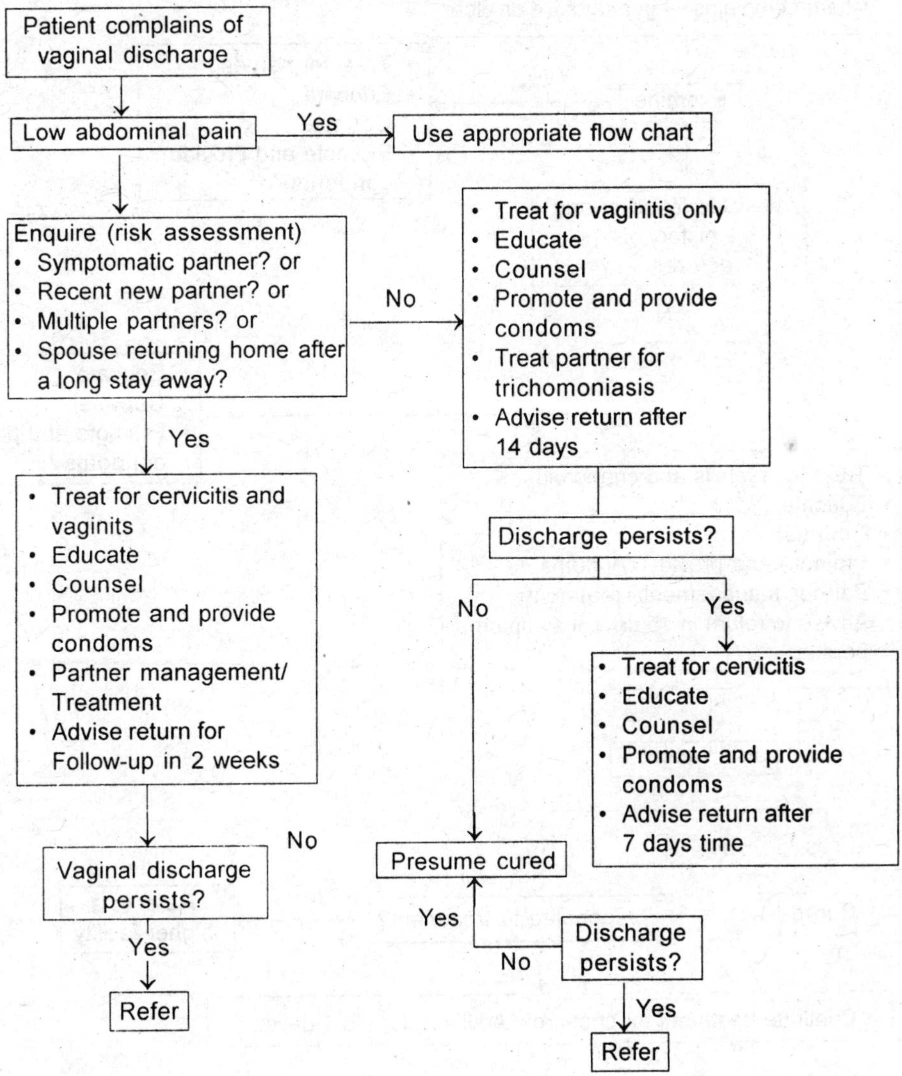

Appendix 7E: Genital Ulcers

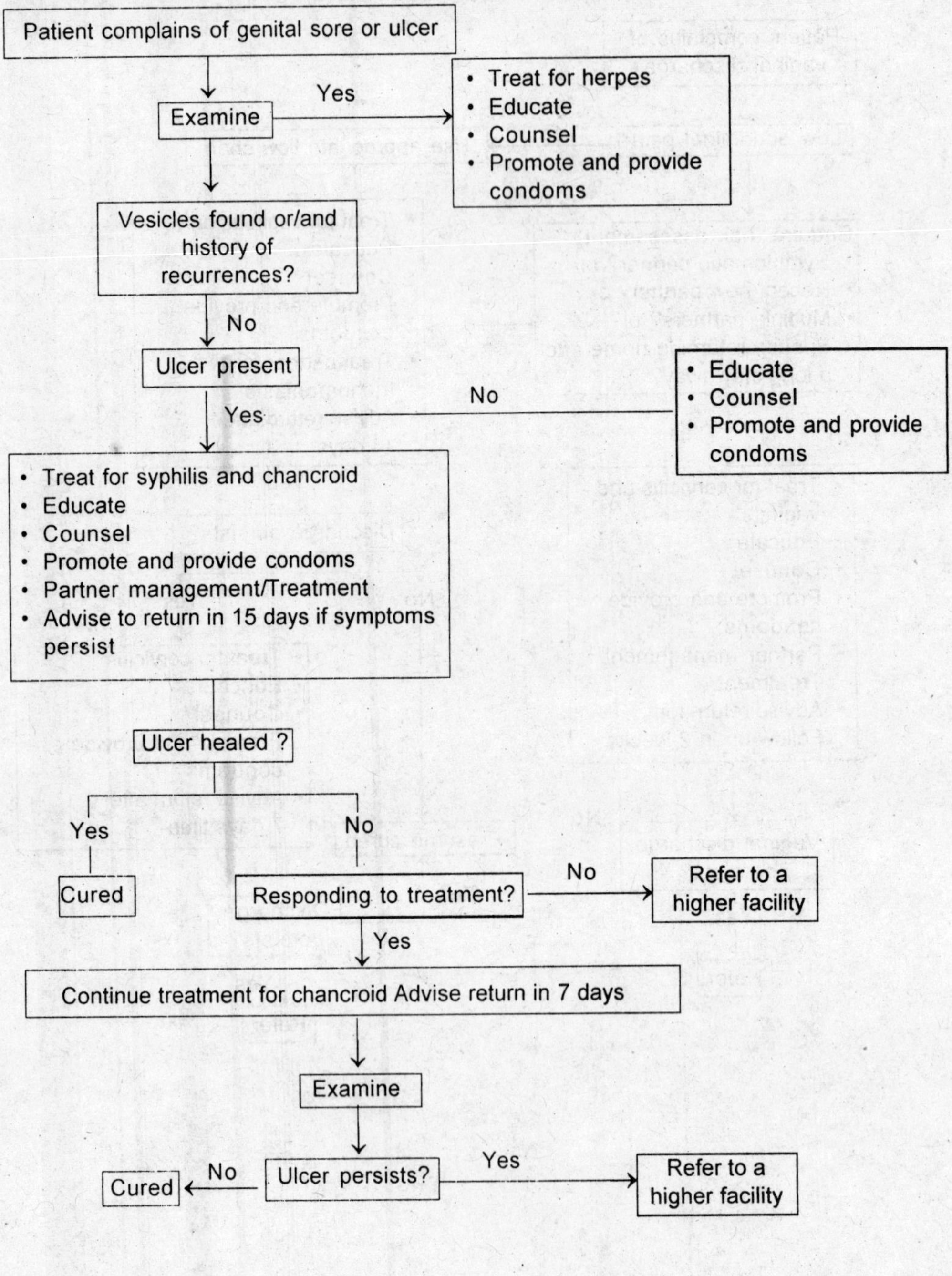

Appendix 8: Contents of Maternity Care Kit

	Item	*Nos.*
1.	Umbilical (cotton 0.3 cm × 25 cm)	2
2.	Blade with holder	1
3.	Cotton swab 7.5cm x 7.5 cm (2.5 gm)	3 pieces
4.	Surgical gauze pieces 5 cm × 7.5 cm- 12 ply	2 pieces
5.	Sanitary pad no. 4	1
6.	Drape—polyethylene sheet 75 cm x 100 cm	1
7.	Trolley cover	1

Appendix 9: Contents of Dais Kit

	Item	*Nos.*
1.	Aluminum kit box	1
2.	Stainless steel straight scissors (blunt–pointed)	1
3.	Stainless steel teaspoon	1
4.	Enamel irrigator with rubber tubing and ebonite nozzle	1
5.	Enal bowl (large)	1
6.	Aluminum bowl	2
7.	Mackintosh sheeting (90 cm square)	1
8.	Hand towel	2
9.	Soap dish with soap	1
10.	Nail brush	1
11.	Absorbent cotton wool (sterilized)	1 packet
12.	Gauze (sterilized)	1 packet of 12 pieces
13.	Umbilical cord tape (sterilized)	6 pieces
14.	Dusting powder in a plastic container	1
15.	Antiseptic lotion	1 bottle

Appendix 10: Contents of the Kit for Health Guides

List of contents

S.No	*Item*	*Quantity*
*1.	Foetoscope	1
2.	Stainless steel straight scissors (blunt-pointed)	1
3.	Sterile cotton wool	1 packet
4.	Sterile gauze	1 packet
5.	Roller bandage	1
6.	Triangular bandage	1
7.	Adhesive plaster	1
8.	Soap dish and soap	1
9.	Towels	2
10.	Clinical oral thermometer	1
11.	Slide box containing 10 glass slides	1
12.	Cloth for cleaning slides	1
13.	Hagedorn needle	1
14.	Graduated medicine glass	1
15.	Suitable containers for drugs	18
16.	Stainless steel teaspoon (9 ml)	1
17.	Spring scale (hanging)	1
18.	Mid-upper arm circumference strip	1
19.	Measuring tape	1
20.	Exercise book (200 pages)	1
21.	Pencil	1
22.	Forms for reporting blood smears	
23.	Health education materials	
24.	Kit bag	

* Not to be included in the kits meant for Male Health Guides.

Appendix 10 Contd.

Medicines and Contraceptives

A. Essential

	S.No. Name of drug/contraceptive	Source of supply
	1. Chloroquine phosphate tablets	From National Malaria Eradication Programme
*	2. Primaquine tablets	
	3. Iron and Folic acid tablets (for adults and children)	From Family Planning Programme
*	4. Vitamin A Sodium	
*	5. Dapsone tablets	From Leprosy Programme
*	6. Multivitamin tablets	
	7. Nirodh-Depot Holder pack (in case 'Depot Holder Supply' is not available, Free Supply Pack may be provided)	From Family Planning Programme
	8. Oral Contraceptive pills	
	9. Oral Rehydration Solution packets	From Health Guide Programme

**Note:* Supplies of Primaquine tablets, Dapsone tablets and Multivitamin tablets will be kept with the Health Guide for distribution to confirmed cases of malaria and leprosy. Treatment of these cases will be carried out under the instructions of the Health Assistant or Health Worker.

B. Optional

Note: This list can be modified by the State Government according to their requirements. In case the list is modified, the detailed instructions for the use of these medicines should be provided by the State Government to the Health Guides.

1. For Internal use

i. Kaolin pectin suspension
ii. Magnesium hydroxide tablets
iii. Paracetamol tablets
iv. Jatiphaladi Vati
v. Lashunadi Vati
vi. Mehayogaraj Guggulu
vii. Belladonna 30 and Merc Sol 30
viii. Colocynth 6 and Mag phos 6x
ix. Cina 30

2. For External use

x. Antiseptic ointment
xi. Benzoic salicylic ointment
xii. Benzyl benzoate emulsion
xiii. Menthol and eucalyptus oil ointment
xiv. Sulphacetamide eye and ear drops
xv. Terramycin eye ointment
xvi. Zinc boric acid dusting powder

Appendix 11: Contents of Kit for Community Health Worker

1. Slides (5) in slide Hagedorn box
2. Cloth for cleaning slides
3. Hagedorn needle
4. Pencil
5. Clinical oral thermometer
6. Graduated medicine glass
7. Scissors
8. Razor blade
9. Cotton wool
10. Gauze
11. Roller bandage
12. Triangular bandage
13. Adhesive plaster
14. Soap dish and soap
15. Towels (2)
16. Nirodh packets (50)
17. Suitable containers for drugs (17)
18. Forms for reporting of blood smears.
19. Franked envelopes addressed to the Primary Health Centre
20. Exercise book (200 pages)
21. Diary
22. Health Education Materials (flip chart on family welfare. set of contraceptives)
23. Manual for Community Health Worker
24. Kit-bag

Medicines to be carried by Community Health Worker

For Internal Use

1. Aspirin, Phenacetin and Caffeine (APC) tablets
2. Chloroquine tablets
3. Cough mixture
4. Kaolin powder
5. Magnesium hydroxide tablets
6. Rehydration powder (chorosol)

For External Use

7. Antiseptic lotion
8. Benzyl Benzoate emulsion
9. Menthol and eucalyptus oil ointment
10. Mercurochrome 2 per cent
11. Methylated Spirit
12. Methyl salicylate ointment
13. Potassium permanganate crystals
14. Sulphacetamide eye and ear drops 10 per cent
15. Sulphanilamide skin ointment
16. Sulphonamide dusting powder
17. Whitfield ointment

Additional material to be kept with selected members of the community

1. Bleaching powder in pots

Appendix 12: Suggested List of Medicines for Inclusion in Health Worker's Kit

For Internal Use:

1. Acetyl salicylic acid tablets
2. Belladonna and phenobarbitone tablets
3. Chlroquine phosphate tablets
4. Cough mixture
5. Dried aluminium hydroxide tablets
6. Ergometrine maleate tablets
7. Iron and folic acid tablets
8. Kaolin pectin suspension
9. Magnesium hydroxide tablets
10. Magnesium sulphate
11. Mepyramine (antihistamine) tablets
12. Mebendazole tablets (Pantelmin)
13. Oral rehydration powder
14. Paracetamol tablets
15. Phthalyl sulphathiazole tablets
16. Piperazine citrate/ Piperazine adipate tablets
17. Sulphadimidine tablets
18. Vitamin A solution

For External Use

19. Acriflavine ointment
20. Antiseptic lotion
21. Benzoic salicylic ointment
22. Benzyl benzoate emulsion
23. Chloromycetin eye ointment (Applicaps)
24. Gentian violet 2%
25. Menthol and eucalyptus oil ointment
26. Mercurochrome 2%
27. Methyl salicylate liniment
28. Sulphacetamide eye and ear drops 10%
29. Tetracycline eye ointment
30. White Vaseline

Reagents

31. Chemistrips (Miles India Ltd.)
32. Litmus paper (blue and red)

Medicines to be kept at Subcentre

For Internal Use

1. Bephenium hydroxy naphthoate granules
2. Calcium gluconate tablets
3. Liquid paraffin
4. Mist alkaline
5. Mist carminative
6. Mist chloral hydrate
7. Mist sedative expectorant
8. Multivitamin tablets (A,B,C,D)
9. Prochlorperazine tablets (Stemetil)
10. Syrup ferric citrate
11. Vitamin C tablets
12. Injection methyl ergometrine maleate (Methergen)

For External Use

13. Boric acid powder
14. Calamine lotion
15. Methylated spirit
16. Tincture benzoin co.
17. Tincture iodine
18. Zinc boric dusting powder

Appendix 13: List of Drugs to be Supplied to Subcentre

List of Essential Drugs to be Supplied to Subcentre

For Internal Use

1. Acetyl salicylic acid tablets
2. Belladonna and phenobarbitone tablets (Antispasmodic tablets)
3. Chloroquine phosphate tablets
4. Ergometrine maleate tablets (Methergen tablets)
5. Iron and folic acid tablets
6. Liquid paraffin
7. Mebendazole tablets (Pantelmin)
8. Mepyramine (Antihistamine) tablets
9. Oral rehydration salt packets
10. Paracetamol tablets
11. Prochlorperazine tablets (Stemetil)
12. Sulphadimidine tablets
13. Syrup ferric ammonium citrate
14. Vitamin A solution
15. Injection methyl ergometrine maleate (Methergen injection)

For External Use

16. Acriflavine ointment
17. Antiseptic lotion (Savlon/Dettol)
18. Benzyl benzoate emulsion
19. Boroglycerine
20. Gentian violet 2%
21. Sulphacetamide eye and ear drops 10%
22. Tetracycline eye ointment
23. Zinc boric dusting powder
24. Absorbent cotton wool
25. Absorbent gauze
26. Roller bandage (98 X 61 cm)
27. Reagent strips (URISTIX)

List of Optional Drugs to be Supplied to Subcentre

For Internal Use

1. Bephenium hydroxyl naphthoate granules
2. Calcium gluconate tablets
3. Cough mixture
4. Dried aluminium hydroxide tablets
5. Kaolin pectin suspension
6. Magnesium hydroxide tablets
7. Magnesium sulphate
8. Mist alkaline
9. Mist carminative
10. Mist chloral hydrate
11. Mist sedative expectorant
12. Multivitamin tablets (A B C D)
13. Phthalyl sulphathiazole tablets
14. Piperazine citrate/ Piperazine adipate tablets
15. Vitamin C tablets

For External Use

16. Benzoic salicylic ointment
17. Boric acid powder
18. Calamine lotion
19. Chloromycetin eye ointment (Applicaps)
20. Menthol and eucalyptus oil ointment
21. Mercurochrome 2%
22. Methyl salicylate ointment
23. Methylated spirit
24. Tincture benzoin co
25. Tincture iodine
26. White vaseline

Appendix 14: List of Contents of Kit for Health Worker Female

General Kit

Sr.No.	*Item*	*Quantity*
1.	Kit bag (brown) with nylon tray, rectangular aluminium tray, side pocket, rear pocket, cover flap and shoulder strap	1
Cover flap		
2.	Spring type dressing forceps-stainless steel (150 mm)	1
3.	Surgical straight scissors (blunt-stainless steel) (140 mm)	1
4.	Pencil with eraser	1
5.	Teaspoon – stainless steel	1
Side pocket		
6.	Nail brush	1
7.	Soap dish	1
8.	Soap	1
9.	Nail clipper	1
Rear pocket		
10.	Clear vinyl plastic sheeting (910 mm wide)	1 metre
11.	Huck towel (430 × 500 mm)	2
12.	Folding aluminium shield (BCG)	1
13.	Polythene self-sealing bag (125 × 200 mm)	12
14.	Sterile gauze pads (12 ply) (76 × 7 6mm square)	6
15.	Arm circumference scale	1
16.	Nylon tray	1
17.	Absorbent non-sterile cotton wool (113 gm)	1 roll
18.	Vinyl-coated fiberglass tape measure (1.5 metre/60")	1
19.	Safety pins (medium/40 mm)	1 bag of 12
20.	Adhesive zinc oxide tape (25 mm × 0.9 metre)	1 roll
21.	Alcohol lamp with screw cap-metal (60 ml)	1
22.	Safety razor blades (double edge)	1 pkt of 5
23.	Clinical oral thermometer (35 to 42°C)	1
24.	Clinical rectal thermometer (35 to 42°C)	1
25.	Gauze bandage (non-sterile) (25 mm × 9 metres)	1 roll
26.	Triangular cloth bandage (910 mm slides)	1
27.	Microscope slide box	1
28.	Microscope slides (plain) (75 mm × 25 mm)	1 pkt of 10
29.	Cloth for cleaning micro slides	1
30.	Stick swabs	1 bag

Contd.

Contd.

31.	Rubber solid stopper (bottom 16 mm top 20 mm)	1	for hagedorn needle
32.	Specimen tube-glass (1900 × 75 mm)	1	
33.	Keith abdominal suture needle (44 mm)	1	
34.	Anaemia recognition card (English/Hindi)	1	
35.	Nelaton solid-tip one eye urethral catheter (12 Fr)	1	
36.	Urinalysis outfit (test tubes/bottle/clamp)	1	set
37.	Mayo Ochsner haemostat straight forceps- stainless steel (160 mm)	1	
38.	Umbilical tape (non-sterile)	1	
39.	DeLee tracheal catheter with glass mucus trap	1	
40.	Rectangular aluminium tray	1	
41.	Medicine cup – polypropylene (30 ml)	1	
42.	Lubricant jar – plastic	14	
43.	Amber dropping bottle – glass (10 ml)	3	
44.	Wide—mouth screw cap square bottle – polyethylene (60 ml)	9	
45.	Screw cap sputum container	4	
Immunization kit (one for each Subcentre)			
46.	Rubber ring	2	
47.	File for BCG ampoules (6mm × 50 mm)	1	
48.	Wooden block for ampoules	1	
49.	Sharpening stone (50 mm × 19 mm × 6.3 mm)	1	
50.	Bifurcated needles—stainless steel (65 mm)	12	
51.	Luer hypodermic needles (0.90 mm × 25 mm/20 G × 1")	1	box of 12
52.	Luer hypodermic needles (0.60 mm × 25 mm/23 G × 1")	2	boxes of 12 each
53.	Luer hypodermic needles (0.45 mm × 10 mm/26 G × 3/8")	1	box of 12
54.	Luer nylon hypodermic syringe (2 ml × 0.1ml)	2	
55.	Luer glass hypodermic tuberculin syringe (1ml × 0.01ml)	2	
56.	Test tube holder—two piece plastic	1	
57.	Vacuum insulated thermocontainer (300 ml)	1	
58.	Aluminium box (180 mm × 100 mm × 40 mm)	1	

Appendix 15: List of Contents of Midwifery kit (Type 3) Supplied by UNICEF

UNICEF Kit

Sr.No	*Item*	*Quantity*	
1.	Instrument sterilizer – stainless (222 × 82 × 41 mm)	1	
2.	Kidney basin—stainless steel (825 ml/28 oz)	1	
3.	Sponge bowl—stainless steel (600 ml)	2	
4.	Irrigator – stainless steel (1.5 litre)	1	
5.	Opaque plastic utility apron (900 mm × 1 metre)	1	
6.	Open tip funnel end DeLee tracheal catheter (16 Fr)	1	
7.	Nelation solid tip one eye urethral catheter (12 Fr)	2	
8.	5-in-1 connector for 5.4 to 10.9 mm nylon tubing	1	
9.	3-in-1 connector for 6 to 8 mm nylon tubing	1	
10.	Clear polypropylene pouch (250 × 380 mm long)	1	
11.	Clear vinyl plastic sheeting (910 mm wide)	2	
12.	One eye funnel end rubber rectal tube (22 Fr 500 mm)	1	
13.	Latex rubber tubing for irrigator (1.5 metre length)	1	
14.	Amber glass dropping bottle (10 ml)	1	
15.	Amber glass round screw cap bottle (N/M) (60 ml)	1	
16.	Amber glass round screw cap bottle (W/M) (60 ml)	1	
17.	Clinical oral thermometer (Dual Celsius/Fahrenheit scale)	1	
18.	Clinical rectal thermometer (Dual Celsius/Fahrenheit scale)	1	
19.	Surgeon's hand brush with white nylon bristles	1	
20.	Aluminium case with lid for midwifery kit	1	
21.	Metal case for one 2ml syringe and needles	1	
22.	Absorbent non-sterile cotton wool (100 gm)	1	roll
23.	Sterile gauze pads (12-ply 76 x 76 mm square)	20	
24.	Metal alcohol lamp with screw cap (60 ml)	1	
25.	Safety pins (medium size/40 mm)	12	
26.	Two piece hinged plastic soap box	1	
27.	Unwrapped toilet soap (113 gm)	1	
28.	Baby spring scale (10 kg 100 gm graduations)	1	
29.	Vinyl coated fibre glass tape measure (1.5 metre/60")	1	
30.	Huck towel (430 × 500 mm)	2	
31.	Urine analysis outfit for albumen (test tubes, bottle, clamp)	1	set
32.	Binaural complete stethoscope	1	
33.	Rochester Pean straight haemostat forceps—stainless steel (160 mm)	2	
34.	Vaughn sterilizer (utility) forceps—chrome plated (200 mm)	1	
35.	Luer hypodermic needles (0.70 × 32 mm/22G × 1¼")	1 12	box of needles
36.	Surgical straight scissors (blunt/blunt)-stainless steel (140 mm)	1	
37.	Luer hypodermic nylon syringe (2ml × 0.1ml)	1	
38.	Hoffman tubing regulating clamp (13 × 19 mm)	1	
39.	Ergometrine maleate tablets BP (0.2 mg)	1	vial of 10 tablets

Appendix 16: Pesticide Residues in Foods

Pesticides help in high yields of food but not without toxic effects. Their safety limits are laid down through

ADI (Acceptable Daily Intake)

MRL (Maximum Residue Limits

PL (Permissible Limits)

ADI Values mg / kg		*PFA Limits mg / kg*		*PL (WHO / FAO) mg / kg*		*MRL (FAO) mg/kg*	
Parathion	0.005	**Endusulphon**		**HCH**	0.3	**Synthetic**	
Aldrin	0.001	Fruit, veg	2.0	**Endusulphon**		**Pyrethroid**	
Endosulphon	0.008	Oil	0.2		0.5	Veg	1.0
HCH	0.01	**Monocrotophos**		**Phosphine**	0.05	Oil	0.2
Lindane	0.01	Foodgrain	0.025	**Methyl bromide**		Grain	0.2
Malathion	0.02	**Phosphine**		(foods)	0.01	Meat	0.2
		Foodgrain	0.05			Egg	0.05
						Milk	0.05
						Pea	0.05

Appendix 17: Check list of Epidemiological investigation of Poliomyelitis

1. Name of the Administrative area and locality ....
2. Date first case reported from the locality ....
3. Period of field investigation from ....to ....
4. Number of paralytic polio cases detected ....
   1. Clinical diagnosis only ....
   2. Laboratory confirmed ....
   3. Type (s) of virus isolated ....
5. Number of deaths from paralytic polio ....
6. No. of paralytic cases of polio by age

   Below 1 year .... 1 to 4 years.......... 5 to 9 years ....
   10 to 14 years.......... 15 to 19 years.......... 20 and above ....
7. No. of contacts of paralytic polio examined ....
   Household contacts ....
   Others (specify) ....
8. Brief description of field investigation ....

   ....
9. History of previous vaccination practice in the locality including the dates of the last community vaccination .... programme, and the type of vaccine used

   ....

   ....
10. Name of the principal investigator and laboratory

    ....

INDEX

U

V

W

Y

Z